Tutorials in Suturing Techniques for Orthopedics

Peifu Tang • Kejian Wu • Zhongguo Fu
Hua Chen • Yixin Zhang
Editors

Tutorials in Suturing Techniques for Orthopedics

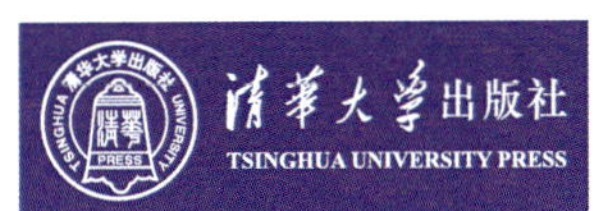

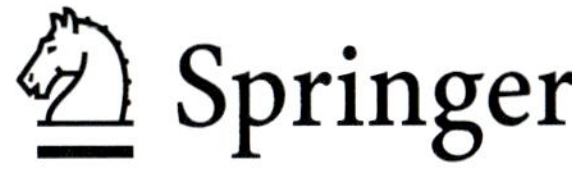

Editors
Peifu Tang
Department of Orthopaedics
Chinese PLA General Hospital
Beijing
China

Hua Chen
Orthopedics
Chinese PLA General Hospital
Beijing
China

Kejian Wu
Fourth Medical Center
Chinese PLA General Hospital
Beijing
China

Yixin Zhang
Plastic and Reconstructive Surgery
Shanghai Ninth People's Hospital
Shanghai
China

Zhongguo Fu
Peking University People's Hospital
Beijing
China

ISBN 978-981-33-6329-8 ISBN 978-981-33-6330-4 (eBook)
https://doi.org/10.1007/978-981-33-6330-4

This Springer imprint is published by the registered company Springer Nature Singapore Pte Ltd.
The registered company address is: 152 Beach Road, #21-01/04 Gateway East, Singapore 189721, Singapore

Preface I

Surgical science has witnessed rapid clinical changes in both theory and technology. Hospitals attach great importance to and are actively engaged in surgeries of all types, and it has become an indicator of the technical strength of a hospital whether it is able to perform various surgical operations and how proficient it is in this respect. Exposure, separation, hemostasis, ligation, incision, and suture are six basic surgical techniques, which often determine the style and quality of the surgery. Surgical suture is one of the major operations in a surgery, and the correct and appropriate selection of sutures and suturing methods has to do with smooth union of the organs and tissues and affects success of the surgery and the quality of life of the patient. At present, inappropriate selection of sutures or suturing methods is still found in clinical practice, which tends to result in a lower rate of success or even failure of the surgery. With the development of economy and the improvement of living standards, the patients' needs for better appearance get stronger and the quality of suture is directly related to the development of postoperative scars. Therefore, it is critical for the surgeons to attach more importance to surgical suturing techniques.

It is said in the book written by Pu Songling (a writer in the Qing Dynasty) that "People who like to read can write good articles with their pens, and people who are obsessed with a craft must have very good skills." Practice makes perfect. Some highly difficult suturing methods will not be used freely unless they are practiced for thousands of times. Attention should be paid to the technical training of doctors, especially standard technical training of young surgeons, so as to meet clinical needs and the requirements for the development of surgery. In order to improve the general quality of doctors and their proficiency in clinical diagnosis and treatment and reinforce potential development of medical science, the Capacity Building and Continuing Education Center (CBCEC) of the National Health Commission (NHC) has introduced new mechanisms and initiatives and formulated effective standard training action plans in a technique-centered manner, with a focus on precision, minimal invasion, and intelligence technology, in recent years, which has achieved remarkable progress. The "Orthopedic Suture Training," led by Professor Tang Peifu and Professor Gu Liqiang, is one of the training programs of CBCEC Professional Committee of Orthopedics of NHC. *Tutorials in Suturing Techniques for Orthopedics*, the first textbook exclusively for the training of orthopedic capacity, provides a panoramic view of suturing techniques by tissue characteristics and surgical sites. It aims to address clinical needs and build technical capacity, with "sufficient" coverage of "practical" knowledge. Theories are closely combined with the clinical practice of orthopedics, with due consideration of practical guidelines for surgical orthopedic suturing in arranging the structural system of knowledge based on the laws of cognition, which fully reflects the integration of applicability with basic theories and sufficiency-oriented selection of contents according to the continuity of knowledge. Highlighted features include:

1. Practicality of contents. The principle of integrating orthopedic theories with clinical practice is followed throughout the textbook, with emphasis on the application of theoretical knowledge, to achieve greater pertinence and practicality of suturing techniques. The development trends at home and abroad are also reflected as far as possible.
2. Innovation in structural arrangement. Combined with the technical theory, teaching method, and teaching mode of orthopedics and cosmetic and plastic surgery, this textbook explores

many new teaching methods, such as the introduction of case online video teaching and on-site practical operation teaching, supplemented by the analysis of surgical tissue structure characteristics, focusing on the operation details that are easy to be ignored in the surgical suture, so as to improve the actual surgical suture ability.

3. The authors' rich experience. All the authors of the textbook are the front-line backbone and lecturers of AO Lecturer Mission selected from qualification examination of the Editorial Committee after recommendations by experts, with rich teaching and clinical experience.

The textbook is excellent in the presentation of both illustrations and texts and explains difficult theories in easy-to-understand language with proper conciseness and elaboration. It can be used as a textbook for interns, residents, and junior attending doctors in orthopedics or as a reference book in surgery or by doctors of plastic or vascular surgery.

We are delighted to prepare the preface to this textbook. We hope that the textbook will help the innovative talent with a full range of quality required in the development of orthopedics in China. We believe that this goal will be achieved and that this textbook will provide fine quality in all respects and become popular among orthopedic doctors.

Shijiazhuang, China Zhang Yingze
Beijing, China Jiang Baoguo

Preface II

Tutorials in Suturing Techniques for Orthopedics will soon be published by Tsinghua University Press, and we are delighted to write this preface for the distribution of this standard textbook, which will standardize the education of orthopedic suturing techniques in China and provide guidance for orthopedic surgeons in fulfilling suturing and improving their suturing skills to enable more effective clinical treatment and push forward overall development of orthopedics.

This work is the product of painstaking efforts of the authors, the experience of the colleagues in clinical practice, and the best essence of the lecturers' courseware in their devotion to basic education. It is filled with memories of scenes how the lecturers are ready to share whatever experience and knowledge they have with the readers conscientiously and how practitioners in local community-level hospitals are learning with great thirst and hunger and keep asking every question they have for fear that they might miss something. It is true that the education of orthopedic suturing techniques has been an important part of our education in orthopedics for many years. In 2006, a decision to create a Trauma and Orthopedics Lecturers' Mission was made at the beginning of the general election of the Trauma and Orthopedics Group of the Chinese Orthopedic Association (COA) to popularize fracture treatment principles, provide professional training, improve technical proficiency, reduce medical errors, and improve the outcome of the treatment for the patients with trauma, and in view of the uneven distribution of healthcare resources, the lagging continuing education of medical science, and the ongoing lack of education in orthopedics, social resources were made full use of to build a basic education platform to provide basic education activities among physicians engaged in trauma and orthopedics nationwide. Unremitting and effective efforts in specialized education have resulted in greatly improved theoretical and technical level of the orthopedists in general, enabling the patients to receive proximate, on-the-spot proper treatment as soon as possible. The benefits the Chinese patients enjoy are tangible! In 2009, the Trauma and Orthopedics Group held a meeting in Nantong and decided to cooperate with the Ethicon Sutures Division of Johnson & Johnson Medical (Shanghai) Ltd. to establish a special lecturers' mission to engage in education of orthopedic suturing technology for the purpose of emphasizing the suturing techniques and the prevention of surgical site infection and improving the quality of tissue repair and wound healing. It is a general principle in the surgical treatment of traumatic orthopedics that "detail determines success" and every step of the surgery should be fulfilled carefully. Complications will occur and the treatment will be less effective if the "degree of difficulty" of the surgery is overemphasized while basic skills and techniques are ignored. In fact, perfect union needs effective blood supply at the edge of the wound, correct matching, and proper tension of each layer of tissues as well as clean wounds to prevent infection, all of which are closely related to suturing techniques. The *Basic Training Handbook on Orthopedic Suturing Techniques* was prepared after the meeting, with Tang Peifu, Gu Liqiang, Fan Cunyi, Zhu Qingsheng, Chen Hua, and Liu Xinghua playing a leading role. Preliminary lectures were provided after a centralized review of the draft, which was followed by a process of addendum filling, error correcting, and improving. Lecturers were trained before standard suturing technique training programs were provided in different places, where theoretical knowledge was integrated with practical operation, with facilities in Johnson & Johnson's Education Base used in demonstration and operation. All these efforts resulted in great popularity among the trainees and remarkable achievement in education. The feedback from the trainees and the deliberation of the lecturers greatly improved the contents of the program and enriched the courseware of the textbook. Then Professor Fu Zhongguo and Professor Wu Kejian led the compilation and publication of *Orthopedic Sutures and Knots*, which, it is safe to say, laid the foundation for *Tutorials in Suturing Techniques for Orthopedics*. As the education of orthopedic suturing techniques has been included in the orthopedic capacity training approved by CBCEC of NHC, the Professional Committee of Orthopedics organized a larger mission of even more lecturers to compile *Tutorials in Suturing Techniques for Orthopedics*, which has come out in full success after several revisions of the draft as a result of the academic teamwork.

The overall design of the textbook follows the principle to make four things easier, i.e., enriched suturing methods in orthopedic surgery, broadened vision of orthopedic surgeons being trained, standardized operation of surgical suturing, and improved suturing proficiency. It succeeds in presenting the core concepts of operation technologies and reflecting the value in the training of standard suturing. The program is arranged and sorted by scenarios and objects, with three-dimensional objectives established: the way in which the contents are presented as well as the framework, so that a general picture is available to all the lecturers; the number of required class hours; and specific form of teaching and practical operation of the suturing techniques that need to be defined, together with assumptions and practice of assessment and evaluation.

Thanks to the authors of the textbook, who have systematically consulted Chinese and foreign materials on suturing techniques during the composition of the textbook. Based on their own experience, they not only elaborate on the operation techniques of the specifications on suturing but also share with the readers their own experience of technical difficulties and solutions to achieve the better training effect. Excellent creation and efforts of all make this work highly theoretical, innovative, instructive, and practical; the chapters and sections are designed in good coherence and order, and the structure is arranged in a proper and eye-catching manner. With concise titles of all the chapters and sections as well as subtitles at all levels as well as the excellent illustrations and texts, the textbook is very easy for orthopedists to quickly view and consult and obtain guidance from it. We have reasons to believe that this textbook will be a blueprint in the education of orthopedic suturing techniques as well as a guideline and tool for orthopedic surgeons in clinical practice. The readers will benefit much from the textbook as long as it is read carefully and observed strictly in practice. They will not only improve their own proficiency but also bring more benefits to the patients, making contribution to the health of the people.

At the time of the publication of the textbook, we would also like to extend our gratitude to Ethicon Sutures Division of Johnson & Johnson Medical (Shanghai) Ltd. and Tsinghua University Press for their full support and assistance, without which the textbook could never have come out before the orthopedic colleagues and readers across the country in such high speed and good quality.

Medical science never stops. As time elapses, new surgical techniques and treatment options will emerge. The experience and techniques in surgical suturing will also keep pace with the times and grow day by day. Technical education, accordingly, will also get richer and keep updating. We hope that all the colleagues throughout the country work together to achieve new findings and creations in the practice of education on orthopedic suturing techniques while using this textbook to provide feedback and recommendations for further improvement of the textbook.

Shanghai, China Zeng Bingfang
Beijing, China Wang Manyi

Introduction

Suturing, the matching of tissues and organs cut open or ruptured due to trauma or the reconstruction of channel, is a basic condition to ensure effective union. As one of the major surgical procedures, it has been a basic skill for the surgeons to practice since their internship as medical students. The selection of ideal suturing materials and appropriate suturing methods varies with treatment objectives and tissue structures. Suturing materials and suturing techniques are related to the successful union of the organs and tissues being sutured and also affect the success rate of surgery and the quality of life of patients.

It is a general principle in the surgical treatment of traumatic orthopedics that "detail determines success" and every step of the surgery should be fulfilled carefully. Complications will occur and the treatment will be less effective if the "degree of difficulty" of the surgical operation is overemphasized while basic skills and techniques are ignored. The education of orthopedic suturing techniques is an important part in the education of orthopedics. Especially today, when medical reform is going on, we make full use of social resources to enable fruitful education and training activities in view of the uneven distribution of health resources, the lagging of continuing medical education, and the lack of orthopedic education. In 2006, a decision to create a Trauma and Orthopedics Lecturers' Mission was made at the beginning of the general election of the Trauma and Orthopedics Group of the Chinese Orthopedic Association (COA), and in 2009, dozens of AO lecturers met in Nantong, Jiangsu Province, for the first "Orthopedic Suturing Training" Workshop following the call of Professor Wang Manyi and Professor Zeng Bingfang, and a special lecturers' mission was created to engage in the education of orthopedic suturing techniques. The *Basic Training Handbook on Orthopedic Suturing Techniques* was prepared after the meeting, with Tang Peifu, Gu Liqiang, Fan Cunyi, Zhu Qingsheng, Chen Hua, and Liu Xinghua playing a leading role. Training activities of integrated lecturing of theories on standard suturing techniques with practical operations are provided in different places, which have proven to be very effective. The training materials were fantastically applauded by the trainees, with ever-expanding contents and increasingly sufficient courseware. In 2018, the education of orthopedic suturing techniques has been included in the orthopedic capacity training approved by CBCEC of NHC. With coordination of the Professional Committee of Orthopedics, we organized a larger mission of even more lecturers and fulfilled compilation of *Tutorials in Suturing Techniques for Orthopedics* on the basis of the *Basic Training Handbook on Orthopedic Suturing Techniques* in time.

Tutorials in Suturing Techniques for Orthopedics strives to be novel and practical in contents. While presenting the basic knowledge of surgical sutures, the selection of suturing materials for various secondary specialties of orthopedics, as well as the most critical points in the suturing of different tissue structures, it focuses on new methods and approaches, such as the key steps in drainage tube fixation, in addition to methods commonly used in suturing skin. It also elaborates systematically on common suturing methods and techniques in surgical operations of traumatic orthopedics. We hope that all these contents can impress the readers in a new way, so as to improve the clinical treatment in orthopedics and promote the overall development of orthopedics.

We hereby extend our thanks to all the authors who participated in the composition of this book in their spare time. We would also like to extend our gratitude to Ethicon Sutures Division of Johnson & Johnson Medical (Shanghai) Ltd. and Tsinghua University Press for their full support and assistance, without which the textbook could never have been published as scheduled.

I sincerely hope, on behalf of the authors of this book, that our readers will, as always, put forward valuable feedback on the book, regardless of its form or the contents, which is extremely important and precious. Sincerest thanks!

Tang Peifu
Gu Liqiang

Contents

Contributors

Editors

Peifu Tang Department of Orthopedics, The First Medical Center of PLA General Hospital, Beijing, China

Kejian Wu Department of Orthopedics Trauma, The Fourth Medical Center of PLA General Hospital, Beijing, China

Zhongguo Fu Peking University People's Hospital, Beijing, China

Hua Chen Department of Orthopedics, The First Medical Center of PLA General Hospital, Beijing, China

Yixin Zhang Shanghai Ninth People's Hospital, Shanghai JiaoTong University School of Medicine, Shanghai, China

Deputy Editor

Liqiang Gu The First Affiliated Hospital, Sun Yat-sen University, Guangzhou, China

Weishi Li Peking University Third Hospital, Beijing, China

Yuqiang Sun Shanghai Sixth People's Hospital, Shanghai, China

Jian Qi The First Affiliated Hospital, Sun Yat-sen University, Guangzhou, China

Yimin Chai Shanghai Sixth People's Hospital, Shanghai, China

The History of Knots and Surgical Suturing

1

Kejian Wu and Peifu Tang

Abstract

As one of the oldest materials used by human, many evidences show that ropes are closely related to human evolution. Due to perishability, few ropes remain intact after thousands of years. Even if there are few intact ropes found, most of them are collected in museums. Therefore, ropes may be "the most remarkable invention of human." One piece of fiber is of no use. But when these fibers are spun into yarns, yarns are twisted into strands, and strands are woven into ropes, such a trivial thing will become strong and flexible, creating unlimited possibilities.

Long time ago, our ancestors collected grass, vines, and bamboo and twisted them into a knot to thread through, tie up, and bundle up fruits and prey. These knots are the most original ones. As early as the end of the Paleolithic Age, the remains of the Caveman culture in Zhoukoudian were found to have "bone needles." Since needles appeared at that time, there might have been threads and ropes, from which we can infer that the simple techniques of knot tying and sewing should have begun to take shape.

The earliest records of surgical suture can be traced back to 3000 B.C. in ancient Egypt, where a Greek physician Hippocrates, known as the "Father of Medicine," described the basic suture technique. Surgical sutures have evolved from plant-derived materials (flax, hemp, and cotton) or animal-derived materials (hair, tendons, arteries, muscle strips or nerves, silk, catgut) or animal body parts (ant's head and mandibles) to metal materials (silver, copper, aluminum, and bronze wires) to various synthetic materials in nowadays.

K. Wu
Department of Orthopedics Trauma, The Fourth Medical Center of PLA General Hospital, Beijing, China

P. Tang (✉)
Department of Orthopedics, The First Medical Center of PLA General Hospital, Beijing, China

Keywords

History · Rope · Knot

1.1 The History of Ropes

1.1.1 Overview

The bone needle unearthed in 1933 in the upper cave of Dragon Bone Hill at Zhoukoudian, Fangshan County, Beijing (700,000–200,000 years ago) was a sewing tool [1, 2] used in the Paleolithic Age. Though the thread used was merely the tendon of an animal, it proved to be the prototype of simple ropes. The stone axe unearthed in Banpo Village of Xi'an [3] also supports the use of ropes by our ancestors. The murals [4] from tombs in ancient Egypt also show the state-of-the-art rope-making methods and use of ropes in large-scale constructions.

Ancient ropes were mostly made of tendons and vines, making them incredibly difficult to be preserved physically to the present day. Thanks to the unremitting efforts of archeologists, we are now able to see many. In Wadi Gawasis, an ancient Egyptian port, a large number of ropes preserved intact about 4000 years ago [5] have been found with skilled rope making technique. Archeologists infer that these exquisite ropes are used for navigation.

1.1.2 Materials of Early Ropes

Rope in simplified Chinese is "绳," originally meaning snake-shaped flexible strap fabric made of twisted ramie threads or other fibers (Fig. 1.1). The left part of the character indicates the twisting of grass, ramie, or silk. Humans started making rope using grasses or small branches when they started using the simplest tools. Small branches, willows, weeds, or vines were the earliest materials for making ropes. When our ancestors began to open up the world, they

P. Tang et al. (eds.), *Tutorials in Suturing Techniques for Orthopedics*, https://doi.org/10.1007/978-981-33-6330-4_1

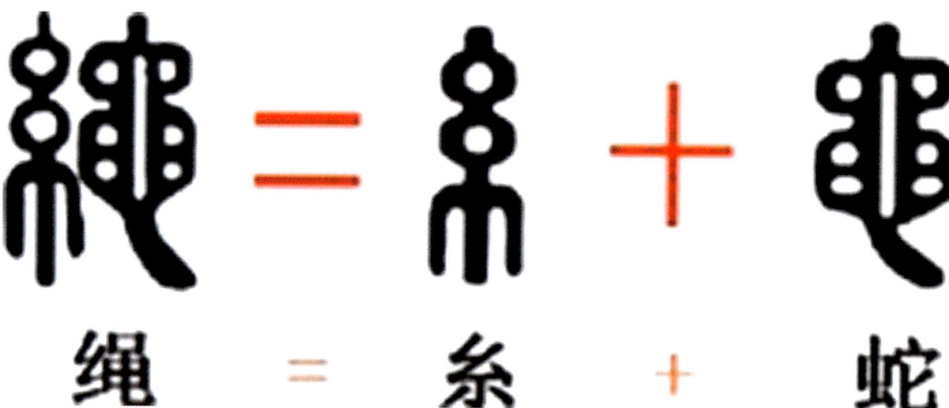

Fig. 1.1 "Rope" in seal script, an earlier writing system of Chinese characters

used such stuff to make tools by tying a stone onto a wooden stick. These rough materials were the ancestor of the modern ropes. With the development of human cultures, ramie, cotton, palm leaves, silk, hardware, and the chemical fiber of today, nylon, have been used as materials in making ropes.

Ramie, the best material for making ropes, was discovered and used in China and Egypt 3000 years ago. Traditionally ropes were made of natural fibers, including cotton, ramie, linen, jute, sisal, Manila hemp, straw, silk, wool, and other hairs. Modern synthetic fibers used to make ropes include polypropylene, nylon, polyester, polyethylene, rayon, etc. Those similar to ropes in structure and function but thinner and weaker in strength are yarns, threads, and strings.

1.1.3 Rope Making Methods

1.1.3.1 Basic Structure of Ropes

Ropes are strips of cotton, hemp, palm, or other fibers or steel wires twisted together. Ropes are twisted from several strands to 2, 3, 8, 16, 24, 32, and 48 strands, making the surface of the ropes increasingly delicate and beautiful [6] with strands twisted together in one or more colors regularly. The simplest way to make a rope is "twisting": single fibers are twisted first; several twisted single fibers are twisted again in reverse into threads; several threads are twisted again in reverse into yarns; several yarns are twisted again in reverse into bundles; several bundles are then twisted into cords (Fig. 1.2); and several cords twisted into thicker ropes (Fig. 1.3).

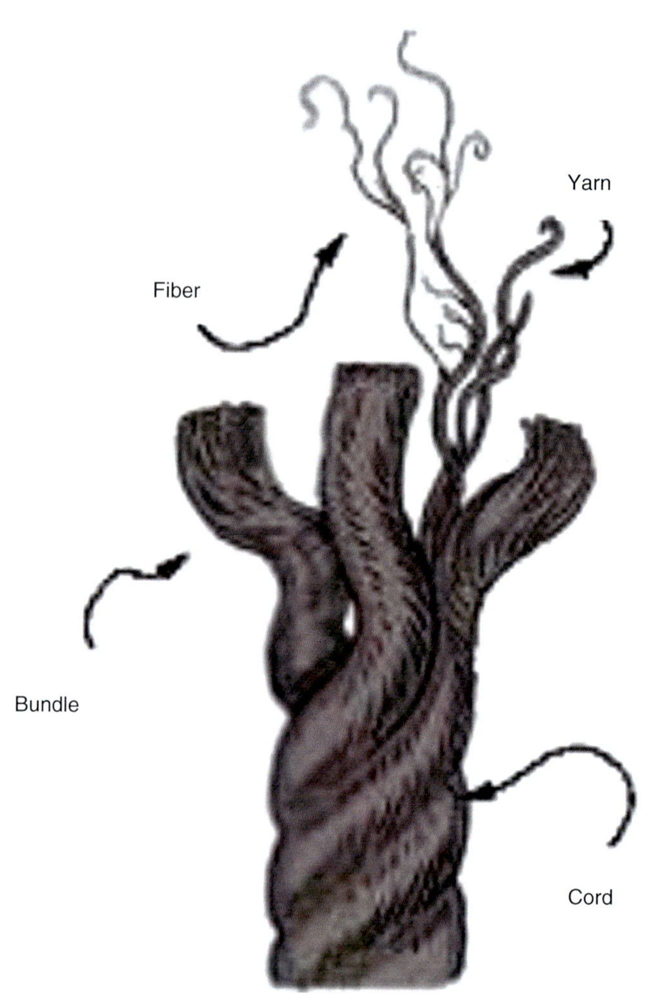

Fig. 1.2 Basic structure of cords

1.1.3.2 General Classification

Ropes can be classified in different ways. They can be divided into natural-fiber ropes and chemical-fiber ropes according to the type of the fiber used. For instance, flax ropes and linen ropes are natural-rope fibers, whereas Kevlar ropes and Vectran ropes are chemical-fiber ropes; and ropes made of steel wires are called steel wire ropes. Ropes are divided into twisted ropes, braided ropes, and parallel fiber ropes according to the manufacturing process; ropes, cords, and cables according to the diameter; marine ropes and agricultural ropes according to the industry they are used in; and military ropes and civil ropes according to the purpose they are used for.

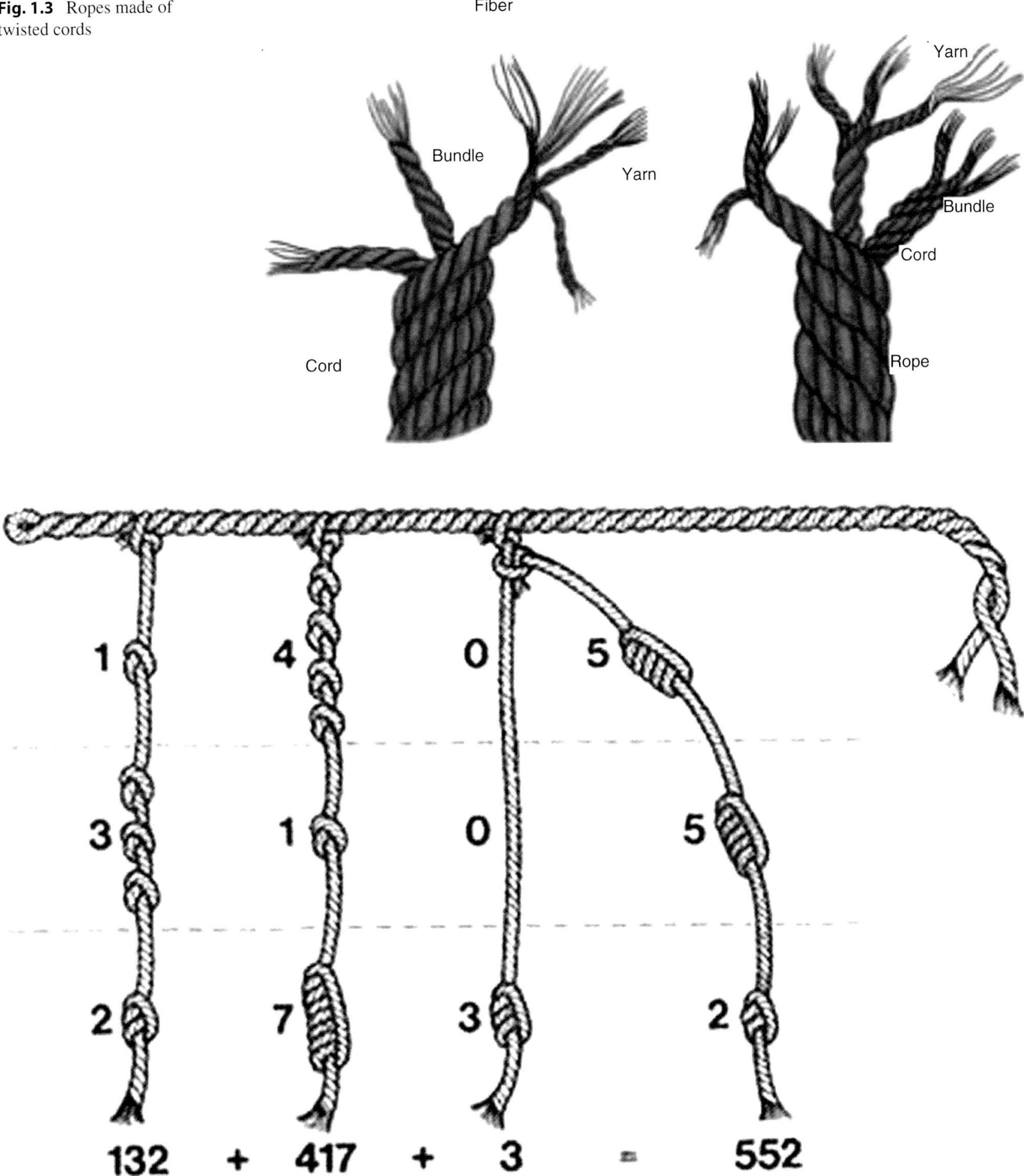

Fig. 1.3 Ropes made of twisted cords

Fig. 1.4 Recording events (number) with tied knots

1.1.3.3 How Ropes Were Made

Early humans used ropes to tie animals, build thatched huts, and make belts to fasten the straw skirts... Later, they kept records of events by tying knots, i.e. one after another knots in varied sizes. "People in ancient times tied knots in a string for record-keeping, and later generation did this by writing," said in the ancient Chinese book—"周易·系辞下"—written in Warring States Period. The Incas in South America tied the knots in the most developed and complex way in the history of the world. Quipu, i.e., a single knot of the rope (Fig. 1.4), was used by people living in Lapa Village of Lima, Peru to count numbers and record events [7]. They already knew the decimal system and even the use of "zero" (represented by a vacancy).

The ropes used in ancient times were made by twisting the grasses or small branches with the palm against the bare thigh (Fig. 1.5). Firstly, the fibers were sorted out and spun into yarns; multiple yarns were twisted together into a thread, and then multiple threads were twisted into ropes. Each twisting step was done in opposite directions to secure tightness. Both ends of the rope should be fastened separately; otherwise, the rope would fall apart.

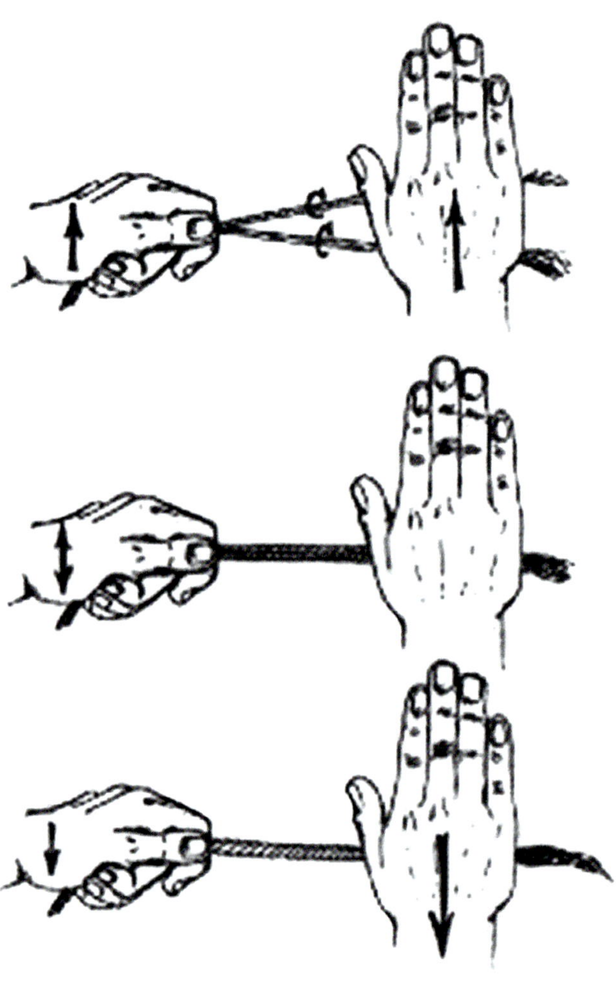

Fig. 1.5 Twisting of a rope

Due to the emergence of canoes and the need of large-scale constructions, manual twisting of ropes has far cannot satisfy the needs for the usage and strength of ropes. Ancient Egyptians began to make ropes with simple tools (Fig. 1.6) and even by means of a division of labor, with reeds and hemp as the most commonly used materials (Fig. 1.7). With the accumulation of experience and advancement in technology, the ropes produced were more and more exquisite and practical. Ropes were generally made in the following steps: carding, spinning, twisting, and braiding [8]. Each step was assisted by appropriate tools, which greatly improved production efficiency.

1.2 The History of Knotting

1.2.1 Overview

Lubbock, a British archeologist, was the first who fulfilled the division of Paleolithic Age and the Neolithic Age (about 10,000 years ago) in 1865, believing that one of the basic characteristics of the Neolithic Age was the manufacture and use of ground stone tools [9]. A sickle made of ground stone slab unearthed in Shuiquan, Jia County, Henan Province in 1989 which is a unique tool representing the Peiligang culture of the Neolithic Age. When it was practically used, the sickle needed to be mounted onto a wooden handle, and fixed with ropes and other materials. Tools in the Neolithic age were no longer simple ground tools but combined with wooden handles, which were more in line with the principles of mechanics, more labor-saving, and more efficient. The connection between the ground stone tools and the wooden handles was fulfilled by means of ropes. The end of the rope was an incipient rope knot although its structure cannot be seen today.

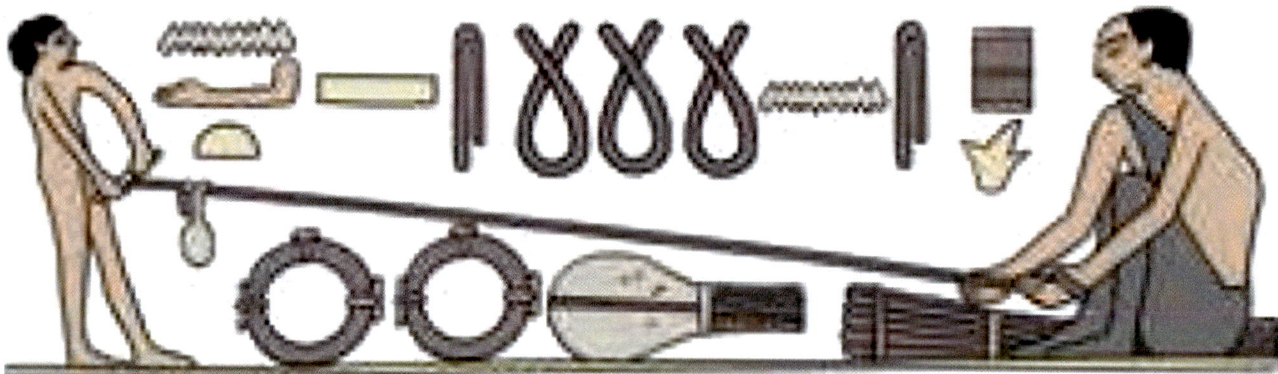

Fig. 1.6 Rope twisting by two people (part of a mural in a tomb of ancient Egypt)

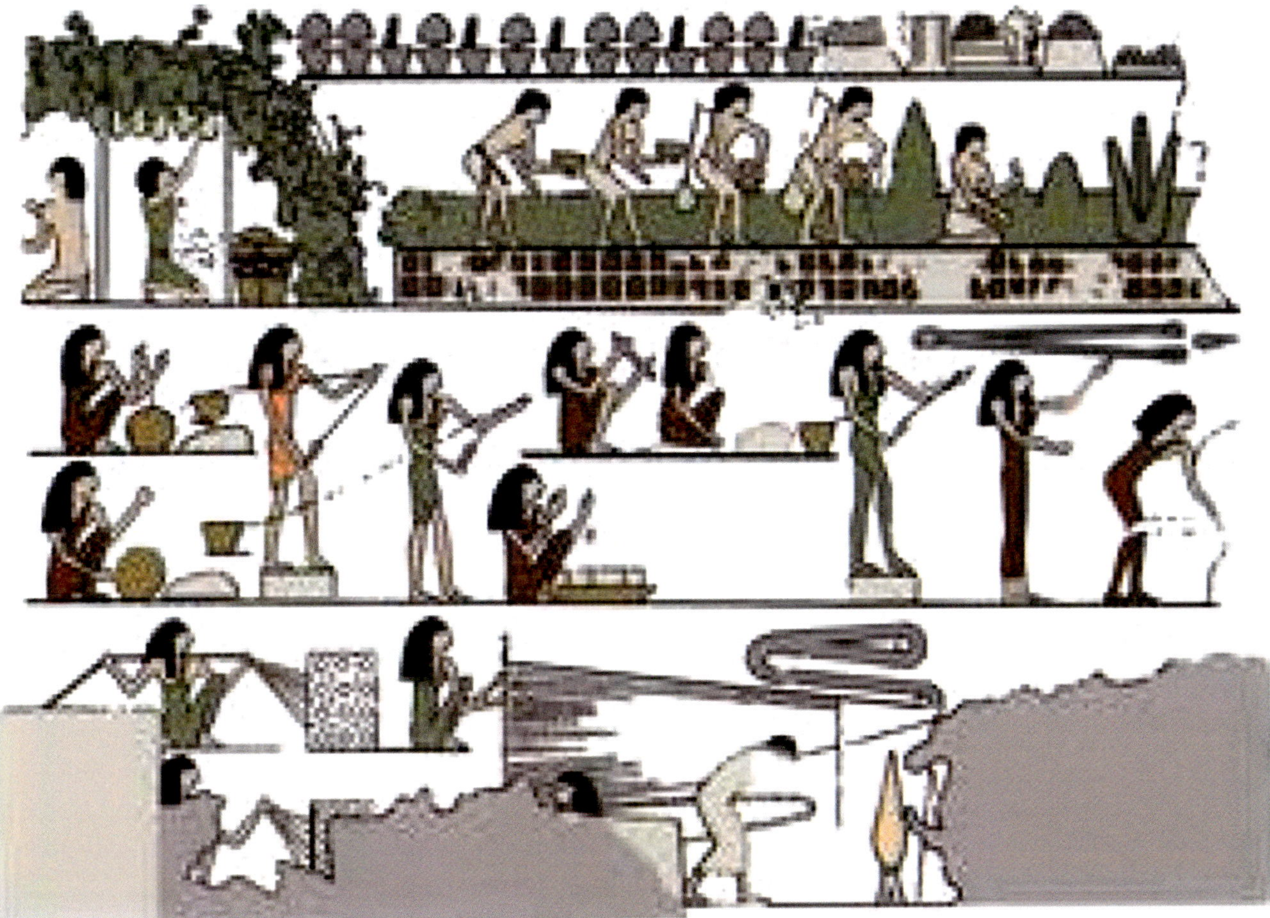

Fig. 1.7 Rope twisting by means of division of labor among more people (part of a mural in a tomb of ancient Egypt)

1.2.2 Development of Knotting

A knot is the product of the knitting, winding of one or more segments of one-dimensional flexible materials for appreciation and application, and the action that leads to a knot is called knotting. In ancient times, the rattan and grasses would fold and gather up during people's collecting and carrying, leading to a growing awareness of the increased strength of the rattan and grasses put together and hence the beginning of rope making was kicked off. With increasing knowledge on the forms of ropes and the way in which ropes were made, human beings strode towards a new era for the invention and manufacturing of tools. Ancient people dragged a long rattan and rotate their wrists, and a wristband would come into being. The rattan would also wrap up the wrist into a wristband when it was pulled by the hands alternately. A single knot would appear when such wristband was tightened up. There would also be knots when someone was eager to get out of a tangle. Due to the complex interlocking of the rattan, the greater the effort to pull the rattan was, the tighter the tangle would become, which would resulting knots. Such experiences developed from unconscious and accidental actions to conscious "knot making." People continued to connect and tie things by means of these ropes and knots. Single knots did exist in ancient times though they are no longer seen today. It took merely a small step for single knots to evolve into figure-of-eight knot, the second basic knot. With the progress of the times and the increasing knowledge of human beings, the invention has become more and more complex. To tackle the increasingly complicated work, many new knots, of which reef knot might be the first, were created. Reef knots were decorative graphics commonly used by Egyptians as ornaments 5000 years ago.

Net, a vital tool in the evolution of mankind, appeared in the era when "substitution of record-keeping by means of knotting." Nets were used for hunting and fishing as an important tool to obtain a wide variety of food in the sky, on the earth, and in the water. They helped reduce the casualties of animals and fish, not only preventing starvation but enabling breeding as a result of the surplus of food.

Nets had been used during the Banpo period 6000 years ago. Square and conical fishing nets painted on the earthenware unearthed in Banpo reflected that Banpo people had been able to fish with nets in different shapes according to different water areas. In addition, a large number of stone and pottery net sinkers were found across sites of the Neolithic Times, indicating that fishing nets were widely used in the primitive society. Fishing nets in primitive society were also recorded in early ancient Chinese books. "In ancient times, Fuxi ruled the empire by making nets with ropes and knots and using them in hunting and fishing as an effective instrument," said in the ancient Chinese book—"易经·系辞下."

In the world's history of navigation, some ancient Egyptians sailed alongside the Mediterranean Sea to Lebanon as early as 2500 B.C.; in the second half of the fourth century B.C., the Greek navigator Pytheas started from the Greek colony of Massalia (now Marseille in France), navigated along the Iberian Peninsula and the coast of France and then northward along the east coast of the Island of Great Britain to the Orkney Islands, and then moved eastward to the mouth of River Elbe. It was the earliest long-distance sea voyage in the west. Before such voyage, navigation had been remarkably active in the Mediterranean with outbreak of naval wars. During the famous Greco-Persian War in 490 B.C., Greece fought against the Persian fleets with hundreds of warships about 130 ft. long with three levels of oars.

The compass invented in China was introduced into Europe by the Arabs and Egyptians around the fourteenth century. Great achievements were made in the navigation activities of the maritime countries in Europe. Columbus, the Italian, sailed across the Atlantic Ocean and arrived in the America in 1492; Vasco da Gama, the Portuguese, sailed around the Cape of Good Hope to India in 1497; Magellan, the Portuguese, sailed westward for a voyage around the world, which was also included in the history of world navigation. The Age of Discovery was the age when countless brave adventurers sailed small boats to challenge the mysterious open sea; and it was the age when they bravely challenged the unknown areas and brought countless discoveries and hopes to Europe. The Age of Discovery refers to the extensive transoceanic activities and major geographic breakthroughs all over the world, which were initiated from Europe, in the fifteenth to seventeenth centuries. These ocean-going activities had promoted the communication among different continents and resulted in a large number of new trade routes.

Sailors' knots, as essential skills of ancient sailors, have a history of over a thousand years. They have been widely used as basic means of strapping, binding, and fastening in maritime life. According to different purposes and habits, sailors' knots are made in more than a hundred different ways. Sailors' knots are generally secure and look gorgeous. A good use of sailors' knots also makes lifer much easier and interesting. Sailors' knots must withstand wind, exposure to the sun and soaking in the water, endurable and secure, easy to make and unfold, and not easily to get loose. Sailor's knots represent the wisdom of ancient sailors who had safeguarded thousands of years of navigation history. There would not have been a glorious navigation history without the sailors' knots.

Clifford Warren Ashley is an American famous painter, sailor, and the most important master of knots in the history [10]. He sorted out more than 3000 knots in his lifetime, and invented many new ways of knotting. His creatively use his painting skills to vividly depict the knotting techniques collected from around the world in a manual on knots, *The Ashley Book of Knots*. The book was published in 1944 after 11 years of great effort.

The book presents the culture and history of knots, as well as the methods, purposes, and classification of all knots, from the simplest to the most complicated, available to you, which enables us to find that many knots are related to navigation, and the development of knots is closely related to navigation.

1.3 A Brief History of Surgical Suture

The earliest surgical suture we can see today was on the ancient Egyptian mummies in 3000 B.C. Ancient Egyptians believed that their soul would survive after their death but would be attached to the body or the statue. Therefore, after Pharaohs and others died, people made them into mummies, as the hope for immortality and deep remembrance of the dead. Mummies found in Egypt were the largest in number, the earliest in time, and the most complex in technique. When making a mummy, the Egyptians pulled out part of the brain marrow from the nostrils of the dead body first with an iron hook and injected some medicine into the brain for cleaning, then cut open the side of the abdomen with a sharp stone knife, took out the viscera completely, cleaned the abdomen, filled it with coconut wine and mashed spices, and sewed it up as it was.

Sushruta, an Indian doctor, 150 years earlier than Hippocrates [11], was the first person who had recorded wound suturing and the materials used in 500 B.C. His nose reconstruction operation in north India is till prestigious all around the world today, with skin flaps on the forehead cut and moved for reconstruction of the nose [12]. In Sushruta's time, criminals were often punished by cutting their noses. With an elaboration on 650 medicines, 300 kinds of operations, 42 surgical procedures, and 121 devices, *Sushruta Samhita*, his medical book, is highly respected by the following generations.

In *On Head Wounds*, the most famous surgical book of Hippocrates, a Greek physician known as the "Father of Medicine," injuries on the skull and the nomenclature of "cranial suture" were described in detail, and the surgical and suturing methods were provided. Operations were recorded very carefully in precise wording, which proved that the book was a summary of his personal experience.

Aulus Cornelius Celsus, a doctor in ancient Rome, and Galen, a Roman doctor in the second century A.D., had, respectively, described catgut suturing techniques, which became very mature by the tenth century. The development of catgut suturing techniques benefited from the manufacturing technology of catgut. In addition to surgical suturing, catgut is also widely used in making strings for violins and tennis rackets.

Catgut was originally made of ovine intestine, and later it was found that the quality of catgut made of the chorionic membrane of bovine intestine was better. We still call it catgut because we have been used to the nomenclature already. There are two kinds of catgut, i.e. plain catgut and chromic catgut. It takes less time for plain catgut (4–5 days) to be absorbed than chromic catgut (14–21 days). The advantage of catgut is its absorbability without foreign matter, which had been favored by surgeons at that time. However, the tissue reaction to catgut was great during the absorption. The absorption of catgut varies with human tissues, and the quality of catgut also affects the absorption by human tissues. Catgut often led to infection due to the lack of knowledge on disinfection and sterilization techniques at early stage. In 1866, Lister invented the disinfection method, and surgical infection declined dramatically [13]. Lister advocated that surgical sites and devices must be disinfected (Fig. 1.8), and took the lead to disinfect plain catgut and chromic catgut with carbolic acid (phenol). The use of phenol to disinfect catgut had lasted for nearly 20 years until 1906 when it was replaced by iodine disinfection.

With the development of chemical industry, a wide diversity of absorbable and non-absorbable synthetic sutures has been developed rapidly. The first synthetic suture was made of polyvinyl alcohol in 1931. Polyester sutures were developed in the 1950s. The sutures of mixed catgut and polyester greatly reduced the adverse reactions of original catgut, and radiation sterilization begun to be used. Polyglycolic acid was synthesized in the 1960s and used in the manufacturing of sutures in the 1970s. At present, most sutures are made of polymer fibers. Catgut and silk threads used at early stage are rarely used today due to the stimulation of sutures to tissues and potential zoonotic infection.

Abu al-Qasim Khalaf Ibn Abbas al-Zahrawi, also Albucasis, a descendant of the Arabs born in Zalagh city near Cordoba, Spain, was known as one of the greatest doctors in Arab countries, particularly excellent in internal medicine, surgery, and ophthalmology. *Al-tasreef liman ajiza an al-taaleef*, commonly referred to as *Al-Tasreef*, the best known work written by him, is an encyclopedia of medicine, which consists of 30 chapters, including two parts of surgery, internal medicine, orthopedics, ophthalmology, pharmacology, nutrition science, etc. [14]. Zahrawi's book describes in detail the use of the ant mandibles to close the wound as they work like two serrated and sharp teeth with an amazingly great strength to close. Doctors of Zahrawi's time used the ant mandibles to close the wound. They separated the chest of the ant from the head, and left the mandibles closing the wound, similar to the skin suturing device today [15]. The chest and abdomen of the ant were discarded [16], and the action must be done quickly; otherwise, the ant would eject formic acid from the gaster, and spray it on the wound, which would cause severe pain and even inflammation and swelling if it is not inhibited with drugs in time.

Before the discovery of microorganism by Pasteur and the invention of disinfection by Lister, silver products were widely used for antisepsis and preventing against infection. Very small amount of silver ions can be decomposed from the silver products in water to adsorb microorganisms in water and cause the enzyme that enables breathing of microorganisms to lose its function, thereby killing the microorganisms. In mid-nineteenth century, J. Marion Sims, an American gynecologist, succeeded easily in treating vaginal fistula [17, 18] with silver sutures but would likely fail with other sutures. In 1852, Sims published his results and shared this repair and suturing technique in Germany and France, so that the results were accepted in Europe. Wounds were still sutured with silver sutures till World War I.

For thousands of years, sutures have evolved from botanical (linen, hemp, and cotton) or animal materials (hair, ten-

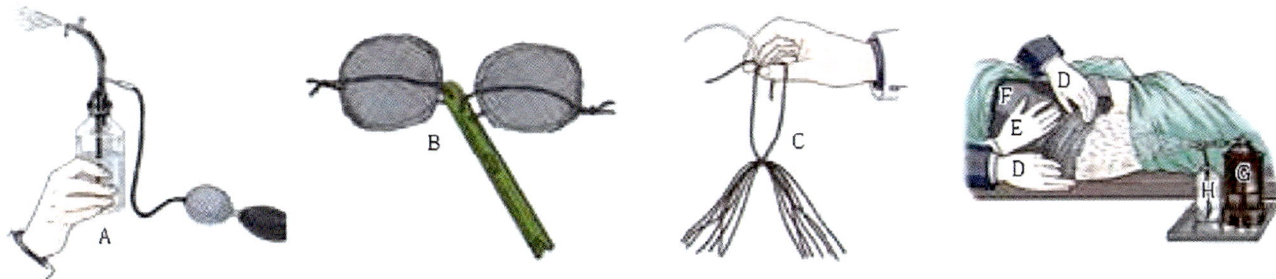

Fig. 1.8 Aseptic surgery advocated by lister. (A) Phenol sprayer, (B) dressing and surgical device disinfection, (C) suture needle and catgut disinfection, (D) surgeon hand disinfection, (E) assistant hand disinfection, (F) surgical area disinfection, (G) heating sprayer, (H) phenol

don, artery, muscle strip or nerve, silk, catgut) and animal parts (ant mandibles) to metals (such as silver, copper, aluminum bronze wire), and to all sorts of synthetic materials today, all representing the human wisdom.

Search Terms

Ropes, History, Knots, Rope making, Sailors, Navigation, Surgical suture, Catgut, Suture, Carbolic acid, Chromic catgut, Clifford Warren Ashley, Sushruta, Hippocrates, Pasteur, Lister

References

1. d'Errico F, Doyon L, Zhang S, et al. The origin and evolution of sewing technologies in Eurasia and North America. J Hum Evol. 2018;125:71–86.
2. Chia L-p. The cave home of Peking Man. Foreign Languages Press Peking; 1975. First edition 1975 Printed in the People's Republic of China, p. 16–18.
3. Liu L. The Chinese neolith trajectories to early states. Cambridge; 2005. p. 37–9. First published in print format.
4. De Meyer M, Willems H. The regional supply chain of Djehutihotep's Ka-Chapel at Tjerty. CRIPEL. 2016–2017;31:33–56.
5. Borojevic K, Mountain R. The ropes of pharaohs: The source of cordage from "rope cave" at Mersa/Wadi Gawasis revisited. J Am Res Center Egypt. 2011;47:131–41.
6. Verrill AH. Knots, splices and rope work. 21 Sept 2004 [eBook]. www.free-ebooks.net/fiction-classics/Knots-Splices-and-Rope-Work
7. Zepp RA. Numbers and codes in ancient Peru: The Quipu. Arithmetic Teach. 1992;39(9):42–4.
8. Teeter E. Techniques and terminology of rope-making in ancient Egypt. J Egypt Archaeol. 1987;73:71–7.
9. Pumphrey RJ. The forgotten man: Sir John Lubbock, F.R.S. Notes Rec R Soc Lond. 1958;13(1):49–58.
10. Williams NJ. "Whalecraft": Clifford Warren Ashley and whaling craft culture in industrial New Bedford. J Mod Craft. 2018;11(3):185–217.
11. Champaneria MC, Workman AD, Gupta SC. Sushruta father of plastic surgery. Ann Plast Surg. 2014;73(1):2–7.
12. Mazzola IC, Mazzola RF. History of reconstructive rhinoplasty. Facial Plast Surg. 2014;30:227–36.
13. Brand RA. Biographical sketch: Baron Joseph Lister, FRCS, 1827–1912. Clin Orthop Relat Res. 2010;468(8):2009–11.
14. Noras MR, Hajzadeh M, Arianpoor A. A short review on Albucasis achievements in dentistry based on his book: Al-Tasrif li man Ajaz an-il-Talif. J Res Hist Med. 2015;4(1):3–8.
15. Schiappa J, Van Hee R. From ants to staples: history and ideas concerning suturing techniques. Acta Chir Belg. 2012;112:395–402.
16. Davis HE. Leaf-cutter ants in wound closure. Wilderness Environ Med. 2019;30(4):469–70.
17. Bissell D. J. Marion Sims, M.D. LL.D. surgeon and humanitarian. Am J Surg. 1929;6(4):560–5.
18. Sims JM. On the treatment of vesico-vaginal fistula. Am J Med Sci. 1852;45:59–82.

2 Basis for Soft Tissue Repair and Healing

Kejian Wu, Peifu Tang, and Yanbin Lin

Abstract

Soft tissue repair or healing refers to a series of pathophysiological processes in which tissues are repaired by regeneration, repair, and reconstruction after soft tissue defects (such as wounds, incisions, and wound surfaces) caused by trauma or other reasons. In essence, soft tissue repair is an inherent defensive adaptive response to the injury and defect of tissues and cells caused by various injury and pathogenic factors. Soft tissue injury and tissue defect caused by wound or tissue missing caused by extensive necrosis and tissue destruction usually needs to be repaired by regeneration and reconstruction of surrounding histocyte or by proliferation of other histocytes (usually connective histocytes) to replace the original tissue. These wounds are common in peacetime and wartime and generally can be divided into mechanical (such as incised wound and surgery), physical and chemical (such as thermal burn, frostbite, chemical skin injury, and radiation skin ulcer), inflammatory (such as abscess), ischemic (such as infarction) and metabolic (such as diabetic skin ulcer) wounds, etc., which are characterized by the formation of compensatory tissue.

The body has great and amazing ability to repair and restore the damage and defect of tissues and cells, which is manifested by the recovery of tissue structure and partial recovery of its function. As mentioned before, the defect or injury of tissues can be "completely restored" by the regeneration of original histocytes, that is, completed by the proliferation of its original substantial components or by the proliferation of non-specific fibrous connective tissue to replace the original histocytes and become the fibrogenic focus or scar, that is, "incomplete restoration." For the traditional concept of pathology, the former is called regeneration, and the latter is called repair. Repair of damaged or defect tissues, whether regeneration or repair, involves the same or similar principles and pathological processes.

Keywords

Soft tissue · repair · heal

2.1 Soft Tissue Repair Pathology

2.1.1 Basis for Wound Repair–Regeneration

2.1.1.1 Concept and Classification of Regeneration

Soft tissue healing refers to the histocyte injury and defect caused by various injury and pathogenic factors and can be repaired through regeneration of allogeneic or xenogeneic cells in the damaged site, finally achieving the purpose of wound closure. In other words, regeneration is the initiation and basis of wound soft tissue healing, repair is the process of wound healing, and healing is the wound outcome. Regeneration is defined as "compensation for the loss of tissues or cells." In the normal physiological process, some tissues and cells are continuously consumed, aged, and disappeared and are continuously supplemented by division and proliferation of allogeneic cells. This kind of regeneration is called physiological regeneration. For example, the keratinocytes of the skin continuously fall off, and the basal cells continuously proliferate and differentiate; endometrium falls off periodically (menstruation), then will proliferate and repair from the fundus; after aging and consumption, blood cells constantly regenerate and replenish, all belong to this category, its characteristic is the cells and tissues after regeneration can completely maintain the original structure and

K. Wu (✉)
Department of Orthopedics Trauma, The Fourth Medical Center of PLA General Hospital, Beijing, China

P. Tang
Department of Orthopedics, The First Medical Center of PLA General Hospital, Beijing, China

Y. Lin
Fuzhou Second Hospital Affiliated to Xiamen University, Fuzhou, Fujian, China

P. Tang et al. (eds.), *Tutorials in Suturing Techniques for Orthopedics*, https://doi.org/10.1007/978-981-33-6330-4_2

function, so it is also called complete regeneration. In the pathological state, the regeneration of cells or tissues after defects caused by injury is called pathological regeneration, also called reparative regeneration. When the defects are superficial or slight, they can be repaired by division and proliferation of allogeneic cells, which also have the original structure and function (i.e., complete pathological regeneration); however, when the defects are deep or serious, they can only be filled by another substitute tissue (usually fibrous connective tissue), losing the original structure and function (i.e., incomplete pathological regeneration).

1. Physiological regeneration: According to the characteristics of the frequency and time of regeneration compensation in a lifetime, it can be divided into:
   (a) One-time physiological regeneration: A certain tissue or cell is compensated only once in a certain period of human development in a lifetime, for example, deciduous teeth are compensated by permanent teeth.
   (b) Periodic physiological regeneration: A certain tissue or cell is repeated for many times in a lifetime with a fixed time interval and periodically compensated, such as endometrial regeneration after menstruation in women.
   (c) Persistent physiological regeneration: Some tissues or cells are often consumed, died. and disappeared in a lifetime; meanwhile, they are compensated and renewed constantly and frequently, which are mainly found in tissues with cell division cycle, such as epidermis, columnar epithelium of mucosa, vascular endothelium, spermatogenic epithelium, and blood cells.
2. Pathological regeneration (reparative regeneration): It can be divided into the following two categories:
   (a) Complete pathological regeneration: After a certain tissue or cell defect, the original normal structure and function are reconstructed through the regeneration of homospecific cells in the tissue. Such regeneration is mainly found in the following situations: When the basement membrane of epidermis and epithelium is still intact (such as complete regeneration of superficial epidermal abrasions); when the vascular or perivascular connective tissue scaffold (reticular fiber scaffold) is still preserved (if there is only central lobular necrosis or single hepatocyte necrosis in the liver, and when the reticular fiber scaffold is preserved, it is completely regenerated by the mitosis of hepatocytes around or adjacent to the lobule). As the integrity of basement membrane is a guide rail for regenerative cells, complete pathological regeneration can be carried out as long as the basement membrane is intact, no matter the regeneration of skin, mucosa, or vascular endothelium, or the regeneration of parenchymatous organs such as liver, kidney, and lung or glandular organs.
   (b) Incomplete pathological regeneration: In most cases, as the regeneration ability of human and other higher animals' tissues and cells is mostly limited, it is often impossible to restore the original structure and function through regeneration of allogeneic cells and tissues when some tissues with weak regeneration ability or lacking regeneration ability are damaged and defective. Especially when the tissue defect is serious, the scope is relatively large, and the basement membrane and surrounding reticular scaffold are damaged, complete regeneration cannot occur, and it can only be replaced by fibrous connective tissue or scar. Most of the wound, extensive soft tissue necrosis, or destruction can only be compensated and repaired by incomplete pathological regeneration, that is, scar formation [1].

From this, it can be seen that the wound repair healing process belongs to incomplete pathological regeneration in most cases.

2.1.1.2 Regeneration Ability of Histocytes

The regeneration, repair, and healing of soft histocytes after wound are realized by the division and proliferation of adjacent living cells, which depends on the regeneration ability and proliferation process of tissues and cells. However, various histocytes in the body have different regeneration abilities. In general, the regeneration ability is related to the degree of biological evolution, i.e., the regeneration ability of histocytes in low-grade animals is stronger than that of histocytes in high-grade animals; it is also related to its differentiation degree, i.e., the regeneration ability of histocytes with high differentiation degree and complex structure and function is weak, but on the contrary, it is strong; it is also related to the proliferation ability and metabolic state of tissues and cells, i.e., the tissues and cells with active division and vigorous metabolism (i.e., vigorous DNA synthesis) have strong regeneration ability, but on the contrary, it is weak; it is also related to age, i.e., tissues in infancy, especially in early development (including fetus), have stronger regeneration ability than those in old age. At present, according to the regeneration ability of cells, human's histocytes can be roughly divided into three categories (Fig. 2.1).

1. Labile cells: Also known as continuously dividing cells [2]; refer to the cells that divide and proliferate continuously in a lifetime to replace and supplement declining and depleting cells, which is the case under normal circumstances. Such cells have very strong regeneration ability, mainly including skin, mucosa (such as mucosa of

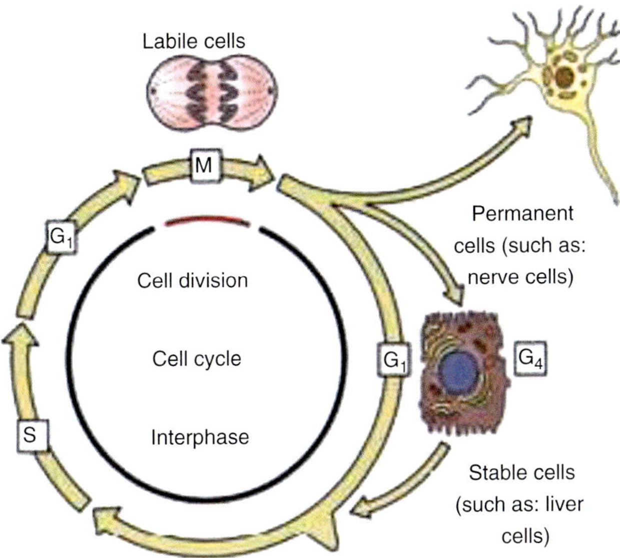

Fig. 2.1 Characteristics of three types of tissues and cells

oral cavity, digestive tract, respiratory tract, and urogenital tract), hematopoietic cells, lymphocytes, embryonic cells, and spermatogenic epithelial cells.

2. Stable cells: Refer to cells that have reduced or stopped proliferation after puberty and organ development, but still maintain potential division and proliferation ability throughout adulthood, but after the tissues and cells are damaged or defective, they show stronger or even extremely strong regeneration ability. Such cells mainly include all kinds of parenchymal cells of glandular epithelium and glandular organs, such as hepatocytes, pancreas, salivary gland, endocrine glands (thyroid, adrenal gland, etc.), sweat glands and sebaceous glands of skins, renal tubular epithelial cells, and all kinds of submucosal glands (such as mixed acinar epithelium of trachea and esophagus). The classic example is that a large number of hepatocyte mitotic figures can be seen in the residual liver several days after 80% liver resection in experimental rabbits, and the liver weight can even restore to its original state at about 100 days.

   In particular, it should be pointed out that the body's mesenchymal tissue and its differentiated tissues and cells also belong to stable cells, among which fibroblasts and primitive mesenchymal cells (or mesenchymas) have strong regeneration ability, especially primitive mesenchymal cells have stronger proliferation and differentiation ability, and can differentiate into many specific mesenchymal cells, such as osteoblasts, chondroblasts, fibroblasts, and myofibroblasts, which also have strong regeneration and differentiation ability. In addition, smooth muscle cells have weak regeneration ability at ordinary times, but can also have obvious regeneration figures under the action of certain diseases (such as chronic gastritis) or estrogen (such as uterine smooth muscle).

3. Permanent cells: Refer to cells that have lost ability of division and proliferation after birth, mainly nerve cells, including central nerve cells and ganglion cells of peripheral nervous system. This is because the nervous system has complete neurons at birth, it lacks the regeneration ability. When it is destroyed, it becomes permanently absent because the preserved nerve cells cannot divide and proliferate; however, limited regeneration can still take place in peripheral nerves, especially on the premise that nerve cells themselves are not damaged, and their axons still have strong or very strong ability to grow and lengthen, that is, regeneration ability. It is observed that the axons can grow at a rate of 3–4 mm/day.

There is still controversy about the regeneration and repair ability of muscle tissue and its classification. The common view is that mitotic figures are rare or absent in striated muscle, cardiac muscle, and smooth muscle cells after birth, which have very weak regeneration ability. When the striated muscle is only slightly damaged, the undamaged muscle fiber stump can stretch, in which the muscle fiber stump can grow into the residual endomysium (if the endomysium of the damaged site still exists), and the muscle satellite cells of the damaged site become myoblasts, to divide, and then differentiate into muscle fibers, and gradually fill the damaged site. However, when the muscle is damaged in a wide range and more seriously, the damaged site can only be repaired by connective tissue scar. Although myocardial fibers have a lot of mitosis in embryonic stage, it is very difficult to see nuclear division after birth, so their regeneration ability is extremely weak. Interestingly, in animal experiments, myocardial fibers in the damaged site regenerate to a certain extent, but in humans, there is no real regeneration figure of myocardial fibers. The necrotic myocardial fibers can only be proliferated, grown, and replaced by the surrounding connective tissues, forming permanent scars. Therefore, striated muscle cells and cardiomyocytes are classified as "permanent cells." As for smooth muscle cells, although their regeneration ability is very weak at ordinary times, they show strong regeneration ability in the process of wound healing of vascular wall or visceral wall. Although the origin of regenerated smooth muscle cells is unclear (most scholars believe that they are from the differentiation of undifferentiated mesenchymas in connective tissues, and some scholars believe that they are derived from fibroblasts close to them), it is more appropriate to classify smooth muscle cells as "stable cells."

2.1.2 Formation of Granulation Tissue and Its Significance

In the process of wound soft tissue repair and healing, one of the key steps is the formation of granulation tissue. The quality of granulation tissue directly affects the degree of wound repair and healing and its prognosis. The granulation tissue is an immature connective tissue with exuberant proliferation and vitality [3]. The name of granulation tissue is due to capillary ingrowth in the open wound of skin, visual observation shows bright red, granular, rich in blood vessels, soft in texture, easy to bleed when being touched, and looks like fresh granulation (Fig. 2.2).

2.1.2.1 Formation and Structure of Granulation Tissue

The essence of granulation tissue is a large number of capillaries and micro-vessels and abundant fibroblasts. The formation process of granulation tissue is as follows:

1. Early stage of granulation tissue formation: Within 48 h after injury. Immediately to 30 min after injury, there are aggravating congestion, blood stasis, micro-thrombosis, edema, a small amount of cellulose exudation, mild hemorrhage and blood clot formation, and gradually increasing neutrophils and monocytes infiltration under the wound. 24 h after injury, the situation is basically the same as above; however, the exudate increases, the blood circulation disorder intensifies, and the inflammatory cells increase, but granulation tissue has not yet appeared.
2. Initial stage of granulation tissue formation: 48–72 h after injury. Based on the above lesions, early granulation tissue can be observed 48 h after injury [4]. At this time, the visual observation only shows that the wound surface is relatively clean, and there is no typical granular granulation. However, few new fibroblasts and capillary "buds" are observed under the microscope. The former has a large cell body, enhanced basophilic cytoplasm, more mitotic figures, obvious nucleoli, double nucleoli, increased free ribosomes, and mild to moderate expansion of rough endoplasmic reticulum; the latter is made up of new endothelial cells, manifested as parallel arrangement of bulky endothelial cells, solid cords, no lumen or luminal stenosis, and lack of the capillary "bud" of basement membrane. Most scholars believe that it is derived from the original small vessels and capillaries growing outward by germination, and some new capillaries may be from the reconstruction of proliferative fibroblasts. 60–72 h after injury, the above early granulation tissue has increased significantly. One of the remarkable characteristics of granulation tissue at this stage is that new capillaries and fibroblasts mostly grow vertically toward the wound, in which the endothelial cell cords of new capillaries are not connected to each other or are not completely connected, and the basement membrane of endothelial cells is often absent or incomplete. Another characteristic is that the wound is accompanied by more neutrophils (microphages) and monocytes (macrophages) and more lymphocytes and other inflammatory cell infiltration. At the initial stage of granulation tissue formation, there are mostly liquid components among cells, including exudative plasma protein and cellulose, and there are a few or very few collagen fibers formed by fibroblasts and acidic mucopolysaccharides.
3. Peak period of granulation tissue formation: A large number of granulation tissues are formed, which can be observed 72–144 h after injury. Fresh, clean, and vibrant typical granular granulation tissue protruding from the wound can be observed macroscopically. Microscopically, with the arterioles as the axis, a large number of loop-like curved capillary networks are formed around the arterioles and form small masses together with abundant and proliferative fibroblasts with more mitotic figures, which evenly distribute and grow vertically towards the center of the wound or defect, and protrude out of the wound, that is, which are the granular granulation tissues observed macroscopically. During this period, the typical capillary structure has formed, that is, it has a complete basement membrane, fibroblasts have become adventitial cells, lumens vary in size, in which red blood cells and white blood cells are filled, and some capillaries gradually develop into real micro-vessels, arterioles, and venules, which may be caused by their respective differentiation according to the difference in intracavitary pressure and blood flow. During this period, the number of fibroblasts increases dramatically; fibroblasts arrange densely and grow towards the wound and superficial site and grow into blood clots together with capillaries. It is reported that the forward speed is 0.2 mm every day. Under electron microscope, fibroblasts show "active protein synthesis figure," that is, more abundant rough endoplasmic reticulum, with mild to moderate expansion, denser free ribosomes, increased mitochondria and dense matrix, and

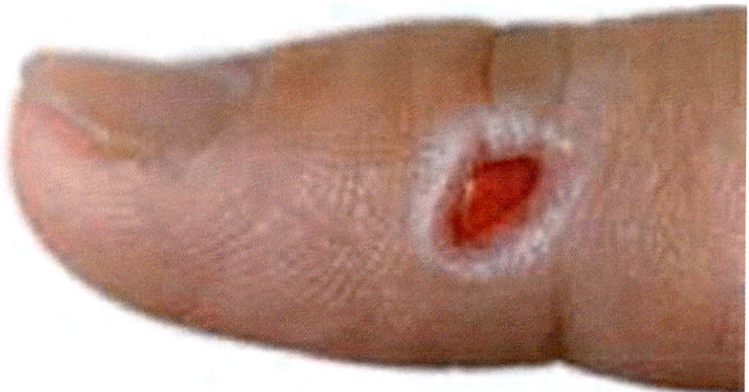

Fig. 2.2 Granulation tissue formation after finger injury

gradually increased collagen fibers and microfilament structure in cytoplasm. After 4–5 days, the "secretion" figures of collagen fibers into the extracellular matrix are common. 5–6 days after injury, fibroblasts in granulation tissues begin to produce collagen fibers, and the formation of collagen fibers is most active within 1 week. Starting from day 5, it can be seen that the contractile apparatus containing myofilaments formed in the cytoplasm of fibroblasts may be used as the myofibroblast with the function of producing fibers to strengthen wound closure and tear resistance, and is beneficial to wound contraction.

At the peak period of granulation tissue formation, the liquid components among cells have gradually reduced and are replaced by collagen fibers formed by fibroblasts and acidic mucopolysaccharides. The amount of collagen fibers in granulation tissue depends on the balance of synthesis and decomposition. The matrix component of granulation tissue is mainly proteoglycan, which is synthesized and secreted by fibroblasts and myofibroblasts, mainly chondroitin sulfate and hyaluronic acid, and then gradually forms Type I and Type II collagen with tear strength. However, the mechanism of its synthesis and secretion and the relationship with collagen secretion are still unknown. In this period, there is no nerve growing into granulation tissue, so there is no pain. However, some scholars have reported that vasomotor nerves were observed in the arterioles of granulation tissue 5–7 days after injury, and such vessels were found to have contraction phenomenon. Since then, such autonomic nerve fibers gradually formed, increased, and formed a network. Only after granulation tissue fibrosis and collagenization, nerve tissue gradually decreased.

4. Reduction period of granulation tissue: Usually, granulation tissue decreases gradually 7–14 days after injury, while fibroblasts produce collagen fibers most actively and produce fibronectin more and more. Some fibroblasts gradually become elongated stationary fibrocytes, with obviously reduced mitotic figures, and the new capillaries no longer increase, but gradually close, degenerate, and reduce, and are replaced by more arterioles and venules with thickened walls, that is, granulation tissues show reduction figures. Especially after week 3 after injury, granulation tissues gradually disappear, the growth of collagen fibers become less obvious. Instead, collagen fibers gradually mature and thicken, with increased reticular fibers, showing fibrous hyperplasia figures, and are mainly composed of Type I collagen fibers with tensile strength and tear strength. In this period, fibrous connective tissue changes from hyperplastic metabolism to functional metabolism, and the appearance shows that the tissue defects have been gradually filled up. The liquid components and various inflammatory cells in granulation tissue also decrease gradually.
5. Disappearance period of granulation tissue: Usually, granulation tissues gradually disappear completely 3–4 weeks after injury and are replaced by scar tissues with gray color, hard texture, lack of elasticity, and slight bulge. The original immature and active fibroblasts perpendicular to the wound and new capillaries disappear gradually and are replaced by mature and stationary fibrocytes parallel to the wound and arterioles and venules with thickened wall and complete structure, respectively. The collagen fibers become thicker, with hyalinization, the reticular fibers are collagenized, the elastic fibers are scarce, the liquid components in the interstitium extremely reduce, and the infiltrated neutrophils, lymphocytes, plasma cells, and phagocytes almost completely disappear, so the scar tissue volume significantly reduces, forming the so-called scar contraction, especially the bigger the scar, the more obvious the contraction. It often leads to the surface depression of organs and tissues, organ deformation or cavity stenosis (such as intestinal tube), and the scar contraction near the joint will lead to dyskinesia and affect the motor function.

Although collagen fibers in granulation tissues or scar tissues are derived from fibroblasts and fibrocytes, the amount depends on not only the synthesis and secretion of collagen, but also the decomposition of collagen. It is known that the enzymes involved in collagen decomposition mainly include collagenase and lysosomal enzyme. The former may be formed by epidermal basal cells and fibroblasts, while lysosomal enzyme can be produced by macrophages and secreted out of cells after phagocytizing collagen.

The formation process of above post-traumatic granulation tissues is basically the mode of every wound healing, but there are often differences in various injury and pathogenic factors and different tissues and organs. For example, local infection, foreign matters, blood circulation, innervation, drugs, physical and chemical factors, systemic nutrition, age, endocrine and special environmental factors (such as hypobaric hypoxia at high altitude, seawater immersion, and low temperature environment), and pathogenic factors will affect the quantity, quality, and formation rate of granulation tissues.

2.1.2.2 Significance of Granulation Tissue

In the process of wound repair and healing, the formation of granulation tissue has special and important functions, mainly including:

1. Filling up the defects of the wound and other tissues and organs;
2. Protecting the wound, preventing bacterial infection, reducing bleeding;
3. Organized blood clots and necrotic tissues, and other foreign matters, etc.
4. It is the basis of wound healing and scar formation.

2.1.3 Basic Pathophysiological Process of Wound Healing

As far as the wound of skin and subcutaneous tissue is concerned, although there are many causes of wound, and the degree of injury (range, depth, etc.) also varies greatly, the basic process of wound healing is similar or the same, that is, the complex combination of skin tissue regeneration and proliferation of granulation tissue, showing the synergistic effect of various processes.

The wound repair process of skin tissue is mainly related to the depth of injury, which can be roughly divided into three categories: The mildest and shallowest injury only affects the epidermis of skin, which is epidermal exfoliation (Class I, i.e., epidermal); the more serious and deeper injury, the epidermis and subcutaneous tissue layer (dermis) of the skin are broken or damaged (Class II, i.e., dermal); the most serious and deepest injury can also cause the disrupt of muscles, tendons, fascia, nerves, and blood vessels and even be accompanied by fractures (Class III, i.e., full-thickness).

For repair and healing of Class I injuries, when the wound is small, it is realized by migrating upwards after division, proliferation, and differentiation of basal cells; when the wound is large, it is realized by the division, proliferation, and differentiation of normal basal cells around the wound, which grow from the periphery to the center and finally cover the wound. Usually, it can be completed 2–4 days after injury, and the original structure and function are completely restored without any structural and functional disorders, which belongs to the process of "complete pathological regeneration." However, Class II and Class III injuries have the basic common repair and healing process which is different from Class I injury.

With regard to the basic process of repair and healing of Class II and Class III injuries, different scholars perform different descriptions and staging. Some scholars divide it into three stages: early changes after injury, wound contraction, proliferation of granulation tissue, and scar formation (Fig. 2.3). Some scholars also divide it into: (1) Inflammatory reaction, dissolution, and necrotic tissue removal in the early

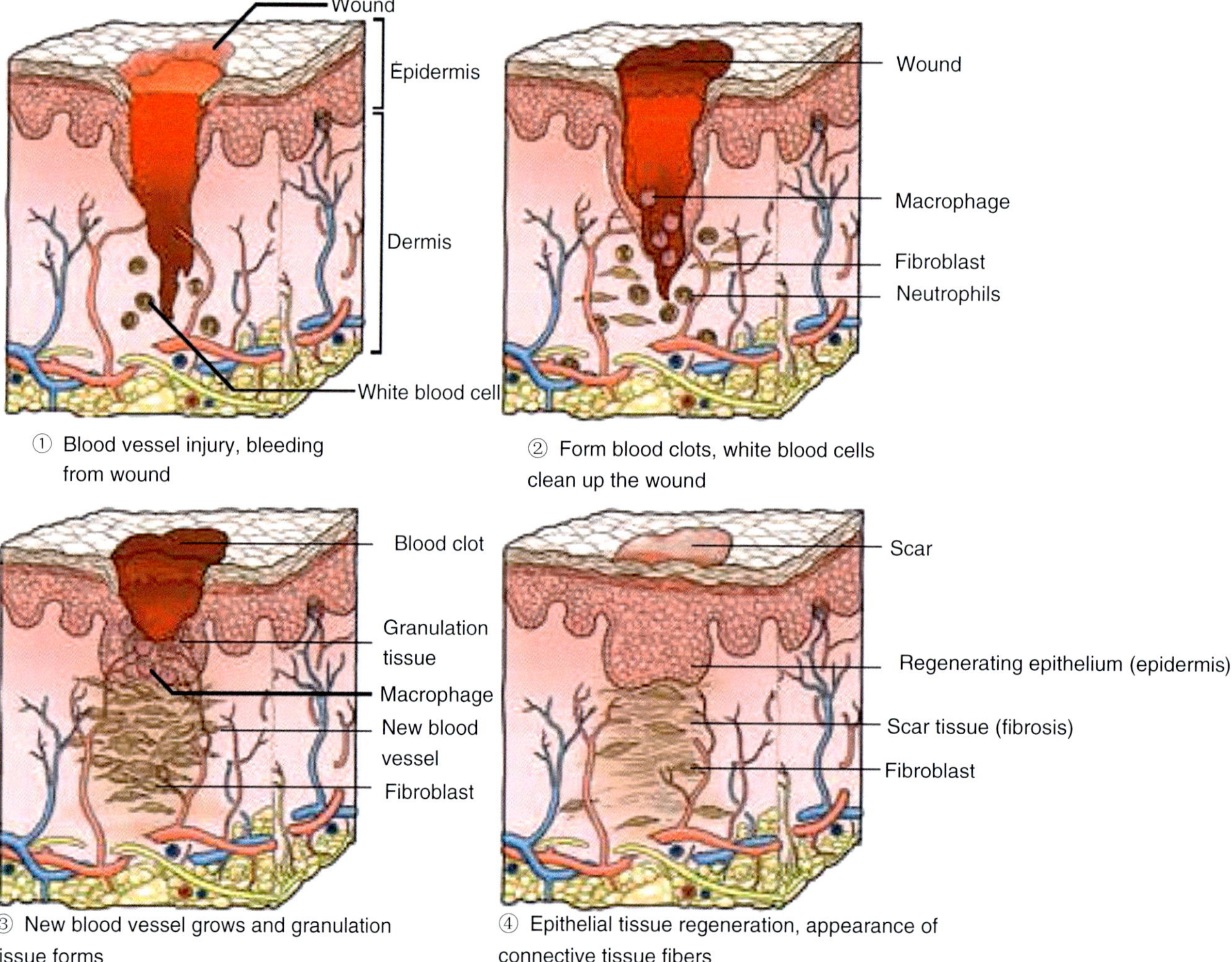

Fig. 2.3 Basic process of wound repair and healing

stage of wound; (2) Connective histocytes and vascular endothelial cells proliferate, swim, and form granulation tissues, or the original tissue regenerates; (3) Deposition of new connective tissue matrix and transformation and reconstruction of new tissue. According to dynamic experimental observations, from the perspective of pathology, wound healing is divided into five stages [5] that are differentiated, interrelated, and overlapped, which can more accurately reflect its essence.

1. Exudation and denaturation phase: From the moment of injury, fresh wound (or wound surface) has blood, exudate, necrotic broken tissue, and other fillings, as well as degeneration of epidermal and dermal tissues at the wound margin, in which blood comes from broken blood vessels, exudate consists of plasma proteins and lymph flowing into wound from blood vessels and tissue spaces of damaged wound margin, with exudation of white blood cells (mainly neutrophils and monocytes). The fibrinogen in these blood and exudates coagulates rapidly in the thromboplastin-rich wound environment to form a clot or scab to protect the wound. At this phase, dilation and congestion of blood vessels and degeneration of epidermal cells (especially basal cells and spinous cells) at the wound margin quickly appear, so many scholars call this phase as "early stage of inflammatory reaction." Some tests have shown that from the moment of injury, K^+, Na^+, Ca^{2+}, Cl^-, and other electrolytes accumulate in the wound immediately, resulting in the increase of moisture content in tissue space, the decrease of oxygen content in local tissues, while the increase of hydrogen ions, lactic acid, and other organic acids, which provides a good condition for the activity of own acid hydrolase. In addition, the injury and the accompanying infection will inevitably cause inflammation of the dermal tissue at the wound margin (obviously, this is caused by the inflammatory mediators sourced from the local blood and exudate of the wound), and then the blood flow of undamaged blood vessels is slow, congested, and even stagnant, resulting in edema in the affected area (i.e., edema at the wound margin), while the permeability of blood vessels increases, so that serous exudate containing immunoglobulin quickly enters the wound and forms molecular infection immunity. The exudation and denaturation phase usually starts from injury and lasts for several hours to more than ten hours, and its pathological findings are basically the same as the early changes of "early stage of granulation tissue formation."
2. Exudate absorption phase: Usually 6–48 h after injury, neutrophils enter the wound area under the influence of activated complement system to carry out "cellular infection defense," that is, phagocytosis and elimination of pathogenic bacteria, and gradually form the boundary zone of inflammatory cells. 18–24 h after injury, monocytes and lymphocytes also enter the wound area and gradually increase and can become histocytes with obvious phagocytosis function (its characteristic prominent change is that rough endoplasmic reticulum and ribosome increase significantly, indicating that protein synthesis is vigorous and active), which can not only phagocytize bacteria, but also phagocytize tissue residues, foreign bodies, and even the whole cell, so that exudates in the wound area are gradually absorbed and reduce.

   During this phase, due to the enzymatic hydrolysis of infectious pathogenic bacteria and damaged tissues, tissue injury acidosis can occur at the wound margin area, thus activating protease and promoting plasma exudation, which is a beneficial and important "culture medium" for inflammatory cells entering the wound area. In the subsequent proliferative phase, the pH value of the wound area is reduced, thus accelerating the wound healing process.

   At the early phase of this stage, the epidermal cells at the wound margin still show reactive alteration, and at the later phase, the basal cells migrate to the wound and become larger, with thicker chromatin, clear nucleolus, and more mitotic figures, showing early proliferation figures.
3. Granulation proliferation and epidermal migration phase: About 3 days after injury, the main findings are granulation tissue proliferation and epidermal cell proliferation and migration. The proliferation figures of granulation tissues are same as the early phase of granulation tissue formation, but its quantity and rate are related to the scope and types of injury. During this phase, granulation proliferates in the "in situ" proliferation of fibroblasts, and hypoxia often occurs in the wound center as a result of active metabolism. Therefore, under the action of hypoxia and various cell growth factors, there is not only fibroblast proliferation, but also a large number of new capillaries growing into the wound area. It should be pointed out that most of these new capillaries come from adjacent blood vessels, which first form capillary buds, then grow into the wound area in a loop shape, form branches through the proliferation of their cells, and finally connect with each other to form capillary networks, that is, germination; other capillaries are formed by "autogenous" reconstruction, that is, their occurrence has nothing to do with the original blood vessels, but new capillaries are directly formed after regeneration and differentiation of mesenchymal cells in dermis, which is similar to angiogenesis in embryonic period, that is, fibroblasts proliferate and arrange in parallel to form small cracks and then communicate with the surrounding capillaries, blood flows through, and new capillaries are formed.

   At this stage, the epidermis at the wound margin enters the migration phase. There is tensile strength among cells of intact epidermal tissue through the connection of intercellular bridges and tonofibrils. About 3 days after injury, the connection between the basal cells at the wound margin and the acanthocytes at the base becomes loose. Such epidermal cells temporarily lose their keratinization ability and form a contractile device containing actin, which can actively participate in the phagocytosis and degradation of wound necrosis substances and fibrin clots. After 3 days of injury, cells begin to proliferate under the influence of local chalone loss, epidermal and platelet-derived growth factor (PDGF), and local inflammatory exudate stimulation and activation and migrate under the scab and above fibronectin-fibrin liner along the wound margin with amoeboid movement. After several days or 1–2 weeks, the wound is finally closed.

4. Wound contraction phase: 5–6 days after injury, with the formation and gradual maturity of granulation tissues, being pulled by proliferating myofibroblasts, and the whole skin tissue (including epidermis and subcutaneous tissue) at the wound margin regenerating and migrating towards the center along the margin and bottom of the wound, the wound gradually shrinks and disappears. Although the synthesis of intercellular substances starts in the early phase of granulation tissue formation and early in the peak phase, fiber synthesis and connective tissue regeneration, which play a decisive role in quantity and maturity, start only after a large number of granulation tissues fill the tissue defects, thus enhancing the mechanical stability.

   A large number of studies have shown that the epidermal repair and healing of skin wounds are similar to the epithelium of other organs and can be divided into four stages: epidermal (epithelial) migration, cell division and epidermal (epithelial) differentiation, and epidermal recovery. The basic process is: several hours after the skin is damaged, the basal cells at the broken end of epidermis around the defect site first begin to migrate to the wound surface and gradually cover the exposed surface, side surface of the wound or blood clot surface. After several hours, the basal cells of epidermis begin to divide and proliferate. It is observed that such division and proliferation begin at about 1 mm away from the broken end of epidermis and then becomes more and more extensive, mitosis is also very active, and the wound surface is gradually covered in Phases III–IV. Once the moving epidermal cells meet with each other, the proliferation of epidermal cells stops due to contact inhibition, and the immigrated epidermal cells begin to differentiate further and gradually appear typical stratified squamous epithelium with normal thickness and cell arrangement accompanied by keratinization; meanwhile, intercellular bridges and ultrastructure with tensile strength reappear, so that the skin surface gradually regains its mechanical, chemical, and physical damage resistance. However, when the wound is too large (generally considered that its diameter exceeds 20 cm), it is difficult for the regenerated epidermis to completely cover the wound, and the skin grafting is often required. This stage is usually completed within 2–3 weeks after injury.

5. Scar formation phase (final phase): The final outcome of skin wound repair and healing is scar formation, in which wounds with small defect, neat wound margin, no infection, and neat coaptation (such as surgical incision) can form scars 2–3 weeks after injury, while those with large defect, incomplete wound margin or split, no neat coaptation, or with infection often take 4–5 weeks or longer to form scars. Usually, the former is an inapparent scar like a line and does not affect function, while the latter forms a broader and esthetically objectionable scar, which is easy to cause function limitation in contraction. Such scars are often white-pink due to lack of melanocytes; because its collagen fibers are mainly composed of Type I collagen fibers with tear resistance but almost no elasticity, scar tissue tends to shrink, distort, and deform the surrounding skin. At the same time, because of the deep defects, its hair follicles, sweat glands, seborrhea, and other skin appendages are completely destroyed, which cannot completely regenerate or regenerate. Scar is the final outcome of wound healing, and its main function is to connect the wound margin firmly, with strong tensile strength. The material basis of tensile strength is that Type I collagen fiber is the main component of scar, and its strength mainly depends on collagen fiber, especially the quantity and arrangement of Type I collagen and is also related to elastic fibers, reticular fibers, and other components. Although the local tensile strength of the wound appears at the initial phase of granulation tissue formation 3–4 days after injury and begins to increase at the peak phase of granulation tissue formation about 1 week after injury (especially wound contraction phase), the tensile strength increases most rapidly and obviously on weeks 3–5; after that, although it continues to increase, it gradually slows down, and the tensile strength usually reaches its peak about 3 months after injury, and no longer increases; finally, its tensile strength can only reach 70–80% of normal skin strength. Due to the poor elasticity of scar itself, if the scar is thin, its tensile strength is low, which can often cause scar complications, such as ventral hernia, ventricular aneurysm, and aneurysm.

The formation and regression of scar mainly depend on the balance state of collagen fiber synthesis and decomposition. In the initial phase and fibroplasia phase of wound healing, because the synthesis of collagen fibers is dominant, the local collagen fibers increase continuously; when synthesis and decomposition are in balance, the size of scars has no change; however, when collagen fibers are decomposed and absorbed by collagenase, and they are dominate, the scars gradually soften and shrink, and the time varies depending on the size of scars, usually after several months.

2.2 Types of Skin Healing and Healing Disorders

2.2.1 Types of Skin Repair and Healing

The way of wound healing mainly depends on the degree of injury and whether there is infection. Based on clinical reasons, wound healing is usually divided into three types. The skin wound is taken as an example as follows [6]:

1. Healing by first intention is the simplest wound healing and is also caused by the direct combination of tissues. It can be seen in wounds with few tissue defects, neat wound margin, no infection, tight coaptation, and close contact of the wound surface and is common in sutured or bonded surgical incisions (Fig. 2.4). In the past, it has long been mistakenly believed that the healing of such wound was formed by new epidermal cells, capillary endothelial cells, and connective tissues on both sides crossing the wound in a short time. At present, the dynamic observation of animal experiments has confirmed that a small amount of granulation tissue also involves in such healing by first intention, and its basic process is: due to the less blood clots, weak inflammatory reaction, and mild cell injury at the wound margin in these wounds, the epidermal basal cells on both sides of the wound develop reactive thickening several hours after injury, with increased mitosis, and migrate into the wound; on the one hand, they migrate along the surface layer of dermis, on the other hand, they grow downward, between blood clot and wound margin, separating dermis from blood clot; they proliferate actively after more than 10 h and cover the wound at 24–48 h; at 48–72 h after injury, granulation tissues begin to grow and fill the wound rapidly, and new collagen fibers form at 5–6 days after injury (usually sutures can be removed at this time), and the wound can completely heal at 2–3 weeks after injury, leaving only a linear scar. Therefore, the healing by first intention time is short, with less scars and no dysfunction. It has been reported in the literature that epidermal (epithelial) cells are the first to be activated and proliferated after skin wound, which causes the response of connective tissues such as granulation tissue, and the formed granulation tissue can inhibit the growth of epidermal cells in feedback way.
2. Healing by second intention can be seen in the skin wound which is too large and accompanied by infection. Because the wound is too large, new cells cannot cross. Because of infection, inflammation and tissue necrosis often exist at the same time, its healing can only be filled by granulation tissues, and then its surface is covered by new epidermis (Fig. 2.5). Studies have confirmed that the healing process of such wound is not to form granulation tissues first, but to regenerate epidermal cells first, and then stimulate the formation and proliferation of granulation tissues, thus healing the wound. The basic process of its healing is as follows: the epidermal basal cells at the wound margin proliferate actively, migrate down along the wound margin, isolate the dermis from the blood clot, and extend to the center of the wound, at the same time stimulate the proliferation of peripheral fibroblasts and endothelial cells, and new capillaries appear and form granulation tissues at the bottom and margin of the wound; then granulation tissues gradually increase, pushing the new epidermal cells upward, and epidermal cells gradually cover the granulation tissues completely; finally, scars form, and the wound heals completely.

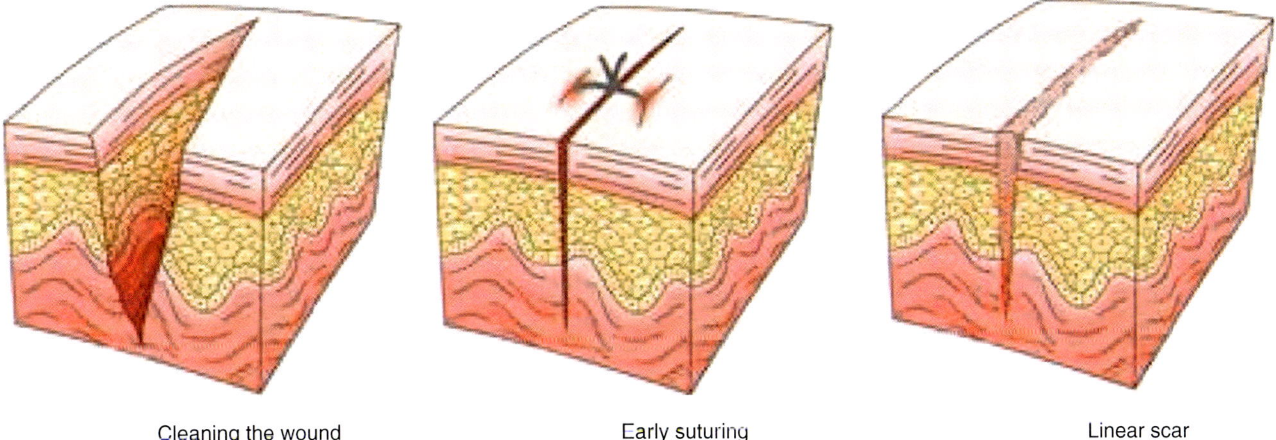

Fig. 2.4 Healing by first intention of wound

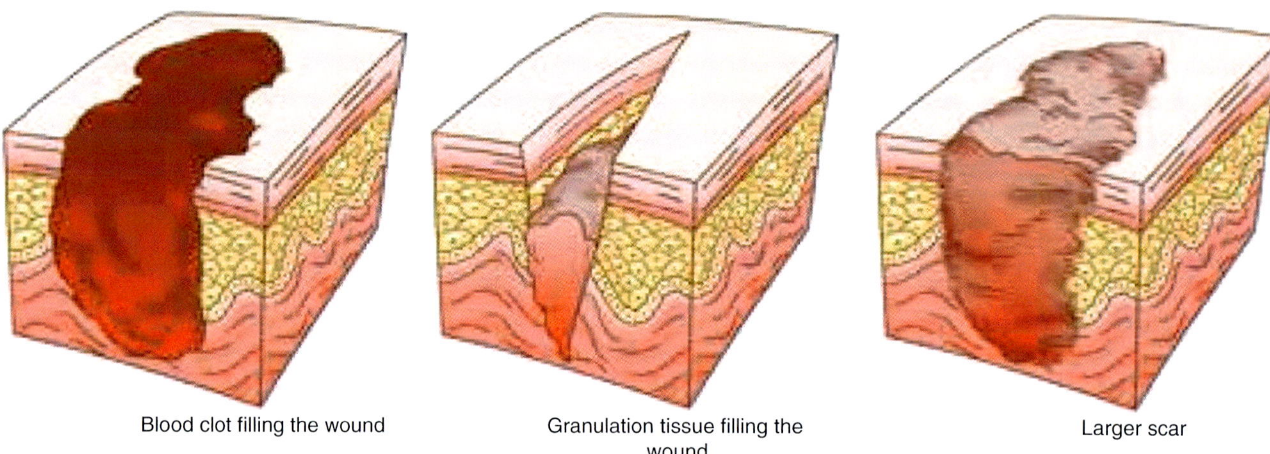

Fig. 2.5 Healing by second intention of wound

Compared with healing by first intention, the characteristics of healing by second intention are as follows: (1) The start time of epidermal regeneration delays, because there are many necrotic tissues, and infection is easy to induce local tissue degeneration, necrosis, and serious inflammatory reaction; only when infection is controlled and necrotic tissue is basically cleared, can epidermal regeneration begin. (2) There are many granulation tissues and the scars formed are large, which are caused by large wounds. (3) The healing time is longer, usually more than 4 weeks, because the wound is too large, infection is more common, bacterial toxins are easy to cause tissue necrosis and suppuration, and the plasmin in pus destroys the fibrin scaffold (which is an extremely important structure for fibroblast and neovascularization to grow inward), resulting in delayed healing; meanwhile, bacterial toxins may cause thrombosis and affect the blood supply for healing tissues.

3. Healing under scab is a repairing and healing way of special wounds under special conditions, which refers to the above-mentioned healing by second intention under a dark brown hard scab formed on the wound surface after drying exudate, blood and exfoliated necrotic tissue, such as the healing process under leather-like hard scab after deep second- or third-degree burns. Although scab is not conducive to the growth of cells because of its dryness and has a certain protective effect on wounds, when there is more exudate under scab, especially when there is bacterial infection, scab becomes an obstacle for exudate drainage and a "medium" under scab. Bacterial infection is often aggravated, which affects its healing process. Therefore, it is often necessary to perform "escharectomy" or "tangential excision" to expose wounds and accelerate healing. Generally, scab cannot fall off until the regeneration of epidermis is completed. Healing under scab is also the proliferation of epidermal basal cells at the wound margin first, which migrate to the wound center under scab, following by granulation tissue proliferation. The speed of healing under scab is generally slower than that without scab, with long healing time. This is because when the epidermis regenerates, the scabs encountered must be dissolved before it can grow forward. Such healing under scab is not only often encountered in skin wounds, but can also be seen in respiratory tract mucosa burns such as trachea and nasal vestibule.

2.2.2 Skin Healing Disorders

The regeneration mode, healing time, repair degree, and size of cicatrix after wound are not only related to the degree of injury (wound size and depth) and tissue regeneration ability, but also affected by systemic and local conditions. Although some favorable factors, treatment measures and various growth factors can promote the regeneration and repair of wound tissue, other unfavorable factors, especially aging, undernutrition, and infection, often cause wound healing disorders and even cause some serious complications.

2.2.2.1 Factors That Cause Wound Healing Disorders

Systemic Factors

1. Aging: Aging is one of the main factors that cause wound healing disorders. The regeneration ability of each tissue and cell itself in the elderly has significantly weakened, and the blood supply reduces due to the aging of blood vessels. Meanwhile, with the increase of age, the cell cycle of fibroblasts of tissues obviously prolongs, resulting in delayed healing, even nonunion, and the mechanical enhancement of wounds also significantly delays.
2. Undernutrition: Serious protein deficiency can cause hypoplasia or slow regeneration of tissues and cells, espe-

cially when sulfur-containing amino acids (such as methionine) are deficient, which often leads to the growth disorder of tissues and cells in wounds, poor granulation tissue formation, failure of fibroblasts to mature into fibrocytes, and reduction of collagen fiber synthesis. Vitamin deficiency has a greater impact. For example, vitamin C deficiency does not affect the proliferation of fibroblasts, but hinders their collagen synthesis function (including hydroxylation disorder of proline) and affects their transformation into fibrocytes, making less scar formation and weak in tensile strength; the deficiency of vitamin A1, B2, and B6 leads to poor fibrosis; the decrease of the systemic and local zinc content also leads to delayed healing.

3. Improper medication: Large dose of adrenocortical hormone can obviously inhibit the formation of new capillaries, the proliferation of fibroblasts and collagen synthesis, and accelerate the decomposition of collagen fibers, resulting in poor healing; penicillamine has a similar effect and weakens its tensile strength, because it can combine with aldehyde group on collagen α-peptide chain and interfere with the formation of intramolecular and intermolecular crosslinking of collagen, which leads to the instability of collagen fibers and accelerates the decomposition and absorption of collagen fibers.

Local Factors

1. Infection and foreign bodies: Wound infection is very common and easy to cause suppuration, and 100 bacteria are enough to cause subcutaneous abscess. There are a lot of exudates after infection, which can increase the local tension of the wound and lead to the wound dehiscence (including healing and healed wounds). Especially, some toxins and enzymes produced by pyogenic bacteria can cause cell necrosis, collagen fibers, and collagen dissolution, thus aggravating tissue damage and hindering healing.
2. Poor local blood circulation: Good local blood circulation can not only ensure the required nutrition and oxygen, but also facilitate the absorption and transportation of necrotic substances and the control of local infection. On the contrary, it will affect the regeneration and repair of tissues and cells and delay healing; for example, in patients with varicose veins of lower extremity or atherosclerosis. Especially when the blood circulation disorder of tissues occurs, its lower PO_2 also easily promotes the growth of anaerobic bacteria (such as Bacillus fusiformis), which can cause gas gangrene and tetanus.
3. Impaired innervation: Impaired autonomic nerve can cause local blood supply disorder and affect the regeneration of tissues and cells. Leprosy skin ulcer will not heal for a long time, which is caused by nerve involvement.
4. Irradiation: All kinds of irradiation (including γ-ray, X-ray, α-ray, and β-ray, electron beam, etc.) can directly cause refractory skin ulcer, and combined irradiation can also hinder wound healing caused by other reasons, because rays can damage small vessels, inhibit fibroblast proliferation and collagen synthesis and secretion, and directly damage all kinds of cells, and finally prevent scar formation. The factors causing wound healing disorders and their complications are listed in Table 2.1.

Table 2.1 Factors of wound healing disorders

Disorder factors	Pathogenesis	Complications
Advanced age	Prolonged cell cycle of fibroblasts	Healing retardation, wound dehiscence
Nutrition disorders	Systemic cell growth disorder	Healing retardation, prolonged unhealed
Blood circulation disorder	Local cell growth disorder	Healing retardation, prolonged unhealed
Vitamin C deficiency	Collagen synthesis disorder	Wound dehiscence and healing retardation
XII factor deficiency	Coagulation disorder	Wound infection, seroma
Anticoagulant drugs, fibrinolytic drugs	(Fibrinopeptide)	Wound infection, seroma
Corticosteroids, ACTH	Inhibition of exudation process and fiber formation	Wound infection, wound dehiscence
Cell inhibitor	Hyperplasia disorder	Prolonged unhealed ulcer
True diabetes	Excessive glucose, granulocyte dysfunction, bacterial growth	Wound infection
Irradiation	Hyperplasia disorder	Prolonged unhealed, accompanied by canceration
Contamination	Effects of pyogenic bacteria, anaerobes, and toxins	Gas gangrene, tetanus

2.2.2.2 Types of Skin Wound Healing Disorders

In the process of skin wound healing, healing disorders can be caused by different factors, resulting in various complications.

1. Wound dehiscence: Refer to the dehiscence of a healing wound or a wound that has been surgically sutured (Fig. 2.6). It is more common in elderly patients or wound infection, resulting in delayed healing.
2. Granuloma formation: Refer to the foreign bodies that cannot be absorbed in the wound or the foreign body granuloma (Fig. 2.7) or lipophagic granuloma formed

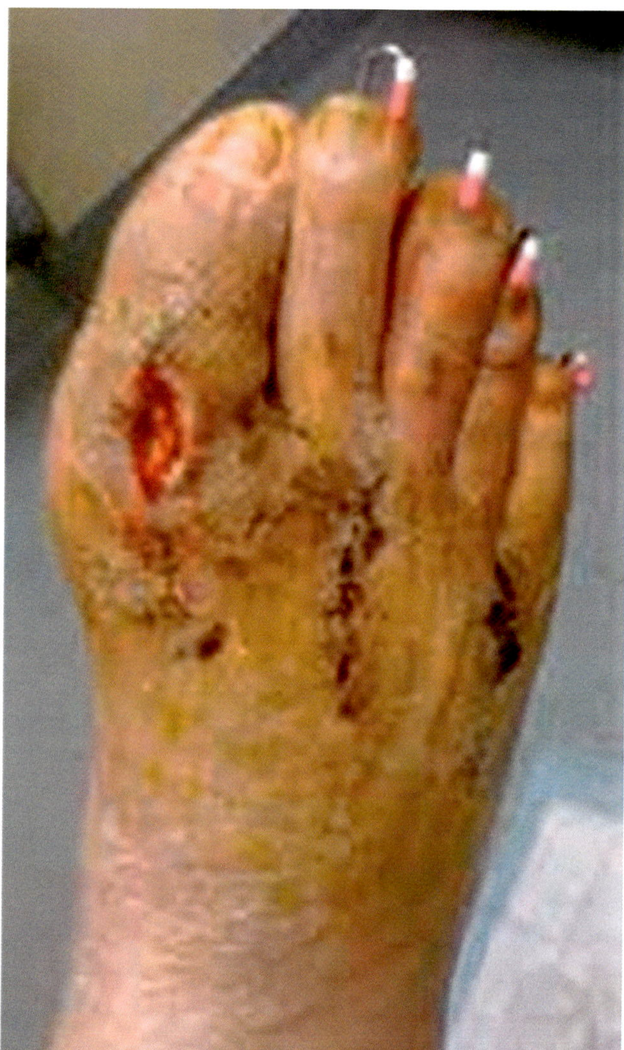

Fig. 2.6 Poor healing and wound dehiscence

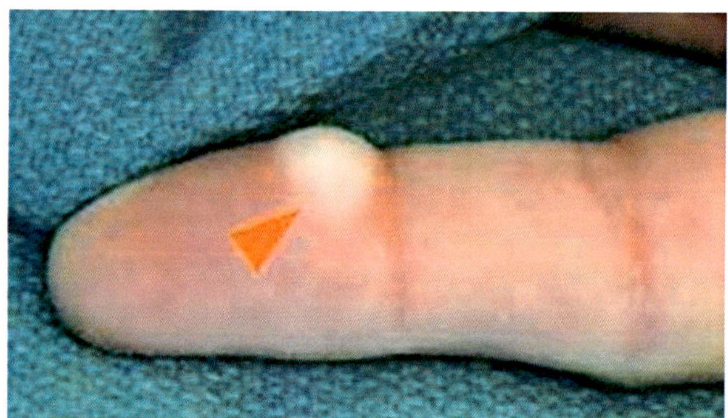

Fig. 2.7 Foreign body granuloma of finger

around the necrotic adipose tissue. It can delay the wound healing of some patients.

3. Traumatic epidermoid cyst: Refer to some germinal layers (such as basal cells and deep spinous cells) of the skin epidermis that are brought into the deep site of the wound by injury during the wound, in which they can continue to grow and product keratocysts (Fig. 2.8) and can cause chronic granulomatous inflammation, hindering wound healing.
4. Proud flesh: Refer to tumor-like neoplasm formed by excessive growth of granulation tissue during wound healing (Fig. 2.9). It is more common in skin (telangiectatic granuloma) and gums (granulomatous epulis).
5. Seroma formation: Refer to a "cyst" formed in a large cavity in the tissue of the wound area, which is filled with blood, serum, and lymph. When blood cells disintegrate, the liquid is light yellow or yellowish brown (Fig. 2.10). This cavity is surrounded and covered by fibrous connective tissues and cells (i.e., fibrous "epithelium"), which affects the continuous healing of wounds.

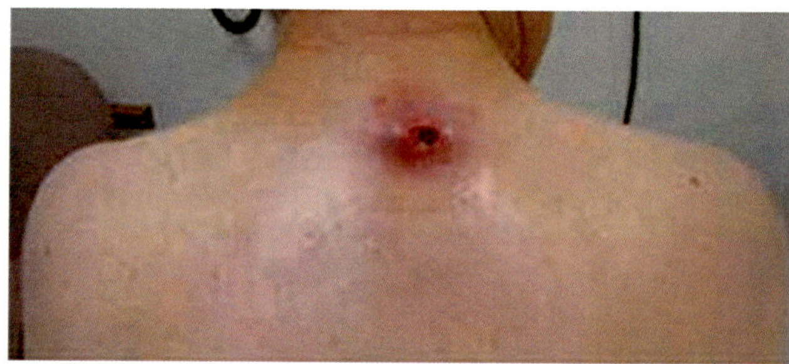

Fig. 2.8 Traumatic epidermoid cyst

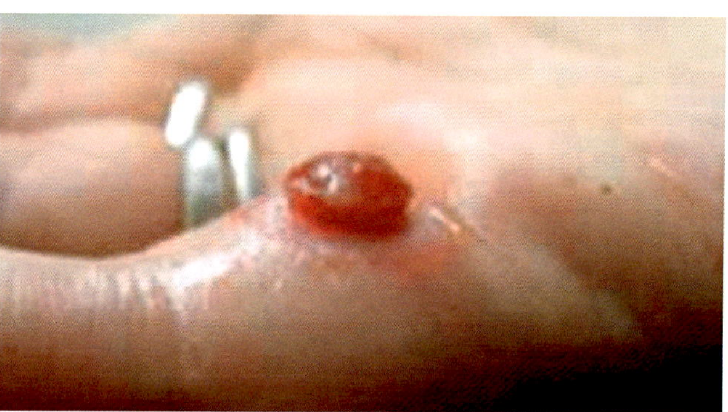

Fig. 2.9 Tumor-like neoplasm of hand

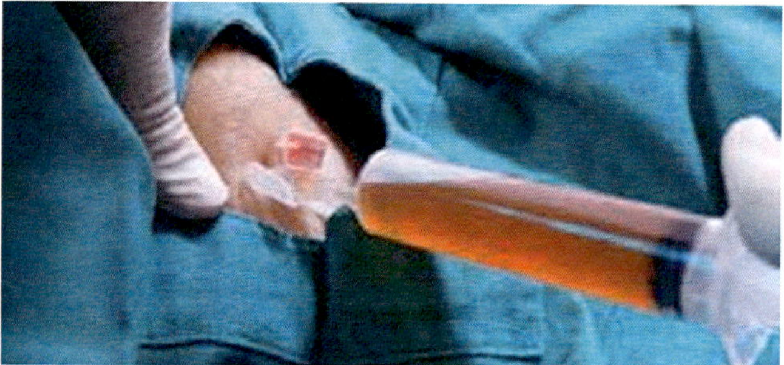

Fig. 2.10 Seroma puncture liquid

6. Keloid formation: Refer to excessive scar formation in the process of wound healing, which can be divided into two categories.
   (a) Hypertrophic scars: Refer to hyperplastic scar formation only limited to the local site of the wound (Fig. 2.11). In this case, the crosslinking process of collagen is obstructed, and only a few collagen fibers gather into fiber bundles. If fibers of hypertrophic scars are rotated by 90° (i.e., Z-plasty), the excessive collagen will be decomposed in a short time.
   (b) Keloid: Refer to hyperplastic scar formation beyond the wound area and spreading to the surrounding skin. Keloids are more common in chest and limbs (Fig. 2.12). Colored people (especially the black and yellow races) have a greater tendency to develop keloids than the white. The formation conditions and mechanism of keloids have not been clarified. The main viewpoints are heredity, endocrine, constitution, neurotrophic disorder, blood circulation disorder, and ethnology theories. Recently, some scholars think that it is caused by local connective tissue formation disorder, because myofibroblasts (accounting for 50–75% of all cell components in dermis) cannot differentiate into fibrocyte and proliferate for a long time, during which collagen fiber crosslinking disorder occurs. Collagen fibers randomly deposit in tissues and are bonded together through the increase of proteoglycan components to form keloids. Its morphology is characterized by dense arrangement of a large number of collagen bundles, with messy directions, each with a whorled or curve-like structure, accompanied by obvious vitreous degeneration; abundant small blood vessels and good blood supply; lack of skin appendages structure, most atrophy of epidermis covering keloids, so it is easy to be damaged. Presumably, it may also be one of the reasons why squamous cell carcinoma often occurs in keloid areas, and many eosinophils can be found in the lesions.
7. Formation of intractable refractory skin ulcer: Refer to the recurrent intractable skin ulcer caused by some chemical, physical, and metabolic disorders, etc. (Fig. 2.13), especially the latent period of radiation skin ulcer can be as long as several years or even decade(s), which is characterized by recurrent, prolonged unhealed, and accompanied by canceration.
8. Ulcer canceration: Refer to canceration occurred during wound healing (Fig. 2.14). For example, the canceration rate of radiation skin ulcer can reach 5–28%.

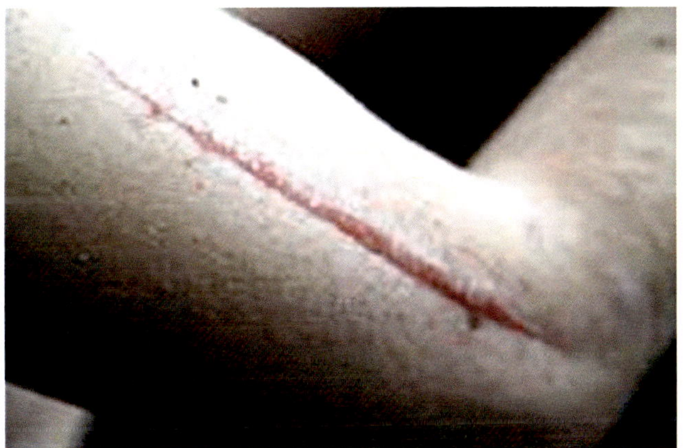

Fig. 2.11 Hypertrophic scars of incision

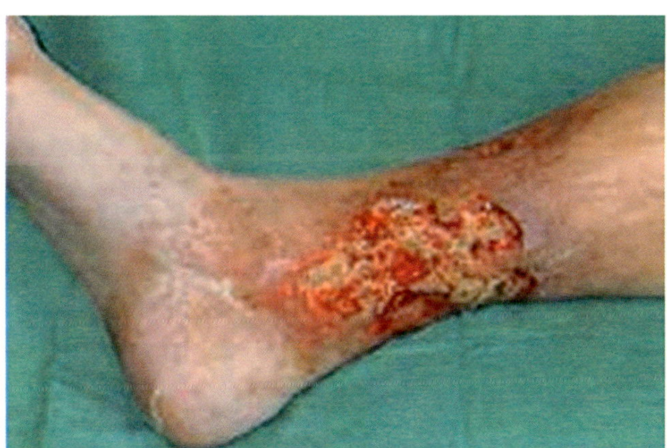

Fig. 2.13 Intractable refractory skin ulcer

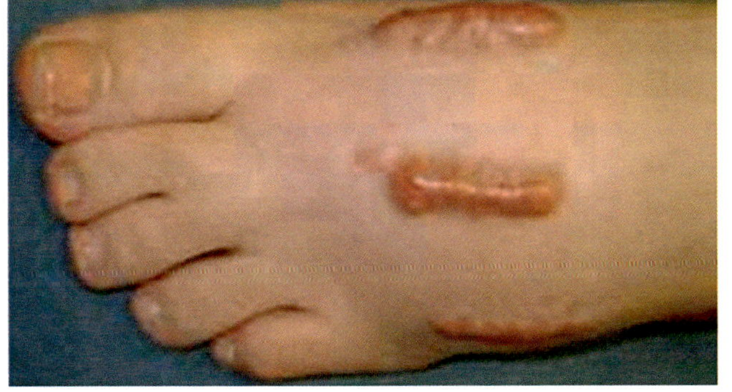

Fig. 2.12 Keloid

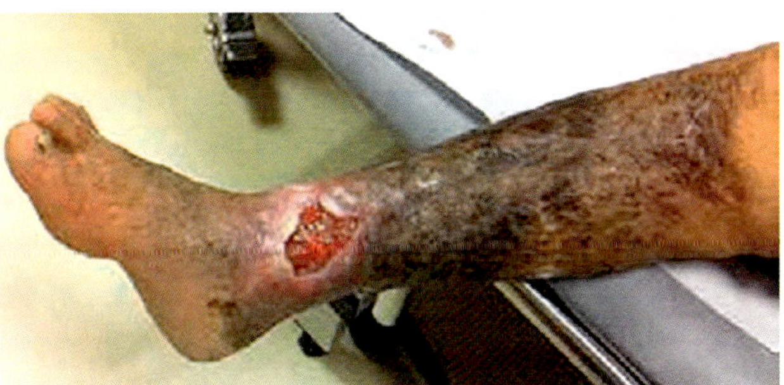

Fig. 2.14 Ulcer canceration

Search Terms

Soft tissue repair, Regeneration, Physiological regeneration, Pathological regeneration, Regeneration ability, Labile cells, Stable cells, Permanent cells, Granulation tissue, Repair of class I injuries, Repair of class II injuries, Repair of class III injuries, Healing by first intention, Healing by second intention, Healing under scab, Scar, Keloid, Ulcer canceration

References

1. Thorne CH. Wound healing: Normal and abnormal. In: Grabb and Smith's plastic surgery. 6th ed. Philadelphia: Lippincott Williams & Wilkins, a Wolters Kluwer Business; 2007. p. 15–22.
2. Rubin E, Reisner HM. Essentials of Rubins pathology, 6th revised ed. Philadelphia: Lippincott Williams and Wilkins; 2013. p. 64–5.
3. Flanagan M. The characteristics and formation of granulation tissue. J Wound Care. 1998;7(10):508–10.
4. Lanza R, Langer R, Vacanti JP. Principles of tissue engineering, 2nd ed. Academic; 2000, p. 862–8.
5. Thiruvoth FM, Mohapatra DP, Kumar D, et al. Current concepts in the physiology of adult wound healing. Plast Aesthet Res. 2015;2:250–6. https://doi.org/10.4103/2347-9264.158851.
6. Trott AT. Wounds and lacerations: emergency care and closure. 3rd ed. Mosby; 2005. p. 19–27.

Measures for Prevention and Control of Surgical Site Infection

3

Kejian Wu, Jie Sun, and Xinghua Li

Abstract

Surgical site infection (SSI) is the most common nosocomial infection in surgical patients. Surgical operation will inevitably bring injury to the skin and tissues of the surgical site. When the microbial contamination of the surgical incision reaches a certain degree, SSI will occur. It not only increases the pain and the economic burden of patients, prolongs the hospital stay, but also leads to the mortality and re-hospitalization rate significantly higher than those of uninfected patients. SSI includes incision infection and infection of organs or spaces involved in surgery, and the risk factors of SSI include both patient and surgical aspects. The main factors in patient aspect are age, nutritional status, immune function, health status, etc., and those in surgical aspect are preoperative hospital stay, skin preparation method and time, skin disinfection at surgical site, operating room environment, sterilization of surgical instruments, aseptic operation during surgery, surgical technique, duration of surgery, antimicrobial prophylaxis, etc. Medical institutions and medical personnel should strengthen the prevention and control of SSI in response to risk factors.

Keywords

Surgical site infection · Knotless suture · Incision scar

K. Wu (✉)
Department of Orthopedics Trauma, The Fourth Medical Center of PLA General Hospital, Beijing, China

J. Sun
Tianjin Hospital, Tianjin, China

X. Li
Department of Lower Extremity Orthopedics, Zhengzhou Orthopedics Hospital, Zhengzhou, China

3.1 Diagnosis of Surgical Site Infection and Incision Classification

3.1.1 Definition and Diagnostic Criteria of Surgical Site Infection

Surgical site infection (SSI) refers to the infection (such as incision infection, brain abscess, and peritonitis) that occurs in the incision or deep organ or space of the surgery in the perioperative period (after the perioperative period, in some cases). SSI accounts for about 15% of all nosocomial infections, and 35–40% of nosocomial infections in surgical patients. The concept of SSI is wider than that of wound infection, because it includes the infection of organs and spaces once involved in surgery; it is narrower and more specific than the concept of "postoperative infection," because it does not include infections that are not directly related to surgery, such as pneumonia and urinary tract infection. SSI can be divided into the following categories: (1) Superficial incisional SSI (infection involves only skin or subcutaneous tissue of the incision); (2) Deep incisional SSI [involving fascial and/or muscular layers]: deep incisional primary (DIP)-SSI refers to one or more primary incisional SSI in patients undergoing surgery, and deep incisional secondary (DIS)-SSI refers to one or more secondary incisional SSI in patients undergoing surgery; (3) Organ/space SSI (infection involves any part of the anatomy, other than the skin, fascia or muscular incision, which is opened during an operation). The diagnostic criteria for SSI [with reference to the revision opinion of the US Centers for Disease Control and Prevention (CDC)] [1] are listed in Table 3.1.

3.1.2 Classification of Surgical Incisions

The occurrence of SSI is related to the degree of contamination of the surgical field during the operation. In the past, surgical incisions were divided into three categories: Class I/Clean Incision, Class II/Potentially Contaminated Incision,

P. Tang et al. (eds.), *Tutorials in Suturing Techniques for Orthopedics*, https://doi.org/10.1007/978-981-33-6330-4_3

Table 3.1 Diagnostic criteria for SSI

Superficial incisional SSI
Infection occurs within 30 days after the operation, and infection involves only skin or subcutaneous tissue and at least one of the following:
1. Purulent discharge from the superficial incision;
2. Presence of bacteria growth in the discharge from the superficial incision;
3. At least one of the following symptoms: pain or tenderness, swelling, redness or heat, so the incision is deliberately opened by surgeon;
4. Determined as superficial incisional infection by a surgeon but not includes the abscess and infection at and around the suture and stitches
Deep incisional SSI
Infection occurs within 30 days after the operation (within 1 year if implant is in place), and infection involves deep fascia and muscular layer of incision, and at least one of the following:
1. Purulent drainage from the deep incision: A deep incision spontaneously dehisces or is deliberately opened by a surgeon when the patient has at least one of the following symptoms or signs: (1) Fever (>38 °C); (2) Localized pain or tenderness;
2. An abscess involving the deep incision is found during the operation, or by histopathologic or radiologic examination;
3. Diagnosis of deep incisional SSI by surgeon. Infection that involves both superficial and deep incision sites shall be listed as deep incisional SSI
Organ/space SSI
Infection occurs within 30 days after the operation (within 1 year if implant is in place) and infection involves organs or spaces of surgical site, which is opened or manipulated during an operation and at least one of the following:
1. Purulent drainage from a drain that is placed into the organ/space;
2. Pathogenic bacteria isolated from culture of fluid or tissue in the organ/space;
3. An abscess involving the organ/space that is found during the operation, or by histopathologic or radiologic examination;
4. Diagnosis of an organ/space SSI by a surgeon

Note: Artificial implants refer to prosthetic heart valve, vascular graft, hip prosthesis, etc.

and Class III/Contaminated Incision; the healing and infection situation of the incisions are classified into Level A, Level B, and Level C. This classification has been used for a long time as one of the indicators of medical quality assessment in surgical departments. In practice, it is found that this classification method is not perfect. In order to better evaluate the contamination of surgical incisions, incisions are generally divided into four categories [2] (Table 3.2).

According to the above classification, the infection rates of different incisions were significantly different: 1% for clean incision, 7% for clean-contaminated incision, 20% for contaminated incision, and 40% for dirty-infected incision. Therefore, the classification of incisions is an important basis for determining whether antimicrobial prophylaxis is required.

Table 3.2 Classification of surgical incisions

Category	Classification criteria
Class I: Clean incision	An uninfected operative wound in which no inflammation is encountered and the respiratory, alimentary, genital, or urinary tract is not entered
Class II: Clean-contaminated incision	An operative wound in which the respiratory, alimentary, genital, or urinary tracts are entered without obvious contamination, e.g., non-infected and successfully completed operations involving the biliary tract, gastrointestinal tract, vagina and oropharynx.
Class III: Contaminated incision	Fresh, open wound surgery; operations enter the area of acute, nonpurulent inflammation, with gross spillage from the gastrointestinal tract, and major breaks in sterile technique (e.g., open cardiac massage)
Class IV: Dirty-infected incision	Old traumatic wounds with retained devitalized tissue and those that involve existing clinical infection or perforated viscera

3.2 Measures for Prevention and Control of Orthopedic Surgical Site Infection

In recent years, the concept of enhanced recovery after surgery has been rapidly promoted and applied in orthopedic surgery, and has achieved remarkable results. Surgical incision complications often affect the enhanced recovery process. Common surgical incision complications include postoperative incision exudate, bleeding, swelling, blisters, ecchymosis, infection (superficial or deep), poor healing, scars, etc. The incision complications of traumatic orthopedic patients can reach more than 10%, among which there are many types of pathogenic bacteria detected in patients with incision infection, and there are many multi-drug resistant strains; the incidence of incision complications after spinal surgery is 1.6–12%; that of deep infection in joint surgery, such as total knee arthroplasty and total hip arthroplasty, is 1–2% within 2 years after the surgery, but poor incision healing and incision infection (superficial and deep infection) are the main reasons for unscheduled secondary surgery, accounting for more than 50%. Therefore, the incision complications of orthopedic surgery are serious complications that affect the surgical effects. Paying attention to incision complications is as important as paying attention to surgical technique itself. Evidence-based medical evidence shows that preoperative evaluation and scientific management of incisions is an effective measure to prevent incision complications, which can reduce the incidence of incision complications, reduce patients' discomfort and tissue injury, accelerate patients' postoperative recovery, shorten hospital stay, reduce treatment expenses, and save medical resources.

3.2.1 Evaluation of Risk Factors for Orthopedic Surgical Incision Complications

- Comorbidities: For example, patients with hypertension, diabetes, malnutrition, rheumatoid disease, connective tissue disease and other immunodeficiency diseases, hemophilia, vascular disease of the affected limb, psoriasis, radiation injury, gangrene, genetic disease, gout, obesity and, other diseases [3].
- Poor living habits: Smoking and drinking for a long time, etc.
- Surgical technical factors: Multiple operations at the surgical site, prolonged use of tourniquet, long operation time, rough operation, etc. Local factors are related to aseptic operation technique, suture material selection, intraoperative suture technique, etc.
- Medication: Knowing whether the patient has a history of using such drugs as corticosteroids, anticoagulants, immunosuppressants, and local drug injection [4], and evaluating and dealing with the lesion degree of related diseases according to medication.

Therefore, the evaluation of preoperative risk factors is very important. It is necessary to optimize the controllable factors before the operation and take corresponding measures, so as to achieve the purpose of reducing incision complications.

3.2.2 Incision Suture Techniques in Orthopedic Surgeries

In order to achieve the ideal effect of enhanced recovery, the scientific management of surgical incision is a very important factor, and the correct selection of suture techniques and suture materials for surgical incisions is very important for the good healing of surgical incision [5].

3.2.2.1 Selection of Suture Methods

The suture methods for orthopedic surgical incisions follow the principles of sterility, minimally invasion, restoring the patient's anatomical structure, and ensuring good blood supply. Incision suture is mainly divided into two categories: continuous suture and interrupted suture. On this basis, it has evolved into buried suture, purse-string suture, relaxation suture, knotless suture, etc. [6]. The simple interrupted suture, simple continuous suture, continuous horizontal mattress suture (intradermal suture), and knotless suture are most commonly used in orthopedic surgeries; sometimes, vertical mattress suture (eversion suture) and relaxation suture are also used.

1. Simple interrupted suture (Fig. 3.1): It is the most commonly used suture method, which is suitable for suture of joint capsule, deep fascia, superficial fascia, and skin. Interrupted suture can reduce the dead space and ensure good alignment. The spacing of interrupted suture is generally 5–8 mm, and the needle distance and spacing are slightly different according to different suture tissues. Generally, the spacing between tissues with high tension such as joint capsule and deep fascia can be appropriately reduced, and the needle distance should also be slightly smaller; however, the spacing of subcutaneous and skin tissues during suturing can increase appropriately. After completion of suture, whether the suture gap is tight should be checked, and the suture should be added if necessary.
2. Simple continuous suture (Fig. 3.2): It is often used for suture of fascia and joint capsule. Simple continuous

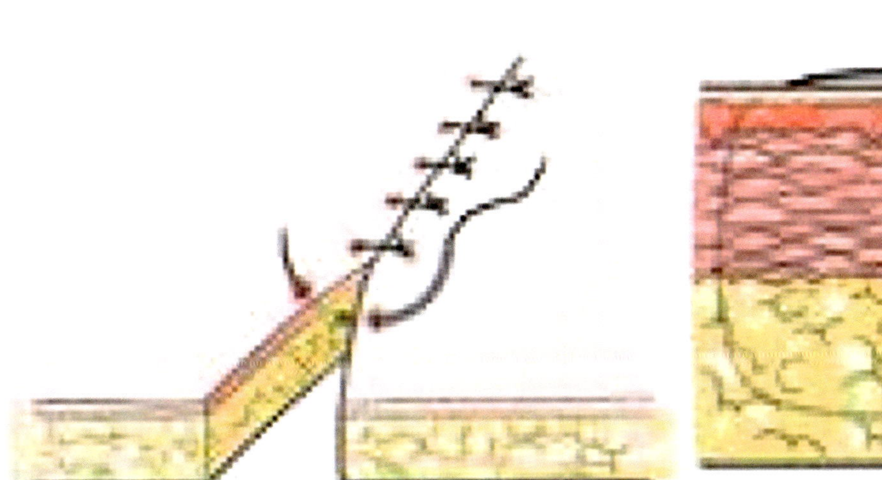

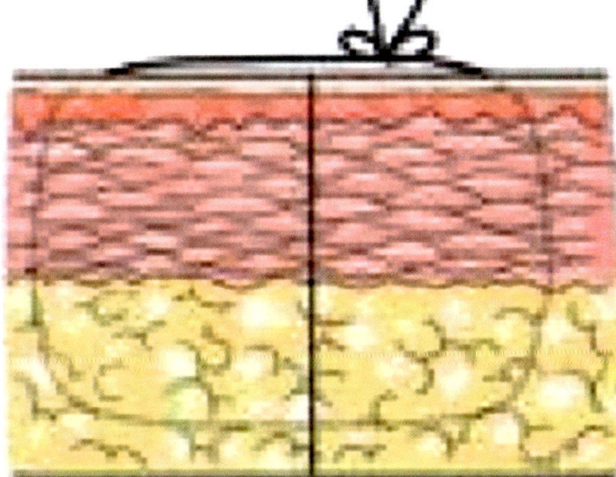

Fig. 3.1 Simple interrupted suture

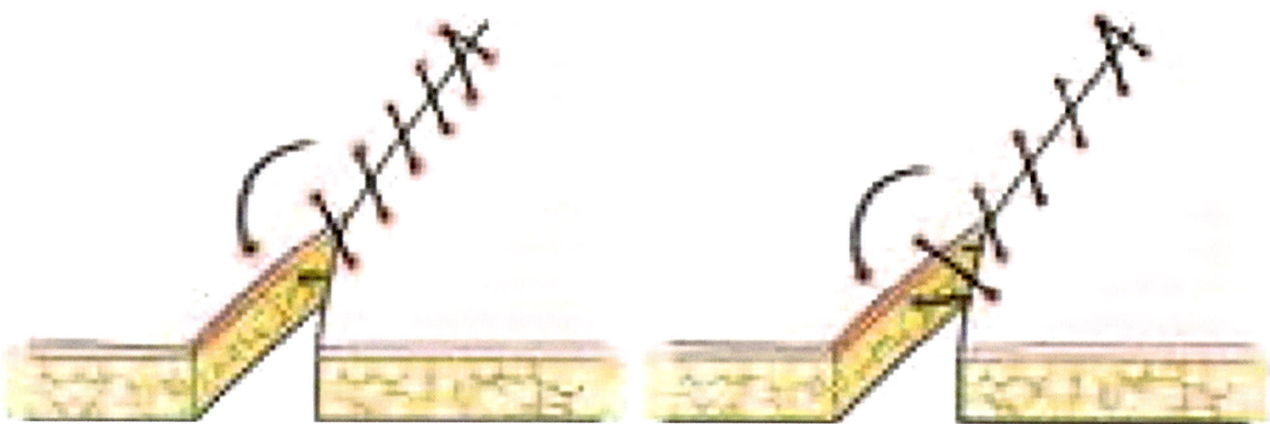

Fig. 3.2 Simple continuous suture

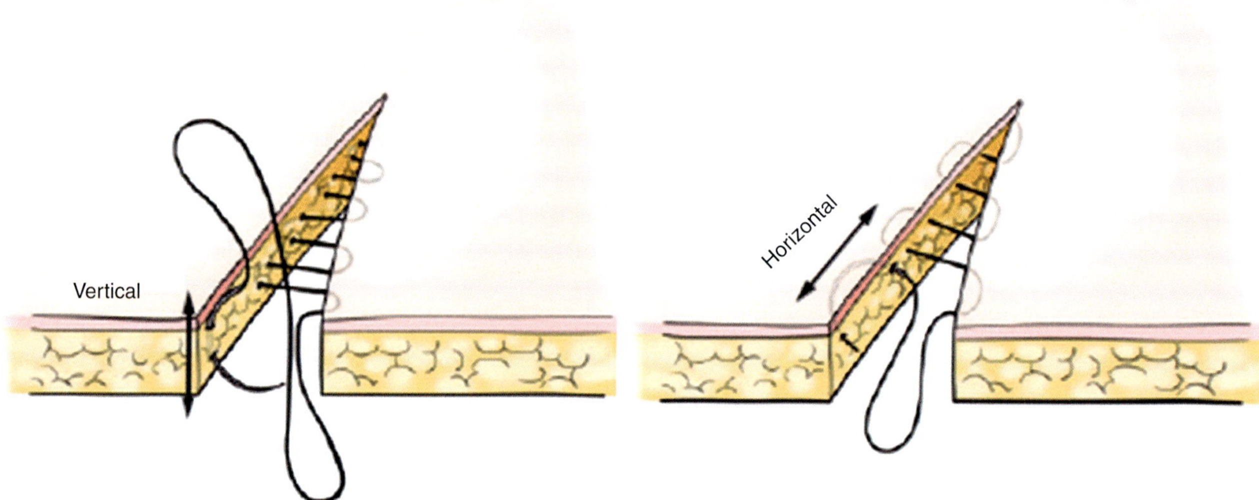

Fig. 3.3 Continuous horizontal and vertical mattress suture

suture has the advantages of fast time and reduced suture knots. When suturing, the suture is not loose or tight, ensuring good blood supply. After completion of suturing, whether there is any leakage should be checked. If there is any leakage, it should be reinforced by interrupted suture.

3. Continuous horizontal and vertical mattress suture (Fig. 3.3): It is mainly used for subcutaneous and intradermal suture. It is beneficial to aligning the skin edge, and intradermal suture can reduce the scar of the needle of skin and the trouble of suture removal, and improve the aesthetic effect of the skin. It can be used for some patients who have higher requirements for surgical scars.
4. Knotless suture: It is an emerging suture method, which uses special "barbed" suture (Fig. 3.4), with enough large tension support, strong and even grip on the tissue, so it can be done quickly by a single person. It is necessary to pay attention to the appropriate tightness and not too tight during suturing, with cross set-back suture for 2–3 stitches (Fig. 3.5) when finishing, and the suture is cut along the

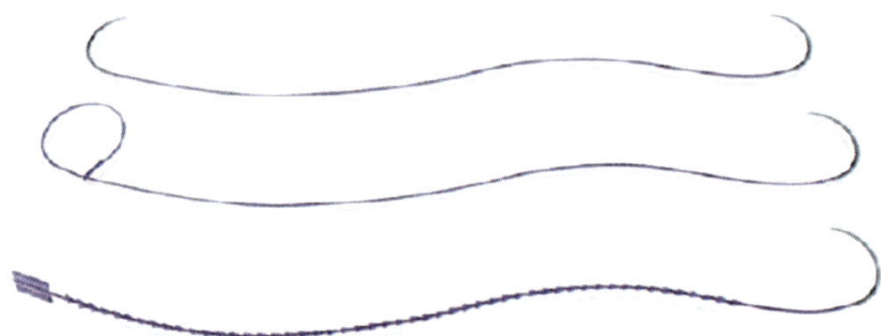

Fig. 3.4 Knotless suture with "barbed" suture

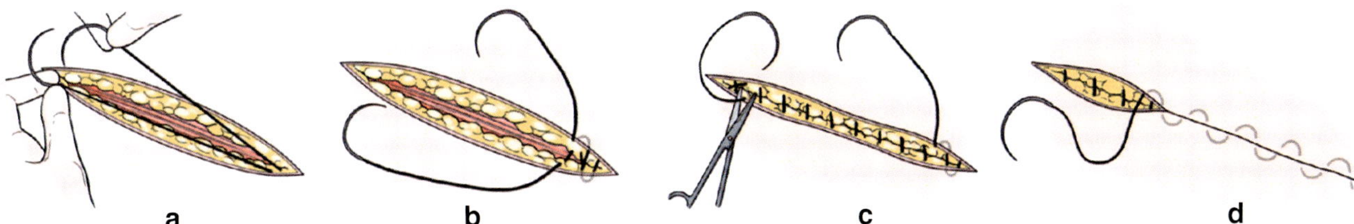

Fig. 3.5 Common methods of knotless suture. (**a**) Stitch the needle from either end, start suture from the unilateral fat layer at one end of the incision, stitch through the tissue and pull over the suture until the barb on the other side of the suture is felt to stick to the tissue, or pull both sides of the suture to the same length; (**b**) Continuously suture the fat layer with the needle for two stitches under the fat layer, and then suture the dermis layer with the needles for two stitches above the fat layer, tighten the suture to the desired anastomosis. The barbs on the suture surface will fix the tissue and keep the incision closure; (**c**) Suture the fat layer by continuous suture method till the other end of the incision, and at the opposite of the needle exit, add two stitches backward, cut the suture close to the needle eye after tightening the suture, without knotting during the whole process; (**d**) Continuously suture the dermis layer at the other side with the needle, suture in the opposite direction for one stitch after suturing, or suture on the edge of the incision for two stitches and pass through the epidermis, cut the suture against the epidermis after pressing the tissue slightly, at this time, the incision has been completely closed, and there is no need to knot during the whole process

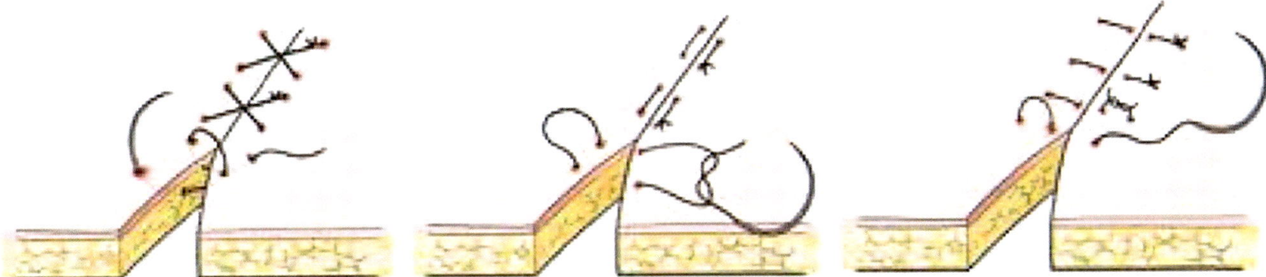

Fig. 3.6 "Figure of 8" suture

tissue to prevent the suture ends from damaging the surrounding local tissue.

5. "Figure of 8" suture (Fig. 3.6): For tissues with high tension, such as deep fascia or tendon, the "Figure of 8" suture can be used, so as to ensure that the tissues are not cut and torn due to high alignment tension and promote healing; it is also often used to reinforce the residual leakage site after continuous suture.
6. Vertical mattress suture: It is often used for suturing the tissues with wounds of large span and tension, and divided into horizontal and vertical mattress sutures (Figs. 3.7 and 3.8).
7. Relaxation suture: It is commonly used to suture skin incision with high tension, and the edge distance is usually more than 1 cm. It can be combined with vertical mattress suture to further increase the suture tension (Fig. 3.9). If possible, the new skin adhesive with mesh can be used to provide extra high tensile strength to the incision on the skin surface and keep the skin beautiful. It can be used for some patients with higher requirements for surgical scars.

3.2.2.2 Selection of Suture Materials

At present, the suture materials can be divided into two categories: absorbable and non-absorbable. In addition to the highly-inert non-absorbable materials for tendon and ligament repair, triclosan-coated absorbable sutures are basically recommended for incision of orthopedic surgery, so as to reduce infection caused by implants (sutures) and foreign body reaction caused by silk threads (Fig. 3.10). For the selection of absorbable sutures, it is necessary to understand the two most critical elements: tension support time and absorption time [7]. The tension support time refers to the

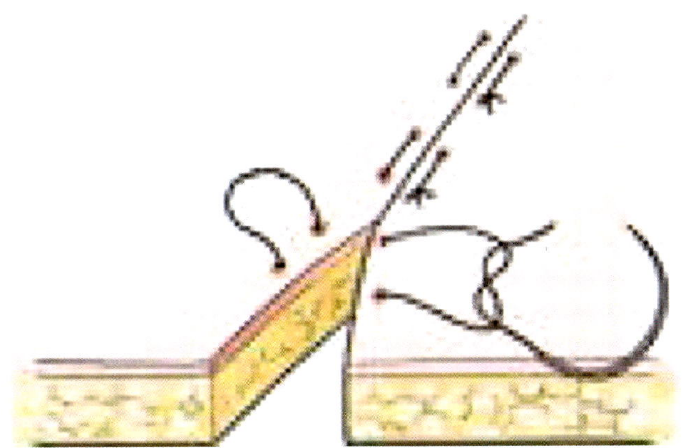

Fig. 3.7 Horizontal mattress suture

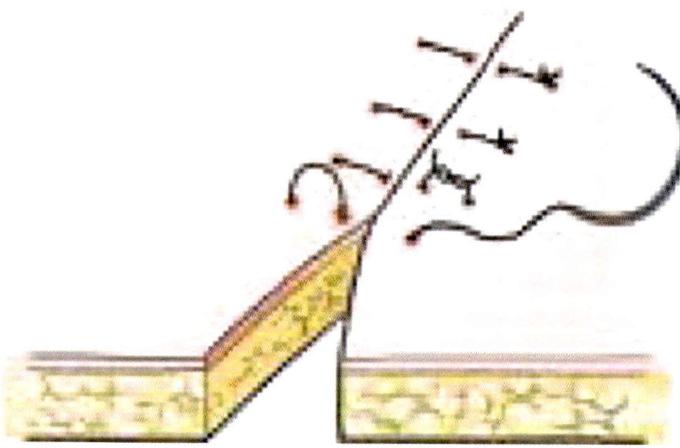

Fig. 3.8 Vertical mattress suture

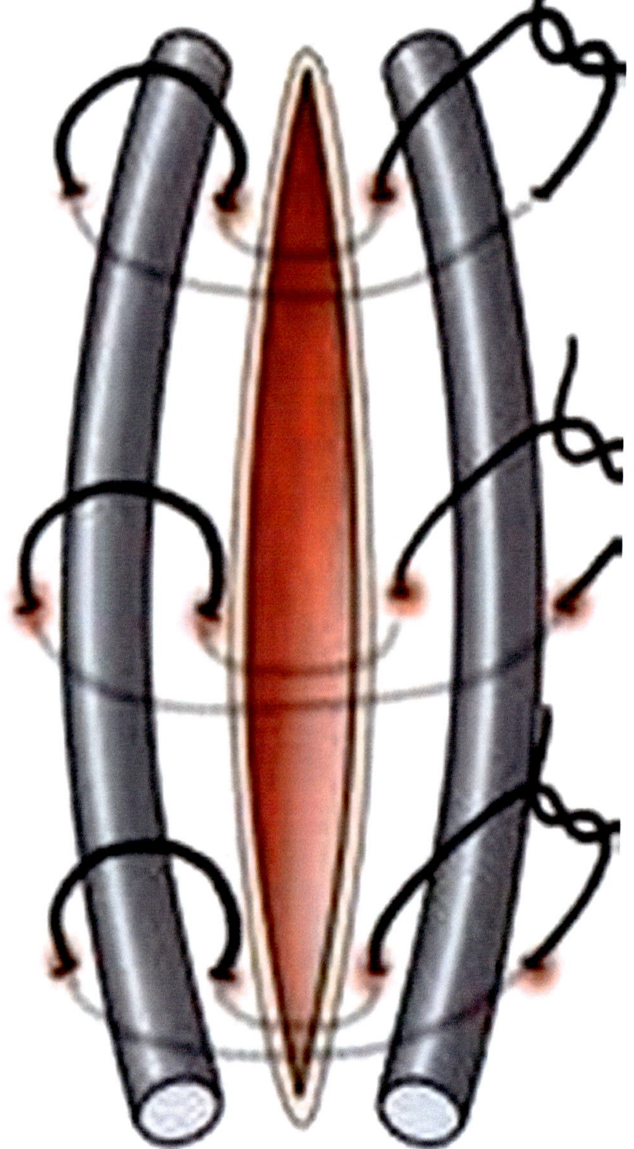

Fig. 3.9 Relaxation suture

time that the absorbable suture can maintain the tension required to align the incision well; the absorption time refers to the time when the absorbable suture is completely degraded and absorbed in human tissue. Principles of selecting suture materials: (1) Non-absorbable suture with small tissue reaction and strong inertia, such as suture made of polypropylene and polyester, should be selected for tissues with slow healing, such as tendon and ligament, and the suture has strong tension and can last for a long time; (2) Absorbable suture should be selected as far as possible for incision tissue with healing time within 2–6 weeks to reduce the risk of infection caused by foreign body residues; (3) The healing time of wound tissue at different sites should be known, the tension support time of absorbable suture must be greater than the complete healing time of tissue. If the patient's systemic and local high-risk factors are considered, the absorbable suture with longer tension support time and antimicrobial agent should be selected; (4) In order to reduce the formation of skin scars, the method and material that does not penetrate the epidermis should be selected as far as possible to suture the incision, and continuous intradermal suture should be performed when the situation allows; (5) Most suture materials now are equipped with needles. Selecting as thin needles as possible without damaging strength and sharpness is also in line with the concept of minimally invasive. During the operation, the rigidity is enough to resist bending, while the toughness is enough to resist fracture. Chord length and radian should be considered for needle type, and different needle types should be selected according to the depth of sites and tissue thickness.

3.2.2.3 Suture of Incisions of Special Types

1. Suture of incision of knee surgery in patients with rheumatoid diseases: Because of long-term use of glucocorticoid, subcutaneous superficial fascia and dermal layer of skin are very thin, it is difficult to suture smoothly and tightly; moreover, the incision healing speed of patients with rheumatoid diseases is slower than that of general patients, and the risk of postoperative exudation is also higher. For example, the poor alignment of subcutaneous and skin sutures can easily lead to repeated exudation of postoperative incision, leading to delayed incision healing and even infection. For the suture of incision of knee surgery in patients with rheumatoid diseases, it is suggested that the simple interrupted suture should be used for subcutaneous superficial fascia with 2-0 absorbable suture, the edges of incision should be aligned neatly, and then the continuous horizontal mattress suture should be used for intradermal suture to ensure smooth alignment of skin edges.
2. Suture of high tension incision: If the tension of the patient's incision is too high during suturing, suturing should be started from the site with the lowest edge ten-

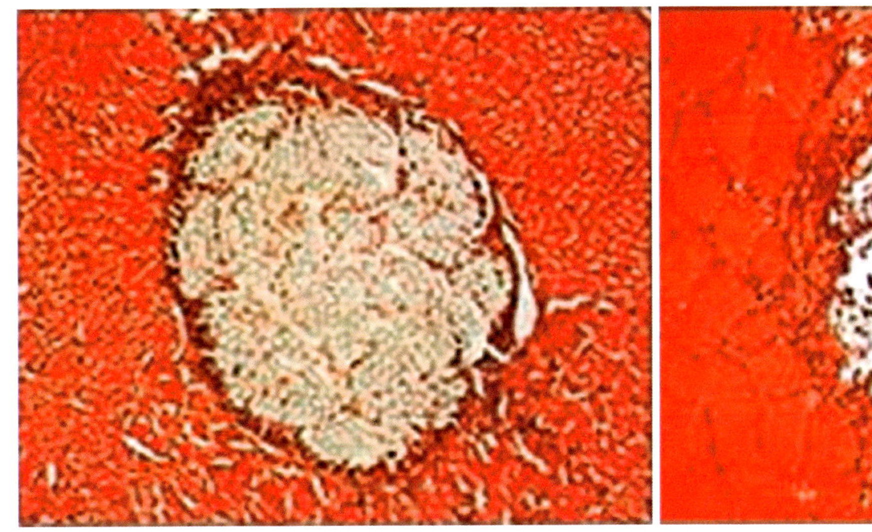

Triclosan-coated absorbable sutures

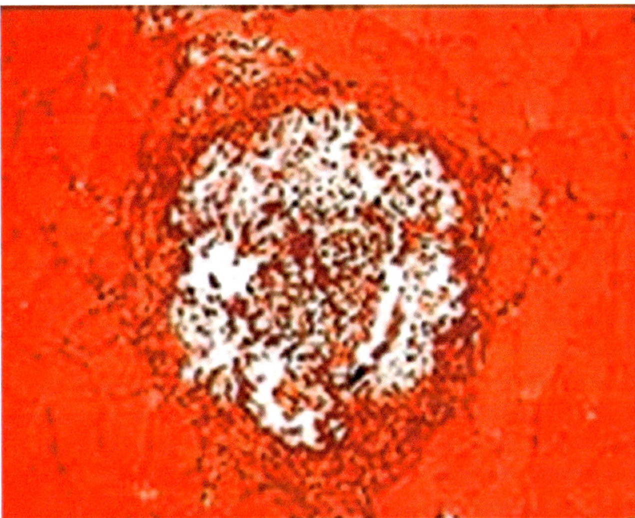

Silk

Fig. 3.10 Suture comparison, more serious foreign body reaction in silk thread

sion at both ends of the incision. The simple interrupted or internal "Figure of 8" suture may be chosen. If the skin tension is too high, the simple interrupted or vertical mattress suture can be used with relaxation suture at a wide margin distance.

3. Suture of incision of flabby skin: For patients with flabby skin, when suturing subcutaneous and skin, remember not to stretch excessively when knotting, so as to avoid overlapping skin edges. Continuous horizontal mattress method can be used for intradermal suture, with moderate tightness, so that the skin edges can be aligned smoothly.

3.2.2.4 New Incision Suture Method

As a biological adhesive, biological hydrogel is an organic material (such as PRINEO®). It can provide a certain incision tension under the condition that the skin is sutured perfectly, isolate incision from the external environment, and has bactericidal effect. The literature has confirmed that bioglue can not only provide sufficient safety and effectiveness, but also improve the scar after incision and feeling [8]. Without changing drugs/dressings and removing sutures/nails, patients can take a bath immediately after the operation. When the wound is fully healed, the mesh tape is easier to be torn off, with less pain (Fig. 3.11).

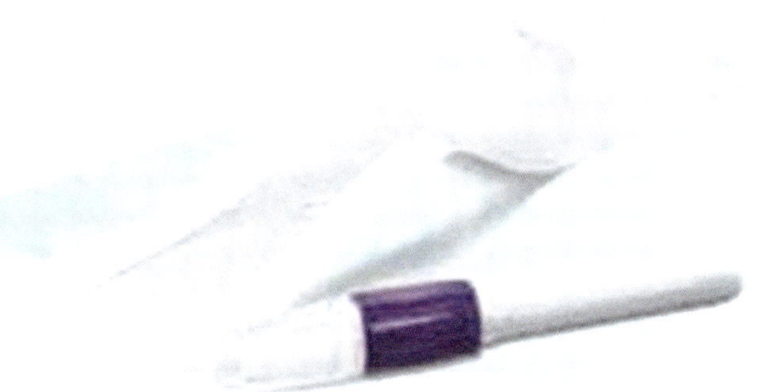

Fig. 3.11 Medical skin tissue adhesive. Staple: As a type of wound closure device that can save operation time, staple is also widely used in clinic

3.2.3 Common Incision Complications as Well as Prevention and Treatment in Orthopedic Surgery

Most elective surgical incisions in orthopedics are Class I incisions, and most incisions can achieve Level A healing. However, due to comorbidities or other risk factors [9] in the patients undergoing orthopedic surgeries, complications such as exudation, blood oozing, ecchymosis, blisters, infection, and poor healing may occur in surgical incisions, which affect incision healing. Therefore, prevention and treatment of incision complications should be strengthened to accelerate incision healing and promote enhanced recovery.

3.2.3.1 Incision Exudate

1. Definition: Postoperative fluid exudation from incision, which is a liquid component leaking into body tissues from capillaries, plays an important role in wound healing process, but excessive exudate will not be conducive to incision healing. The main component of exudate is water, in addition to water, it also includes electrolytes, nutrients, proteins, inflammatory mediators, protein digestive enzymes (such as matrix metalloproteinase (MMP)), growth factors, metabolic wastes, and various

cells, such as neutrophils, macrophages, and platelets. Although the exudate often contains microorganisms, it does not mean that the incision has been infected.

2. Causes: There are many reasons that can cause incision exudate. (1) Causes of operation: Rough operation, excessive traction of soft tissue due to the pursuit of small incision, irregular use of electric knife, etc. (2) Early stage of infection: Wound and inflammation will increase the permeability of capillaries, resulting in excessive fluid flowing into the incision and continuous exudate; (3) Hypoproteinemia: Patients with hypoproteinemia have decreased plasma albumin, and the effective osmotic pressure is reduced, so that too much water is retained between tissues and wound exudate appears; (4) Ischemia reperfusion after the tourniquet is applied in limb surgery causes swelling and exudate around incision; (5) Poor incision healing; (6) Use of anticoagulants: If patients receive excessive anticoagulation after major orthopedic surgery such as joint replacement, the incidences of hidden blood loss, limb swelling, subcutaneous ecchymosis, wound exudate, and hematoma will increase; (7) Thick fat layer of obese patients, wide release and separation during surgery and space left during wound suture are also one of the influencing factors of wound exudate.
3. Prevention and treatment: Excessive exudate of incision will affect the healing of incision and easily lead to postoperative incision infection. The non-use of tourniquet in limb surgery can reduce swelling and pain caused by ischemia reperfusion injury, and may reduce exudate. The debridement of subcutaneous fat particles before incision closure in obese patients is beneficial to wound healing and reducing exudate. The application of tranexamic acid can reduce bleeding in the incision, reduce ecchymosis around incision, inhibit inflammatory reaction, and promote wound healing. The following prevention and treatment measures should be adopted: (1) Reasonably using minimally invasive technology; (2) Removing subcutaneous fat particles, so that the edge of incision shows fibrous septa with good blood oozing, so as to facilitate the healing of incision; (3) Improving the suture technique, using suitable suture materials and new techniques when conditions permit, reducing excessive pull for soft tissues, and closing the tissues tightly to minimize gaps or dead spaces; (4) Using tranexamic acid to reduce bleeding in the incision, and inhibiting inflammatory reaction at the same time; (5) Reasonably using anticoagulants, and adjusting according to specific conditions; (6) Selecting the dressings capable of absorbing exudate and the preventive negative pressure incision therapy technology when conditions permit, so as to effectively manage exudate; (7) Improving the systemic condition of patients with poor general conditions (such as anemia, malnutrition, and hypoproteinemia) before surgery, actively treating the primary disease, and making corresponding adjustment for medication due to primary disease before surgery, and then performing surgery after the primary disease is reasonably controlled and the constitution is enhanced; (8) Actively treating hypoproteinemia occurred after surgery; (9) Performing wound debridement for continuous incision exudate if necessary.

3.2.3.2 Incision Bleeding

1. Definition: Postoperative bleeding caused by various reasons flowing out of the incision or continuous bleeding in the incision leads to joint swelling, limited mobility, pain, and other complications, and bleeding in the incision can lead to localized superficial hematoma or deep hematoma.
2. Causes: The incidence of hematoma after orthopedic surgery is 2–4%. Potential risk factors of hematoma formation include the followings. (1) Underlying diseases: Hemophilia (factor VIII deficiency, etc.), thrombocytopenic purpura, BMI > 25 kg/m^2, etc. (2) The electrocoagulation block of dermal layer of incision falling off or bleeding when suturing; inadequate hemostasis of blood vessels in incision or release of suture of ligated blood vessels. (3) Increased blood pressure and reperfusion of collapsed blood vessels after surgery. (4) Bleeding caused by early over-activity after orthopedic surgery. (5) Perioperative use of anticoagulants, which mainly includes long-term use of anticoagulants and antiplatelet drugs in patients with preoperative history of deep vein thrombosis and atrial fibrillation; deep vein thrombosis (DVT) or pulmonary embolism (PE) after surgery, which requires prolonging the time of anticoagulants or increasing the dose of anticoagulants.
3. Prevention and treatment: (1) Every possible bleeding point is treated properly before incision closure (if there is a tourniquet, it may be loosened to stop bleeding at the bleeding point); (2) After limb surgery, the pressure dressing method with pressure bandage can be applied to the affected limb; (3) If bleeding tendency is found during surgery, the drainage tube should be placed to observe postoperative drainage; (4) The time to prevent DVT after surgery should be based on the patient's personal physical condition, previous medical history and intraoperative situation to choose the appropriate drugs and use time; (5) Coagulation time, prothrombin, and international normalized ratio should be monitored; (6) Bleeding and extravasation formed after surgery usually requires reinforced suture or pressure dressing within 24 h; (7) Localized superficial hematoma usually can be absorbed by itself without surgical removal. If necessary, the wound is sutured after suture removal, drainage, and hematoma removal; (8) Complications such as joint swelling, limited mobility, severe pain, persistent bleeding, and exuda-

tion caused by deep hematoma often require hematoma removal. If it is clear that there are greater arteriovenous injuries, the emergency exploratory surgery is required.

3.2.3.3 Swelling Around Incision

1. Definition: Refer to the increase in volume of soft tissues such as muscle, skin or mucosa around incision due to congestion, edema, bleeding, and inflammation. Swelling around the incision generally involves the limb far from the surgical incision, which can lead to tension blisters, induce DVT, and even develop the osteofascial compartment syndrome.
2. Causes: (1) Direct surgical trauma leads to reactive edema, hematoma formation, and joint effusion after tissue injury. Long operation time and tourniquet use time are the influencing factors of swelling. (2) It is related to stimulation of incision edge, such as foreign body, coagulated necrotic material, large ligature, excessive wound tension (too tight suture, malposition of wound edge), etc. (3) The superficial vein and lymphatic return of limbs are blocked due to various reasons. (4) Prolonged bed rest, decreased activity, and slowed lower limb blood return. (5) Excessive activities in the early stage after surgery, such as too frequent flexion exercises and too long weight-bearing walking time.
3. Prevention and treatment: Swelling around incision will aggravate pain, reduce the strength of surrounding muscles, reduce the range of motion of joint after surgery, change gait, and delay recovery. Therefore, the following prevention and treatment measures should be taken to prevent swelling: (1) Reasonably using minimally invasive technology, manipulating gently during surgery, reducing the tourniquet use time, and shortening the surgery time; (2) If there is no contraindication, intravenous application of tranexamic acid before skin incision and after surgery is beneficial to reduce postoperative bleeding, tissue inflammation, and swelling; (3) The drainage tube can be placed according to the intraoperative situation, the extubation time is determined according to the postoperative drainage volume, the extubation should be performed as early as possible (within 24 h after surgery), and prophylactic negative pressure wound therapy technology can be used for high-risk patients; (4) After anesthesia recovery after surgery, the patient should be instructed to conduct the ankle pump exercise; (5) When conditions permit, the incision is sutured with knotless sutures, especially the deep fascia layer (joint capsule, muscle fascia layer), which provides tension support for the fascia layer for up to 6 weeks. Compared with the continuous and interrupted suture with traditional sutures, it has stronger tension and tissue grasping power, which can meet the needs of functional exercise as soon as possible after surgery; (6) In clinical treatment, the common methods to reduce postoperative incision swelling include proper elevation of the affected limb, cold compress therapy, application of pressure bandage, early functional exercise and physical therapy using dressing with high compliance and stretchability, which is beneficial to patients' joint activities, etc. If acute deep hematoma formation is accompanied, it is necessary to find the cause and actively deal with it.

3.2.3.4 Blister Around Incision

1. Definition: Blister is herpes higher than skin surface, containing liquid. Most of the blisters are caused by inflammatory reactions. The blisters after orthopedic surgery are usually allergic blisters and tension blisters, with different sizes.
2. Causes: Generally speaking, there are few blisters occurred in postoperative wounds. However, once it appears, it may cause pain, discomfort, continuous exudate of the wound and the risk of infection at the incision site. The causes of blisters around incisions are related to many factors. (1) Patient factors: Age, gender, drug treatment method, comorbidity, allergy to dressing or adhesive tape, skin condition, allergy to skin disinfectant (such as iodine allergy), etc.; (2) Surgical factors: Type of incision, swelling of incision, and movement of incision site lead to friction between skin, which makes the dressing produce shear force. In addition, pressure unevenly applied by pressure bandages around some incisions can also lead to blister formation.
3. Prevention and treatment: When observing and evaluating incisions, attention should be paid to the surrounding skin conditions, such as whether there are vulnerable and damaged conditions, whether there are traumatic scars, and whether there are rheumatoid arthritis, long-term use of glucocorticoids, chronic skin diseases, skin allergies, and other potential medical conditions that may affect the patient's skin. The following preventive actions should be taken: (1) For patients with allergic history of adhesive tape, other ways of fixing dressings should be used; (2) To prevent blister around incision, the dressing with high compliance and stretchability can be selected as the incision dressing, which does not damage the skin around the incision, especially when the joint part moves, the dressing with high compliance and stretchability can reduce the occurrence of blisters; (3) The flexibility and adhesion performance of wound dressing are very important, especially for orthopedic surgical incisions which are prone to swelling. Dressings with good compliance, easy covering and easy uncovering, good exudate absorption ability and protection ability can be used, which can reduce the frequency of dressing changes, and is beneficial to observing incisions, changing dressings, and active motion of joints of patients after surgery. (4) The new type of skin adhe-

sive with mesh can be used when conditions permit, which can keep a mild and moist environment on the wound surface, and reduce the poor wound healing caused by the friction between wound dressing and skin.

3.2.3.5 Ecchymosis Around Incision

1. Definition: Subcutaneous or submucosal hemorrhage caused by increased vascular permeability due to various injuries, poisoning, infection, allergy or thrombocytopenia, etc.
2. Causes: The ecchymosis around the incision after orthopedic surgery is the subcutaneous plaque-like hemorrhage around the incision caused by surgical injury, tourniquet use, long surgery time, thrombocytopenia, coagulation dysfunction and the use of anticoagulants or antiplatelet drugs.
3. Prevention and treatment: (1) The medication history of patients should be evaluated before surgery, especially the use of anticoagulants or antiplatelet drugs. For patients with thrombocytopenia and coagulation dysfunction, surgery should be performed only after thrombocytopenia and coagulation dysfunction have been treated and the coagulation function is normal. The tourniquet is avoided to be used or the use time should be shortened during surgery. The surgical operation should be gentle, with reduced surgery time. (2) There is no clear standard on how to balance the use of anticoagulants to prevent venous thromboembolism (VTE) and the risk of bleeding. Many studies have reported that if patients receive excessive anticoagulation after major orthopedic surgery, it will increase the probability of hidden blood loss, limb swelling, subcutaneous ecchymosis, and wound hematoma, to which attention should be paid. (3) It is suggested that the use principles of antithrombotic drugs after surgery are: comprehensive prevention of high-risk VTE (three-in-one combination), using drug prophylaxis cautiously for high bleeding risk; consideration on the balance between VTE prevention and bleeding risk; minimized application of anticoagulants.

3.2.3.6 Incision Infection in orthopedic Surgery (Superficial and Deep)

1. Definition: See Sect. 3.1 of this chapter for details.
2. Causes: There are many risk factors causing incision infection. (1) Patient factors: Complicated with diabetes, malnutrition, rheumatoid diseases, connective tissue diseases, and other immune deficiency diseases, hemophilia, vascular diseases of affected limbs, psoriasis, radiation injury, gangrene, glucocorticoid use history, local hormone or Chinese herbal medicine injection history, organ transplantation, AIDS, previous infection history, concurrent infection (urinary system, oral cavity, skin, and soft tissue infection), obesity, etc.; (2) Surgical factors: Soft tissue injury, superficial infection spread, deep hematoma, wound dehiscence, long surgery time, long postoperative drainage time, etc. (3) Environmental factors of operating room: There are too many personnel and personnel flow, and the skin disinfection at the surgical site, laminar airflow operating room, surgical gown, etc. do not comply with requirements.
3. Prevention and treatment: Deep infection, including infection around implant or prosthesis, is disastrous. Literature reported that the incidence of infection around implant or prosthesis was about 0.1%.
   (a) Prevention principle
      I Preoperative preventive actions
         (a) Evaluate the nutritional status and infection defense of patients, carry out comprehensive and detailed preoperative examinations, improve the systemic condition for patients with poor general conditions (such as anemia and hypoproteinemia) before surgery, actively treat the primary disease, and perform surgery after the patient's constitution is strengthened; (b) Screen the coexisting infection foci before surgery, and treat the potential infection foci in vivo: thoroughly cure the infection foci by using antimicrobial agents for patients with tonsillitis, upper respiratory tract infection, urinary tract infection, tinea pedis infection, etc.; (c) Evaluate whether there are scars, surgical history, skin psoriasis plaques, and vascular diseases in the surgical area; (d) For preoperative skin preparation, it has been proved in clinical practice that the shower effect is better, and chlorhexidine bath and hair removal are not recommended; (e) Try to shorten preoperative and postoperative hospital stay and reducing the incidence of nosocomial infection.
      II Preventive actions in operating room
         (a) Principle of minimizing the flow of operating room personnel: Strictly limit the number of surgical visitors and reduce the flow of personnel in the operating room; (b) Normally operate laminar airflow system, maintain aseptic environment; (c) Rinse the incision repeatedly, remove the scar as much as possible when suturing, and pay attention to the skin tension and alignment; (d) Use sutures containing triclosan antimicrobial agent when conditions permit (Fig. 3.12); the literatures prove that it can reduce the incidence of SSI by about 30%, and is recommended by the WHO, ACS, and CDC guidelines for fighting SSI; (e) Use knotless sutures when conditions permit, reduce suture and surgery time, and make the incision tension uniform and alignment well; (f) When conditions permit, choose bacteria-proof and

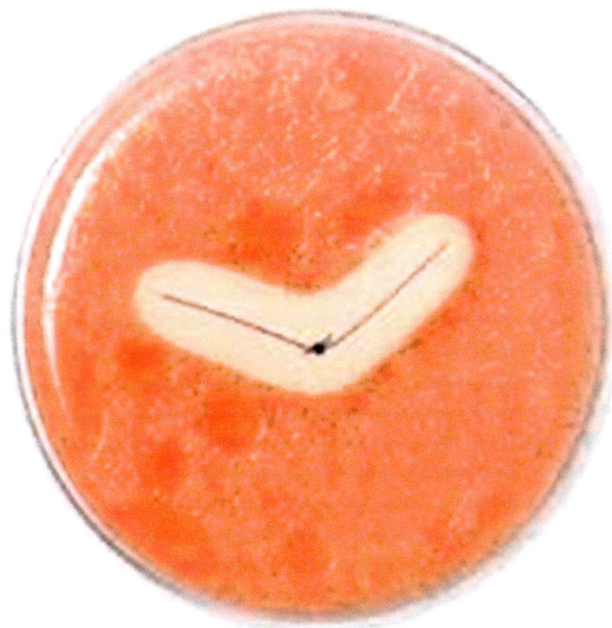

Fig. 3.12 Bacteriostatic zone formed around suture containing triclosan

waterproof dressing with membrane absorbent pad or visual waterproof foam dressing to separate the external environment, and take a shower; (g) Use a new type of skin adhesive with mesh when conditions permit, which can form a bacteriostatic barrier on the incision surface to prevent the entry of bacteria on the skin surface and external bacteria without the need for additional dressings; (h) Use drainage tubes as appropriate, which can be placed routinely in patients with bleeding tendency or wound near epidural, and should be kept unobstructed to reduce hematocele (effusion) and infection; (i) Use prophylactic negative pressure wound therapy system when conditions permit.

III Postoperative preventive actions

(a) Observe the postoperative incision, and reduce the occurrence of hematoma. The early incision with a small amount of exudate can be bandaged with suitable dressing; (b) Improve postoperative nutrition and correct anemia, and enhance human body anti-infection ability; (c) Correctly administer prophylactic anti-infective drugs, and keep sufficient concentration of anti-infective drugs in the surgical field from skin incision to incision suture; the administration time is 30–120 min before incision of the surgical site, and anti-infective drugs should be used as appropriate after surgery.

(b) Treatment suggestion: The infection in the superficial site of the incision can be cured by treatment with anti-infective drugs, disinfecting the incision regularly and changing the dressing, etc. Drug treatment, debridement and preservation of implant, or removal of implant and staged surgery are carried out for deep infection according to specific conditions.

3.2.3.7 Poor Healing of Incision

1. Definition: Incision healing refers to the reaction and repair process of tissue to wound. Incision healing is a complex biological process, which can be divided into three stages: inflammatory phase or exudation phase; fibrous tissue hyperplasia phase; scar formation and repair phase. In clinical practice, it is also referred to as debridement phase, granulation phase, and epithelialization phase. Poor healing of incision refers to the obvious stagnation or delay of three biological stages of incision healing, which leads to long-term incision nonunion or even incision dehiscence, and obvious infectious or non-infectious exudation in the incision, with or without necrotic tissue; the other situation is the hyperproliferation of Type I collagen granulation, which causes hyperplasia and contracture of scar.
2. Causes: The influencing factors include systemic and local factors. Systemic factors include the followings. (1) Age: The older the age, the slower the incision healing. (2) Obesity: Slow healing and increased risk of infection. (3) Smoking. (4) Malnutrition: Mainly hypoproteinemia, vitamin deficiency is mainly B and C families, trace elements zinc, iron, copper, manganese, etc. are also related to incision healing. (5) Metabolic diseases: Diabetes, hypertension, arteriosclerosis, cirrhosis, uremia, etc. (6) Immune diseases: Organ transplantation, chemotherapy, radiotherapy, HIV infection, allergic diseases, leukemia, etc. (7) Connective tissue diseases: Diseases with collagen synthesis disorder. (8) Vascular factors: Local vasculopathy and poor blood circulation will increase the risk of poor incision healing. Local factors include the followings: (1) Mechanical injury: Excessive pull during surgery and tight dressing at the surgical site make the skin edge of the incision ischemic and anoxic, which have adverse effects on the incision healing. The electrocoagulation hemostasis and suture are used unreasonably. (2) Infection: When the incision is infected, the exudate increases, which increases the local tension of the wound and easily causes the wound dehiscence. (3) Edema and hematoma of incision. (4) Ischemic necrosis of the skin edge of the incision. (5) Foreign body residue. (6) Suture method. (7) Local multiple surgeries, poor skin blood circulation.
3. Types and treatment of poor healing of incision

(a) Incision hematoma: Refer to the aforementioned "incision bleeding."
(b) Soft tissue necrosis.

Definition: Soft tissue necrosis occurs when injury or congestion causes ischemia and hypoxia of incision edge or soft tissue. In the early stage of incision healing, soft tissue necrosis is characterized by pale skin or cyanosis gradually turning to brown, with larger necrosis scale, poor tissue growth, which is easy to be complicated with infection.

The causes of soft tissue necrosis are: (a) Excessive pull; (b) Unreasonable use of electric knife and suture technology; (c) Poor blood supply of transplanted skin flap or "vascular crisis" of free skin flap.

Prevention and treatment: (a) Early drug administration to improve circulation; (b) The necrotic epidermis should be kept intact as far as possible, and that with clear demarcation of necrotic tissues should be removed. If it is wet necrosis, it should be removed immediately, so as to avoid the formation of local infections. (c) It is suggested to use knotless sutures to reduce suture reaction and the traction to the soft tissue.

(c) Definition of incision dehiscence: It refers to the incision that is correctly sutured but still has part of its surface not being stitched that becomes the boundary of the surrounding tissues. Incision dehiscence usually occurs 1–2 days after suture removal, that is, 8–10 days after surgery, but it can occur 2–14 days after surgery. According to the speed of dehiscence, it can be divided into acute dehiscence and chronic dehiscence.

Causes: (a) Elderly and infirm, anemia, hypoproteinemia, vitamin C deficiency, obesity or chronic internal medicine diseases such as nephritis, diabetes, jaundice, and long-term use of glucocorticoids, such patients have weak tissue regeneration ability, slow healing speed, and easy dehiscence of incision; (b) Excessive incision exudate also directly affects incision healing; (c) Early infection, there are toxins produced by bacteria in the incision, which hinder the healing of the incision and cause its dehiscence; (d) Suture technique; (e) Poor healing of incision.

Prevention and treatment: (a) Local dehiscence caused by poor alignment in suture of dermis layer is treated conservatively by changing dressings. (b) Patients with acute incision dehiscence should undergo emergency debridement suture. (c) For patients with chronic incision dehiscence, the incision should be kept dry and clean, the dressing should be changed every day to prevent infection, and the secondary suture should be considered after new granulation grows. (d) Suture method: The deep fascia layer, as the main layer bearing tension, should be tightly closed. It is recommended to use knotless sutures for suture, with reliable tension; the tension is fully relaxed during subcutaneous suture, and the dermal layer is recommended to be sutured intradermally by using barbed suture, and the incisions should be well aligned to reduce incision displacement. (e) Prophylactic negative pressure wound therapy system can be used when conditions permit.

3.2.3.8 Incision Scar

1. Definition: The scar is a general term for the appearance, morphology, and histopathological changes of normal skin tissues caused by various kinds of wounds, and is an inevitable product in the process of human body wound repair. When the scar growth exceeds a certain limit, various complications will occur, such as appearance damage, pruritus, pain, and dysfunction, which will bring physical pain and mental pain to patients. Severe scar (contracture) will affect joint activities.
2. Classification of scars: (1) Mature scar: Slight pigment change, smooth. (2) Immature scar: Redness, accompanied by occasional pain and itch, and slightly prominent. It usually becomes smooth over time, with slight pigment changes. (3) Hypertrophic scar: Redness, prominent, usually itchy, confined to the original wound range, usually occurred several weeks after surgery. It can increase rapidly within 3–6 months, and then enter the decline phase after the stable phase. It usually forms a protuberant, rope-like appearance when it matures. (4) Keloid.
3. Causes: The incidence of the scar in the population is not clear, the scar has a certain genetic tendency, and its occurrence may be the result of interaction between multiple genes and exogenous factors. Necrosis of skin edge of incision, fat liquefaction, infection of incision, excessive local tension of incision, delayed healing, poor alignment, and excessive joint movement are the important causes of scar formation.
4. Prevention and treatment: High-risk population are the patients with previous history of hypertrophic scar or keloid. Prevention of scar: (1) Early application of silicone rubber dressings is recommended, which may reduce the formation of hypertrophic scar; (2) For severe cases, hormones can be injected locally at the same time [10]; (3) For scars that seriously affect joint activity, surgical resection or scar removal therapy and early use of silicone rubber dressings can be considered. (4) According to the specific situation, the pressure therapy, relaxation of skin adhesive incision with mesh, photoelectric tech-

nology, etc. can be selected or the wound center or scar treatment center can be consulted; (5) Tobacco, alcohol, and stimulating food shall be prohibited within half a year.

Search Terms

Surgical site infection, Superficial incisional SSI, Deep incisional SSI, Classification of surgical incisions, Simple interrupted suture, Simple continuous suture, Continuous horizontal mattress suture, Knotless suture, Vertical mattress suture, Relaxation suture, Incision exudate, Incision bleeding, Poor healing of incision, Incision scar

References

1. Woods A. Key points in the CDC's surgical site infection guideline. Adv Skin Wound Care. 2005;18(4):215–20.
2. Devaney L, Rowell K. Improving surgical wound classification-why it matters. AORN J. 2004;80(2):208–23.
3. Ban KA, Minei JP, Laronga C, et al. American College of Surgeons and Surgical Infection Society: surgical site infection guidelines, 2016 update. J Am Coll Surg. 2017;224(1):59–74.
4. Allegranzi B, Zayed B, Bischoff P, et al. New WHO recommendations on intraoperative and postoperative measures for surgical site infection prevention: an evidence-based global perspective. Lancet Infect Dis. 2016;16(12):e288–303.
5. Kang Yan, Zhou Zongke, Yang Huilin, et al. A guideline on the management of incisions for the enhanced recovery after orthopaedic surgery in China. Chin J Bone Joint Surg. 2018;11(1):3–10.
6. Kantor J. Atlas of suturing techniques: approaches to surgical wound, laceration, and cosmetic repair. McGraw-Hill/Medical; 2016. p. 24–155.
7. Bennett RG. Selection of wound closure materials. J Am Acad Dermatol. 1988;18:619–37.
8. Huemer GM, Schmidt M, Helml GH, Shafighi M, Dunst-Huemer KM. Effective wound closure with a new two-component wound closure device (Prineo?) in Excisional body-contouring surgery: experience in over 200 procedures. Aesthet Plast Surg. 2012;36(2):382–6.
9. Ehrlichman RJ, Seckel BR, Bryan DJ, Moschella CJ. Common complications of wound healing. Prevention and management. Surg Clin North Am. 1991;71(6):1323–51.
10. Lee Peng G, Kerolus JL. Management of surgical scars. Facial Plast Surg Clin North Am. 2019;27(4):513–7.

4 Design and Selection of Surgical Suturing Materials

Kejian Wu, Jiangdong Ni, Dankai Wu, and Lei Wang

Abstract

Suture is one of the basic surgical skills. The needle and suture are equally important as basic materials. Surgical sutures retain in the tissues for varying lengths of time, while needles pass through the tissues for only a few seconds. If needles are not ideal, it is difficult for the suture to play its role well. Whether the needle is stable on the needle holder and the size of the wound caused by the needle both influence the suture effect. Hence suture needles are quite important especially for delicate surgeries. Under the premise of ensuring strength, the needle should be as thin and sharp as possible and can be firmly held by the needle holder. The suture needle guided through the tissue under minimum resistance causes minimum damage. The rigidity and flexibility of the needle should be well matched and can resist both bending and breakage. It should also be easy to be disinfected, resist corrosion, and effectively prevent microorganisms or foreign bodies from entering the wound. Suture needles with corresponding shape and diameter can be designed and manufactured according to the suture diameter and different surgical procedures. The sutures are used for suturing tissues and ligating blood vessels, which should have certain tension, easy knotting, minor tissue reaction, no toxicity, no sensitization, no carcinogenicity, and easy sterilization and preservation. The sutures are divided into absorbable sutures and non-absorbable sutures. New suture materials can meet different surgical needs.

K. Wu (✉)
Department of Orthopedics Trauma, The Fourth Medical Center of PLA General Hospital, Beijing, China

J. Ni
Department of Orthopedics, The Second Xiangya Hospital of Central South University, Changsha, Hunan, China

D. Wu
The Second Hospital of Jilin University, Changchun, Jilin, China

L. Wang
Johnson & Johnson, Beijing, China

Keywords

Surgical suturing materials · reverse cutting needle · OS needle · knotless suture devices

4.1 Surgical Suture Needle

4.1.1 Key Points of Ideal Suture Needle

High-quality stainless steel is used as the material. Under the premise of ensuring strength, the needle should be as thin and sharp as possible and can be firmly held by the needle holder. The suture needle guided through the tissue under minimum resistance causes minimum damage. The rigidity and flexibility of the needle should be well matched and can resist both bending and breakage. It should also be easy to be disinfected, resist corrosion, and effectively prevent microorganisms or foreign bodies from entering the wound. Suture needles with corresponding shape and diameter can be designed and manufactured according to the suture diameter and different surgical procedures.

4.1.1.1 Materials of Surgical Suture Needle

The design of suture needle requires detailed analysis for surgical procedures and density of human tissue. Suitable metal alloy is preferable for which heat treatment should be performed to ensure maximum strength and flexibility. For example, Ethalloy needle (Fig. 4.1) uses alloy with super strength and is suitable for surgical sutures requiring high precision, such as cardiovascular, eye, plastic, and microsurgical procedures.

4.1.1.2 Key Points of Suture Needle Design

1. Strength: The strength of suture needle refers to the ability of the needle to resist deformation as it repeatedly passes through the tissue. If the suture needle is bent and deformed when passing through the tissue, it will affect the surgeon's control of the suture needle during suturing,

P. Tang et al. (eds.), *Tutorials in Suturing Techniques for Orthopedics*, https://doi.org/10.1007/978-981-33-6330-4_4

resulting in tissue damage. The higher the strength of suture needle is, the smaller the tissue damage will be. Losing control of the suture needle can also cause difficulty in suturing.

The laboratory method for testing the strength of suture needle (Fig. 4.2) is: bending the suture needle to a large strength of 90°, which is the limit far beyond the clinical bending [1]. During the surgery, the key to the strength of suture needle is: "Surgical resistance" point, which is the angle at which the needle is bent to show permanent deformation. The surgical resistance point is usually between 10° and 30°, depending on the material and technique of suture needle. Exceeding this resistance point will break the suture needle. Combining alloy material and manufacturing process of suture needle makes resistance point and strength perfect.

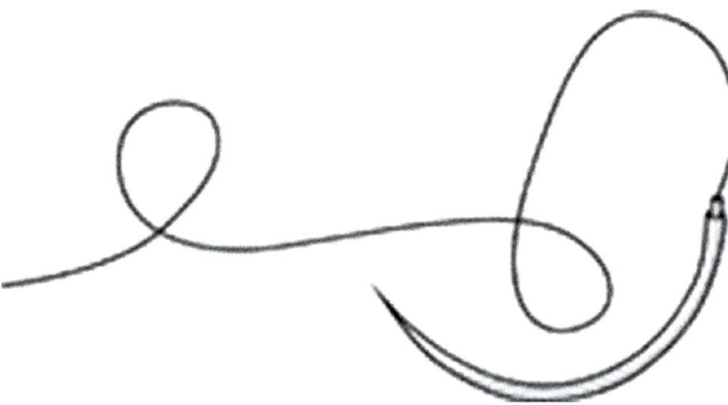

Fig. 4.1 Ethalloy needle

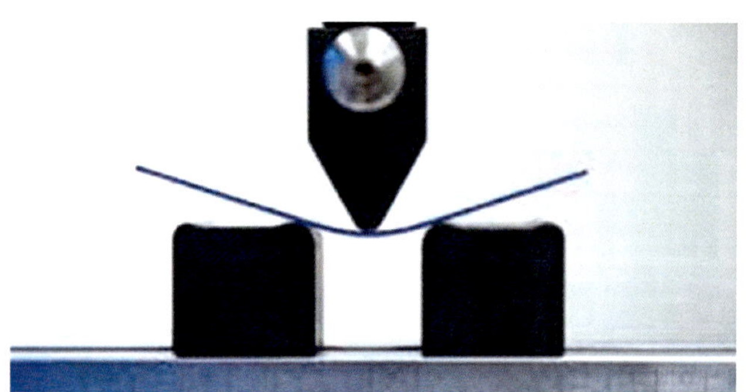

Fig. 4.2 Method for testing the strength of suture needle

2. Flexibility: Flexibility refers to the extent to which the suture needle can resist bending without breakage. The suture needle with good flexibility can only be broken after being greatly bent. During the surgery, the broken suture needle will remain in the tissue, and looking for it increases the tissue damage and the patient's anesthesia time. Failure to find the broken needle may cause injury to patient and lead to medical disputes.
3. Sharpness: The sharpness of suture needle is especially important for delicate surgery or plastic surgery. The sharper the suture needle is, the smaller the scar will be. But the sharpness should be moderate. If the suture needle is too sharp, the surgeon will find it difficult to control when the needle passes through the tissue. The sharpness is related to the angle of needle point and the taper rate of suture needle. The ratio of the taper length to the diameter of taper needle is usually 8:1, 12:1, etc. (Fig. 4.3). Scanning electron microscope shows that among the same type of suture needles, the sharpest one has a thin and long taper with smooth edge, while the blunt one has short and thick taper with its edge being jagged and uneven. The sharpness tester consists of an ultrathin, laminated, and synthetic film that has similar density to human tissue, allowing technicians to precisely measure the force required for the needle to penetrate the tissue.

   Many needles supplied are coated with layer of ultrathin silicone or similar lubricant to allow the needle to pass through the tissue smoothly. Coatings in laboratory tests have the following effects:
   (a) Reduce initial force when the suture needle penetrates the tissue.
   (b) Reduce traction applied to the needle body when the suture needle repeatedly passes through the tissue.
4. Stability in the needle holder: The evaluation for the performance of suture needle also includes its performance in the needle holder. To be better clamped, most curved needles have flat needle holding area. The curved needle has two types of needle holding area, ribbed, and flat. The ribbed type has longitudinal ribs or grooves on both inside and outside of the needle holding area of the curved part (Fig. 4.4), which function to brake crosswise to reduce unnecessary swinging, skewing, or rotation of suture needle in the needle holder.

Fig. 4.3 Taper rate

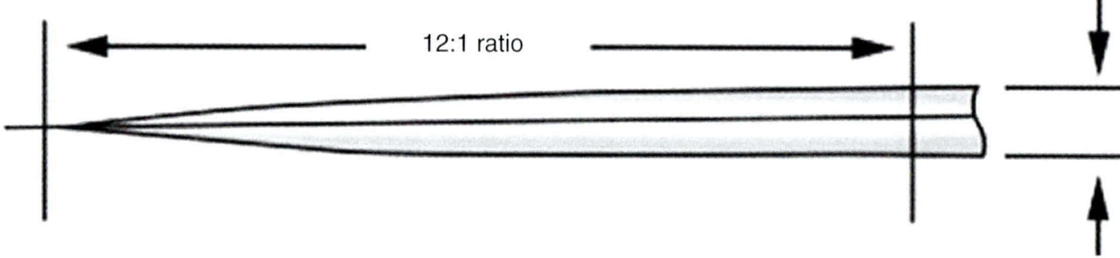

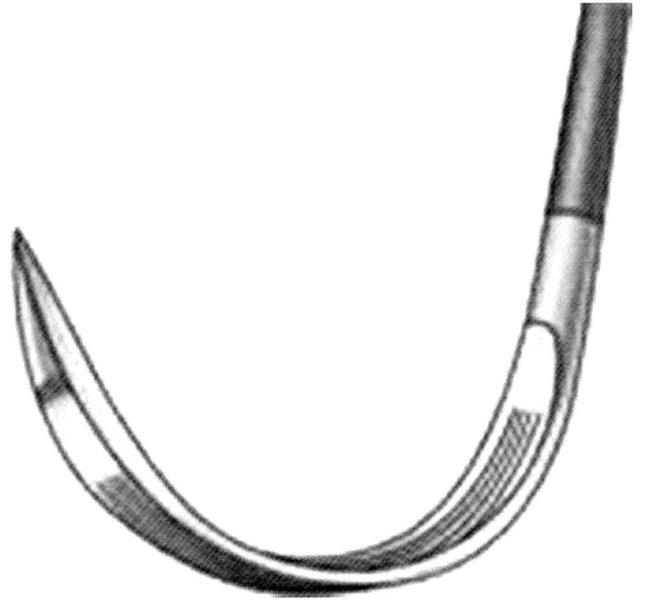

Fig. 4.4 Ribbed suture needle

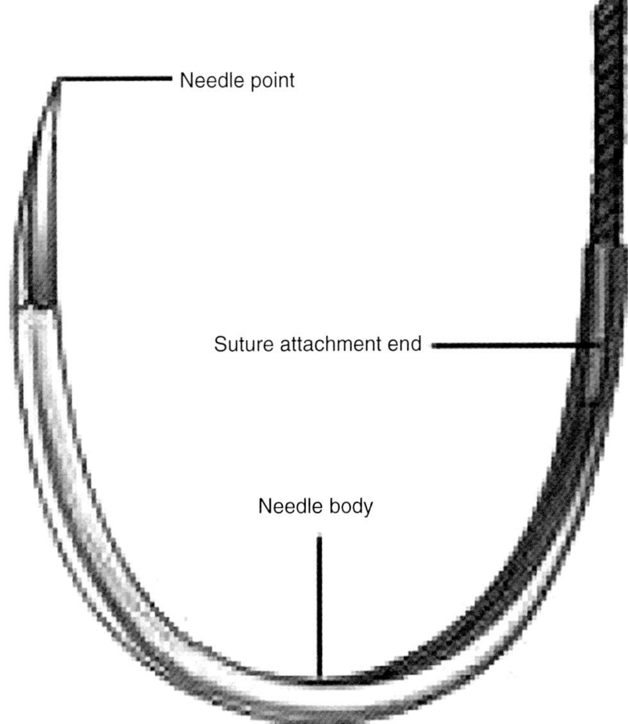

Fig. 4.5 Basic components of suture needle

4.1.1.3 Selection Principles of Surgical Suture Needle

The main function of suture needle is to guide suture passing through the tissue, and the damage to the tissue by the needle should be as small as possible. Refer to the following principles when selecting a suture needle:

1. First consider the tissue to be sutured. In general, the taper needle is most commonly used for tissue that is easy to pass through. The cutting needle or taper needle is more commonly used for suturing tough tissue that is hard to pass through. Taper needles are preferable in most cases except for suturing the skin.
2. Closely observe the surgeon's suturing technique and site. The length, diameter, and curvature of suture needle vary with the requirements for suturing site.
3. Consult the surgeon in time. Even the same surgeon may use different needles under different conditions.
4. When using an eyed needle, note that the needle diameter should match the size of suture. Swaged needle has been fitted with suture, and there is no matching problem.
5. The instrument nurses should accumulate experience, and the physician should focus on the surgical process. When the surgeon does not prioritize the suture needle, the nurse can choose according to the surgical procedures and the tissue to be sutured.

4.1.2 Structure and Type of Suture Needle

4.1.2.1 Basic Components of Suture Needle

The suture needle is composed of three basic parts (Fig. 4.5): suture attachment end (swaged, eyed); needle body; needle point [2]. Different specifications for specific parts determine the most effective function of suture needle.

4.1.2.2 Measurement of Suture Needle

The size of suture needle can be measured by inch or metric unit. The method is as follows (Fig. 4.6). Chord length: Linear distance from needle point to suture attachment end of curved needle. Needle length: Distance from needle point to needle tail measured along needle body. Radius: The needle is extended along the curved part by a broken line to form a complete circle, and the distance from the center of the circle to the needle body is the radius. Diameter: The thickness of suture needle. Microsurgery requires needles with small diameter, and when surgeons suture through the sternum and abdominal wall, large and thick needles are required. There are a variety of extremely thick and extremely fine needles for selection.

4.1.2.3 Suture Attachment End of Suture Needle

The suture attachment end of needle is mainly classified into (Fig. 4.7) swaged type (eyeless), closed type, and French type (split or spring).

1. The closed type is similar to household needles, of which the closed needle eye is round, oblong, or square.
2. The French type has a ridge-like bulging split at the tail end of suture needle to pass and fix the suture.

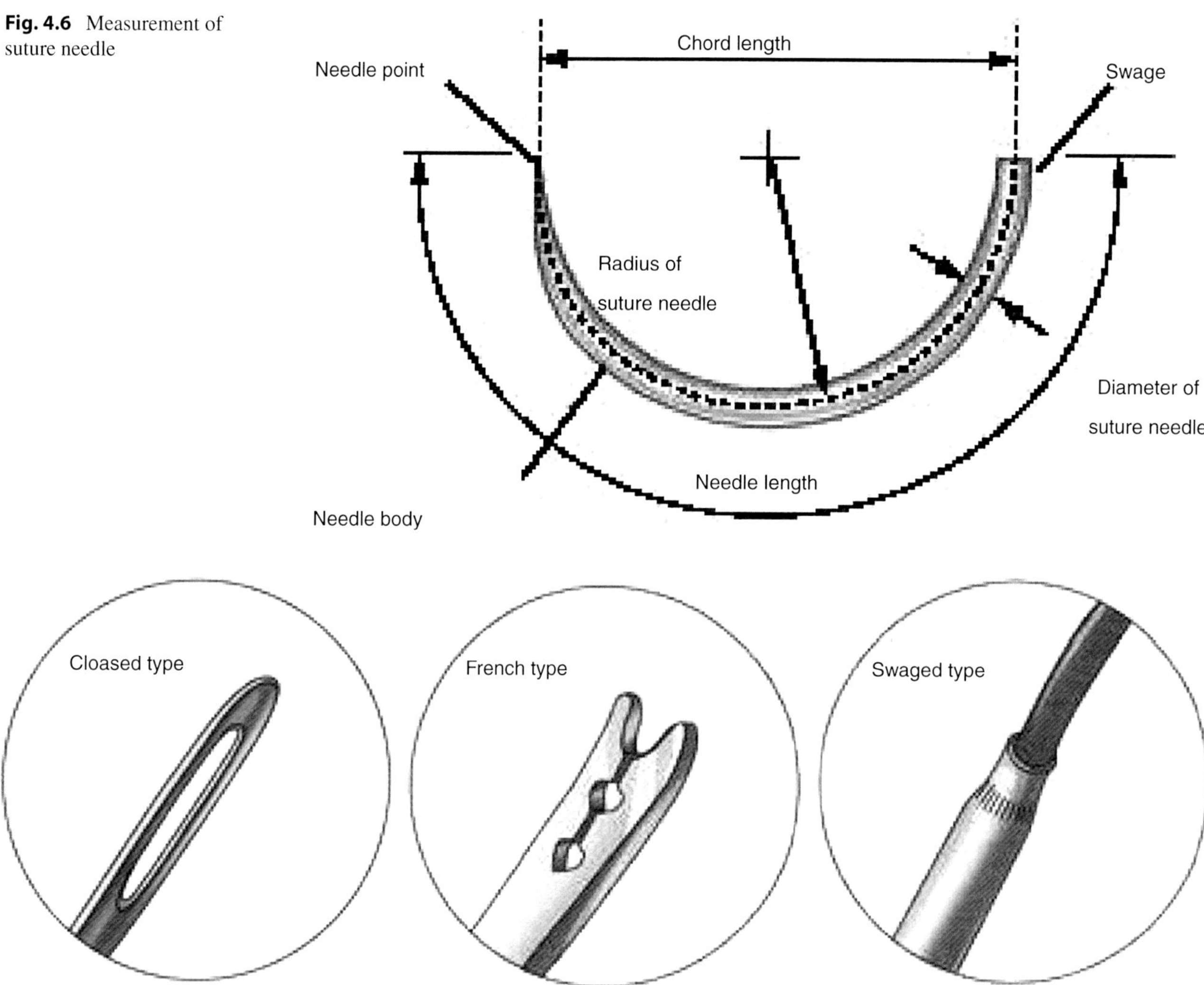

Fig. 4.6 Measurement of suture needle

Fig. 4.7 Types of suture attachment end

3. Most suture needles are swaged, and the needle is integrated with the suture for easy use and minimum damage.

For the instrument nurses, manipulation of an eyed needle is time-consuming. The disadvantage is that when the needle passes through the tissue with a double-stranded suture, it results in a larger needle tract (Fig. 4.8) with additional tissue damage. In addition, the suture may fall off at any time during suturing. Although it can be prevented by knotting at the needle eye, the suture volume will be further increased.

The method of swaging varies according to the diameter of suture needle. For a suture needle with a larger diameter, a small hole can be drilled at the tail end of the needle. For a needle with a smaller diameter, the suture attachment end is made to form a "U" groove, or a laser is used to make a hole in the metal wire. Each hole or groove is specifically designed and manufactured according to the type and size of the suture swaged, in order to tighten and fix the suture. After the suturing is completed, the suture can be cut, or easily removed from the needle, which is the same as the control release.

A laboratory test was conducted to compare taper needles with small diameter and "split" grooves to laser-drilled ones in cardiovascular surgery. Laser-drilled suture needles require less traction force when passing through simulative vascular tissue membranes and may be associated with less damage to the vessel wall.

The control release allows the needle to be easily and quickly removed from the suture based on the surgeon's need. In interrupted suturing, the suture can be quickly replaced. When the suturing is finished, the needle can be pulled out with a slight pull (Fig. 4.9). This integration of needle and suture was first used for abdominal suturing and small bowel resection and has currently been widely used in various operations.

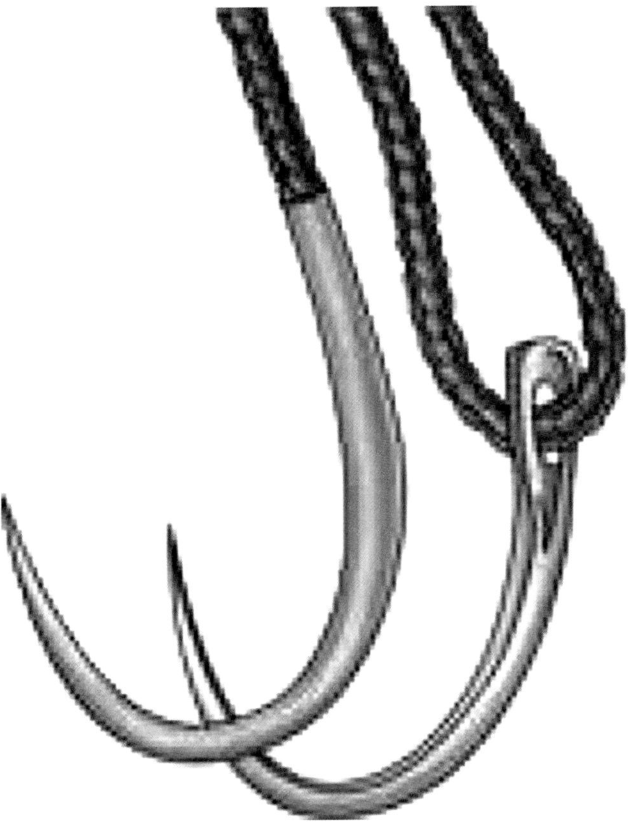

Fig. 4.8 Swaged and closed needles and comparison of sutures diameters

Advantages of Swaged Needle

The diameter of swaged needle matches the diameter of the swaged suture. The 1:1 ratio of the diameter of the suture to that of the needle contributes to the most needed "needle eye closure" in cardiovascular surgery. Swaged needle has the following advantages:

1. The suture is already attached with a needle, so when the surgeon needs a specific suture, the surgical nurse does not need to select the corresponding needle.
2. Reduce the workload of operation and preparation. Needle-attached sutures can be taken directly from the package (Fig. 4.10). It is beneficial to keep the suture intact.
3. Minimize tissue damage, save surgery time, and reduce the anesthesia time of the patient.
4. Each suture is attached with a new, sharp, and intact needle, and it can reduce tissue damage.
5. The suture does not accidentally detach from the swaged needle.
6. With the help of attached suture, it is easy to retrieve the suture needle that accidentally falls into the body cavity.
7. Reusable eyed needles need to be counted, cleaned, and disinfected; swaged needles are disposable, so time is saved.
8. There is a sharp point in the eye of the eyed needle, which may lead to wear or even breakage of suture; the swaged needle eliminates this hidden danger.
9. The needle is corrosion resistant.

4.1.2.4 Needle Body

In surgery, the needle body is the part that the needle holder clamps (Fig. 4.11). The diameter of needle body should be as close as possible to the diameter of suture, which is especially important for cardiovascular, gastrointestinal, and bladder surgeries. The curve of needle body has different shapes, which satisfy the need for different surgeries.

Straight Needle

Straight needles are suitable for suturing tissues that are easily penetrated. Most needles of this type are designed for sites where surgeons can suture directly with their fingers.

1. The Keith needle is a kind of straight needle (Fig. 4.12), which is mainly used in suturing abdominal skin wounds. Keith needles of different lengths can be used to suture the knee meniscus in arthroscopic surgery.
2. Bunnell (BN) needles are often used in tendon repair (Fig. 4.13). Different sizes of round or straight needles can also be used for suturing the gastrointestinal tract. In ophthalmic surgery (Fig. 4.14), a straight transchamber needle protects endothelial cells and facilitates to position lens of the eye.

Half Curved Needle or "Ski" Needle

Half curved needles can be used for suturing the skin. But as it is difficult to be controlled, currently it is very rarely used (Fig. 4.15). Although the curved part of needle body easily penetrates the tissue, the straight part of needle body cannot be bent along with, or it may skew or enlarge needle tract.

Curved Needle

Surgeons can predict where the needle penetrates out of the tissue when using curved needles; therefore, curved needles are widely used. The curved needle requires less space than the straight needle. A needle holder is required when operating the curved needle. The curvature can be 1/4, 3/8, 1/2 or 5/8, etc. (Fig. 4.16).

The taper needle with 3/8 radian is most commonly used to suture the skin. This radian allows surgeons to suture large and superficial wounds easily with only a slight rotation of the wrist. But in the deep and confined region of the body cavity, it is difficult to use a 3/8 radian taper needle because of the large curve required in the operation.

The 1/2 radian taper needle requires a larger rotation of the wrist, and it is designed for confined space. But when operating in the deep region such as pelvic cavity, the point of this needle is also buried in the tissue, so it is much more

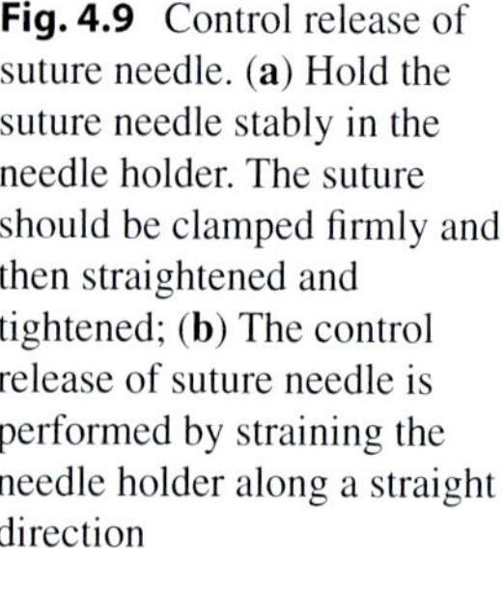

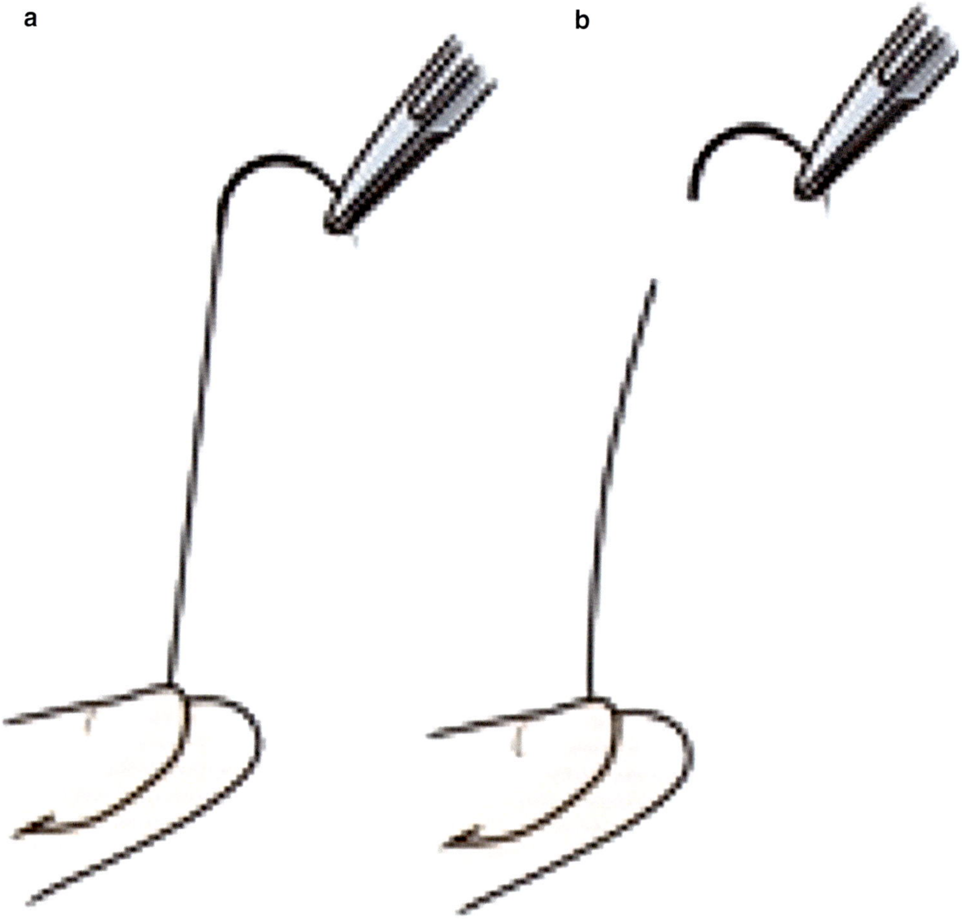

Fig. 4.9 Control release of suture needle. (**a**) Hold the suture needle stably in the needle holder. The suture should be clamped firmly and then straightened and tightened; (**b**) The control release of suture needle is performed by straining the needle holder along a straight direction

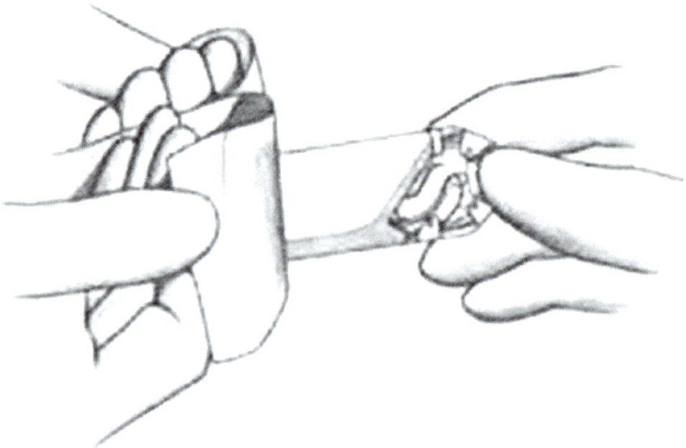

Fig. 4.10 Method for taking out swaged needle

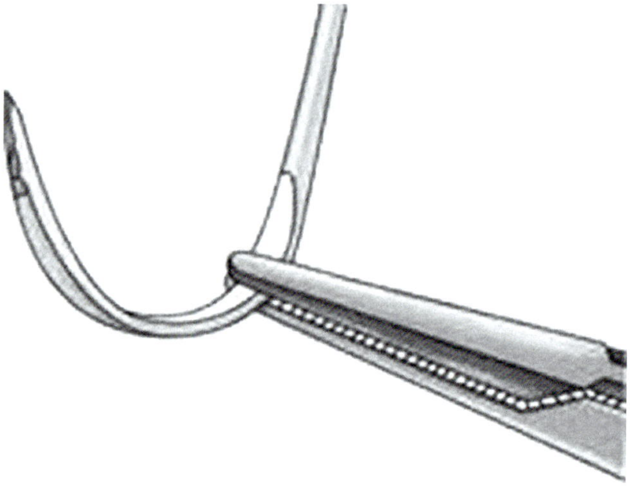

Fig. 4.11 Needle holder holding a suture needle

difficult to pull it out. The 5/8 radian taper needle is more suitable for these parts, especially the anus, genitourinary system, oral cavity, and cardiovascular surgery.

Compound Curved Needle

The compound curved needle is originally designed for surgery of ocular anterior chamber, and the surgeon can use the needle to accurately puncture the tissue. The 80° curvature at the needle point is extended to 45° curvature at the needle body (Fig. 4.17). The curvature of needle point facilitates short and deep tissue puncture, while the curvature of needle body facilitates pushing the needle out of the tissue. The curvature of needle body is conducive to avoiding the edge of the wound, observing the wound, and ensuring that the suture is isometric on both sides of the incision. The stress on both sides of the corneal-sclera junction should be equal, which reduces astigmatism after surgery of anterior oculus.

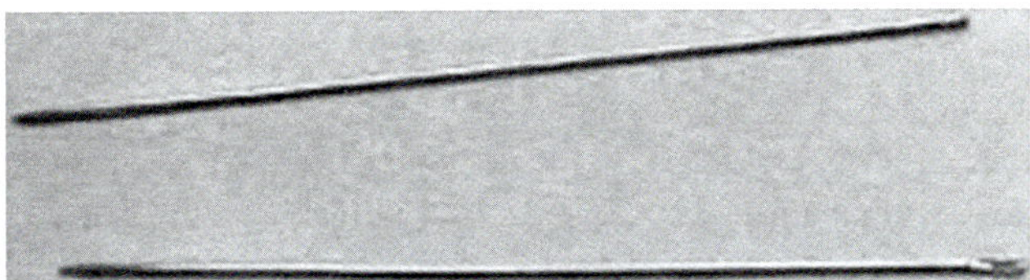

Fig. 4.12 Keith needles

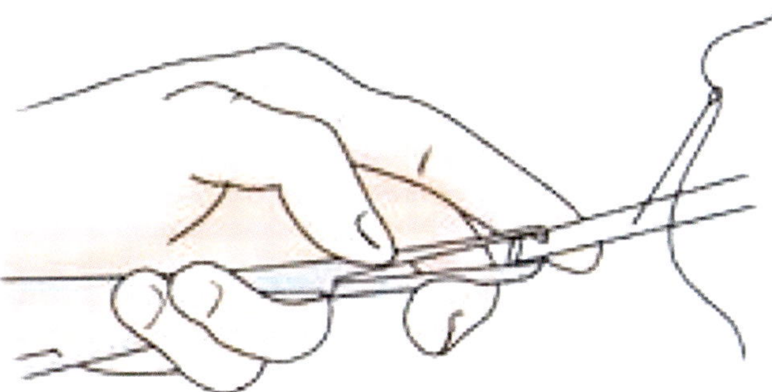

Fig. 4.13 Bunnell needle is used in tendon repair

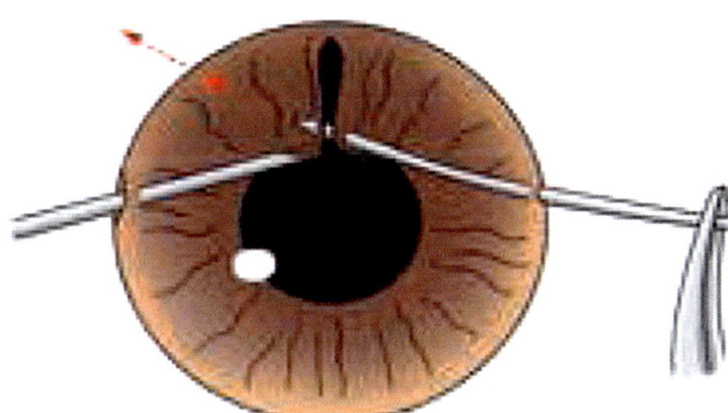

Fig. 4.14 Used in ophthalmic surgery

4.1.2.5 Needle Point

The needle point extends from the tip of suture needle to the largest cross section of needle body. The needle point is designed and manufactured according to the sharpness required to penetrate a specific type of tissue.

4.1.2.6 Needle Tail

It is the joint between needle and suture, which connects the needle and the suture (Figs. 4.18, 4.19, and 4.20).

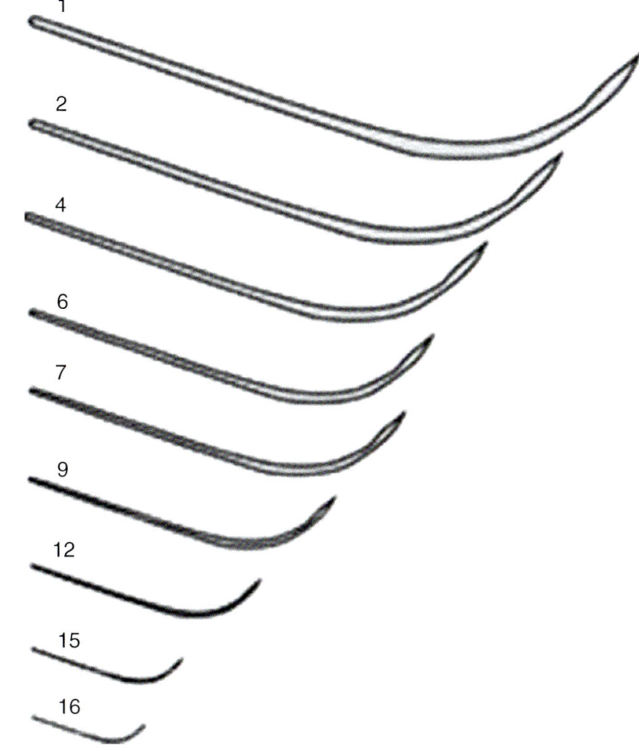

Fig. 4.15 Different sizes of half curved needles

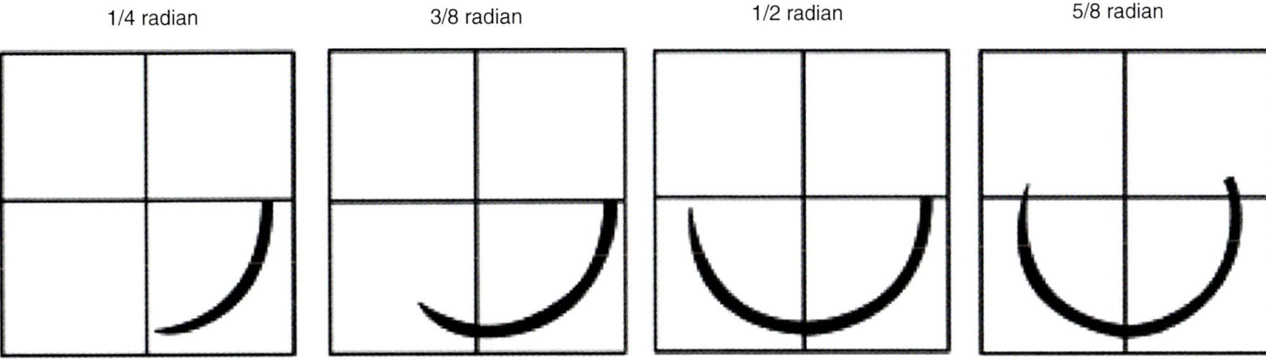

Fig. 4.16 Curvature of curved needle body

4.1.2.7 Material Science of Suture Needle

Stainless Steel Alloy

Martensitic stainless steel: It is easy to be shaped, hard, and relatively brittle; the strength can be enhanced by heat treatment.

Austenitic stainless steel: It contains more nickel and relatively less carbon, and it is easier to be shaped. At the same time, more molybdenum can enhance corrosion resistance, and more silicon improves surface accuracy. Austenitic stainless steels are not magnetic and have high flexibility and plasticity with relatively low strength.

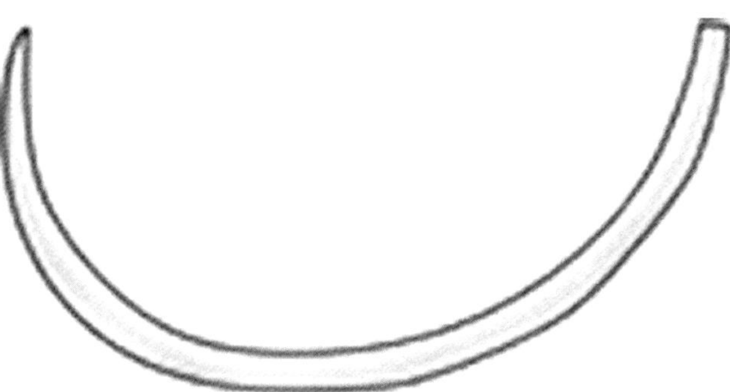

Fig. 4.17 Compound curved needle

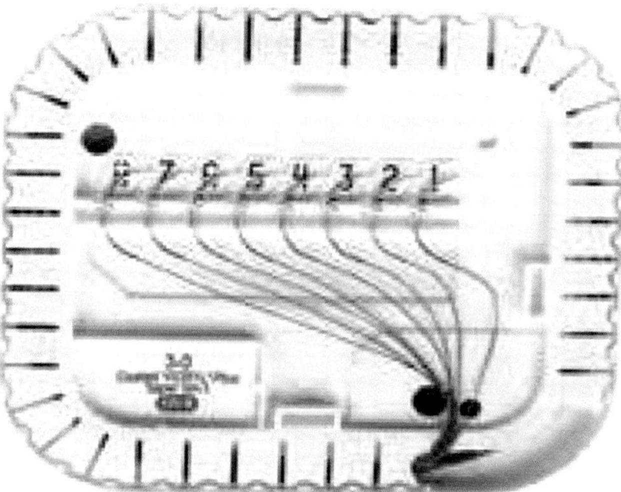

Fig. 4.19 Control release technique in needle tail does n'ot need scissors and allows separation between needle and suture with a slight traction, helping to reduce operation time

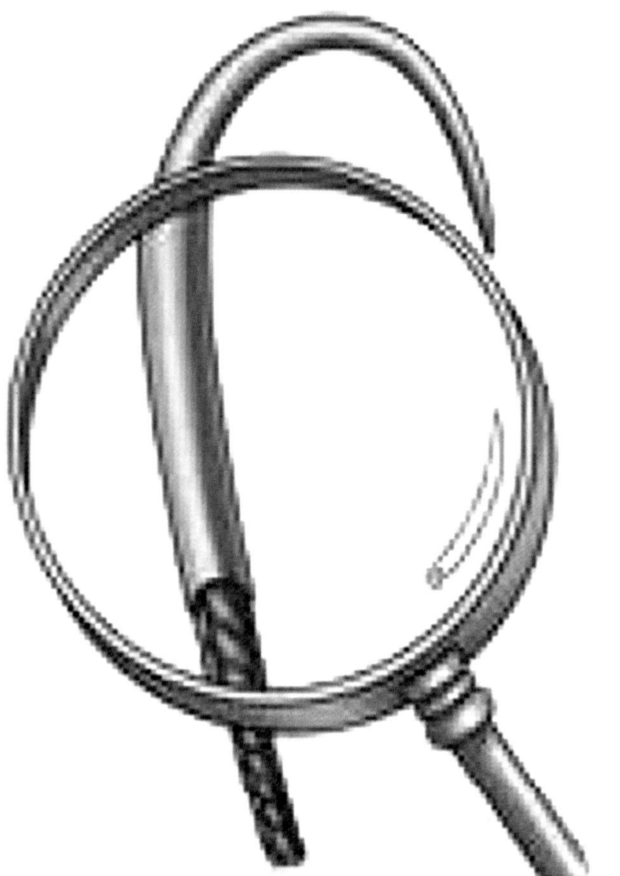

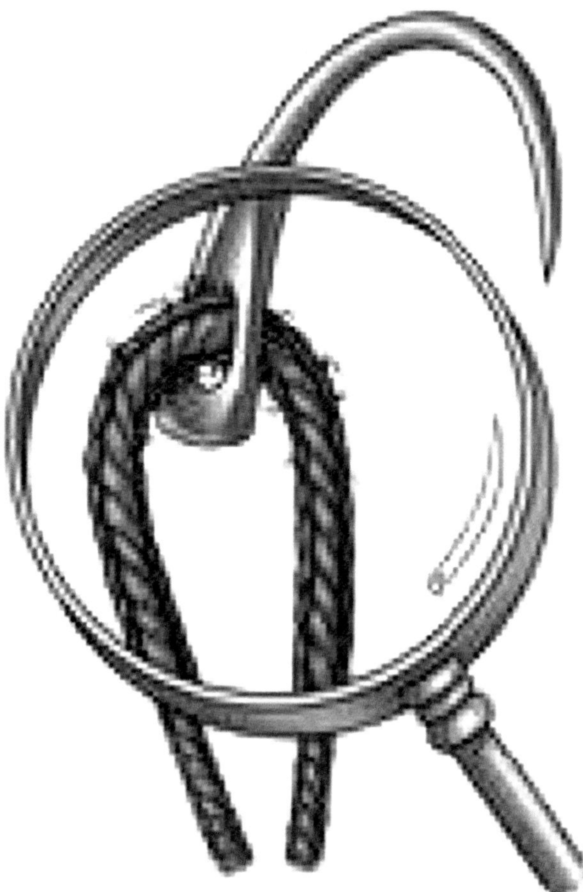

Fig. 4.18 Single-stranded suture tail, free of threading, disposable, compared with burr produced by threading of double-stranded suture, causing less tissue damage, convenient in use

Coating

Ordinary silicone coatings have excellent performance in the first penetration. However, due to the coating falls off, the resistance force increases after the needle passes through the tissue for multiple times. The MultiPass® silicone coating contains polymetric composite material to form a stronger and more stable coating, and it does not compromise the lubrication of suture needle. EVERPOINT® fine spraying multi-layer silicone can better cover the needle point.

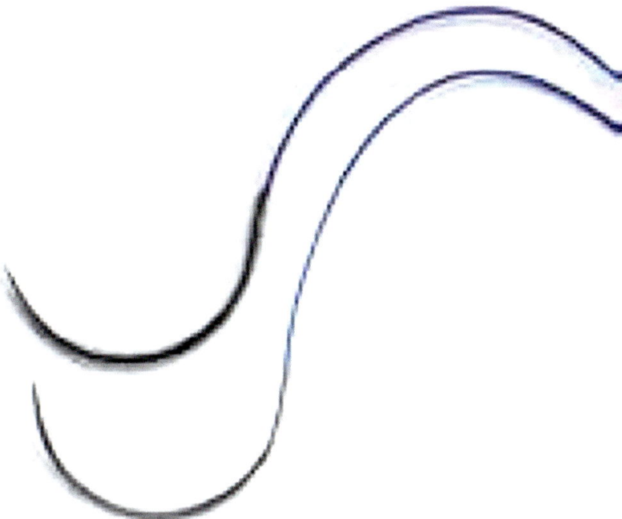

Fig. 4.20 Needle tail with Hemo-Seal technique has almost or totally consistent needle and suture, so as to realize anti-leakage function and reduce intraoperative bleeding

4.1.2.8 Types of Needle

Suture needle is the device used for suturing various tissues. In principle, the needle diameter should be smaller, as it causes less damage. But sometimes the tissue is quite tough, so if the needle diameter is too small, it is easily broken. Therefore, the selection of needle should be reasonable (Fig. 4.21).

Cutting Needle

The cutting needle has at least two opposing needle edges that are sharp enough to pass through tough tissue that are difficult to be penetrated. As for suturing dense, irregular, and relatively thick skin connective tissue, the cutting needle is ideal. Due to the sharpness of the needle edge, surgeons must take care to avoid unnecessary tissue cutting when the needle is passing through certain tissues (e.g., tendon sheath and oral mucosa).

1. Conventional cutting needle: In addition to the two needle edges, the conventional cutting needle has a third edge located on the inside of the concave surface of the curved part. This inner edge cuts the edge of the incision (wound), and it is easy to cut and penetrate tissue.

Types of needle point and needle body	Main applications
Conventional cutting needle (Needle point; Needle body)	Skin suture Sternal suture
Reverse cutting needle (Needle point; Needle body)	Fascia suture, ligament suture Suture of nasal mucosa, oral mucosa, throat mucosa, skin and tendon sheath
Precise cutting needle (Needle point; Needle body)	Skin suture (plastic and cosmetic)
PC PRIME* cutting needle (Needle point; Needle body)	Skin suture (plastic and cosmetic)
MICRO-POINT* reverse cutting needle (Needle point; Needle body)	Ophthalmic suture

Types of needle point and needle body	Main applications
Spatulated needle (Needle point; Needle body)	Ophthalmic routine suture Microsurgical suture Ophthalmic repair and reconstruction suture
CS ULTIMA* ophthalmic needle (Needle point; Needle body)	Ophthalmic routine suture
Taper point (Needle point; Needle body)	Suture of tendon sheath, biliary tract, dura mater, sarcolemma Suture of gastrointestinal tract, laparoscopic suture Suture of muscle, myocardium, nerve and peritoneum Suture of pleura, subcutaneous fat and urethra Suture of blood vessels and cardiac valves
TAPERCUT* surgical needle (Needle point; Needle body)	Suture of trachea, bronchus and calcified tissue Suture of fascia and ligament, laparoscopic surgical suture Suture of cartilage, periosteum and sternum Suture of tendon, nasal cavity, oral cavity and pharyngeal cavity Suture of uterus, cardiac valves and blood vessels (sclerotic)
Blunt taper point (Needle point; Needle body)	Suture of bluntly separated tissue (delicate) Cervix (ligation of cervical insufficiency) Suture of fascia Suture of intestinal tissue, kidney, liver and spleen

Fig. 4.21 Types of suture needle and their main applications

2. PC (precision cosmetic) PRIME needle: It is specially designed for plastic surgery and has conventional needle edges. Due to the high requirements of plastic surgery, the PC PRIME needle has a small needle point, a small suture diameter, and a delicate needle body ratio. The needle edge is very sharp when the needle passes through the soft tissue. In the needle holding area, the inner and outer sides of the curved part of needle body are flat, ensuring that it is more stable to operate by the needle holder.
3. Reverse cutting needle: It is specifically designed for tough tissues that are difficult to be penetrated, such as skin, tendon sheath, oral mucosa, etc. Reverse cutting needles are commonly used in ophthalmology and plastic surgery. These types of surgeries emphasize minimizing tissue damage, with the purpose of rapid tissue regeneration and little scar formation.

The reverse cutting needle is as sharp as the conventional cutting needle, but its design is quite different. The third needle edge of the reverse cutting needle is located on the outside of the convex surface of the suture needle's curved part, and the advantages are as follows: (1) The reverse cutting needle has higher strength than the conventional cutting needle of the same size; (2) It reduces tissue damage; (3) Needle tract in the tissue left by the suture needle is wider, and the suture is easier to be knotted.

MICROPOINT Suture Needle

The MICROPOINT suture needle for ophthalmic surgery has a smooth surface and is extremely sharp, enabling surgeons to easily and accurately suture very tough tissue around the eye. Neat suturing can minimize bumps and the holes, greatly reducing the possibility of local microbial reproduction.

Other Cutting Needles

The OS (orthopedic surgery) needle is a curved and reverse cutting needle with a large needle body. Orthopedic surgeons often use this needle to suture tissues that are very tough and require great force when puncturing, such as fascia.

The side-edge needle, also known as the "spatulated" cutting needle, is flat on both sides of the needle point and the needle tail. The edge of spatulated needle is designed for ophthalmic surgery. This needle edge facilitates the separation or rupture of the thin layer of sclera or corneal tissue and is easy to pass through it. The width, shape, and sharpness of suture needle ensure the maximal precision when the needle penetrates the tissue or passes through it. The direction of needle point varies with the different sizes of each spatulated cutting needle.

The CS ULTIMA ophthalmic cutting needle is the sharpest of its kind and is commonly used to suture the cornea or sclera. This suture needle greatly increases its sharpness as it has a small angle and extended length of tangent plane, therefore can smoothly pass through the tissue.

The TG PLUS cutting needle has a very sharp and slim point. When the TG PLUS cutting needle is used, the penetration resistance encountered is small, and the tactile feedback is excellent. In the suturing of the corneal wound, such needle facilitates the surgeon to control the suture depth and the puncture length.

Taper Cutting Needle

A taper needle that becomes tapered at one end is also called a "taper needle." It penetrates the tissue and extends without cutting. The needle point tapers to form a sharp tip, and the needle body is gradually flattened into an oval or rectangular shape, which prevents the needle from twisting or rotating when held by the needle holder. Taper needles are commonly used in tissues that are easier to pass, such as the peritoneum, abdominal organs, myocardium, dura mater, and subcutaneous tissues. Taper needle minimizes the holes and cutting to the tissues and is therefore preferable. The taper needle is also used for small bowel anastomosis to prevent leakage and to avoid abdominal infections. The taper needle greatly reduces the possibility of tearing the tissue when it penetrates the parallel and staggered fascia.

TAPERCVTCC is a kind of needle used for suturing calcified blood vessels. This kind of suture requires sharp needle point for piercing without tearing the blood vessels. This needle has a longer and thinner geometric shape from the needle body to the needle point than other taper needles, minimizing the risk of leakage of fragile blood vessels and vascular graft materials.

Stab-Prevention Blunt Needle

Needle stabs may expose medical staff to hematogenous viruses, such as hepatitis B virus (HBV), hepatitis C virus (HCV), and human immunodeficiency virus (HIV). According to a paper published in the Association of periOperative Registered Nurses Journal in 2010, more than half of stabs related to suture needles occurred in the process of suturing fascia and muscle [3]. Published studies have shown that the use of blunt-tip suture needles reduced the risk of stabs caused by suture needles by 69% [4]. The use of blunt-tip suture needles in surgery has been recognized and recommended by international government agencies and professional organizations including Food and Drug Administration (FDA), National Institute for Occupational Safety and Health (NIOSH), and Centers for Disease Control and Prevention (CDC) [5].

In fact, a blunt needle separates, rather than punctures brittle tissues. The needle body is round, with its needle point round and blunt, so it is difficult to penetrate gloves, but it can easily penetrate tissues. It can be used to suture the liver and kidney, and surgeons also use the blunt needle in gynecological surgery (Fig. 4.22).

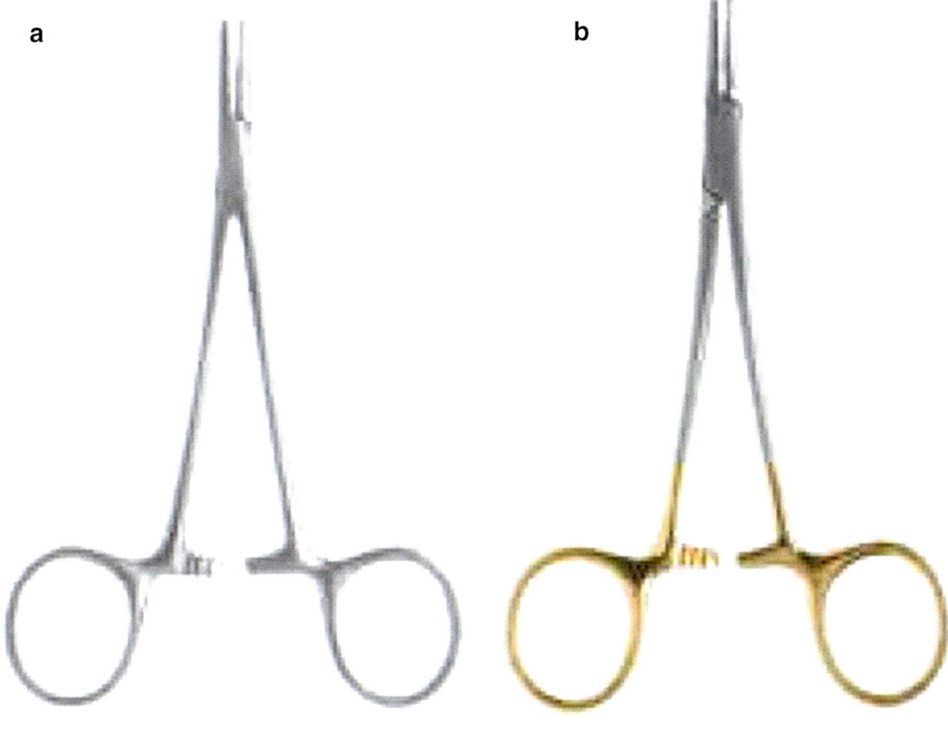

Fig. 4.22 Needle holders. (**a**) Common needle holder. (**b**) Needle holder with tungsten carbide inlaid jaws

4.1.3 Needle Holder: Important Assistant in Suturing

Surgeons use the needle holder when suturing the tissue with curved needle. The needle holder must be made of corrosion resistant, high-strength, and high-quality alloy steel (Fig. 4.22). The jaws are designed to ensure that the suture needles are securely fastened. The jaws of the needle holder have different width, length, and flatness. The clamped jaws can be round and flat, and the clamping part of jaws can be serrated or non-serrated (Fig. 4.23). Needles held by the non-serrated jaws can swing or rotate, while the serrated jaws can tightly clamp needles, but excessive force can easily damage the suture or needle. The needle holder with tungsten carbide inlaid jaws (Fig. 4.24) has two distinct advantages: (1) The jaw surface with fine granule has greater clamping force than the non-serrated jaws; (2) It will not damage the suture or change its breaking strength easily.

The surgical needle is designed according to the maximum stability of the needle holder. The needle holder is the operating tool of suture needle and can greatly influence the whole suturing process. Most needle holders have one tooth. Only when the suture needle is securely held by the needle holder and does not swing when passing through the tissue, can the surgeon accurately suture the tissue. The needle holder, like other surgical instruments, becomes dull after repeated use. Therefore, the surgical nurse should perform examination before each operation to ensure an accurate match of the needle holder jaws and a tight clamping. It is strictly forbidden that surgeons use the needle holder to pull out Kirschner wires or twist down screws. The needle holder can be easily damaged by rule-breaking operations.

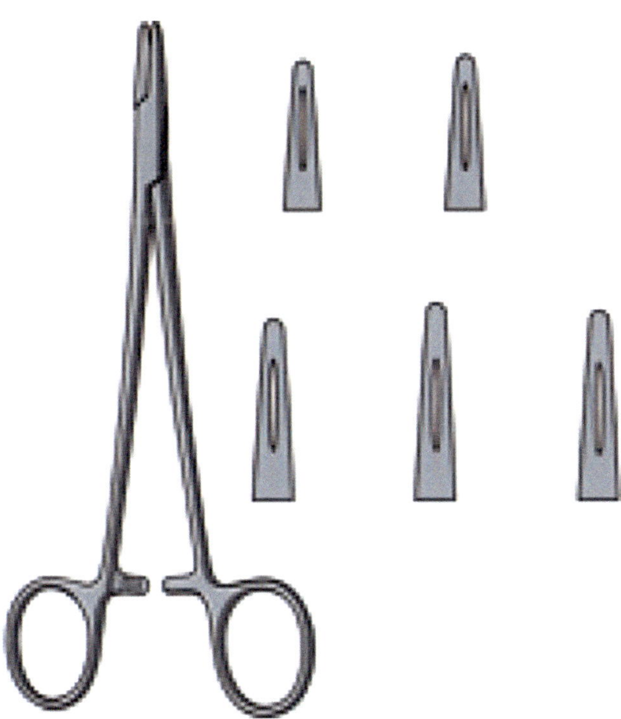
Fig. 4.23 Needle holder with serrated jaws

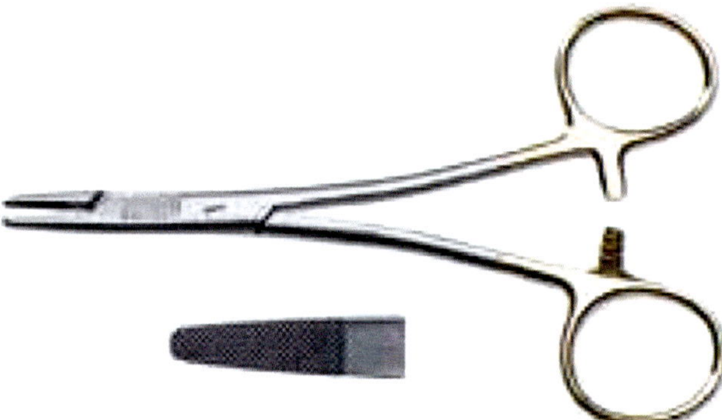

Fig. 4.24 Needle holder with tungsten carbide inlaid jaws

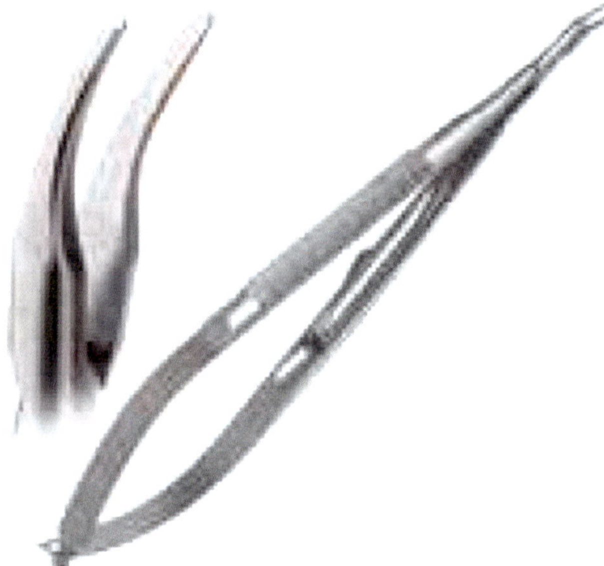

Fig. 4.25 Microsurgical needle holder (with non-serrated jaws)

4.1.3.1 Selection of Needle Holder

1. The size of the needle holder should match the suture needle. When the suture needle is small, the jaws should be correspondingly small; when the suture needle is thick and large, the jaws of the needle holder should be wide.
2. The size of the needle holder should match the surgery. For surgeries in the deep body cavity, a longer needle holder is required. Microsurgery uses fine microsurgical needle holders (Fig. 4.25).

4.1.3.2 Precautions When the Instrument Nurses Use Needle Holder

1. Hold the suture needle with the tips of needle holder jaws, and clamp it at 1/3 to 1/2 from the suture attachment end to the needle point. Avoid the needle holder to be clamped at the suture attachment end, which is the weak part of suture needle.
2. When clamping round or cutting needles, keep it as far as possible from the needle point, to avoid damaging the needle point or cutting edge.
3. Do not clamp the suture needle much too tightly with needle holder jaws, which may cause the suture needle to irreversibly deform, damage, or bend.
4. Frequently check the needle holder jaws to make sure that the needles do not swing, twist, or rotate.
5. Handle the suture needle and the needle holder flexibly as a whole.
6. Pay attention to the direction of the needle holder when passing it, so that the surgeon does not need to make an adjustment again before suturing the tissue; when being passed, the direction of suture needle should be accordant with the direction of use, and the suture should not be entangled.
7. When the suture needle is pulled out of the tissue, make sure that it is passed to the needle holder instead of the hemostatic forceps. Hemostatic forceps or other clamps may damage the suture needle.
8. After use, each needle that is clamped to the needle holder should be returned immediately to the surgical nurse. Use one and pass one, so as to prevent the needle from being lost.

4.1.3.3 Precautions When Surgeons Use Needle Holder

1. When the surgeon takes the needle holder, the needle point should direct the thumb (Fig. 4.26) to avoid unnecessary wrist movement. The surgical nurse pulls the free end of the suture to prevent it from passing through the sterile area and ensure that the suture is not delivered to the surgeon along with the needle holder.
2. The surgeon should pay attention to the entry point when suturing and plan the needle gauge and edge distance.
3. The suture needle passes through the tissue. The surgeon releases the suture needle from the needle holder and then clamps the needle holder again near the needle point and pulls the needle and suture through the tissue. The needle is controlled and released or cut from the suture.
4. The surgeon clamps the suture needle in the same direction and returns it to the surgical nurse. The instrument nurse immediately hands the other suture to the surgeon. Receive one, and pass one.

4.1.4 Correct Tissue Suturing Technique

Improper operation of the suture needle in the patient's tissue can cause additional damage. Pay attention to the following key points when suturing:

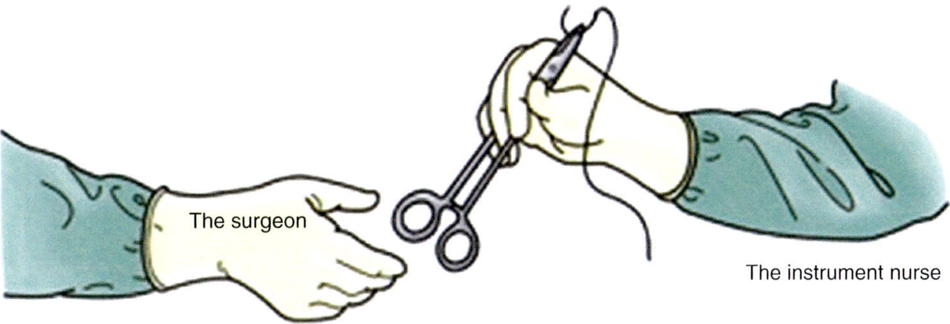

Fig. 4.26 Correct way to pass needle holder

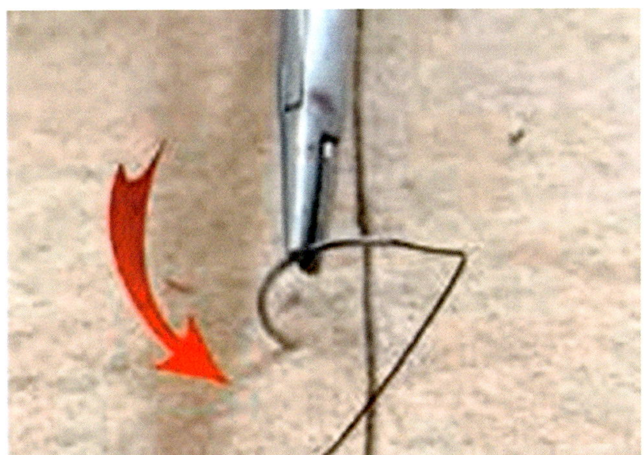

Fig. 4.27 Direction of force when suturing

1. When suturing the tissue, the direction of force should be accordant with the direction of the curvature of suture needle (Fig. 4.27).
2. Do not suture large tissues with small needles.
3. Do not use dull needles to pass through the tissue by violence, but replace it with a new one.
4. Do not pass the suture needle through the tissue by pushing or twisting it. In this case, the suture needle should be completely pulled out and re-inserted into the tissue, or a larger one should be used.
5. When suturing, avoid using the suture needle to pull the tissue to be sutured.
6. Follow the principle of personalized suture. If the sutured tissue is tougher than expected, a larger suture needle should be used. Conversely, weaker tissue requires smaller suture needles.
7. When suturing in deep and confined regions, needles cannot be ideally positioned. In this case, the operation must be cautious. It may be helpful to use a suture needle with a larger size or different curvature.
8. If the gloves are punctured by the suture needle, the needle must be discarded immediately, and the gloves must be replaced to ensure the safety of the patient and the surgical team member.

4.1.5 Using Suture Needle Safely

To use suture needles safely, the following principles should be complied with:

1. Carefully open the needle package and carefully prepare the suture needle to protect its sharpness.
2. Make sure that the suture needle does not rust.
3. If an eyed needle is used, ensure that the needle eye has no rough or sharp edges to prevent the suture from being damaged or broken. Also check the needle eye for burrs or passivation to ensure that the needle penetrates and passes through the tissue smoothly.
4. If the suture needle is defective, it should be discarded.
5. Pass the suture needle in an exchange manner: let the surgeon return one and then pass one to the surgeon.
6. Once the suture needle is used, it should be put away. Do not let suture needles scatter in the disinfection area, or on the operating table, and do not allow suture needles to be close to the gauze or sterile surgical towels to avoid being accidentally pulled into the wound.
7. If the suture needle is broken, each fragment must be completely assembled and properly disposed.
8. According to the surgical routine, all the suture needles should be counted before and after use.
9. Magnetic or non-magnetic disinfected sticky pads or disposable magnetic pads can be used to facilitate to count and safely dispose the needle.
10. Keep the package, as the description on number and size of needles are printed on it and it is convenient to count and ensure each needle is collected. The swaged needle

is inserted into the original bag, and the empty bag indicates a lost needle.

11. Reusable suture needles should be put back in the needle shelf. After the surgery is completed, suture needles should be cleaned and completely sterilized before they are used again.
12. Do not collect used suture needles and put them into containers on the operating table. Otherwise, the gloves may be punctured, and medical risks may be increased.
13. Dispose the used disposable suture needles in a container labeled "Box for Sharp Instruments."

4.2 Surgical Suture

4.2.1 Suturing Materials

4.2.1.1 Ideal Suturing Materials Should Meet the Following Standards

1. Versatile. That is, it can be used in any surgical procedure (of course, the difference in suture size and tensile strength should also be considered);
2. Sterile;
3. Non-electrolytic, with no capillarity, non-allergenic and non-carcinogenic;
4. If stainless steel suture is used, it must be non-magnetic;
5. Easy to handle;
6. Have slight tissue reaction and is not conducive to bacterial growth;
7. Do not loosen when being knotted and the suture itself will not wear or split;
8. Do not shrink within the tissue;
9. Can be absorbed after the aim of suture is achieved and only causes a slight reaction.

However, standards of ideal versatile suture are difficult to be fully met, so the surgeon should choose sutures that are the closest to the ideal one and that have the following characteristics:

1. Uniform tensile strength facilitating the use of thinner suture;
2. The diameter of the suture is uniform and constant;
3. Sterile;
4. Highly flexible, easy to handle, and secure to ligate;
5. Contains no irritating substances or impurities to facilitate tissue compatibility;
6. The suture results are trustworthy.

4.2.1.2 Size and Tensile Strength of Suture

The size indicates the diameter of the suture material. It is universally accepted in surgical practice that the thinnest type of suture that allows safe alignment of the tissue should be selected to minimize the trauma caused by suturing. The size of the suture is represented by numbers: above "0," larger number indicates thicker suture, for example: No.3 is thicker than No.1; starting from "0," more "0" indicates smaller diameter and lower tensile strength.

The tensile strength of a suture is the strength (in pounds) that it can withstand before breaking. The tensile strength of the tissue is a prerequisite for the surgeon to select the suture size and tensile strength. The surgeon should also understand the relationship between the decreasing suture strength and the increasing tensile strength of the wound, and whether the foreign body reaction caused by the implant material affects the healing process of the tissue. It is generally believed that the tensile strength of the suture does not need to exceed that of the tissue, but should be at least the same strong as the normal tissue that it sutures.

4.2.1.3 Monofilament and Multifilament Sutures

The monofilament suture is made of a single bunch of filaments that encounters less resistance as it passes through the tissue, and it prevents bacteria from adhering. Due to these qualities, it is especially suitable for vascular surgery. Monofilament sutures are easy to knot. However, care must be taken during handling and ligating, as folding or curling may cause gaps or weak points in the suture and make it easy to break.

4.2.1.4 Absorbable and Non-absorbable Sutures

Absorbable sutures are produced from collagen of healthy mammals or synthetic polymers. Natural absorbable sutures are degraded by digestion of enzymes in the human body. The synthetic absorbable suture is firstly hydrolyzed to cause the water to gradually permeate into the suture filaments to cause decomposition of the polymer chain. Compared with the natural absorbable suture, the synthetic absorbable suture is hydrolyzed after implantation, only causing a lighter tissue reaction.

In the first stage of the suture absorption process, the tensile strength linearly and gradually decreases, which occurs within a few weeks after surgery. The second stage often overlaps with the first one, and finally the suture almost disappears.

Non-absorbable sutures are not digested by enzymes or hydrolyzed. Its scope of application is as follows:

1. The suture of skin. The suture should be removed immediately after the wound heals;
2. The suture in the body cavity. The suture will remain in the tissue for a long period;
3. Suitable for patients who are allergic and have scar constitution or tissue hypertrophy to absorbable sutures;
4. Used to fix temporary devices such as defibrillators, pacemakers, and drug releasers.

4.2.2 Introduction to Common Suturing Materials

4.2.2.1 Natural Absorbable Sutures

Surgical catgut: It can be divided into normal catgut and chromic catgut. Both are produced from highly purified collagen. The absorption rate of the surgical catgut depends on the type of the suture, the type of the tissue, the condition of the tissue, and the general condition of the patient. Surgical catgut can be used to suture infected wounds, but the absorption rate is significantly accelerated.

Normal surgical catgut is absorbed rapidly. The tensile strength only maintains for 7–10 days after operation and is completely absorbed within 70 days. The catgut is called a chromic catgut after being treated by chromate solution. It can resist the digestion of various enzymes in the body and extend the absorption time to more than 90 days.

4.2.2.2 Synthetic Absorbable Sutures

Due to the shortcomings of the natural catgut, such as antigenicity, strong tissue reaction, and unpredictable absorption rate, people are working hard on the research and development of synthetic absorbable sutures. The latter has a wide range of applications, from the suture of thoracic and abdominal wounds to the application in ophthalmic surgery (Table 4.1). For example, the multifilament braided absorbable suture Polyglactin 910 (VICRYL PLUS®) (Fig. 4.28). The Polyglactin 910 is a copolymer of 90% glycolide and 10% L-lactide. Its advantages are:

1. Passing through the tissue smoothly;
2. Stable knotting and accurate positioning;
3. Reducing the tendency to incarcerate the tissue;
4. Can be used for suturing infected wounds (Tables 4.2 and 4.3).

Table 4.1 Types of sutures

Types of suture	Characteristics	Examples
Natural	Digested by enzymes in human body; greater tissue reaction	Catgut, silk
Synthetic	Greater tension; smaller tissue reaction	VICRYL PLUS® PDS PLUS®
Monofilament	Bacteria are not easy to adhere; little tissue pulling	PDS PLUS®
Multifilament	Easy to knot; good tensile strength; if coated, it has the same advantages of monofilament	VICRYL PLUS®
Absorbable	No foreign body left in body	VICRYL PLUS®
Non-absorbable	Supporting the wound permanently	PROLENE, ETHIBOND

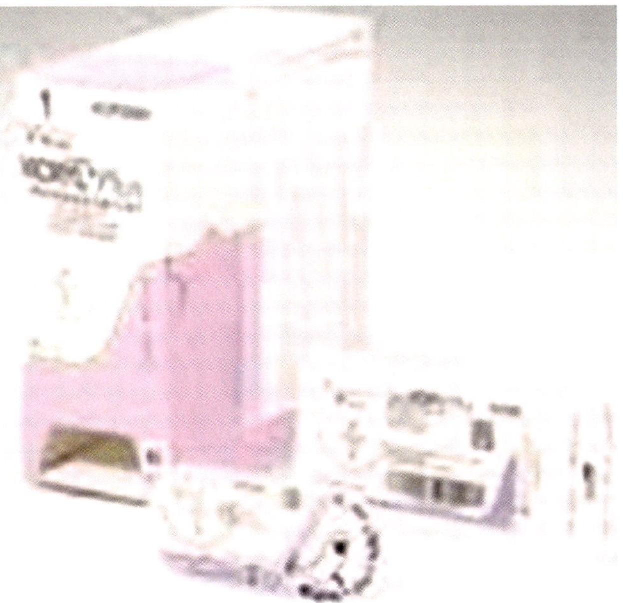

Fig. 4.28 Polyglactin 910 suture (antibacterial VICRYL)

The coating is a blend of lactide and glycolide (Polyglactin 370) copolymer plus calcium stearate. This coating has significant absorbability, adhesion, and lubricity without exfoliation.

At 14th day after suturing, the tensile strength of the VICRYL PLUS® suture maintains about 65%. At 21st day after suturing, the tensile strength of the 6-0 or thicker suture maintains about 40%, while the 7-0 or thinner suture maintains only about 30%. Within 40 days, the suture is hardly absorbed, and it is absorbed between 56th and 70th day. The absorption of the coating is also very rapid, estimated to be between 56th and 70th day.

Antibacterial Polydioxanone (PDS Plus) suture:

Significant advance in representative suture material of monofilament suture [6]. It integrates the characteristics of softness, flexibility, and monofilament structure (Fig. 4.29). It has good absorption performance and can maintain the tensile strength of wound for more than 6 weeks (twice as much as other synthetic absorbable sutures). The tissue reaction is mild, and the affinity for bacteria is low. It is suitable for suturing a variety of soft tissues and can be used in children's cardiovascular, obstetrics, ophthalmic, plastic surgical, digestive tract, and colon surgeries.

Similar to other synthetic absorbable sutures, antibacterial polydioxanone (PDS Plus) sutures are absorbed in the body by hydrolysis. About 70% of the tensile strength is maintained at 14th day after suturing, 50% at 28th day, and 25% at 42th day. The suture is barely absorbed within 90 days after surgery and is completely absorbed after 6 months.

Poliglecaprone 25 (antibacterial MONOCRYL Poliglecaprone 25) suture:

Table 4.2 Types and characteristics of common synthetic absorbable sutures

Suture name	Hand feeling in surgery	Tension left	Firmness of knot	Tissue reaction	Absorption time (days)	Clinical applications
Polyglactin 910 (VICRYL PLUS®)	Good	Tension disappears between 5 and 6 weeks	Good	Slight	56–70	Fascia, muscle, and subcutaneous tissue
Polydioxanone (PDS PLUS® multifilament braided suture/ Symmetric/Spiral)	Fair	Tension retains 50–70% at 4th week	Good	Slight	180–210	Fascia, muscle, and subcutaneous tissue that requires high-strength support or contaminated subcutaneous tissue
Poliglecaprone 25 (MONOCRYL PLUS®/Spiral)	Relatively good	Tension disappears at 4th week	Good	Slight	90–120	Intradermal continuous suture
Copolymer of glycolide and e-caprolactone (ETHICON spiral knotless PGA-PCL suture)	Good	Tension retained 62% at 1st week; 27% at 2rd week	Knotless	Slight	90–120	Intradermal continuous suture

Table 4.3 Types of non-absorbable sutures

Suture name	Type	Hand feeling in surgery	Tension left	Firmness of knot	Tissue reaction	Clinical applications
Natural silk	Braided/twisted	Very good	No tension after 1 year	Good	Moderate	Vascular ligation
Synthetic non-absorbable suture						
Nylon (NYLON), ethilon (ETHILON)	Monofilament	Fair	Tension retains 20–30% after 1 year	Fair	Slight	Skin suture
Polypropylene (PROLENE)	Monofilament	Fair	Permanent support	Poor	Slight	Skin suture
Polyester (ETHIBOND)	Monofilament braided	Very good	Permanent support	Good	Slight	Skin suture
Stainless steel wire	Monofilament	Poor	Permanent support	Good	Slight	Skin suture

Fig. 4.29 Antibacterial polydioxanone (PDS Plus) suture

This kind of monofilament suture is flexible, easy to handle, easy to knot, does not have chemical reaction in the tissue, and can be absorbed as expected. Surgeons often use it in suturing the tissues that require higher tensile strength within 2 weeks after surgery, i.e., subcutaneous sutures, soft tissue alignment and ligation except for nerves, blood vessels, ophthalmic surgery, and microsurgery. At 7th day, 50–60% of the original strength can be retained. At 14th day, it is reduced to 20–30%, and the strength disappears at 21st day. It is completely absorbed between 91st and 119th day (Figs. 4.30 and 4.31).

The absorbable suture made by MONOCRYL material has the characteristics of small tissue reaction, less redness and swelling, and is more suitable for intradermal continuous suture than other materials.

Knotless tissue control device:

The barbed design allows knotless suture devices to have more fixing points than conventional sutures, and it is suitable for sutures with higher tension, such as deep fascia and skeletal muscle (Fig. 4.32).

Symmetric: Fishbone barbs are not produced by incising the core of the suture, and the barbing technique does not affect the tensile strength of the suture core; Spiral: The unique geometric spiral barbs, when passing through the tissue, integrate into the suture core, and when having passed through the tissue, the barbs open again and accomplish safe support. 360° support and fixation reliably close the tissues together.

The unique barbed design provides multiple fixing points along the suture path, allowing the tension of the suture to be maintained during suturing.

Compared with conventional sutures, it allows the surgeon to control tension and pull the tissue more easily each time it passes through the tissue, and there is no need for an assistant to pull during suturing, which may reduce the anesthesia time of the patient [7]. In addition, the Plus antibacterial technology brought by the triclosan coating has been shown in vitro to inhibit bacterial colonization of the suture within 7 days or longer, including bacteria commonly associated with surgical site infections, and can deal with the risk factors associated with surgical site infections.

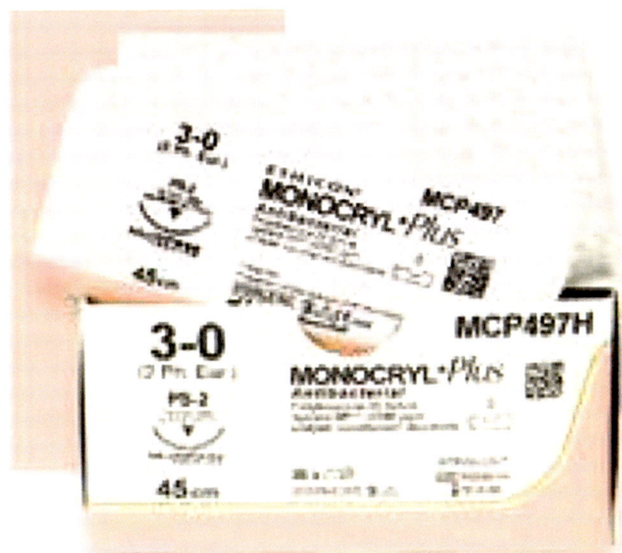

Fig. 4.30 Poliglecaprone 25(MONOCRYL PLUS®, Poliglecaprone 25)

4.2.2.3 Non-absorbable Sutures

The US Pharmacopoeia classifies non-absorbable surgical sutures into the following categories:

- Class I: Silk or synthetic filaments with twisted, braided, or monofilament structure;
- Class II: Cotton or flax filaments, coated natural or synthetic filaments, the coating used makes the suture thicker without increasing the strength;
- Class III: Metal wires with mono- or multifilament structure.

4.2.2.4 Surgical Silk

Due to superior operability of surgical silk, it has become the standard which surgeons use to evaluate the performance of new synthetic materials. Natural monofilament silk can be processed into silk thread by twisting or weaving, and the braided surgical silk has the best performance.

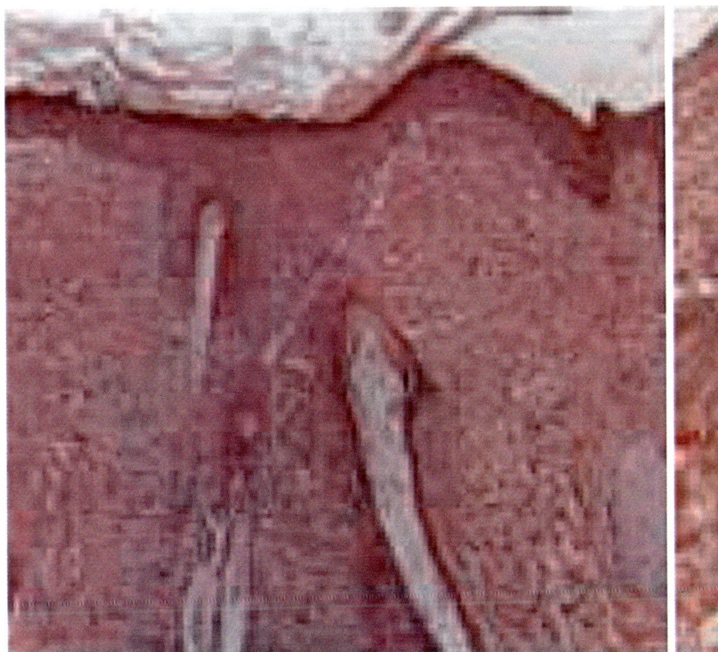

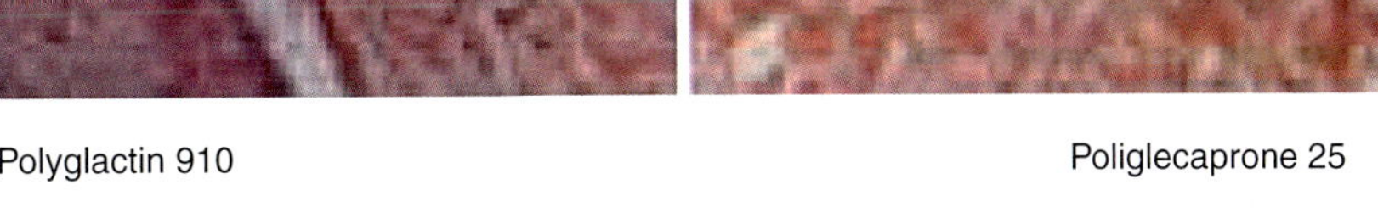

Fig. 4.31 Comparison of tissue reactions of absorbable sutures made by Poliglecaprone 25 material and other materials

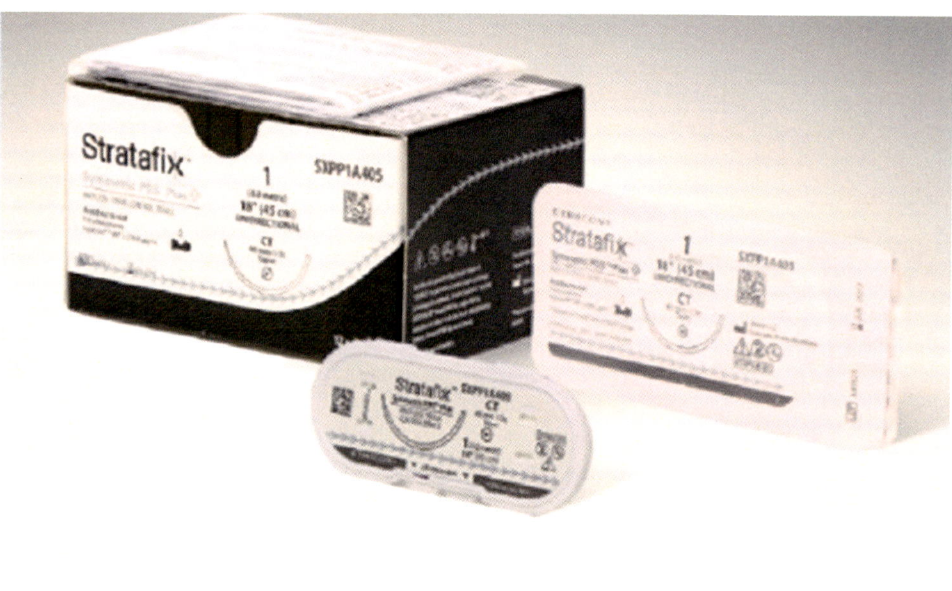

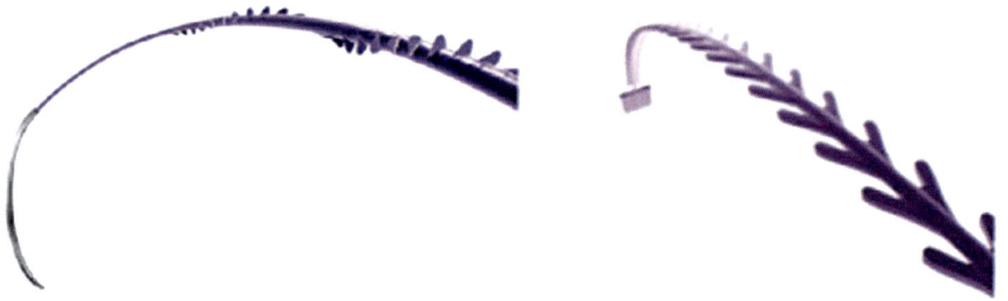

Fig. 4.32 Knotless suture devices

4.2.2.5 Alloy Sutures

Surgical stainless steel sutures: The basic characteristics include being non-toxic, easy to bend, slender, and so on. Both monofilament and twisted multifilament sutures have the advantages of high tensile strength, low tissue reaction, and convenient knotting. As long as the suture does not break, the tensile strength of the tissue changes very little. Stainless steel sutures can be used for suturing the abdominal wall, sternum, skin, relaxation suture, and various plastic and neurosurgical surgeries.

4.2.2.6 Synthetic Non-absorbable Sutures

Nylon suture: It is a chemically synthesized polyamide polymer. Due to its good elasticity, it is especially suitable for relaxation suture and skin suture. Nylon sutures are hydrolyzed at a rate of 15–20% per year in human body. The monofilament nylon suture has the tendency to restore its original straight state ("memory" characteristics), so it is necessary to tie more knots during the ligation compared with the braided nylon suture to ensure safety and reliability.

ETHILON is a nylon suture with high strength and little tissue reaction. Very thin sutures of sizes (9-0, 10-0) are often used in ophthalmic surgery and microsurgery after being stained black (Fig. 4.33).

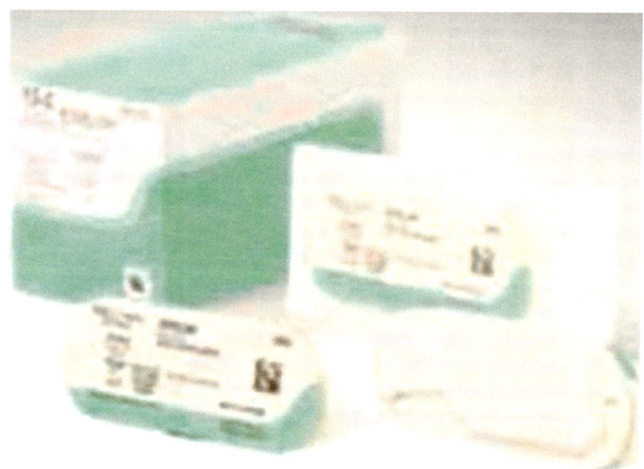

Fig. 4.33 Example of nylon suture (ETHILON)

NUROLON is precisely braided from nylon filaments with a coating to improve its operability. Its appearance, hand feeling, and operation are similar to silk, but the strength is stronger and the tissue reaction is milder. It can

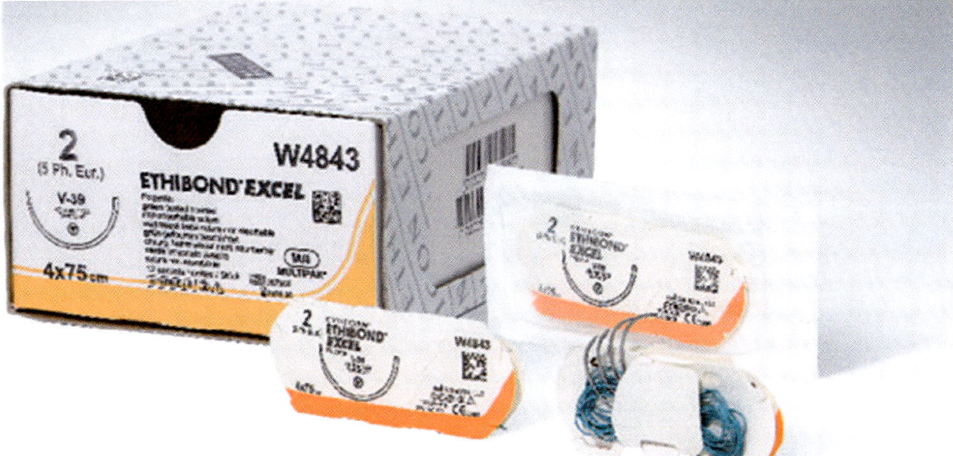

Fig. 4.34 Example of polyester suture (ETHIBOND)

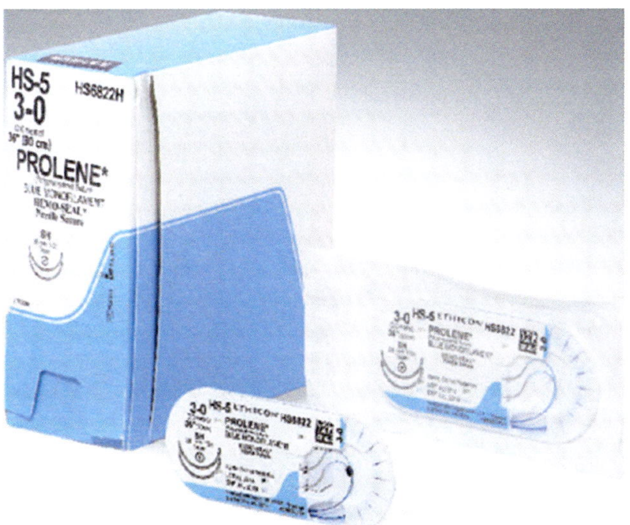

Fig. 4.35 Example of PROLENE polypropylene suture

be used in any tissue that requires multifilament non-absorbable sutures.

Polyester suture: It is a multifilament suture which is tightly woven from benzene-treated polyester filaments (polyethylene terephthalate). It is stronger than natural fiber. Humidification before use does not weaken its strength, and the tissue reaction is slight. Polyester sutures are the best material for suturing artificial blood vessels [8].

MERSILENE polyester sutures are enduringly retained in the body, providing precise and uniform tension with little breakage. There is no need to remove suture stumps due to irritation. After ophthalmic surgery, the MERSILENE suture causes little burning pain and itching. As it is uncoated, the friction coefficient is higher when the MERSILENE suture passes through the tissue. ETHIBOND EXCEL polyester suture is uniformly coated with polybutilate which is the first coating specifically used as a surgical suture lubricant and adheres to braided polyester sutures. This coating enables the braided suture to easily pass through the tissue. It has superior flexibility and operability and can be smoothly ligated and fastened. The pharmacological properties of the suturing material and the coating are not active, and the tissue reaction is slight. The strength can be maintained in the body for a long time. ETHIBOND EXCEL sutures are mainly used in cardiovascular surgery, such as vascular anastomosis, suture of artificial blood vessels or valves. ETHIBOND EXCEL polyester suture can also be used with TEFLON or polyester liners. A small liner acts as a support underneath the suture to prevent avulsion of adjacent fragile tissues. Small liners are routinely used in valvular surgery and are used in the situation where the valve annulus is extremely deformed, distorted, or damaged (Fig. 4.34).

Polypropylene (POLYPROPYLENE) suture:

Polypropylene suture is a stereoisomer of a linear hydroxy polymer. Polypropylene suture manufactured by the patented process has increased flexibility and is easy to use. It is not easily degraded and weakened by tissue enzymes. It has extremely weak activity in tissue and slight tissue reaction, and the tensile strength can be maintained in the body for up to 2 years. Knotting is smoother and firmer compared with other types of monofilament sutures.

PROLENE polypropylene sutures have been widely used in general surgery, cardiovascular surgery, plastic surgery, and ophthalmology. This suture has a weak biological activity, does not stick to tissue, and is easy to remove. PROLENE sutures can be used in contaminated and infected wounds, minimizing later sinus formation and suture removal (Fig. 4.35).

The selection of suture for different tissues and the initial tension of several common sutures are shown in Tables 4.4 and 4.5.

Search Terms

Strength of suture needle, Flexibility, Sharpness, Suture attachment end, Measurement of suture needle, Keith nee-

Table 4.4 Selection and recommendation of sutures for different tissues

	Time for tissue healing (days)	Selection of suturing material	Example
		Absorbable suture	VICRYL PLUS®
Skin	5–7	Monofilament non-absorbable suture	PROLENE
Subcutaneous tissue	7–10	Absorbable suture	VICRYL PLUS®
Fascia	21–28	Absorbable suture	VICRYL PLUS®/PDS PLUS®/Symmetric knotless suture
Joint capsule	21–28	Absorbable suture	VICRYL PLUS®/PDS PLUS®/Symmetric knotless suture
Muscle	14	Absorbable suture	VICRYL PLUS®/PDS PLUS®/Symmetric knotless suture

Table 4.5 Initial tension of several common sutures

	USP 0 (M 3.5)			USP 2-0 (M3)			USP 3-0 (M2)			USP 4-0 (M1.5)		
	Diameter (mil)	Straight Tension (pound)	Knotted Tension (pound)	Diameter (mil)	Straight Tension (pound)	Knotted Tension (pound)	Diameter (mil)	Straight Tension (pound)	Knotted Tension (pound)	Diameter (mil)	Straight Tension (pound)	Knotted Tension (pound)
Poliglecaprone 25 (MONOCRYL)	17.9	28.9	13.9	14.9	20.4	10.4	11.5	13.3	6.6	8.8	8.4	3.8
Polyglactin 910 (VICRYL)	15.8	22.4	11.9	12.7	16.9	8.9	10.1	10.3	5.4	8.1	7.4	3.7
Antibacterial Polydioxanone (PDS Plus®)	17.9	17.2	10.5	14.0	11.5	7.3	11.6	8.5	5.4	8.5	4.8	3.3
Polypropylene (PROLENE)	15.5	13.5	9.0	12.8	10.1	6.8	9.7	6.3	4.3	7.7	4.1	2.9
Polyester (ETHIBOND)	14.5	20.8	8.6	12.6	15.8	7.2	9.5	8.8	4.3	7.3	5.8	2.6

dle, Half curved needle, Compound curved needle, Needle point, Needle tail, Cutting needle, Reverse cutting needle, Side-edge needle, Tensile strength, Monofilament suture, Absorbable suture, Non-absorbable suture, Nylon suture, Polyester suture, Polypropylene suture

References

1. Abidin MR, Towler MA, Rodeheaver GT, Thacker JG, Cantrell RW, Edlich RF. Biomechanics of curved surgical needle bending. J Biomed Mater Res. 1989;23(A1 Suppl):129–43.
2. Chu C-C, von Fraunhofer JA, Greisler HP. Wound closure biomaterials and devices. 1st ed. Boca Raton, FL: CRC; 1996. p. 25–38.
3. Jagger J, Bentley M, Tereskerz P. A study of patterns and prevention of blood exposures in OR personnel. AORN J. 1998;67(5):979–96.
4. Parantainen A, Verbeek JH, Lavoie MC, Pahwa M. Blunt versus sharp suture needles for preventing percutaneous exposure incidents in surgical staff. Cochrane Database Syst Rev. 2011;(11):Art. No.: CD009170.
5. FDA, NIOSH & OSHA Joint Safety Communication: Blunt-tip surgical suture needles reduce needlestick injuries and the risk of subsequent bloodborne pathogen transmission to surgical personnel.
6. Boland ED, Coleman BD, Barnes CP, Simpson DG, Wnek GE, Bowlin GL. Electrospinning polydioxanone for biomedical applications. Acta Biomater. 2005;1(1):115–23.
7. Levine BR, Ting N, Della Valle CJ. Use of a barbed suture in the closure of hip and knee arthroplasty wounds. Orthopaedics. 2011;34(9):e473–5.
8. Ma Z, Kotaki M, Yong T, He W, Ramakrishna S. Surface engineering of electrospun polyethylene terephthalate (PET) nanofibers towards development of a new material for blood vessel engineering. Biomaterials. 2005;26(15):2527–36.

5 Basic Training of Orthopedic Suture Techniques

Wenjun Li

Abstract

In addition to bones, skin, tendon, nerve, muscle, and deep fascia are all important parts of overall combination of the motor nervous system, which will have a great impact on limb function regardless of their single injury or combined injury. Therefore, how to better repair these organ injuries is a very important issue, and is also one of the skills that young doctors must master. Due to the different structural features and functions of each organ, the required repair techniques are also different. In order to better train young doctors, the following training courses are specially set up.

Keywords
Suture · Skin · Tendon · Peripheral nerve · Blood vessel
Muscle · Deep fascia

5.1 Skin Suturing Training

Overview
Skin covers the surface of human body, accounting for about 16% of body weight, and its area can reach 1.2–2.0 m^2. It is one of the largest organs of human body, and is also a beauty organ besides having an important protective effect on human body. The quality of skin suturing after surgical incision or injury is related to its appearance and functional recovery. This section is set for the training of skin and its subcutaneous tissue suturing.

5.1.1 Training Purpose

1. To master basic skin and subcutaneous suturing techniques;
2. To master orthopedic skin and subcutaneous suturing techniques and the selection of sutures;
3. To be familiar with the skills of improving the aesthetics of suturing.

5.1.2 Preparation of Articles

Fresh pig elbow, operating tables and stools, common surgical instruments (tissue scissors, suture scissors, teeth forceps, needle holders, scalpel handles, and hemostats), astral lamps, blades, syringes, cutting needles, taper needles, 3-0 sutures, 4-0 sutures, normal saline, and iodophor (Table 5.1).

5.1.3 Training Process

1. Tutor teaching
   Explain the history and evolution of surgical suturing, suturing methods and indications, suture and needle selection and indications.
2. Operation teaching of skin and subcutaneous suturing
   (a) Lay operating table, prepare surgical instruments, wash hands and wear masks, caps, and gloves;
   (b) Spread towels in the surgical area;
   (c) Cut a 10 cm of incision longitudinally on the pig elbow to the whole layer in depth;
   (d) Select taper needle and 3-0 suture for suturing subcutaneous tissues, pay attention to not leaving dead space, and see the specific suture method later;
   (e) Select cutting needle and 4-0 suture for suturing the skin and subcutaneous tissues, with the needle distance of 6–10 mm and the margin of 5–8 mm, and ensure that the skin edge is aligned with the skin and subcutaneous eversion after suturing;
   (f) Continue to operate the other incision at an interval of 2–3 cm after suturing.
3. Practice in groups
4. Assessment and comment

W. Li (✉)
Beijing Jishuitan Hospital, Beijing, China

P. Tang et al. (eds.), *Tutorials in Suturing Techniques for Orthopedics*, https://doi.org/10.1007/978-981-33-6330-4_5

Table 5.1 Recommendations of sutures for skin and subcutaneous and subcutaneous tissue suturing

Tissue healing time		Selection of suture materials	For example
Skin	5–7 days	Absorbable knotless suture	Absorbable STRATAFIX® Spiral PGA-PCL Knotless Tissue Control Device (PGA-PCL, Ethicon Inc.)
		Absorbable monofilament antibacterial suture	Absorbable MONOCRYL® Plus Suture (Poliglecaprone 25, Ethicon Inc.)
Subcutaneous tissue	7–10 days	Absorbable antibacterial suture	Absorbable VICRYL® Plus Control Release Suture (Polyglactin 910, Ethicon Inc.)

5.1.4 Skin and Subcutaneous Suturing Steps and Common Suturing Methods

1. Explain the suture steps by taking simple interrupted suturing as an example
   (a) When injecting the needle for suturing, hold the teeth forceps with the left hand, lift the skin and subcutaneous edge, and hold the needle holder with the right hand (see the previous chapter for holding methods), spin it in from the outside with the wrist arm force, puncture the skin and subcutaneous tissue along the radian of the needle, and pass through the skin edge of the opposite incision subcutaneously.
   (b) When pulling the needle out, pull the front end of the needle out along the radian of the needle with the teeth forceps, and push it with the needle holder forward from its back.
   (c) When exit and clamping the needle, due to very small resistance when the needle is to be completely pulled out, release the needle holder, and continue to pull needle out only by tweezers, and then quickly shift the needle holder to clamp the needle body (at the back 1/3 arc), pull needle out completely, and knot by the first assistant, and cut the suture by the second assistant to complete the suturing step.
2. Other common suturing methods
   (a) Continuous suturing method: Knot after the first stitch, and then suture the whole wound with this suture, pull out the double tail and leave it on the opposite side before the end to form a double suture, and knot with the double tail.
   (b) Eversion suturing method: Evert the skin edge, and keep the inner surface of the sutured or anastomosed space smooth, for example, suture or anastomosis of blood vessels.
   (c) Intradermal knotless continuous suturing
      I Use absorbable STRATAFIX® Spiral PGA-PCL knotless tissue control device (STRATAFIX® Spiral PGA-PCL SXMD1B402, monocryl, 3-0, tensile strength 4-0, needle length: 17 mm), suture the tissue from one end of the incision, pass the needle through the fixing ring at the tail end of the suture, tighten the suture, and fix the suture on the tissue.
      II After fixation, start continuous suturing at the other end of the incision, and tighten the suture every two stitches to the desired anastomosis.
      III Continuously suture to the other end of the incision. During the whole continuous suturing process, the barbs on the suture surface can stick to the tissue, and will not loosen after tightening.
      IV After suturing, suture at the direction opposite the exit point for one stitch, which is the key step to lock STRATAFIX® Spiral PGA-PCL unidirectional knotless tissue control device, and then cut the suture close to the tissue without knotting.
   (d) Intradermal continuous suturing method
      I Adopt absorbable 4-0 MONOCRYL® Plus suture (Poliglecaprone 25, Ethicon Inc. 4-0 MONOCRYL® Plus MCP426H, 4-0, reverse cutting needle, needle length: 19 mm, 3/8 arc), insert the needle 1 cm away from the top of skin incision on one side, and exit intradermally from the top of this side incision, leaving enough length of suture.
      II Then insert the needle intradermally from the opposite side, exit through the intradermal layer, and tighten the suture to closely align the skin incision at the suturing section.
      III Continue suturing, and tighten the suture while suturing until the whole incision is closed, finally insert the needle intradermally from the top of the incision on the other side, and exit 1 cm away from the incision (on the same side as the entry side).
      IV Cut the suture short close to the skin on both entry and exit sides.
      V Requirements: No suture or dimple on skin surface, neat incision, no skin tag, moderate suture tension, 2 mm entry depth and 5 mm suture spacing.
   (e) Subcutaneous reverse-knotting relaxation suturing
      Suturing and needle traveling steps (deep in shallow out, shallow in deep out at the opposite side):
      I Adopt absorbable 3-0 VICRYL® Plus control release suture (VICRYL® Plus Polyglactin 910, Ethicon Inc., VCP738D, 3-0, taper needle, 8 needles, needle length: 36.4 mm, 1/2 arc), stick the needle to the bottom layer of dermis about 7 mm away from the edge of incision, operate the suturing needle, gently stick the thumb to the needle holder (do not make the thumb deep in the needle holder) and puncture the needle into the fat layer by rotating the wrist.

II Move the thumb to the other side of the needle holder, thus rotate the needle holder in the hand to make it at the shortest distance (about 1 mm) from the upper epidermis at a position about 5 mm away from the edge of the incision, and then pass needle out at a position 2 mm away from the upper epidermis.

III Use the same suturing needle operation skills at the opposite side. Make sure that there is no difference in the thickness of needles across tissues; otherwise, it will cause uneven skin alignment.

IV Complete knotting. In this way, when the skin has not been sutured, the skin edge has been everted, and the tension is small. After the skin is sutured, the cutting effect and tension of the suture on the tissue are correspondingly reduced, which is conducive to reducing postoperative scars.

3. Basic principles of skin and subcutaneous suturing
   (a) Ensuring good alignment of sutured wounds: Suturing should be done in layers according to the anatomical level of the tissue to make the tissue level tight. Do not involve or suture into other tissues, and do not leave residual space to prevent effusion, hematocele, and infection. The distances of sutured wound edges and needles must be uniform, so that it looks beautiful, and more importantly, the stress and shared tension are consistent, and the suturing is tight, so as not to leak.
   (b) Paying attention to the tension at the suturing site: The tightness of ligation suture should be based on the close connection of incision edges, and should not be too tight. In other words, the sooner or later, the better or worse of incision healing is not directly proportional to the tightness, and too tight or too loose can lead to poor healing. Relaxation suturing should be performed when the wound is in tension. If the defect of the wound is too large, flap transposition coverage or skin graft should be considered.
   (c) The selection of sutures and suturing needles should be appropriate: The selection of antibacterial absorbable suture (such as absorbable VICRYL® Plus, Polyglactin 910, Ethicon Inc.) can effectively reduce the risk of infection at the surgical site.

5.2 Tendon Suture Training

Overview

Tendon is an important component of force transmission in the motor system, and the suture method and firmness after rupture are directly related to the healing quality of tendon and adhesion. Tendon suture is a complicated and meticulous surgical technique. This section is set for the training of tendon suture.

5.2.1 Training Purpose

1. To master the basic methods of tendon suturing;
2. To master orthopedic tendon suturing skills and suture selection;
3. To be familiar with the methods of improving the firmness of tendon suturing and reducing adhesion.

5.2.2 Preparation of Articles

Fresh pig's trotters (with joint and tendon), operating tables and stools, common surgical instruments (tissue scissors, suture scissors, teeth forceps, needle holders, scalpel handles, and hemostats), astral lamps, blades, syringes (with needles), cutting needles, taper needles, 2-0 sutures, 3-0 sutures, normal saline (Table 5.2).

5.2.3 Training Process

1. Tutor teaching

   Explain the history and evolution of tendon suturing, suturing methods and indications, suture and needle selection and indications.
2. Operation teaching of tendon suturing
   (a) Lay operating table, prepare surgical instruments, wash hands and wear masks, caps, and gloves;
   (b) Spread towels in the surgical area;
   (c) Cut the tendon of pig's trotters transversely and expose tendon;
   (d) Separate and identify tendon and cut it off;
   (e) Select taper needle and non-absorbable 2-0 ETHIBOND® suture (Polyester, Ethicon Inc.) to suture tendon, use syringe needle to fix tendon broken end, and suture tendon sheath after tendon suturing;
   (f) Re-cut the tendon at an interval of 1–2 cm or remove the suture in situ for re-operation after suturing.
3. Practice in groups
4. Assessment and comment

Table 5.2 Recommendations of sutures for tendon suturing

Tissue healing time		Selection of suture materials	For example
Tendon	21–28 days	Long-term tension support absorbable suture	Absorbable PDS® Plus Suture (Polydioxanone, Ethicon Inc.)
		Non-absorbable suture	Non-absorbable ETHIBOND® Suture (Polyester, Ethicon Inc.)/ Non-absorbable PROLENE Suture® (Polypropylene, Ethicon Inc.)

5.2.4 Tendon Suturing Steps and Common Suturing Methods

1. Bunnell suturing method (Fig. 5.1)
   (a) First, clamp the broken end of tendon with hemostat and tighten it. Cross the tendon with non-absorbable 3-0 ETHIBOND® (Polyester, Ethicon Inc.) at a distance of 1.5 cm from the broken end.
   (b) Run two taper needles obliquely at about 1 mm above the tendon entry point, and exit at 6 mm.
   (c) Cut off the broken end of tendon with a blade at about 5 mm above the exit point of tendon.
   (d) Insert the taper needle obliquely at about 1 mm above the exit point of tendon, and exit at the broken end of tendon.
   (e) Tighten the suture exiting the broken end of tendon.
   (f) Level the other broken end with a blade, then run the two taper needles obliquely, and exit at both sides 5 mm away from the broken end.
   (g) Cross two straight needles obliquely at 1 mm at the exit point, and pierce out at 6 mm, and the taper needle pierces out transversely at 1 mm over the exit point.
   (h) Tighten and knot.
   (i) Characteristics: (1) Suturing is reliable, unlike simple suturing tendon method, which is easy to split; (2) Less rough surface at anastomotic site; (3) The method is cumbersome, and the suture is repeatedly passed through the tendon, causing serious injury, which is easy to cause tendon injury and interfere with tendon blood circulation; (4) At present, it is used to repair flexor and extensor tendons in forearm, but seldom used to repair tendons in fingers, palms, and wrists.
2. Modified Kessler suturing method (Fig. 5.2)
   (a) Fix tendons at both ends with two needles. At 8–10 mm from the broken end, use 3-0 non-absorbable ETHIBOND suture (Polyester, Ethicon Inc., double needle suture) to cross one end of tendon at first, and at 2–3 mm above the exit point on the tendon, insert the double taper needle slightly obliquely into the tendon, and then exit from the tendon section after being parallel to the tendon;

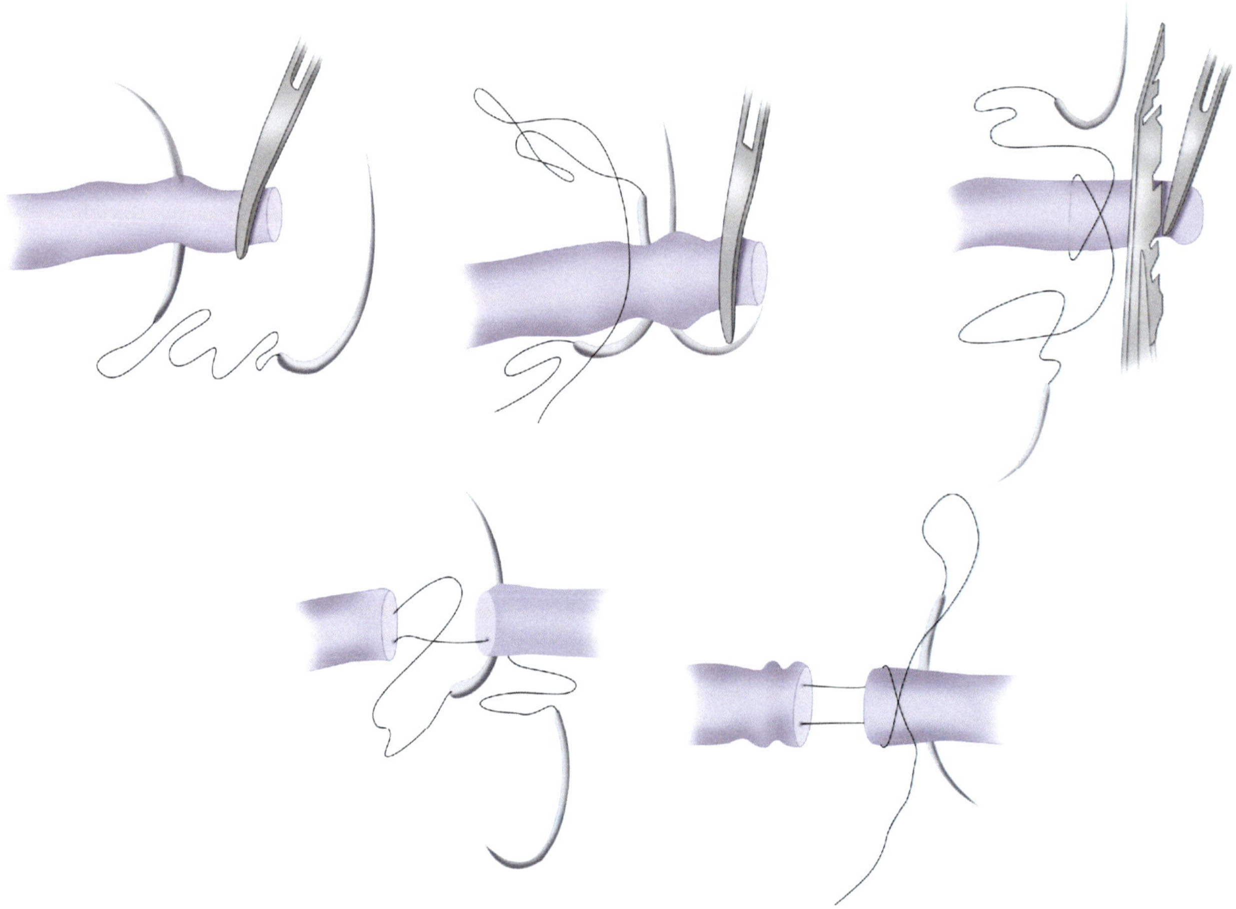

Fig. 5.1 Bunnell tendon suturing method

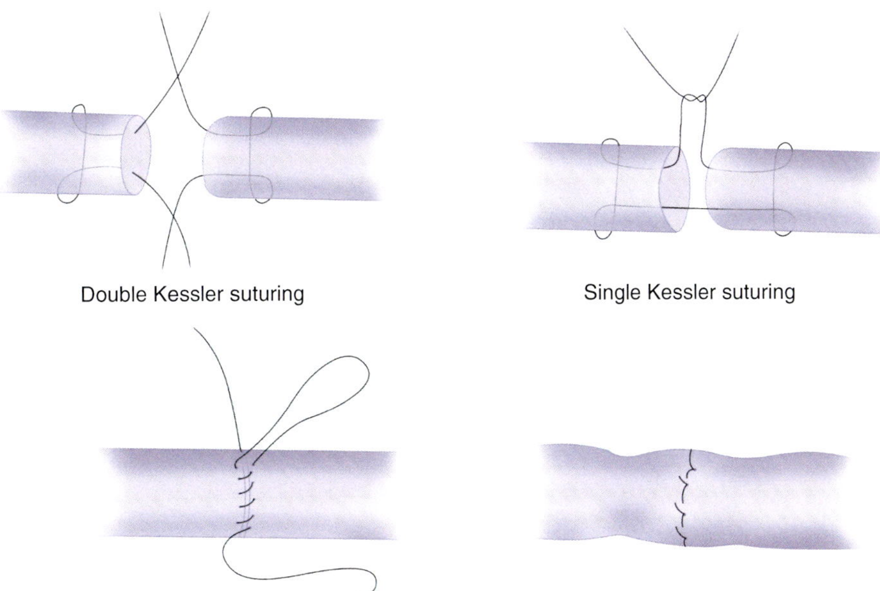

Fig. 5.2 Modified Kessler tendon suturing method

(b) Do the same operation at the other broken end of tendon according to the same steps as above;
(c) Close the two broken ends of tendon, tighten the suture, knot, and bury it in the broken end of tendon;
(d) Also treat the tendon on one side with a continuous suture as described above, and then directly penetrate into the tendon on the other side. After tightening, treat the tendon on the other side as described above, and ligate a single knot at the broken end of tendon.
(e) After the core suturing of tendon, perform continuous peripheral suturing with 5-0 or 6-0 monofilament suture around the anastomotic site of the broken end to make the repaired broken end of tendon flat and smooth.
(f) Characteristics: (1) Simple operation, less injury, less influence on tendon vessel strangulation and blood circulation; (2) The ligature is buried in the broken end of tendon, and the suture connection is smooth, which is beneficial to the early functional exercise of injured toes and reduces tendon rupture and adhesion after operation; (3) Only Kessler suturing is easy to tear, but continuous peripheral suturing around the anastomotic site of the broken end can improve the tensile strength. (4) It can be used to repair flexor and extensor tendons in various areas [1].

3. 6-strand suturing method of single-needle double-strand sutures (Tsai suturing method)

   The double-strand single-needle sutures are adopted, and the suturing is performed according to the suturing method shown below (Figs. 5.3 and 5.4).

   The method has the advantages of simple operation, less time consumption, low learning curve, smooth edge, and high strength of tendon anastomosis after suturing, which is beneficial to postoperative functional training [2].

5.3 Nerve Suture Training

Overview

Peripheral nerve is a channel for uploading effector information and giving central instructions. Its structure is complex and its organization is delicate. After rupture, only by suturing the broken end can it recover its function. Nerve suturing is a complicated and meticulous surgical technique. This section is aimed at how to do well the training of nerve suturing.

5.3.1 Training Purpose

1. To master suturing principles of peripheral nerve injuries;
2. To master microsurgical suturing skills of epineurium and perineurium and suture selection;
3. To understand other methods of microsurgical nerve suturing.

5.3.2 Preparation of Articles

Rubber film (latex gloves can be used instead), bottle caps, rubber bands, fresh chicken wings, operating tables and stools, astral lamps, microscopes, common surgical instru-

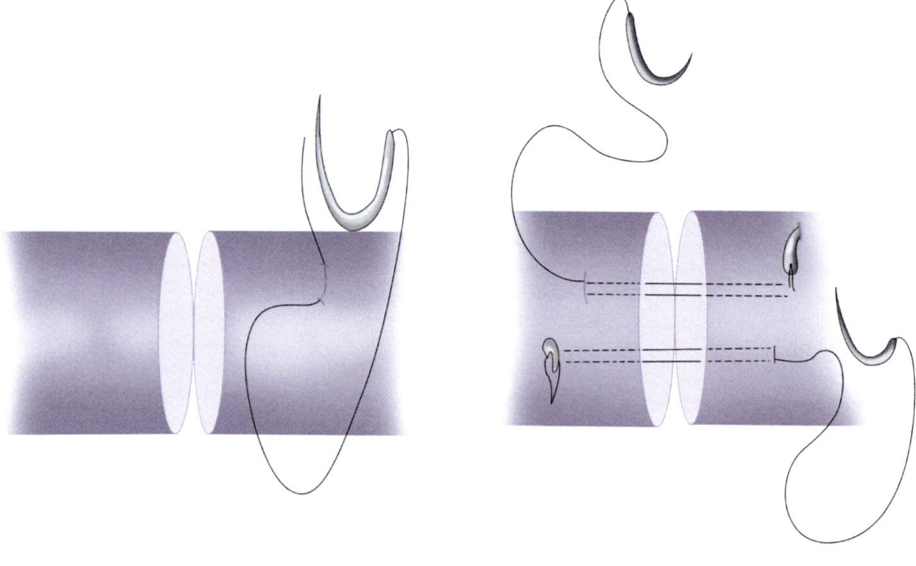

Fig. 5.3 Needle entry point and exit point of double-strand single-needle sutures

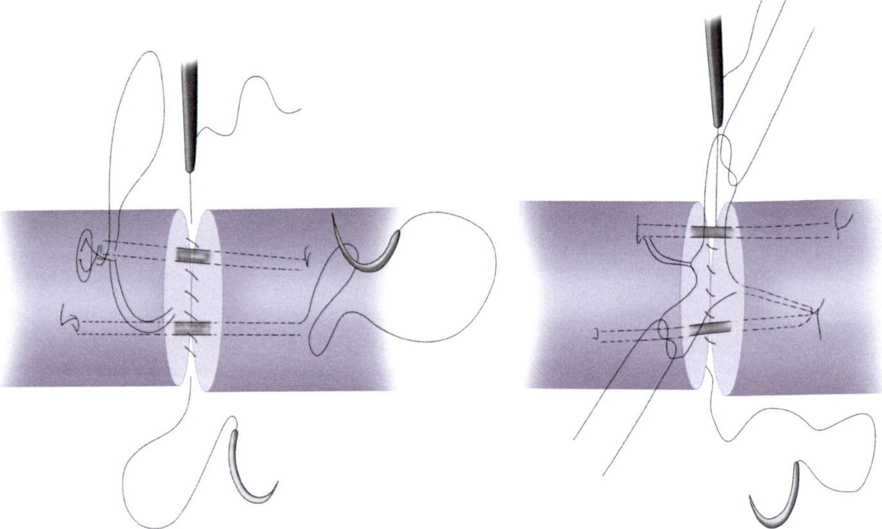

Fig. 5.4 Schematic diagram of removing the needle and knotting after tendon suturing

ments (tissue scissors, suture scissors, teeth forceps, needle holders, scalpel handles, and hemostats), microsurgical instruments (micro forceps, micro scissors, micro needle holders, mosquito forceps, arterial hemoclips, micro rinser), blades, syringes (with needles), 10-0 sutures, normal saline, heparin (Table 5.3).

Table 5.3 Recommendations of sutures for nerve suturing

Tissue healing time		Selection of suture materials	For example
Nerve	20–24 weeks	Monofilament non-absorbable suture	Non-absorbable PROLENE® Suture (Polypropylene, Ethicon Inc.)

5.3.3 Training Process

1. Tutor teaching

   Explain the history and evolution of surgical suturing of nerve injury, suturing methods and indications, suture and needle selection and indications.
2. Micro-suturing practice of adhesive film
   (a) Use bottle cap, rubber film, and rubber band to make "adhesive film suturing practice mold";
   (b) Cut a 1 cm straight incision on the tight rubber film;
   (c) Suture rubber film using micro-suturing technology.
3. Operation teaching of nerve suturing
   (a) Teach nerve exposure of chicken wings and suturing skills by tutors;

(b) Place chicken wings under a microscope, cut the skin through the longitudinal median incision, and search the brachial artery and vein and arm nerve in the shallow layer;
(c) Free brachial artery and vein and nerves;
(d) Cut off the nerve in the middle, and suture the epineurium.

4. Practice in groups
5. Assessment and comment

5.3.4 Key Points of Epineurial ing Technology

1. Preparation of the two broken ends of nerve: The two broken ends of nerve are exposed, the normal nerve bundle is light yellow (living body is shiny), with granular protrusion at the section, and the interfascicular tissues are soft and loose. If there is no normal nerve bundle, continuous cutting is made at every 1 mm using the blade until the normal nerve bundle appears, and then the section is cut off completely.
2. Close alignment of the two broken ends of nerve: Pay attention to the length of the gap between the two broken ends of nerve and require no tension.
3. Alignment arrangement of the two broken ends of nerve: The shape of nerve trunk ends, the distribution of nerve bundles on the section, and the position of nutrient vessels on the nerve surface are taken as marks, so as to make the nerve ends accurately align as far as possible [3].
4. Tension-free suture: The larger nerve is sutured interruptedly with the non-absorbable 8-0 monofilament suture (such as PROLENE® Polypropylene, Ethicon Inc.), and the smaller nerve is sutured with the non-absorbable 10-0 monofilament suture (such as PROLENE® Polypropylene, Ethicon Inc.) (Figs. 5.5 and 5.6).

5.3.5 Key Points of Perineurial Suturing Technology

1. Preparation of the two broken ends of nerve: The two broken ends of nerve are exposed, the normal nerve bundle is light yellow (living body is shiny), with granular protrusion on the section, and the interfascicular tissues are soft and loose. If there is no normal nerve bundle, continuous cutting is made every 1 mm using the blade until the normal nerve bundle appears, and then the section is cut off completely (Fig. 5.7).

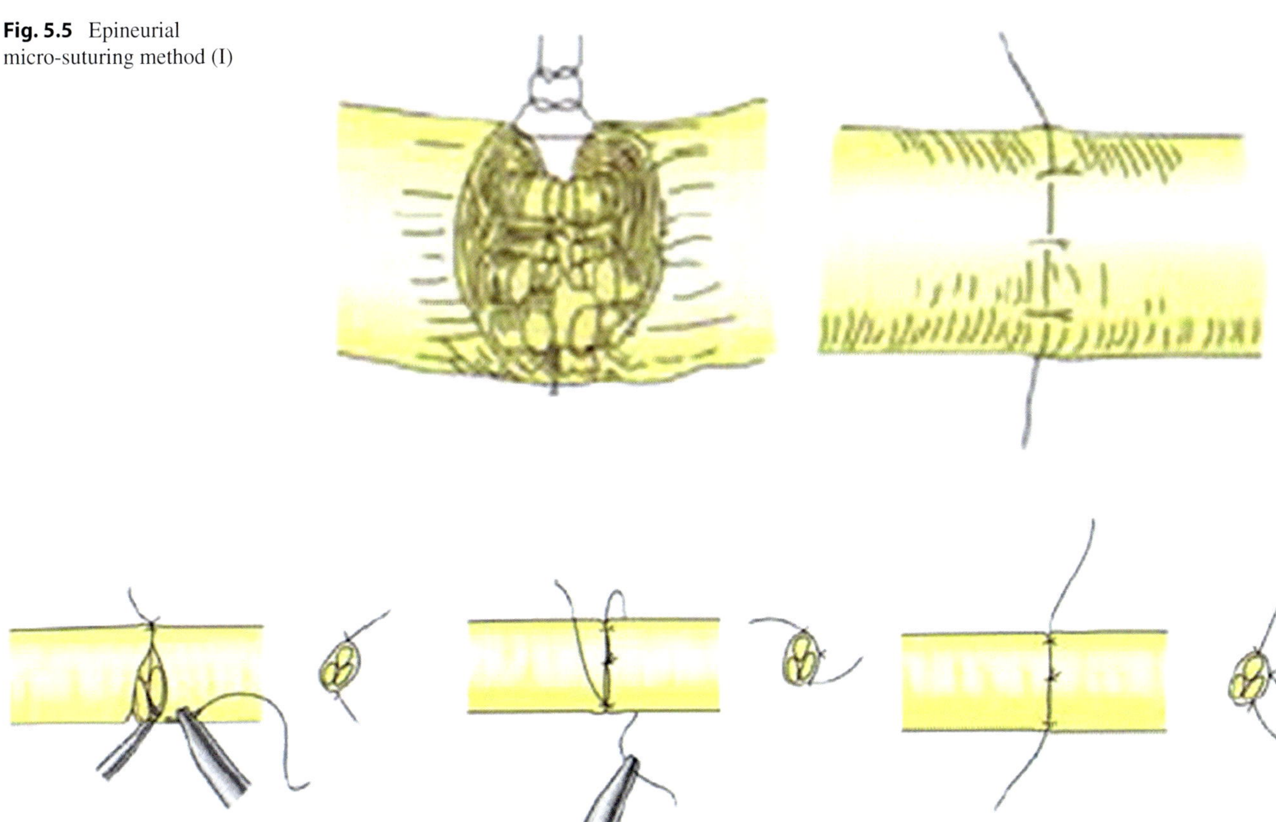

Fig. 5.5 Epineurial micro-suturing method (I)

Fig. 5.6 Epineurial micro-suturing method (II)

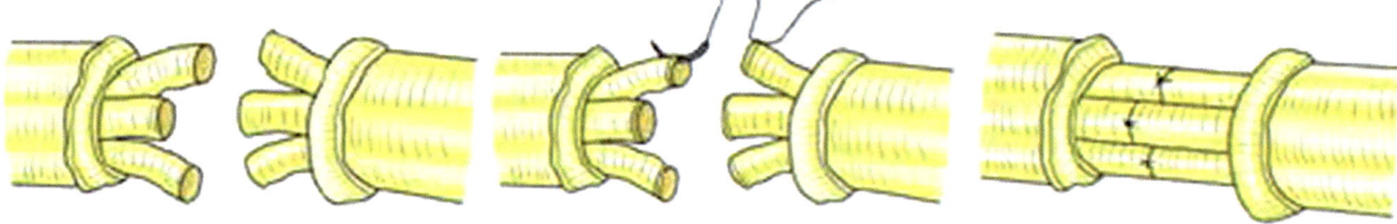

Fig. 5.7 Perineurial micro-suturing method

2. The part of the epineurium is trimmed, the nerve bundle is separated, and the two broken ends of the nerve bundle are closely aligned. Pay attention to the length of the gap between the two broken ends of nerve and require no tension.
3. Alignment arrangement of the two broken ends of nerve bundle: The nerve ends are accurately aligned as far as possible according to the shape of nerve bundle ends and the distribution of nerve bundle section.
4. Tension-free suturing: The larger nerve is sutured interruptedly with the non-absorbable 8-0 monofilament suture (such as PROLENE® Polypropylene, Ethicon Inc.), and the smaller nerve is sutured with the non-absorbable 10-0 monofilament suture (such as PROLENE® Polypropylene, Ethicon Inc.).

5.4 Blood Vessel Suture Training

Overview

Blood vessel is an important organ to maintain life, and it is also the supply channel of limb nutrition. How to better anastomose blood vessels, especially tiny blood vessels of limbs, is a complicated and meticulous surgical technique, and the anastomosis of blood vessels of extremities needs the cooperation of microscope. This section is set for the training of blood vessel suturing.

5.4.1 Training Purpose

1. To master the basic methods of blood vessel suturing;
2. To master orthopedic suturing skills of blood vessels and suture selection;
3. To be familiar with the skills of improving blood vessel reperfusion.

5.4.2 Preparation of Articles

Rubber film (or latex gloves), fresh chicken wings, SD rats, operating tables and stools, astral lamps, microscopes, common surgical instruments (tissue scissors, suture scissors, teeth forceps, needle holders, scalpel handles, and hemostats), microsurgical instruments (micro forceps, micro scissors, micro needle holders, mosquito forceps, arterial hemoclips, micro rinsers), blades, syringes (with needles), 10-0 sutures, normal saline, anesthetic drugs, heparin (Table 5.4).

Table 5.4 Recommendations of sutures for blood vessel suturing

Tissue healing time		Selection of suture materials	For example
Blood vessels	20–24 weeks	Non-absorbable suture	Non-absorbable PROLENE® Suture (Polypropylene, Ethicon Inc.)

5.4.3 Training Process

1. Tutor teaching
   Explain the suturing history and evolution, suturing methods and indications, suture and needle selection and indications of vascular injury surgery, and conduct rubber film suturing training (see "tendon suturing" section).
2. Operation teaching of blood vessel suturing
   (a) Lay operating table, prepare surgical instruments, wash hands and wear masks, caps, and gloves;
   (b) Spread towels in the surgical area;
   (c) Take the rat at the prone position, cut a longitudinal incision of 3 cm in the middle of the dorsal side of the tail, and make transverse incisions at both ends of the incision, open the tail skin of the rat towards both sides to expose the deep structure, and the tail artery is in the middle of the tail;
   (d) Free the tail artery of about 2 cm, trim the connective tissue, put hemoclips on both ends, and cut off the middle with micro scissors to form a broken end of blood vessel injury;
   (e) Trim the adventitia of the broken end of the blood vessel, and trim the broken end to form a smooth section for anastomosis;
   (f) Select non-absorbable 11-0 monofilament suture (such as Non-absorbable PROLENE® Suture, Polypropylene, Ethicon Inc.) to suture the blood vessels under the cooperation of two persons, and see the specific suturing method later;

(g) Loosen the hemoclips, and check the blood reperfusion and leakage;
(h) After suturing, cut off the blood vessels again at an interval of 1–2 cm for operation.

3. Practice in groups
4. Assessment and comment

5.4.4 Two Fixed-Point End-To-End Interrupted Vascular Anastomosis Technique

1. Two fixed-point end-to-end interrupted vascular anastomosis method

It is the basic technique of vascular micro-anastomosis and the gold standard method of vascular suture (Fig. 5.8).

(a) First, the vessel lumen is expanded to make the calibers of vessels at both ends equal (Fig. 5.9).
(b) Heparin normal saline is injected with a blunt needle to rinse the vascular lumen carefully (Fig. 5.10), and the blood vessel to be anastomosed is placed on the vascular clamp of the approximator.
(c) Then the adventitia near the anastomotic site (Fig. 5.11) is cut off, and finally the anastomotic site of blood vessels is leveled to align the two anastomotic sites before anastomosis (Fig. 5.12).
(d) The suture of blood vessels should be carried out strictly according to the two fixed-point interrupted suturing (Figs. 5.13 and 5.14).
(e) Be proficient in holding needles, inserting needles, leading suture, knotting and cutting sutures with tweezers. When entry, pay attention to that the margin of entry is equal to the thickness of artery wall, double for that of vein wall. During entry, the needle should be perpendicular to the outer wall of blood vessel, and the inner surface of blood vessel wall should be padded with tweezers to facilitate entry (Figs. 5.15 and 5.16). Then the needle is punctured into the lumen according to the radian of the needle. Be careful not to hang on the opposite vessel wall. The needle is passed through to the opposite vessel wall and exit according to the same margin, it must be estimated very accurately, and one puncture should be successful (Fig. 5.17). Never puncture repeatedly, so as to avoid damaging the intima of blood vessels. The outer wall of the blood vessel can be gently pressed using tweezers to assist exit.
(f) When knotting, a certain tension must be maintained. It is required that the diameter of the coil knotted for the first time is equal to the thickness of the blood vessel wall, and it should not be tied too tightly. The second knot should be tightened, and three square knots are required. After suturing, the blood vessels should be cut to check whether the quality of each stitch complies with the standard. It is required that each stitch should be parallel to the longitudinal axis of blood vessel, the wall of blood vessel should be aligned smoothly, and the intima is facing the intima, allowing mild eversion, but no inversion. Enter and exit the needle according to the specified margin and needle distance, and the diameter of the coil of the first knot remains equal to the thickness of the vessel

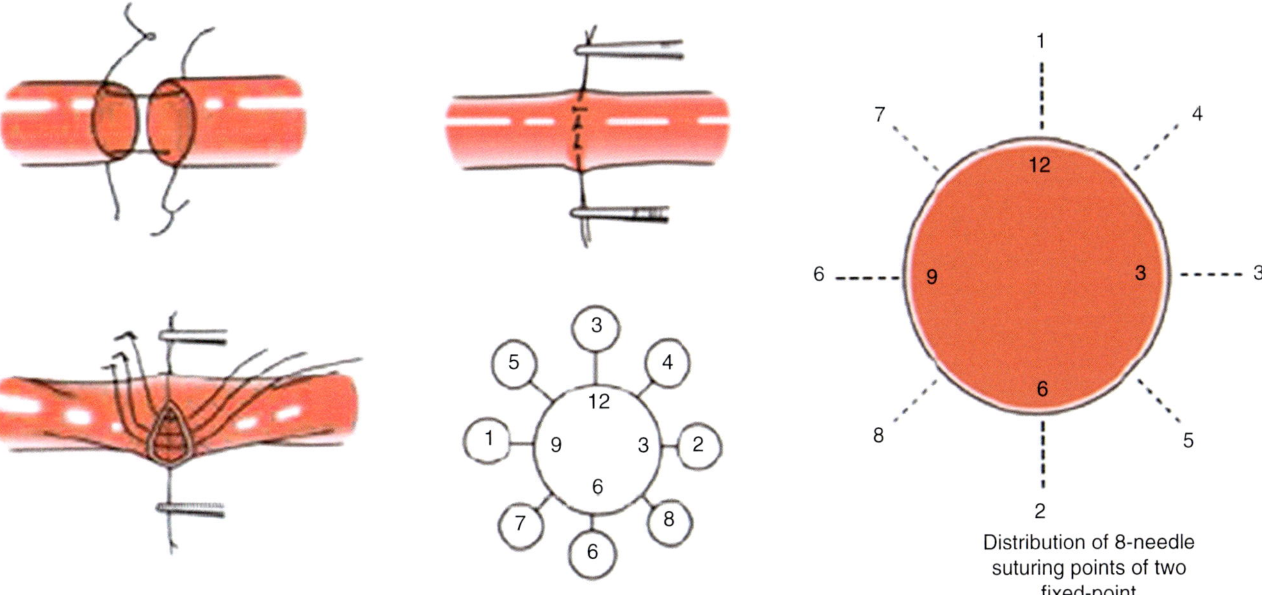

Fig. 5.8 Two fixed-point end-to-end interrupted vascular anastomosis

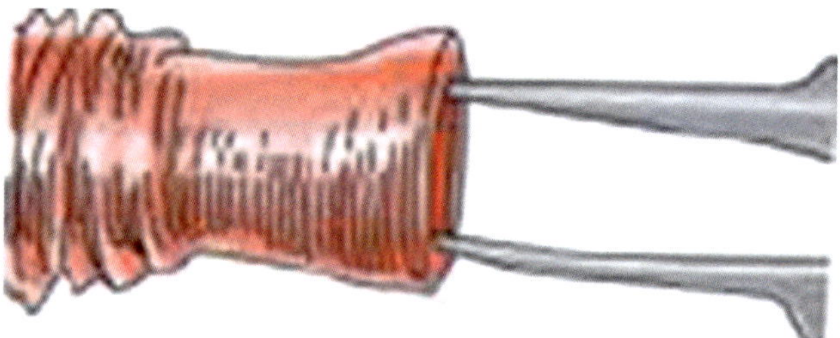

Fig. 5.9 Expand the broken end of blood vessel with a blunt tweezers

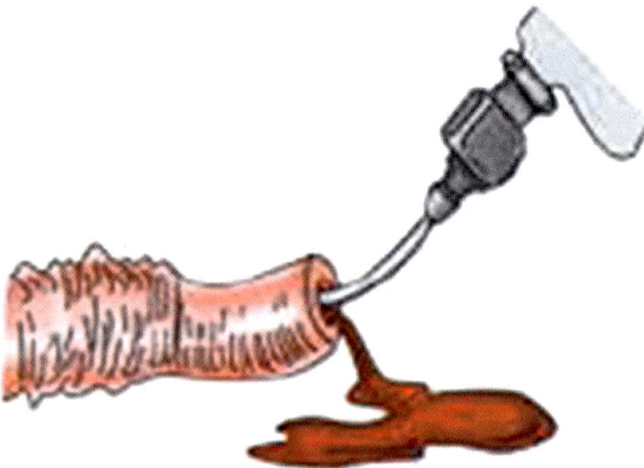

Fig. 5.10 Inject heparin normal saline with a blunt needle to rinse and suck the vascular lumen

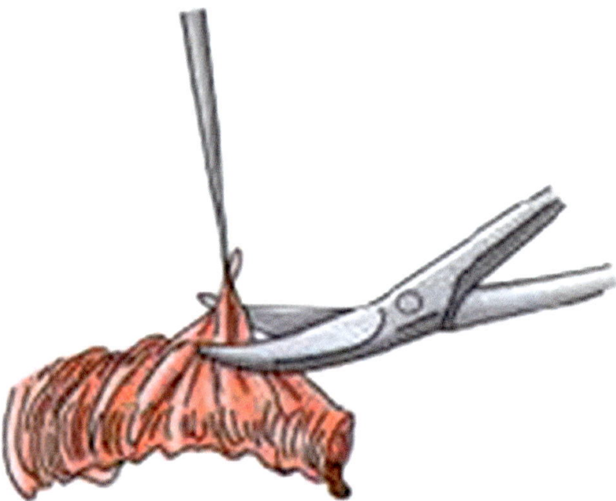

Fig. 5.11 Cut off the 1 cm adventitia of the broken end of the blood vessel

wall. 100% patency rate can be achieved only when every stitch is sutured correctly. On the basis of good quality, it is required to speed up the suturing. To be foolproof.

(g) The anastomosis at 10–20 anastomotic sites is required for each tail artery and vein of rats under

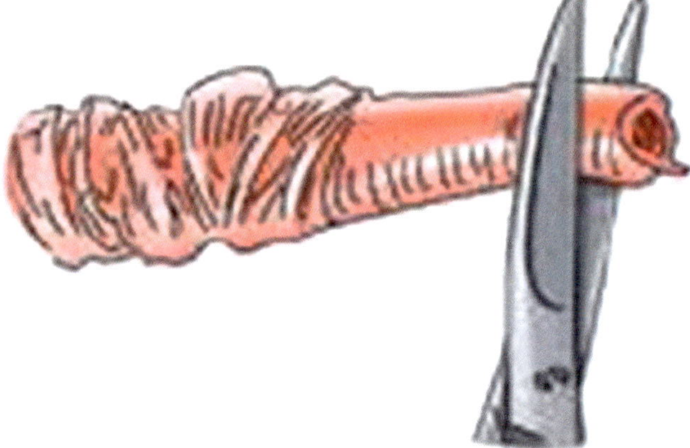

Fig. 5.12 Cut off the two broken ends of blood vessels finally before anastomosis of blood vessels

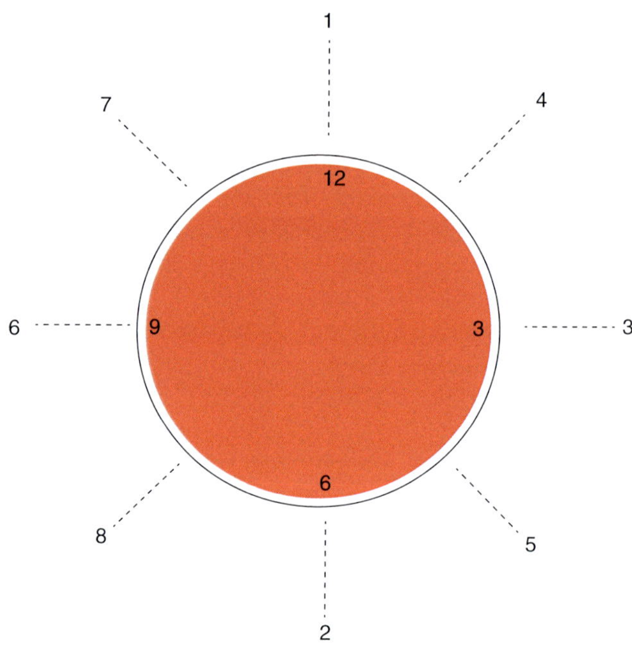

Fig. 5.13 Pattern diagram

microscope. The immediate patency rate of each anastomotic site is 100%. Anesthetizing and fixing animals, as well as depilating and disinfecting, etc., should be learned. The tail artery is exposed under the microscope from separation to use of approximator, with the small yellow backing plate put, and then is suture in situ.

2. Basic principles of blood vessel suturing
   (a) Principles of normal blood vessels: There is no ecchymosis on the adventitia and no cloud-like structure on the intima (exfoliation of the intima).
   (b) Principles of normal blood flow: The proximal artery continuously spurts blood, and water injection in the distal artery lumen is unobstructed; water injection in

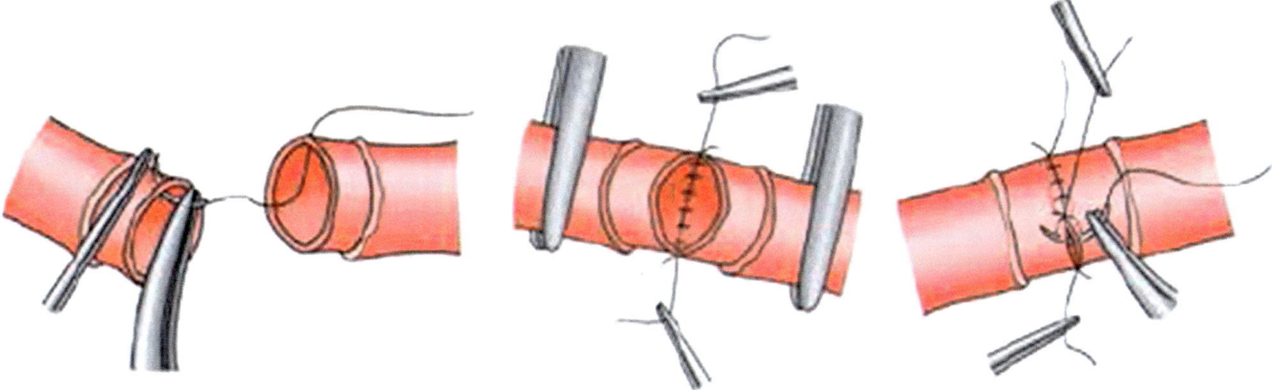

Fig. 5.14 Suturing sequence of two fixed-point interrupted suturing method

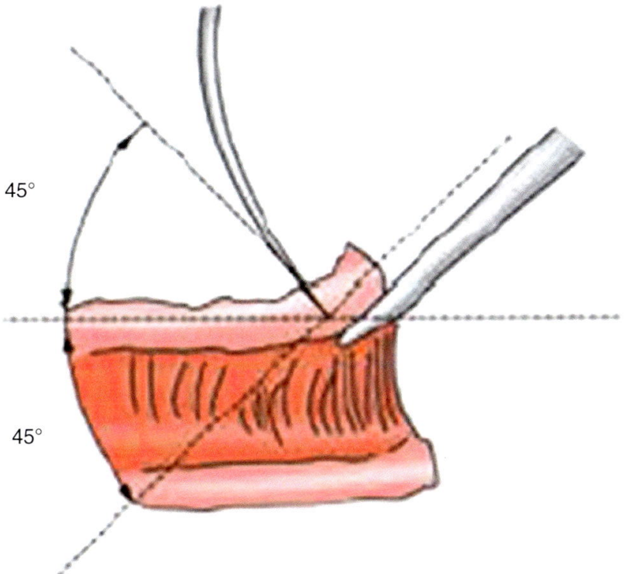

Fig. 5.15 Schematic diagram of entry direction

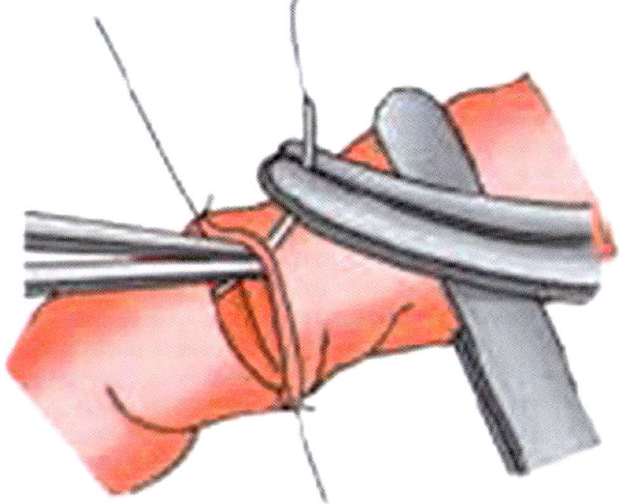

Fig. 5.16 During entry, the needle should be perpendicular to the outer wall of blood vessel, and the inner surface of blood vessel wall should be padded with tweezers to facilitate entry

the proximal vein lumen is unobstructed, and a little or active blood return can be seen in the distal vein.

(c) Non-invasive operation principle: Or minimally invasive operation. Because the vascular tissues are delicate, especially the intima of blood vessels, we should always be vigilant during the whole operation of vascular anastomosis to avoid artificial injury to the vascular tissue, especially not clamping the intima; non-invasive operation also includes selecting suitable non-invasive suture materials to suture blood vessels. Different models of non-coring needles and sutures can be selected for blood vessels with different calibers (Table 5.5) (Fig. 5.18).

(d) Principles of proper tension: The anastomotic tension after anastomosis should be neither too large nor too loose. If too large, the blood vessel will be easily torn, and if too loose, the vascular tortuosity will appear,

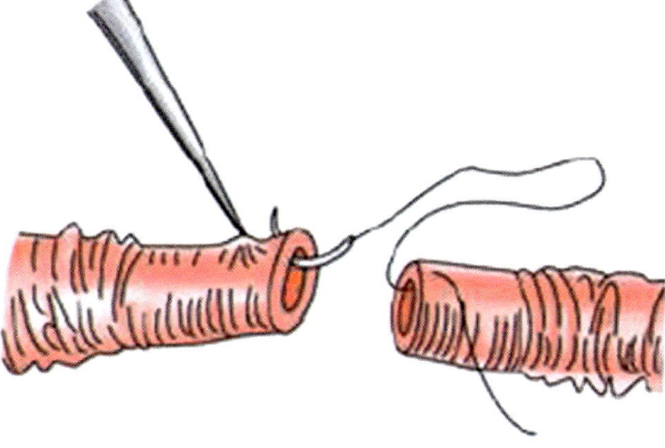

Fig. 5.17 Inject the needle into the lumen according to the radian of the needle, and pass through to the opposite vessel wall and exit according to the same margin

Table 5.5 Blood vessels with different calibers and selection of different models of non-absorbable sutures

Blood vessel diameter	Suture models	Representative blood vessels
Above 5.0 mm	3-0–5-0	Thoracic aorta; Abdominal artery
3.0–5.0 mm	6-0–8-0	Femoral artery; Brachial artery; Popliteal artery
2.0–3.0 mm	8-0–9-0	Radial/ulnar artery; Dorsalis pedis artery
1.0 mm	10-0	Proper digital artery and common digital artery at the root of the finger (toe)
0.5 mm	11-0	Proper digital artery from proximal interphalangeal joint to distal interphalangeal joint
0.2 mm	12-0	Distal branch of artery arch of the finger (toe)

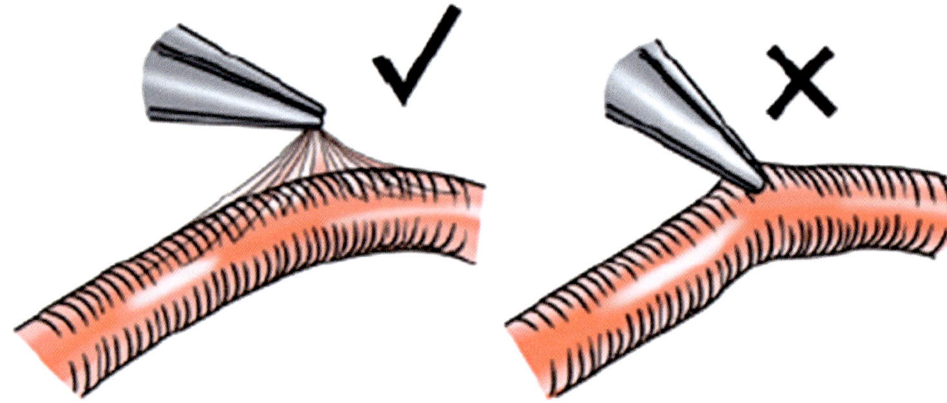

Fig. 5.18 Principles of non-invasive operation of small vessels

all easily leading to anastomotic thrombosis. Besides the proper longitudinal tension of the anastomotic site, rotational tension should also be avoided at the anastomotic site, which requires that the position of blood vessels should be adjusted well before anastomosis, so as to avoid suturing of blood vessels in distortion state.

(e) Principles of approximate calibers: It is required that the calibers of the two broken ends of anastomotic vessels should be approximate; otherwise, the anastomosis is difficult, and it is prone to thrombosis because of vortex formed at the anastomotic site; when there is a big difference between the distal and proximal calibers, the calibers at both ends may become closer by reducing the caliber of the larger end or cutting the caliber of the smaller end obliquely, or the end-to-side anastomosis is adopted between the smaller end vessel and the side wall of the larger end vessel.

(f) Principles of smooth alignment or eversion of adventitia: The eversion suturing of vessel wall should be ensured for vessels larger than 1 mm in diameter, while the smooth alignment suturing of vessel wall is best for small vessels smaller than 1 mm (Fig. 5.19). The basic requirement of both is that the vessel wall cannot be inverted.

(g) Principles of uniform symmetry of margin and needle distance: The anastomosis of large and small blood vessels should be completed with as few stitches as possible, because the more stitches, the greater the injury to blood vessels, thus increasing the chance of thrombosis at the anastomotic site, which is especially important for anastomosis of small blood vessels. The vascular suturing can be completed with as few stitches as possible without obvious blood leakage at the anastomotic site, which is the requirement of high-quality vascular anastomosis. To achieve this, it is a basic premise to maintain the uniformity of needle distance and the symmetry of margin (Fig. 5.20).

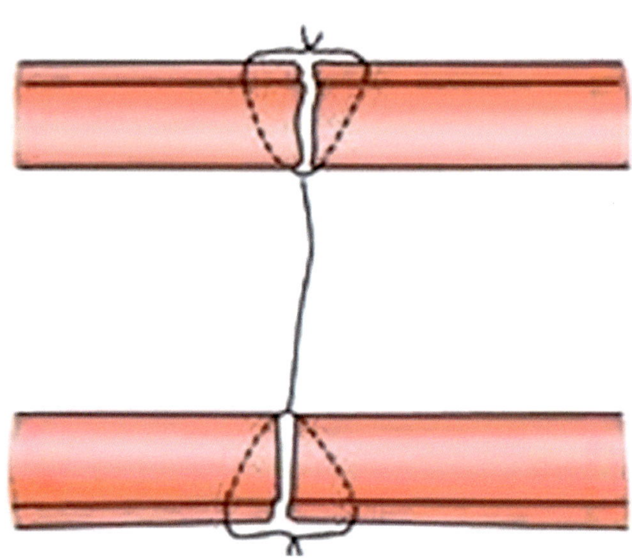

Fig. 5.19 Smooth alignment suturing of small vessel wall with caliber less than 1 mm

5.4.5 Vascular End-to-Side Anastomosis Technique

Vascular end-to-side suturing method is a method of suturing blood vessels. It is suitable for cases where one end of blood vessel cannot be cut off or the caliber difference of two broken ends is too large, that is, the broken end of one blood vessel is sutured on the side of the other blood vessel.

In the operation, an incision with the same circumference as that of the broken end of another blood vessel to be anastomosed is cut at the side wall of blood vessels anastomosed laterally, and then the broken end is sutured on this side incision. When suturing, the upper and lower side corners can be sutured for two stitches first, and the suture end is reserved for traction. Then, a number of stitches are added between the two diagonal traction sutures to complete the vascular anastomosis.

1. Find the blood vessels at donor and recipient areas (Fig. 5.21);
2. Remove the adventitia of the side wall of the blood vessel at the anastomotic site (Fig. 5.22);
3. Open the vascular side wall.

   At the site where the adventitia is removed, suture a stitch with 7-0 micro suture through the whole layer of the blood vessel wall (Fig. 5.23a), and lift the suture end (Fig. 5.23b), and then cut the whole layer of the blood vessel wall with micro scissors to remove the whole layer of the blood vessel wall with appropriate size (Fig. 5.23c, d).
4. Suturing blood vessels

   Adopt the two fixed-point suturing method (Fig. 5.24a–d), and also continuously suture from one side. It is best to use radial suturing method during suturing, so as to prevent blood leakage from corners formed during suturing (Fig. 5.25).
5. Basic principles of end-to-side suturing: (1) The most important thing is to confirm the integrity of the intima of the open side; otherwise, it will eventually lead to blockage at the anastomotic site; (2) When suturing, it must be ensured that the adventitia of each stitch is not inverted; (3) The needle distance and margin should be consistent, and radial suturing should be adopted.

5.5 Muscle and Fascia Suturing Training

Overview

Muscle and its fascia are important parts of generating strength in the motor system. The method and firmness of suturing after rupture are directly related to functional recovery. Muscle and fascia suturing is a complicated and meticu-

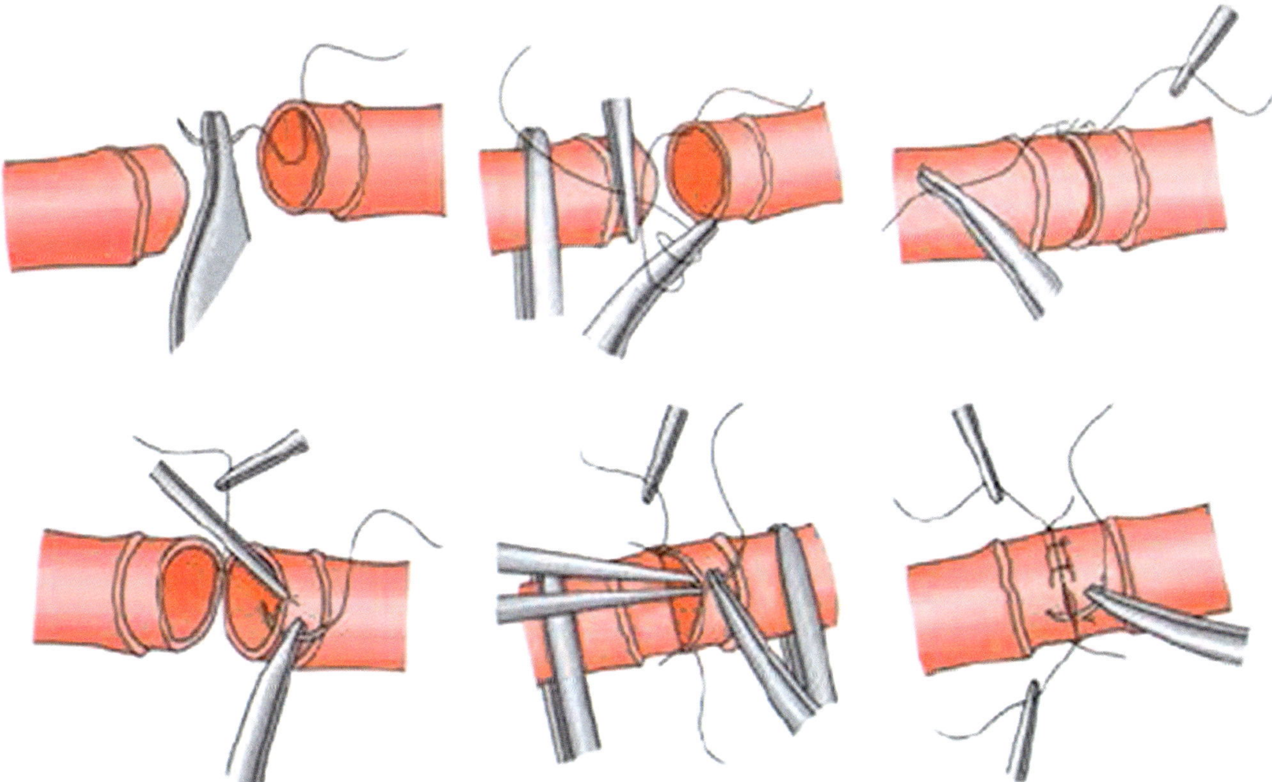

Fig. 5.20 Uniform needle distance and symmetrical margin are beneficial for vascular patency

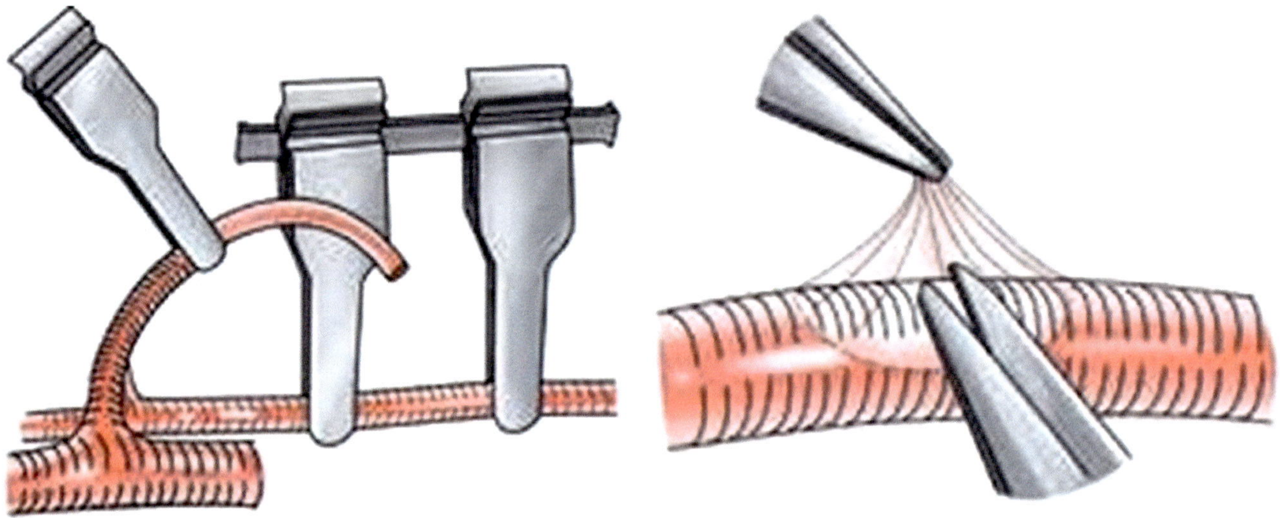

Fig. 5.21 Free the blood vessels at donor and recipient areas for later use

Fig. 5.22 Cut off the adventitia of the side wall of the blood vessel at the anastomotic site

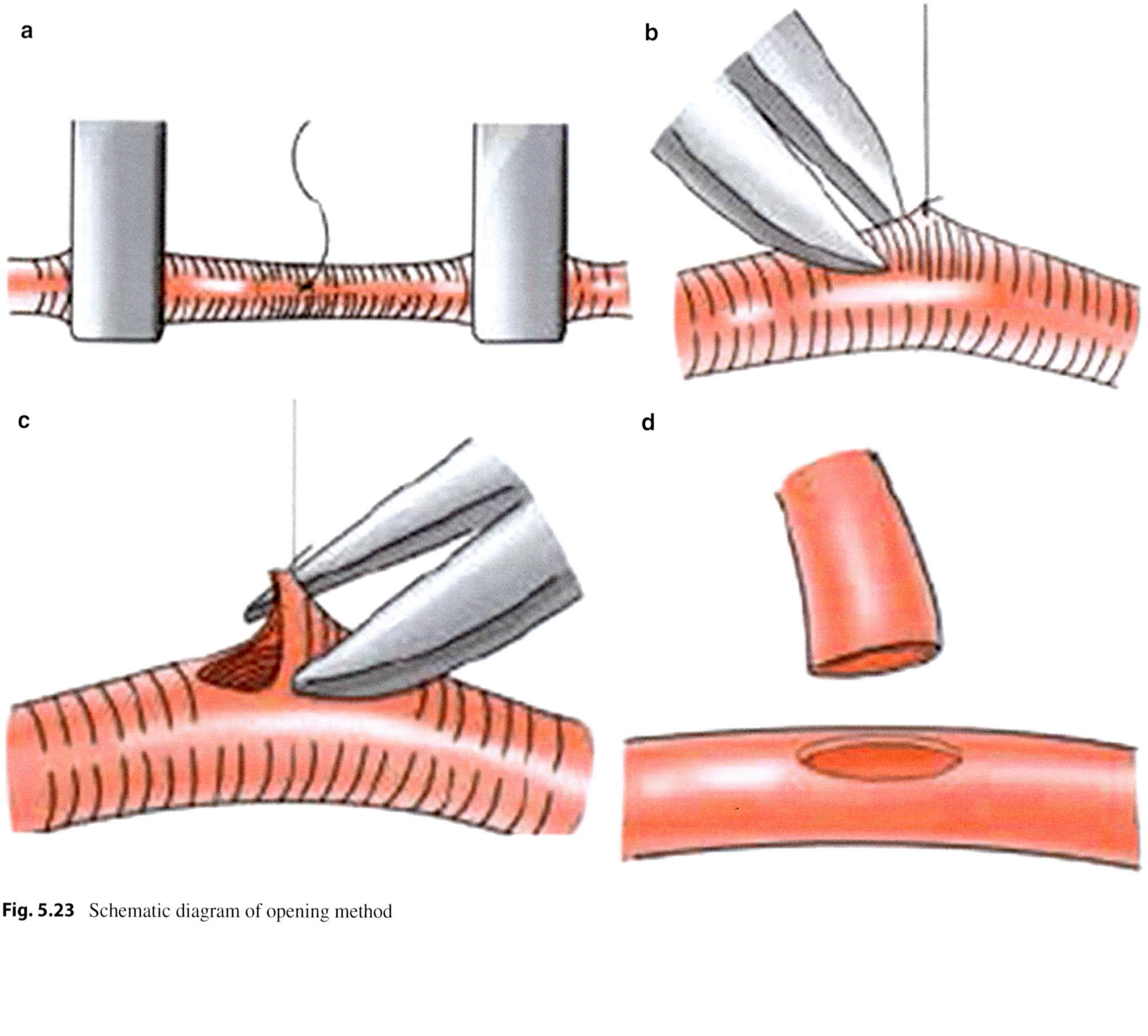

Fig. 5.23 Schematic diagram of opening method

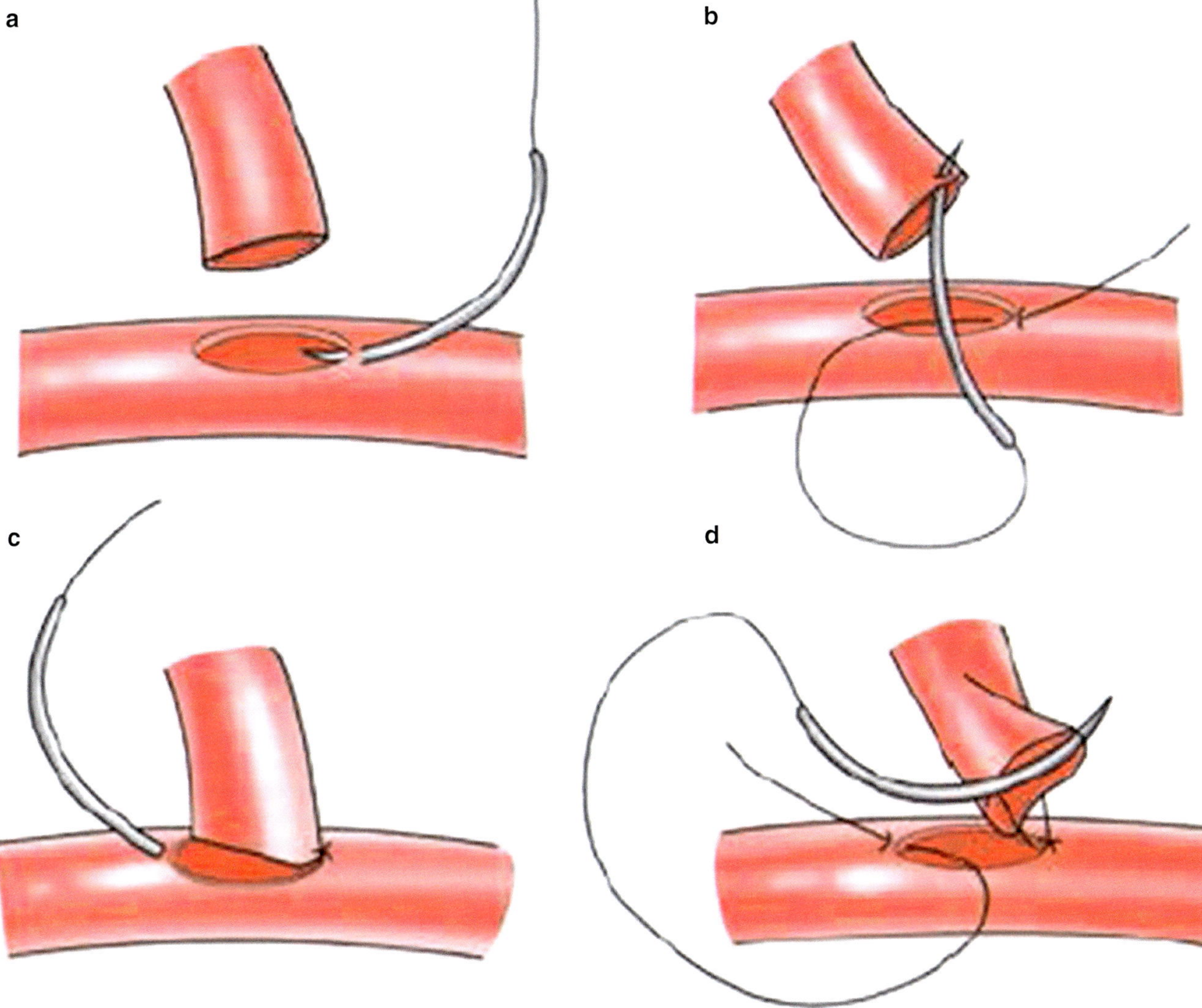

Fig. 5.24 Two fixed-point suturing method

lous surgical technique. This section is set for the training of muscle and fascia suturing.

5.5.1 Training Purpose

1. To master the basic methods of muscle and fascia suturing;
2. To master orthopedic suturing skills of muscle and fascia and suture selection.

5.5.2 Preparation of Articles

Fresh pig elbow, operating tables and stools, common surgical instruments (tissue scissors, suture scissors, teeth forceps, needle holders, scalpel handles, and hemostats), astral lamps, blades, syringes, cutting needles, taper needles, 3-0 sutures, 4-0 sutures, normal saline, and iodophor (Table 5.6).

5.5.3 Training Process

1. Tutor teaching

   Explain the history and evolution of surgical suturing, suturing methods and indications, suture and needle selection and indications.
2. Operation teaching of muscle and fascia suturing
   (a) Lay operating table, prepare surgical instruments, wash hands and wear masks, caps and gloves;
   (b) Spread towels in the surgical area;
   (c) Cut a longitudinal incision of 15 cm on the pig elbow to the whole skin layer in depth, retract the skin, cut the deep fascia longitudinally, and cut off a group of muscle and muscle belly transversely for later use;
   (d) Select the taper needle and 2-0 suture to suture muscle, and then suture deep fascia. See later for specific suturing method.
   (e) After suturing, continue to cut off another group of muscles and repeat the operation.

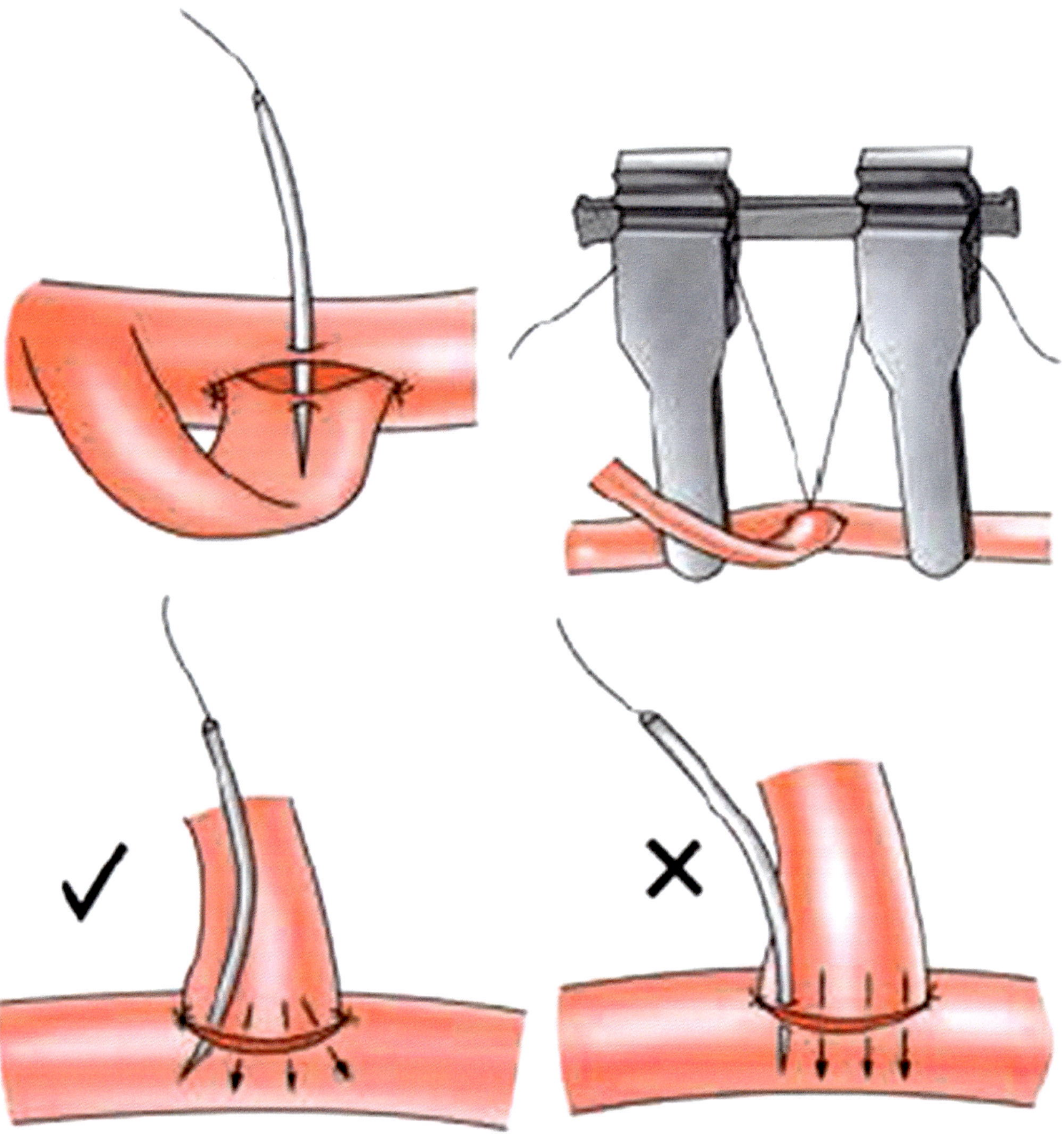

Fig. 5.25 Schematic diagram of suturing skills

Table 5.6 Recommendations of sutures for muscle and fascia

Tissue healing time		Selection of suture materials	For example
Muscle	14 days	Absorbable suture	VICRYL® Plus Suture (Polyglactin 910, Ethicon Inc.)/PDS® Plus Suture (Polydioxanone, Ethicon Inc.)/Symmetric PDS PLUS
Fascia	21–28 days	Absorbable suture	VICRYL® Plus Suture (Polyglactin 910, Ethicon Inc.)/PDS® Plus Suture (Polydioxanone, Ethicon Inc.)/Symmetric PDS PLUS

3. Practice in groups
4. Assessment and comment

5.5.4 Common Suturing Methods and Steps of Muscles

1. Simple figure-of-8 interrupted suture
   (a) When inserting the needle for suturing, hold the teeth forceps with the left hand, lift the edge of the broken end of muscle, preferably find the fascia in muscle fibers, hold the needle holder with the right hand (see the previous chapter for holding methods), spin it in from the outside with the wrist arm force, puncture the surface of muscle belly along the radian of the needle, and exit from the broken end through the deep surface of muscle belly, then inject from the opposite broken end, and exit from the muscle belly surface, and then repeat the entry and exit to form a figure-of-8 suturing (Fig. 5.26)
   (b) When pulling the needle out, pull the front end of the needle along the radian of the needle with teeth forceps, and push it with the needle holder forward from the back of the needle with the trend.
   (c) When completely pulling the needle out, due to very small resistance, release the needle holder, and continue to pull needle out only by tweezers, and then quickly shift the needle holder to clamp the needle body (at the back 1/3 arc), pull needle out completely, and knot by the first assistant, and cut the suture by the second assistant to complete the suturing step.
2. Other common suturing methods

   Interrupted continuous suturing method: Knot after the first figure-of-8 suturing, and then suture part of the muscles continuously with this suture, pull out the double tail and leave it on the opposite side before the end to form a double suture, and knot with the double tail (Fig. 5.27), and then repeat the method, until the suturing is finished.

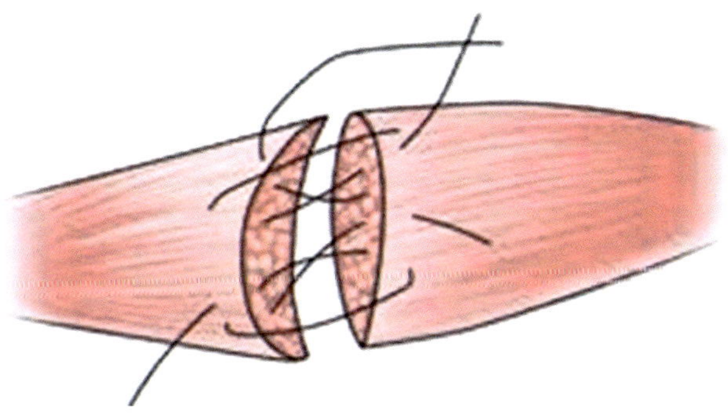

Fig. 5.26 Schematic diagram of muscle figure-of-8 suturing method

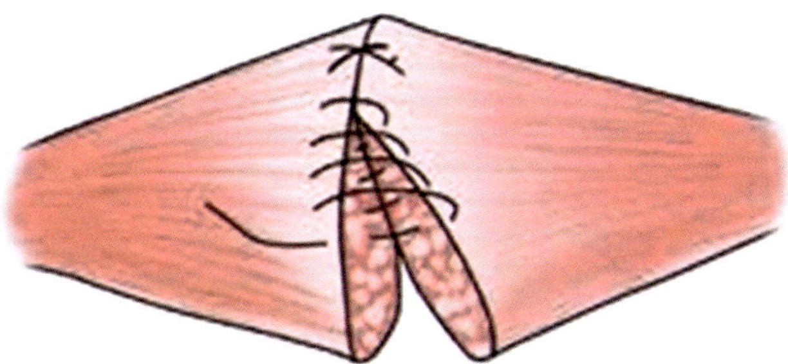

Fig. 5.27 Schematic diagram of continuous suturing of muscles after figure-of-8 suturing

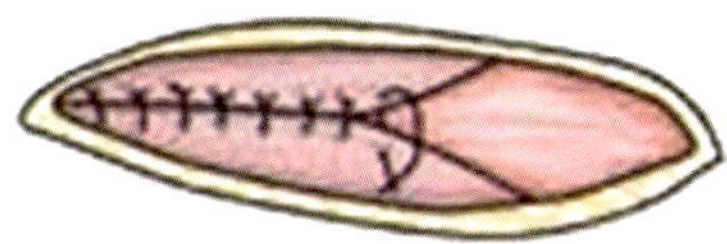

Fig. 5.28 Schematic diagram of interrupted suturing of fascia

5.5.5 Common Suturing Methods and Steps of Fascia (Fig. 5.28)

1. Interrupted suturing
   (a) When inserting the needle for suturing, hold the teeth forceps with the left hand, lift the fascia edge, and hold the needle holder with the right hand (see the previous chapter for holding methods), spin it in from the outside with the wrist arm force, puncture into the fascia along the radian of the needle, insert under the contralateral fascia and exit.
   (b) When pulling the needle out, pull the front end of the needle out along the radian of the needle with teeth forceps, and push it with the needle holder forward from the back of the needle with the trend.
   (c) When completely pulling the needle out, due to very small resistance, release the needle holder, and continue to pull needle out only by tweezers, and then quickly shift the needle holder to clamp the needle body (at the back 1/3 arc), pull needle out completely, and knot by the first assistant, and cut the suture by the second assistant to complete the suturing step.
2. Other suturing methods

   Continuous locking suturing method: Knot after the first suturing, and then suture part of the fascia continuously with this suture, pull the double tail out and leave it on the opposite side before the end to form a double

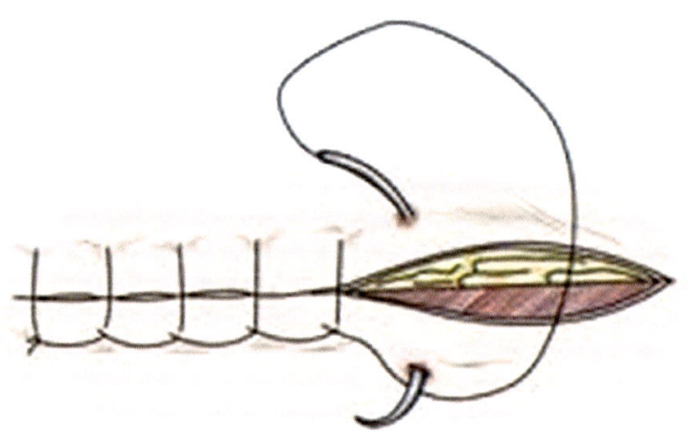

Fig. 5.29 Schematic diagram of continuous locking suturing of fascia

suture, and knot with the double tail (Fig. 5.29), and then repeat the method, until the suturing is finished.

5.5.6 Basic Principles of Muscle Fascia Suturing

1. Ensuring good alignment of sutured muscles and fascia.
2. When suturing muscles, it is best to find the deep fascia between the broken ends of muscles, and then suture through the deep fascia to avoid the suture tearing off the muscles;
3. If there is a defect in fascia, forced suturing may lead to osteofascial compartment syndrome, so it is recommended not to suture;
4. The selection of sutures and suturing needles should be appropriate, and it is best to use absorbable sutures for muscle suturing.

Search Terms

Skin, Tendon, Peripheral nerve, Muscle, Suturing, Suture, Training, Blood vessel, Suture technique, Muscle tissue, Deep fascia

References

1. Gu Y, Wang S, Shi D. Surgery of the Hand. Shanghai: Shanghai Scientific & Technical Publishers; 2002: p. 472–7; 602–8.
2. Liu Z, Zhang B. Surgery of the Peripheral Nerves. Beijing: Beijing Science and Technology; 2004. p. 160–81.
3. Gill RS, Lim BH, Shatford RA, Toth E, Voor MJ, Tsai TM. A comparative analysis of the six-strand double-loop flexor tendon repair and three other techniques: a human cadaveric study. J Hand Surg Am. 1999;24(6):1315–22.

6 Orthopedic Operating Room Settings and Aseptic Techniques

Min Zhuang and Yimin Chai

Abstract

In surgical procedures, improving the utilization efficiency of the operating room, controlling the nosocomial infection of aseptic surgical incision in orthopedics, reducing the infection rate of surgical incision, and ensuring the quality of medical care have always been the goals and key points. Achieving these goals is not one issue, but many, such as the management of operating personnel and environment, the rationality in arrangement of operating rooms, and the technical specifications for surgical instruments and aseptic operations. This chapter will mainly discuss the orthopedic operating room settings and aseptic techniques.

Keywords

Orthopedic operating room · Aseptic techniques

6.1 Orthopedic Operating Room Settings

Concept of clean operating room: A series of measures to ensure the air cleanliness of the operating room, including sterilization, and regulation of temperature and humidity, and fresh air conditioning, by which dust particles in the air are filtered out and microbial particles are removed, maintaining the operating room at a certain cleanliness level with suitable temperature and humidity. Orthopedic surgery should be performed in a clean operating room. The new clean operating room should be built in a quiet, clean location far away from contamination sources in the hospital. The size, quantity, and cleanliness level of the operating room should be determined according to the scale of the hospital and the actual operating conditions. Generally, one room should be set for every 25–30 beds. The architectural layout and regional division of the operating room should comply with the requirements of functional process and aseptic techniques. Clean operating rooms should not be located on the first floor and the top floor of high-rise buildings [1].

6.1.1 Location of Operating Room

Clean operating room should be an area of its own, adjacent to surgical department and ICU and conveniently accessible to relevant departments such as Central Sterile Supply Department, Blood Bank, Imaging Diagnosis Department, and Pathology Department. Logistics transmission system can be built if conditions permit.

6.1.2 Layout of Operating Room

1. The operating room should be divided into restricted area, semi-restricted area, and unrestricted area. The staff access, surgical patient passage, and materials supply passage should be set up in the operating room. The three passages should be easily distinguished to avoid cross-contamination.
2. Clean operating room should be divided into clean area and non-clean area. Buffer room should be set between clean area and non-clean area. Clean area should be divided according to different requirements of air cleanliness level.
3. The internal layout and passages of the clean operating department should be designed to facilitate evacuation, shorten functional flow, and partition clean-and-contaminated items. The passage forms are appropriately selected according to the specific conditions of the hospital:
   (a) Single-passage layout should allow contaminated items to be disinfected and packaged in situ;

M. Zhuang (✉) · Y. Chai
Shanghai Sixth People's Hospital, Shanghai, China

P. Tang et al. (eds.), *Tutorials in Suturing Techniques for Orthopedics*, https://doi.org/10.1007/978-981-33-6330-4_6

   (b) Multi-passage layout should provide personnel passage and material passage;
   (c) The layout of clean-and-contaminated item passage may not be restricted by the above conditions;
   (d) The middle passage should be a clean corridor, and the outer corridor should be a clean corridor.
4. Classes I and II clean operating rooms should be located in the area with the least interference in the Operation Department.
5. The layout of clean operating room is reasonable, and clean area should not be interrupted by non-clean area.
6. Elevators and logistics transmission systems for personnel and materials in clean operating rooms should not be located in clean areas. When it can only be located in a clean area, a buffer room must be set at the exit, and the area of the buffer room should not be less than 3 m^2. There should be a centralized storage location for dirt in the operating room.
7. Surgical hand-washing sink can be set up in clean corridors, and the number should be one for every 2–4 clean operating rooms.
8. The wall in the operating room should be made of materials that are not easy to crack, flame retardant, easy to clean, collision resistant, acid and alkali resistant, and corrosion resistant. The color should be light green and light blue, which can easily eliminate the visual fatigue of the surgeon. The joint between wall and ceiling or floor is semicircle arc, which is convenient for cleaning and reduces dust accumulation. The clear height of the operating room should be 2.8–3.0 m; the clear width of the door should not be less than 1.4 m, and the indoor area should not be less than 40 m^2. Artificial lighting should be used in the operating room without external windows. The orthopedic operating room should be protected by lead plates and marked prominently on the door.
9. Sockets, switches, instrument cabinets, viewbox, etc. set in the operating room and auxiliary rooms shall be embedded in the wall without protruding from the wall. See Fig. 6.1 for the layout flow of the clean operating room.

6.1.3 Basic Facilities of Operating Room

1. Electric induction door should be adopted for the operating room, and a small glass window should be opened on the door to facilitate observation and lighting. The shadowless lamps which are easy to clean and disinfect and do not affect vertical laminar flow are preferred as surgical lighting sources.
2. Operating room should have dual power supply, which can automatically switch when power failures. There should be multiple electric socket groups with multipurpose sockets in the operating room, and the sockets should be provided with earthing system, anti-spark

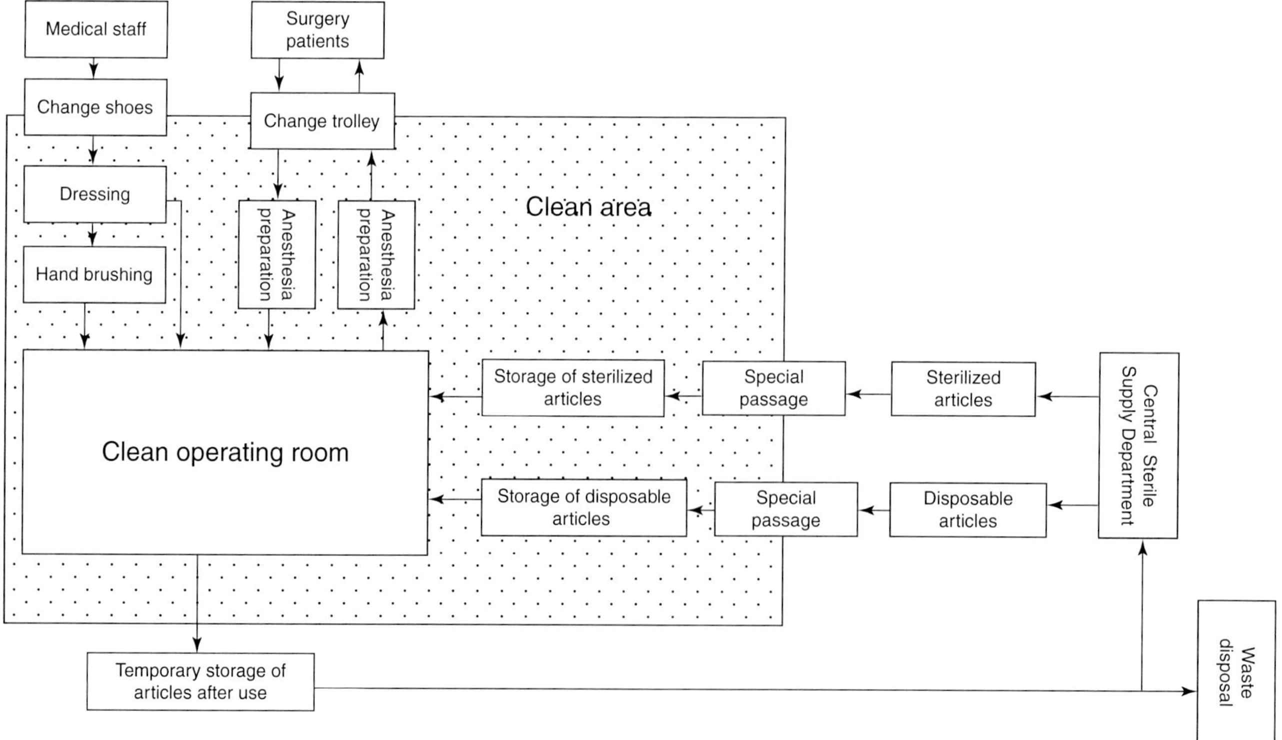

Fig. 6.1 Layout flow of clean operating room

device, and sealing cover. Each operating room should be equipped with an independent distribution box.

3. The operating room shall be provided with central air supply, and each operating room shall be provided with two sets of operation air supply systems, which are, respectively, installed on the ceiling supply units and wall equipment belt. Operation air supply system should be equipped with pipeline terminal interfaces such as vacuum aspiration, oxygen, carbon dioxide, nitrogen, argon, and compressed air. Interfaces should be clearly marked with shapes and colors.
4. The operating room should be provided with central temperature control system with cold and warm air supply equipment. The temperature should be controlled at 18–22 °C and the relative humidity should be controlled at 40–60%. The new hospital can install air purification facilities if possible.
5. Hospitals with teaching tasks should consider setting up digital operating rooms for real-time surgical demonstration such as remote consultation, conference, and teaching.

According to the actual situation of the hospital, it can be considered to build a compound operating room containing DSA, navigation, CT, robot, and other large equipment. The area of the compound operating room should not be less than 80 m^2.

6.2 Aseptic Techniques [2, 3]

6.2.1 Surgical Items

1. Open the sterile instrument package in a clean environment, and the operator's wearing shall comply with requirements. The sterile instrument package should be opened after the operation position placement or covered with sterile towel after opening, and then the operation such as position placement can be carried out.
2. The sterile instrument table should be kept dry, and once the excipients are wet, the sterile towel must be covered again. In case of excessive moisture, the instrument package should be replaced. Do not cross the sterile instrument table during any operation.
3. Before opening the sterile instrument package, check whether the color of autoclave indicator tape has changed; whether the package is damaged or damp; whether it is the required instrument package; whether it is within the validity period.
4. When opening the sterile package, hands and unsterilized articles cannot touch the inner surface of the package and cannot cross the sterile area during operation; hands with sterile gloves can only operate on the instrument table and must not support the edge of the sterile table.
5. Before the operation, instrument nurses and circulating nurses must complete the inventory of all instruments and articles and record one by one.

6.2.2 Surgical Personnel

1. Medical staff can enter the semi-restricted area only after changing sterilized clothes, trousers, caps, and shoes in the unrestricted area. The cap should be fully covered, and the hair should not be exposed. It is best to use nonwoven closed overalls. If split clothing is selected, tuck in the lower hem of the surgical gown to reduce contamination of the sterile area. If the medical staff leaves the operating room midway, they should change their shoes and clothes when returning.
2. Surgical hand antisepsis: The process in which medical staff wash their hands with soap and running water before operation and then use hand antiseptic agent to remove or kill the transient flora and reduce the resident flora in hands. The hand antiseptic agent used can have sustained antibacterial activity. 1) Hand antiseptic agent: Used for hand washing to reduce bacteria, such as ethanol, isopropanol, chlorhexidine, and iodophor. ① Quick-drying hand antiseptic agent: hand antiseptic agent containing alcohols and skin care components, including water aqua, gel, and foam types; ② Rinse-free hand antiseptic agent: It is used for surgical hand antisepsis, without rinsing with water after antisepsis, including water aqua, gel, and foam types. 2) Surgical hand antisepsis principle: Hands are washed first and then disinfected; the surgical hand should be disinfected again between operations of different patients, when the gloves are damaged or the hands are contaminated. 3) Surgical hand antisepsis methods and requirements: ① Before washing hands, wear a cap and mask (Fig. 6.2), remove the hand accessories, and trim the nails, with the length not exceeding the fingertips. ② Take proper amount of cleaning agent to clean hands, forearms, and lower 1/3 of upper arms and knead them carefully. When cleaning hands, care should be taken to clean dirt under nails and wrinkles of hand skin. ③ Flush hands, forearms, and lower 1/3 of upper arms with running water. ④ Dry hands, forearms, and lower 1/3 of upper arms with dry hand articles. 4) Surgical hand antisepsis methods: ① Hand-washing antisepsis method: Apply proper amount of hand antiseptic agent to each part of hands, forearms, and lower 1/3 of upper arms and carefully knead for 2–6 min, rinse hands, forearms, and lower 1/3 of upper arms with running water and dry them thoroughly with sterile towel. The running water shall

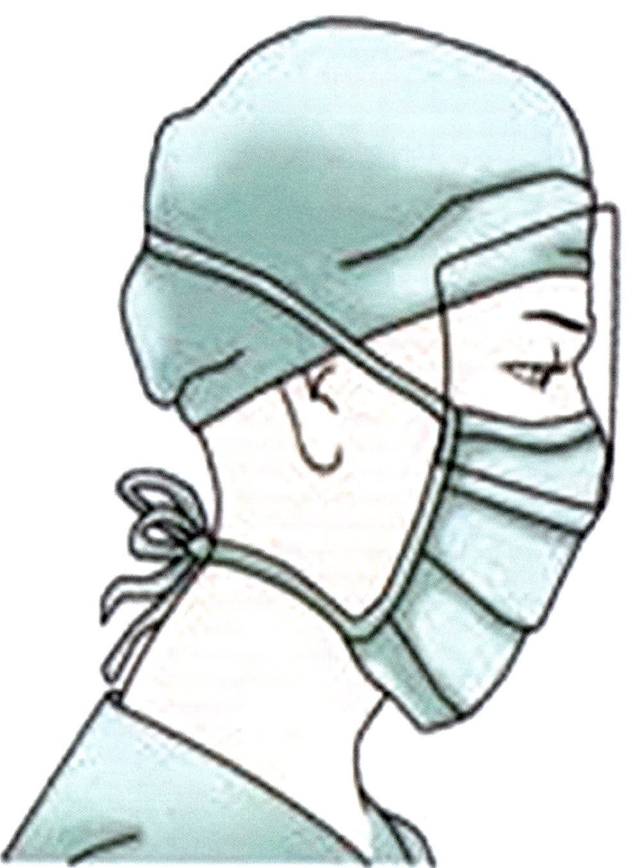

Fig. 6.2 Wear a cap and mask before washing hands

comply with requirements of GB5749. ② Rinse-free hand antisepsis method: Apply a proper amount of rinse-free hand antiseptic agent to every part of hands, forearms, and lower 1/3 of upper arms and carefully knead until the antiseptic agent is dry. The amount of liquid taken from the hand antiseptic agent, kneading time, and method of application should follow the IFU of the product. ③ The steps of brushless hand-washing method in the original Standard for Hand Hygiene of the Ministry of Health (Fig. 6.3): palm to palm kneading (A) → finger crossing, palm to back kneading (B) → finger crossing, palm to palm kneading (C) → bending finger joint and kneading in palm (D) → thumb kneading in palm (E) → fingertip kneading in palm (F). 5) Precautions: ① Fake nails should not be worn, and nails and tissues around nails should be kept clean. ② Hand should be kept on chest and higher than elbow during the whole antisepsis process to make water flow from hand to elbow. ③ The sponge, other kneading articles, or kneading hands together can be used for hand washing and antisepsis. ④ After removing surgical gloves, hands should be cleaned with soap (liquid soap). ⑤After use, nail cleaning appliances and kneading articles such as sponges and hand brushes should be placed in designated containers; kneading articles should be disinfected or used once per person; nail cleaning appliances should be cleaned and disinfected daily.

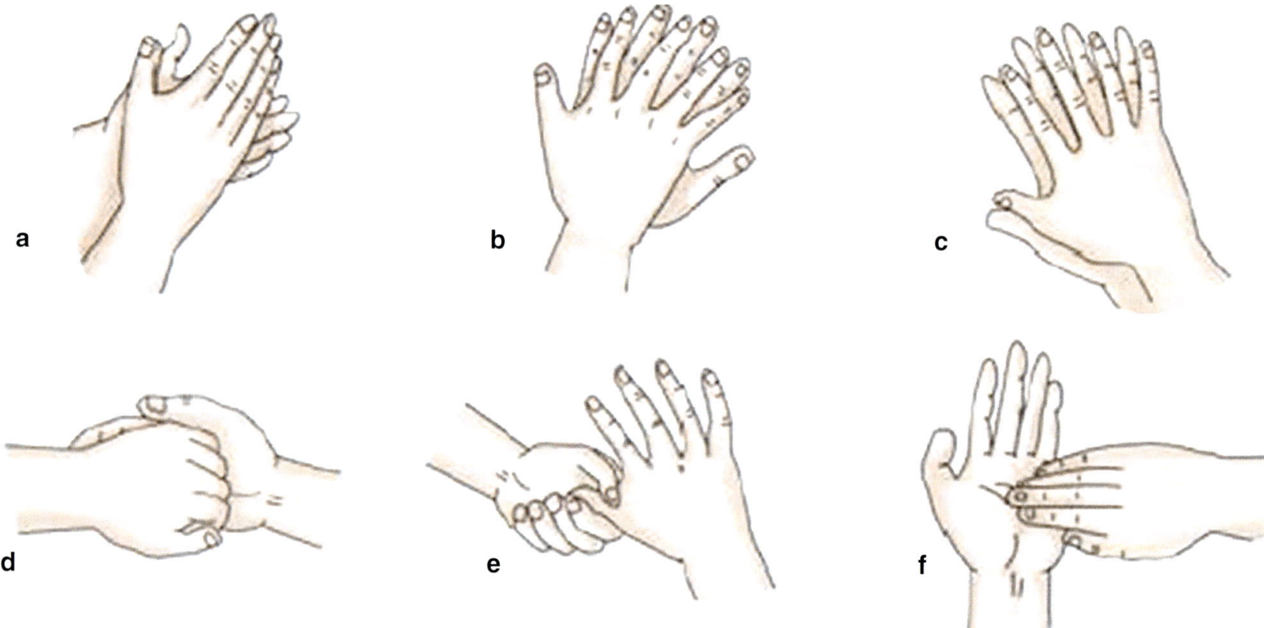

Fig. 6.3 Surgical hand antisepsis method

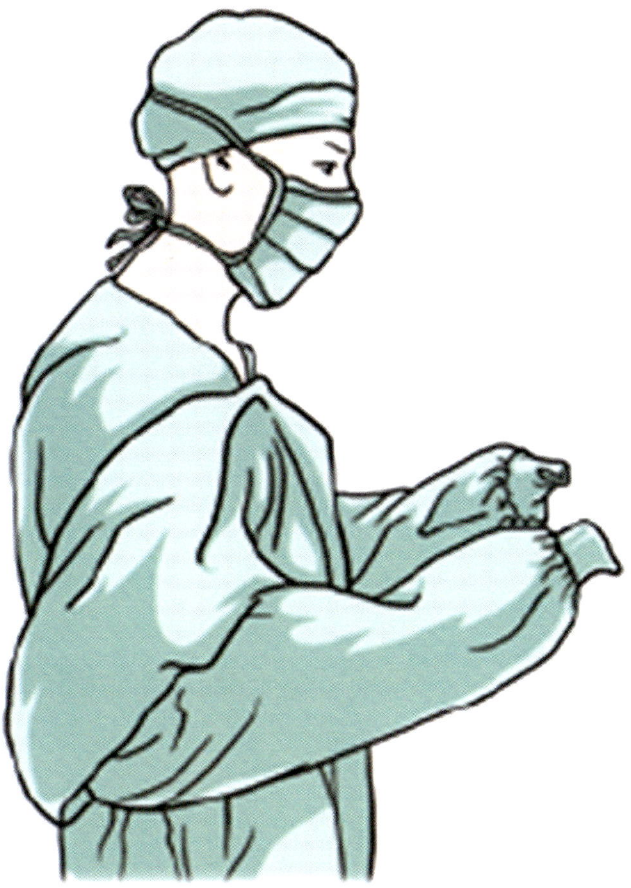

Fig. 6.4 Gowning

3. Principle of putting on and taking off sterile gown: There are two kinds of commonly used surgical gowns: split-type and full cover.
   (a) Method of wearing split-type gown (Fig. 6.4): ① After washing hands, take the surgical gown, lift the collar, and shake it gently. While gently throwing the surgical gown upward, stretch your hands and forearms into the sleeves, and forward in parallel; ② The circulating nurse assists in pulling gown backwards behind wearer; ③ Hand-washing nurse hands cross, do not cross belt, and transfer it to the back; ④ The circulating nurse ties the belt behind him/her; ⑤ Sterile areas of surgical gown are below shoulder, above waist, chest of anterior axillary line and hands.
   (b) Method for wearing full cover gown: ① After washing hands, take the surgical gown, lift the collar, and shake it gently; ② While gently throwing the surgical gown upward, stretch the hands and forearms into the sleeves, and forward in parallel. The circulating nurse stretches the hands into the inside of the surgical gown behind wearer to help pull the gown backward, and the hands cannot touch the outside of the surgical gown; ③ After wearing gloves, pass the belt at the front to the circulating nurse; ④ The circulating nurse clamps the belt around the wearer with sterile holding forceps and then returns it to the wearer; ⑤ The wearer ties the belt on the chest; ⑥ Sterile areas are chest below shoulders and above waist, arms, side chest, and back (Fig. 6.5).
   (c) Precautions: ① Wearing the surgical gown must be carried out in the operating room, with enough space around and the wearer facing the sterile area. When dressing, the surgical gown should not touch any non-sterile items and should be replaced immediately if accidentally touching. ② When the circulating nurse pulls the collar and sleeves back, both hands should not touch the outside of the surgical gown. ③ When wearing a full cover gown, the dressing personnel must wear gloves before taking the belt. ④ Put on the surgical gown and gloves. Waiting for the operation to start, put your hands in the interlayer of the chest of the gown or clasp your hands on your chest. Do not lift hands above the shoulders, hang below the waist, or cross arms and put hands under the armpits.
   (d) The method of changing the surgical gown for continuous operations: When continuous operations are needed, the operators of continuous operations should first wash the blood on the gloves, and then the circulating nurses loosen the back laces and take off the surgical gown and gloves one after another. Hands must be kept free from contamination when the surgical gown is taken off; otherwise, hands must be disinfected again. There are two ways to take off the surgical gown. ① Undressing method assisted by others: With the hands forward and the elbows slightly bent, the circulating nurse faces the undressing people, holds the collar, takes off the surgical gown in turning-over way along elbow and hand, and then the wrist of the glove is turned right at the hand. ② Personal undressing method: The undressing people grasps the outside of surgical gown of the right shoulder with left hand and pulls it down from the front, to make the sleeve of the surgical gown turn over from the inside to the outside; in the same way, pull down the left side and take off the surgical gown, so as to protect the arms and hand-washing clothes from touching the outside of the surgical gown to avoid contamination.

4. Wear sterile gloves: Because surgical antisepsis method can only remove and kill the transient flora on the skin surface, it is ineffective for the resident flora in the deep skin. During the operation, the bacteria in the deep skin

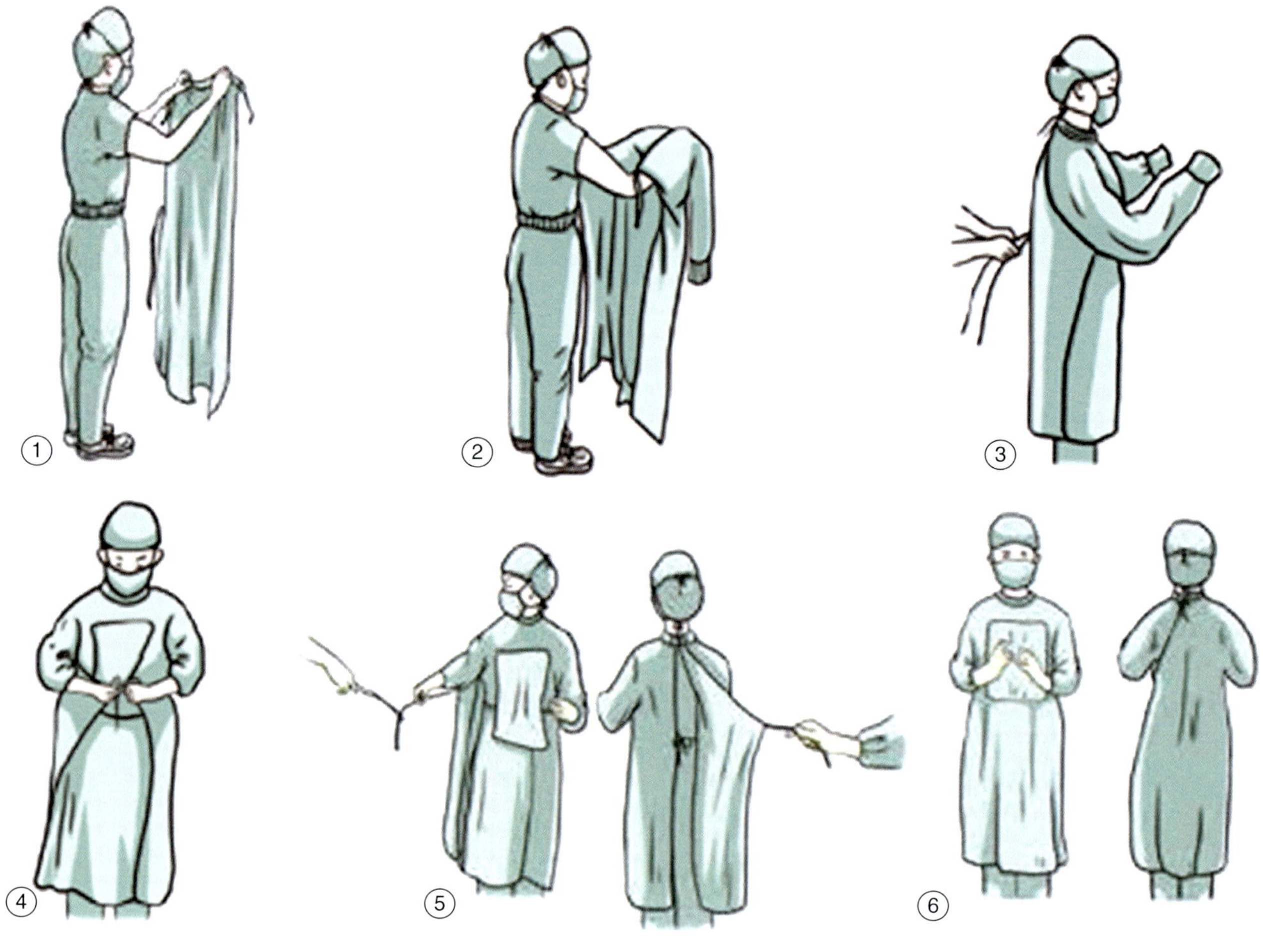

Fig. 6.5 Method for wearing full cover gown

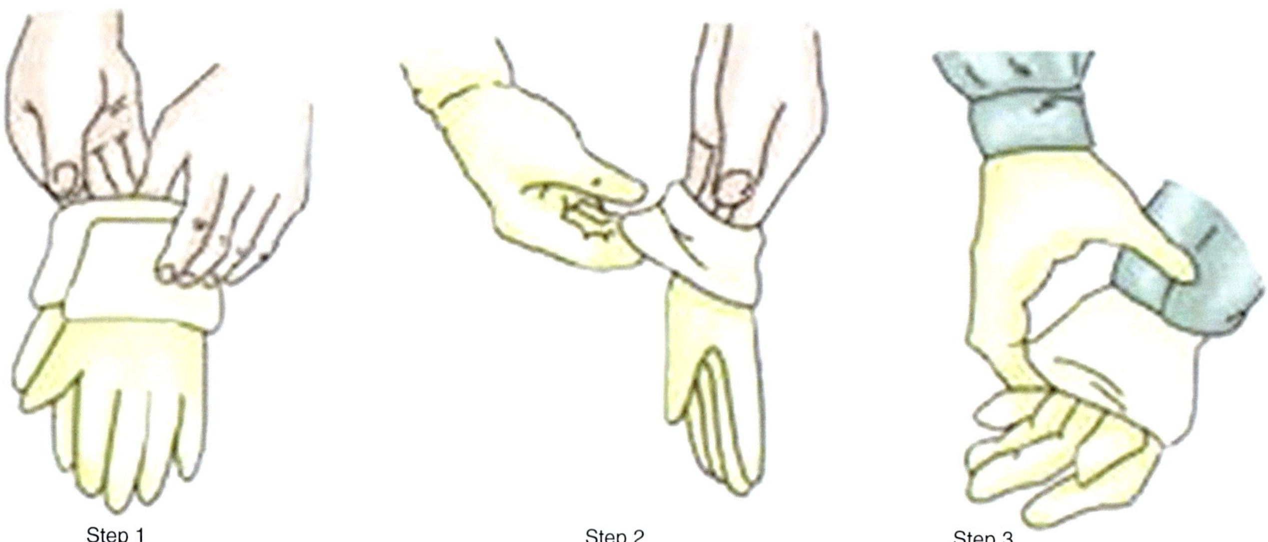

Fig. 6.6 Open gloving method

will be brought to the surface of the hand with the sweat of the operator. Therefore, the surgical personnel must wear sterile gloves.

(a) Open gloving method (Fig. 6.6).
(b) Closed gloving method (Fig. 6.7): Orthopedic surgeons should adopt this method.

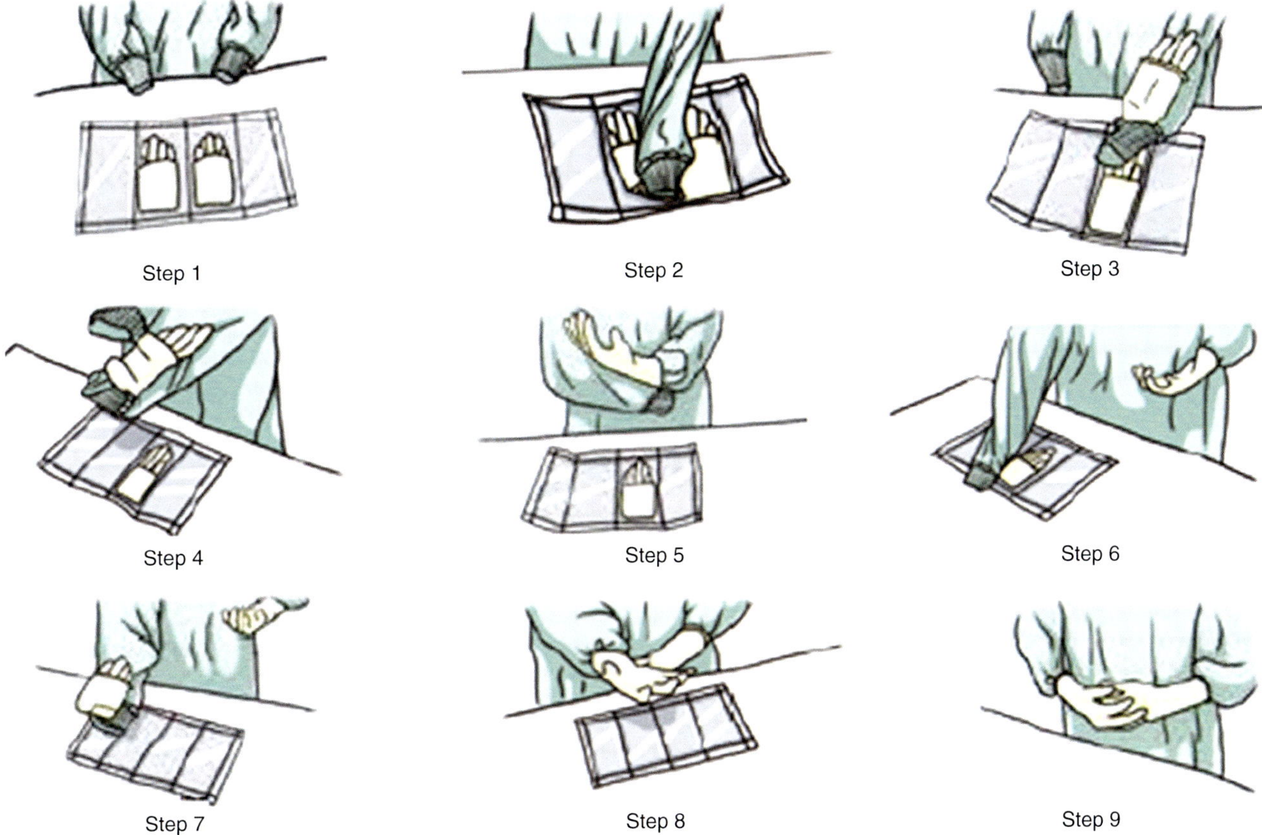

Fig. 6.7 Closed gloving method

(c) Method of assisting the operator to wear gloves (Fig. 6.8): Orthopedic surgeons are recommended to wear double gloves for surgery; the first layer of gloves should be worn by this method with the assistance of the gloved personnel.

(d) Precautions: ① When holding gloves, hands should stretch slightly forward and do not close to the surgical gown. ② When wearing open gloves, ungloved hands should not touch the outside of gloves, and gloved hands should not touch the inside of gloves. ③ After wearing gloves, the folded parts of gloves are turned over to wrap the cuffs, and the wrists should not be exposed; gloved fingers should not touch the skin when turning over. ④ When wearing powdered gloves, the talc on the glove should be rinsed with normal saline before taking part in the operation. ⑤ When assisting the operator to wear gloves, the gloved hand of the instrument nurse should avoid touching the operator's skin.

(e) Degloved method for continuous operation; ①Take off the surgical gown according to the method of tak-

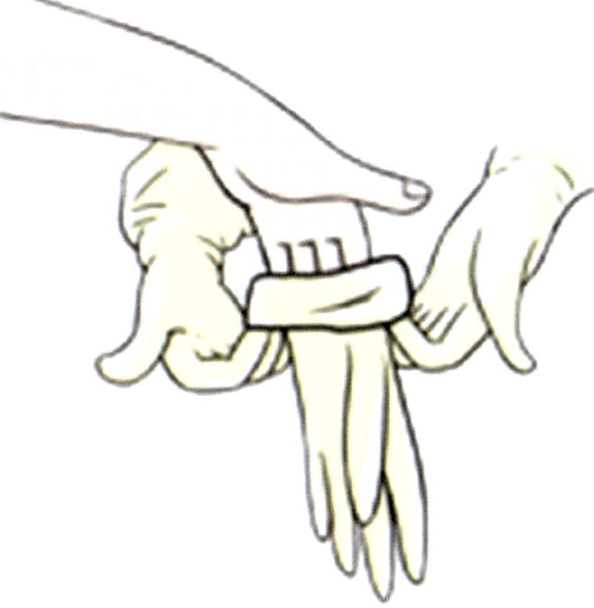

Fig. 6.8 Method for assisting the operator to wear gloves

ing off the surgical gown in continuous operations to make the edge of the glove fold back; ② Insert the gloved right hand into the fold outside the left glove and take off the glove, then stretch the left thumb between the thenar muscles inside the right glove, and take off the right glove downward; ③ Pay attention that gloved hands cannot touch the skin of both hands, and degloved hands cannot touch the outside of gloves to ensure that the hands are not contaminated by bacteria outside the gloves; ④ After taking off gloves, hands should be disinfected again before taking part in the next operation.

6.2.3 Surgical Patients

1. Clearance of the patient's skin: Remove the residual dirt from the patient's skin: 1) Patients who can move freely: Take a bath with bath lotion containing bacteriostatic components (chlorhexidine and alcohols) one day before operation and instruct the patients to clean the skin around the surgical incision and the dirt in the skin folds. 2) Patients with limited activities: Bath in bed with bath lotion containing bacteriostatic components (chlorhexidine and alcohols) before operation, and it is best to bath in bed more than twice if conditions permit (depending on the physical condition of patients and the actual cleanliness of skin).
2. Skin preparation for patients before operation: There are often various microorganisms on the surface of human skin, including transient flora and resident flora. Especially when skin preparation before operation accidentally damages the skin, it is more likely to cause transient flora to colonize and reproduce, which becomes one of the factors of incision infection after operation. 1) Skin preparation method: The depilatory cream, hair remover, etc. are used, and the razor is forbidden to prevent hair follicle damage in the operating field of the patient and secondary postoperative infection. For patients with sparse hair, skin preparation before operation is not recommended, but skin cleaning must be done. 2) Skin preparation time: On the day of operation, the closer to the operation time, the better. 3) Skin preparation location: It is recommended to carry out it in the preoperative preparation room of the operating room; for hospitals that do not have this condition, it can also be conducted in the ward treatment room.
3. Common skin antiseptic agents
   (a) Purpose of skin antisepsis: To kill the transient flora on the skin of the operating field, to kill or reduce the resident flora to the maximum extent, and to avoid postoperative incision infection. Strict skin antisepsis in the operating field is an important link to reduce incision infection.

Table 6.1 Common antiseptic agents

Drug name	Main purpose	Characteristic
2%–3% tincture of iodine	Skin antisepsis (deiodination with ethanol), rarely used clinically	Broad bactericidal spectrum, strong effect, and capability of killing spores
0.2%–0.5% iodophor	Antisepsis of skin and mucosa	The bactericidal power is weaker than tincture of iodine, which cannot kill spores and does not require deiodination
0.02%–0.05% iodophor	Irrigation of mucosa and wounds	Weak bactericidal power and low corrosivity
75% ethanol	Antisepsis of skin in face and skin-taking area; deiodination after using tincture of iodine	Killing bacteria, viruses, and fungi, not effective for spores, not effective for viruses such as hepatitis B
0.1%–0.5% chlorhexidine	Antisepsis of skin	Killing bacteria and inhibiting *Mycobacterium tuberculosis* and spores

   (b) Common antiseptic agents are shown in Table 6.1.
   (c) Precautions: ① The skin is disinfected with iodophor, which should be applied twice for 3 min; ② The antisepsis of skin folds such as umbilicus, armpit, and perineum should be strengthened; ③ In the process of antisepsis, the operator's hands should not touch the operating field or other articles; ④ When performing head-face and posterior cervical approach surgery, eyes should be protected with waterproof eye patches (eye protection pads) before skin antisepsis to prevent disinfectant from flowing into eyes and damaging cornea; ⑤ Once the bed sheet is wet during antisepsis, it should be replaced in time to avoid skin burns caused by prolonged contact with the bed sheet soaked with disinfectant during operation (special attention should be paid to infant surgery); ⑥ After use, dressing forceps should not be put back onto the sterile instrument table.

Search Terms
Orthopedic operating room, aseptic technique

References

1. GB50333-2013 Architectural technical code for hospital clean operating department issued by the Ministry of Health of the People's Republic of China.
2. WS 310.1-2016 Central sterile supply department (CSSD)—Part 1: management standard issued by the Ministry of Health of the People's Republic of China.
3. Guide to Operating Room Nursing Practice, Beijing, People's Publishing House, 2017.

7 Hand Surgery Tendon Suture Techniques

Liqiang Gu, Honggang Wang, and Jian Qi

Abstract

Tendon has excellent sliding mechanism and functions as the transmission for the hand joint movement. Tendon injury will cause severe hand movement dysfunction. In order to restore the functions of limbs and fingers, ruptured or deficient tendons must be repaired in time. Commonly used tendon repair methods include modified Kessler stitching, Bunnell stitching, Tsuge loop stitching, etc. After tendon repair, the major issue is to prevent either tendon adhesion or tendon re-rupture. Therefore, tendon surgery should achieve non-invasive suturing repair. The suturing material should cause less damage to the tendon tissue, and have good tensile strength, so that it could meet the requirements of postoperative rehabilitation training for patients, so as to reduce tendon adhesion and re-rupture. In early postoperative rehabilitation, it is advisable for patients to do active-passive combined exercise or active exercise as primary and passive as supplement, so as to maximize the restoration of the function of each hand joint.

Keywords

Hand surgery · Tendon injury · Tendon suture techniques Tendon repair · Non-invasive suturing repair

7.1 Historical Review of Tendon Repair

As early as the 1920s, hand surgery specialists had proposed non-invasive tendon repair in hand surgery. Because clinical practice has shown that the finger function recovery after tendon injury was poor. In 1944, Bunnell pointed out that tendon injury and repair was quite challenging in hand surgery, proposing the staged tendon reconstruction—wound closure at first stage and tendon graft at second stage—for intrathecal flexor tendon injury [1].

In the 1960s, Potenza, Lindsay, Peacock, and other specialists studied the healing process of tendons. In the 1970s, Matthews, Lundborg, and Manske proposed that tendons have endogenous healing capabilities. Verdan [2], Kleinert [3], and other specialists pointed out that the finger flexor tendons should be repaired early, with postoperative early exercise. The study of Belusa [4] also indicated that early repair of the finger flexor tendons in each area has better outcomes compared to second-stage repair; as long as conditions permit, it should be repaired as early as possible (except for severe infection, severe or extensive crush injuries, and avulsion injuries). In the 1990s, Savage [5], Silfverskiold [6, 7], Tang Jinbo [8, 9], and other specialists proposed that the use of tendon stitching with good tensile strength, with combination of postoperative active and passive or active exercises, could improve the outcomes of tendon repair. In 2007, Elliot, Barbieri, Evans, Mass, Tang, and other specialists pointed out that the incidence of tendon rupture after repair was 3% to 7% [10] (Fig. 7.1a–d).

7.2 Biological Process of Hand Tendon Healing

7.2.1 Hand Flexor and Extensor Tendon Division

Hand flexors are generally divided into five zones, as shown in Fig. 7.2. The specific zones are as follows.

- Zone I: The midpoint of middle segment of finger (proximal segment of thumb) to the tendon insertion (only one tendon);
- Zone II: Distal palmar crease to the midpoint of the middle segment of finger (the tendon is located in the fiber sheath, difficult to treat with poor outcome);

L. Gu (✉) · H. Wang · J. Qi
The First Affiliated Hospital, Sun Yat-sen University, Guangzhou, China

P. Tang et al. (eds.), *Tutorials in Suturing Techniques for Orthopedics*, https://doi.org/10.1007/978-981-33-6330-4_7

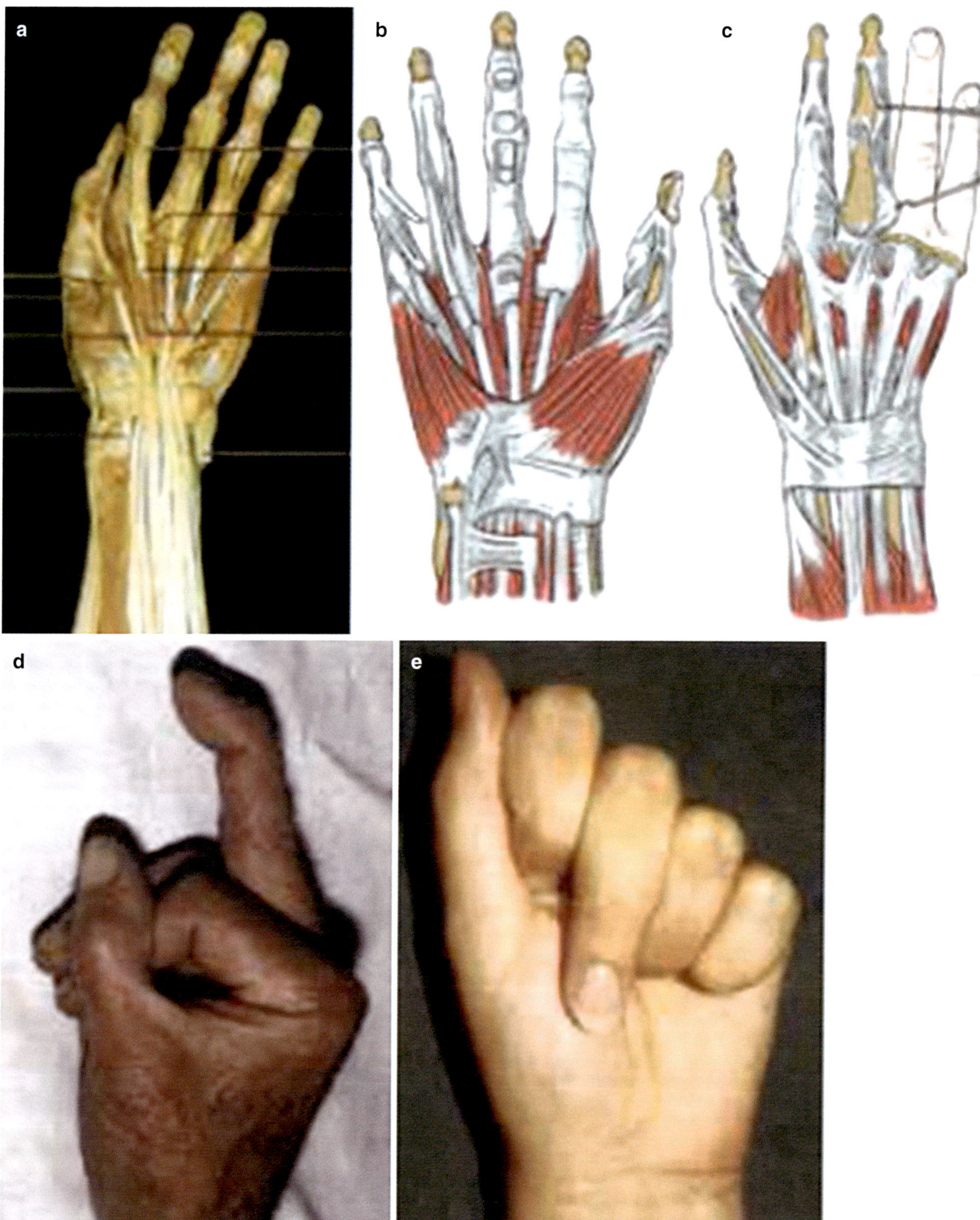

Fig. 7.1 Anatomy of hand tendons and dysfunction after injury. (**a**) Anatomy of the hand flexor tendons; (**b**) Anatomical drawing of the hand flexor tendons; (**c**) Anatomical drawing of the hand extensor tendons; (**d**) Mallet finger deformity and distal extension disorder following the rupture of the extensor tendon insertion; (**e**) Middle finger distal flexion disorder following the rupture of the flexor digitorum profundus (FDP) tendon

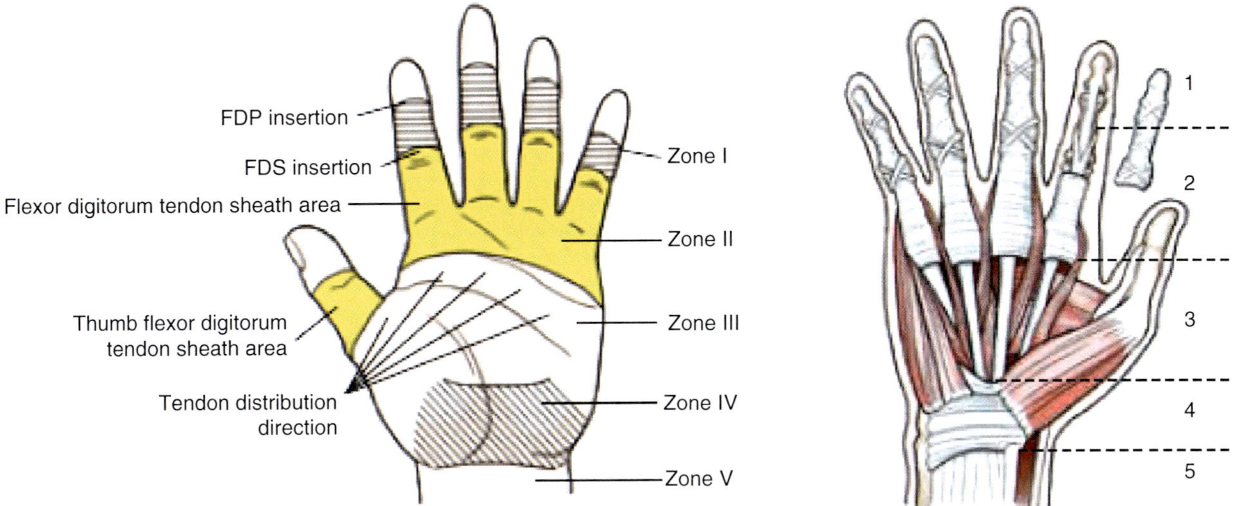

Fig. 7.2 Hand flexor tendon division

- Zone III: The distal edge of the transverse carpal ligament to the distal palmar crease;
- Zone IV: Carpal tunnel zone (nine tendons and median nerve);
- Zone V: The beginning of the tendon to the proximal carpal tunnel (forearm area) [11].

According to the Verdan method, the hand extensor tendons can be divided into eight zones. The odd-numbered zones correspond to joints, and the even-numbered zones correspond to the diaphysis, as shown in Fig. 7.3 [12].

7.2.2 Tendon Nutrition

1. **The tendon sheath area is mainly nourished by synovial fluid**

Synovial fluid is the main nutrition source for the flexor tendons in the tendon sheath area. The tendon blood supply inside the tendon sheath does not play the decisive role in nutrition. How synovial fluid nourishes tendons: active diffusion + synovial fluid passively squeezed into the tissue during finger movement.

2. **Forearm to palm area is mainly nourished by blood supply**

The flexor tendons receive segmental blood supply from the surrounding tissues through peritendinous membrane, and the blood vessels in the tendon distribute longitudinally among tendon bundles (Fig. 7.4).

7.2.3 Biological Process of Tendon Healing

1. **Tendon healing process outside the sheath**

Fibrous scaffold formation period (first week), connective tissue hyperplasia period (second week), tendon collagen fiber formation period (from third week), and absorption period.

2. **Tendon healing process inside the sheath**

The tendon adventitial cells and the tendon cells in the tendon parenchyma have the ability to divide and proliferate. They move towards the rupture end after the tendon is injured, and participate in the healing process; there are also cells from the peritendinous tissue participate in the healing process of the injured tendon. The difference in the degree of participation between the two is closely related to the degree of tendon injury, the nutritional status, and the integrity of the peritendinous tissue. On the one hand, it should be beneficial to tendon healing; on the other hand, it should not form harmful dense adhesions [13].

7.3 Two Major Issues of Tendon Repair

7.3.1 Tendon Adhesion

Clinical studies have found that almost all repaired tendons have formed different degrees of adhesion and joint dysfunction with surrounding tissues, which are closely related to local pathological conditions, surgical operating techniques,

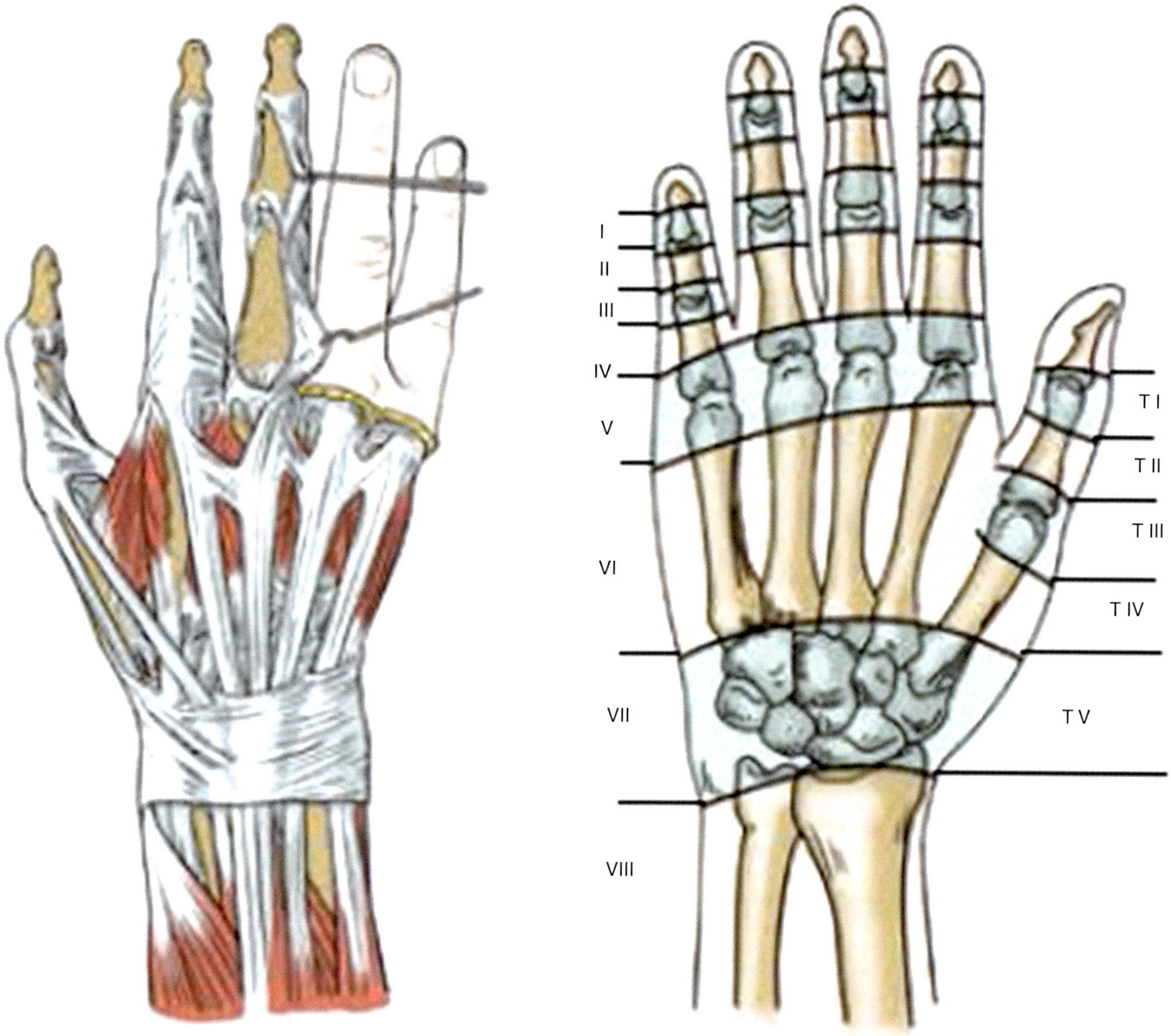

Fig. 7.3 Hand extensor tendon division

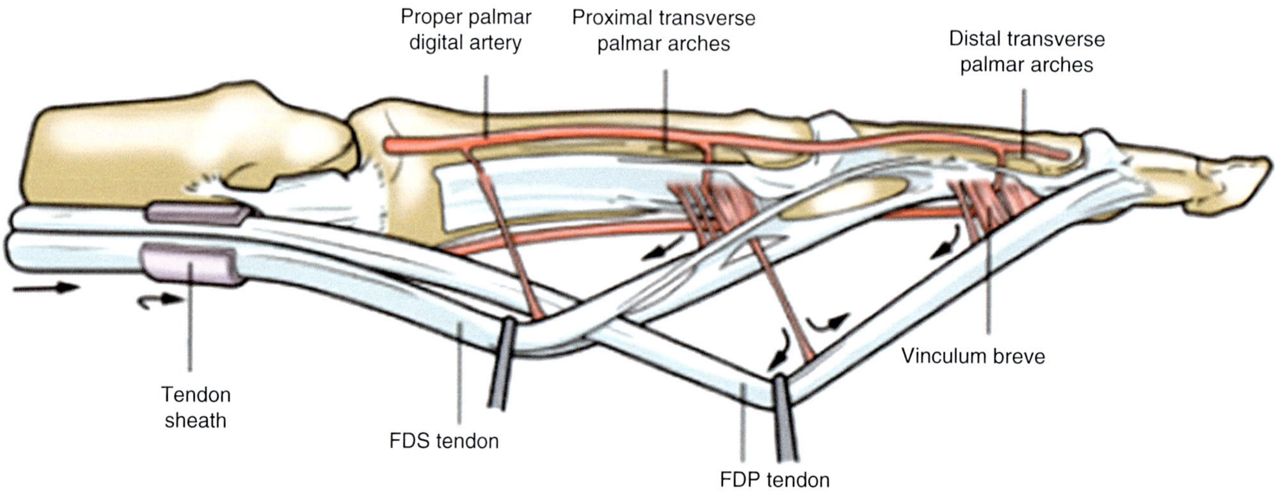

Fig. 7.4 Blood supply and nutrition mode of the tendon

suturing materials, whether the postoperative treatment is correct and other factors, and attention must be paid.

1. **Mechanism**

Tendon cells involved in tendon healing and exogenous cells (mainly fibroblasts) derived from peritendinous tissue grow and connect into a whole tissue.

2. **Prevention: Non-invasive technique procedure (to reduce the damage to the epitendineum) is a reasonable tendon suture technique**

Passive exercise after surgery: To a certain extent, it can prevent tendon adhesion without the risk of repaired tendon rupture.

Postoperative active exercise: Increase the sliding of the tendon and reduce the adhesion between the repaired tendon and the surrounding structure. However, non-absorbable sutures with good tensile strength (such as ETHIBOND or PROLENE) must be used combining with tendon suturing technique, so as to reduce the risk of repaired tendon rupture.

7.3.2 Tendon Rupture

Prevention method: After continuous peripheral suturing around the anastomotic site at the rupture end, the tensile strength can be improved, and multiple sets of stitchings with good tensile strength can be used.

Silfverskiold technique: After completing Kessler stitching, a more endurable cross weaving stitching of epitendineum is applied to the rupture end of the tendon, which greatly increases the suture fastness.

For the hand flexor tendon injury, in the past, it was believed that no repair was performed for postoperative adhesion, and the second-stage tendon transplantation was performed. With the research and understanding of the tendon healing mechanism, it is now advocated for flexor tendon injury at any part, including what was known as "No Man's Land," should be subject to first-stage repair after debridement. If the tendon sheath is intact, it is also advocated to repair the tendon sheath.

For the selection of tendon suturing materials, monofilament non-absorbable 4-0 polypropylene suture (PROLENE) is suitable for suturing hand tendons. It is artificially synthesized, with extremely smooth surface. It passes through the tissue smoothly with less trauma; it has the strongest inertia and less tissue reaction, thereby reducing bacterial adhesion; it is flattened and becomes more reliable after knotting, and is a permanent support.

In short, the tendon repair should consider the biological process of tendon healing, suturing materials, suturing methods, operating techniques, and other factors.

7.4 Principles of Tendon Repair

In the process of hand tendon repair, the principle of non-invasive repair of tendon is mainly followed. Principles commonly used in clinical practice include:

7.4.1 Bunnell Proposed the Principle of Tendon Suture in 1918 [14]

1. Ensure that the tendons heal without separation.
2. No strangulation of the tendon.
3. No knots on the surface of the tendon.
4. Less trauma to the tendon.

7.4.2 Tang Jinbo also Proposed the Principle of Tendon End-to-End Suturing in 2002 [15, 16]

1. The tendon suture must be performed on the premise of one-stage wound healing.
2. The tendon is sutured without obvious tension.
3. It is better to have two or more sets of independent sutures.
4. The suturing materials must have good tensile strength, causing less damage to the tendon, and not be absorbed before the tendon heals. Synthetic non-absorbable sutures, such as PROLENE and ETHIBOND, have good surgical operating feeling, with firm knotting, and can smoothly pass through the tendon tissue to reduce damage. Compared with silk threads, synthetic non-absorbable sutures have fewer tissue reactions.
5. During the suturing process, a non-invasive operation is performed to fully protect the tissues surrounding the tendon and always keep the tendon moist.
6. The suture is relatively smooth, and does not strangulate the tendon, with not much damage to the nutrition of the tendon. The exposure of tendon suture or knot on the surface should be avoided as possible.

7.5 Methods of Tendon Repair

There are many techniques on tendon repairing, such as Bunnell stitching, Kessler stitching, figure-of-8 stitching, double cross stitching, Kleinert stitching, Tsuge loop stitching, etc. (Figs. 7.5, 7.6, 7.7, 7.8, 7.9, and 7.10) [17–19].

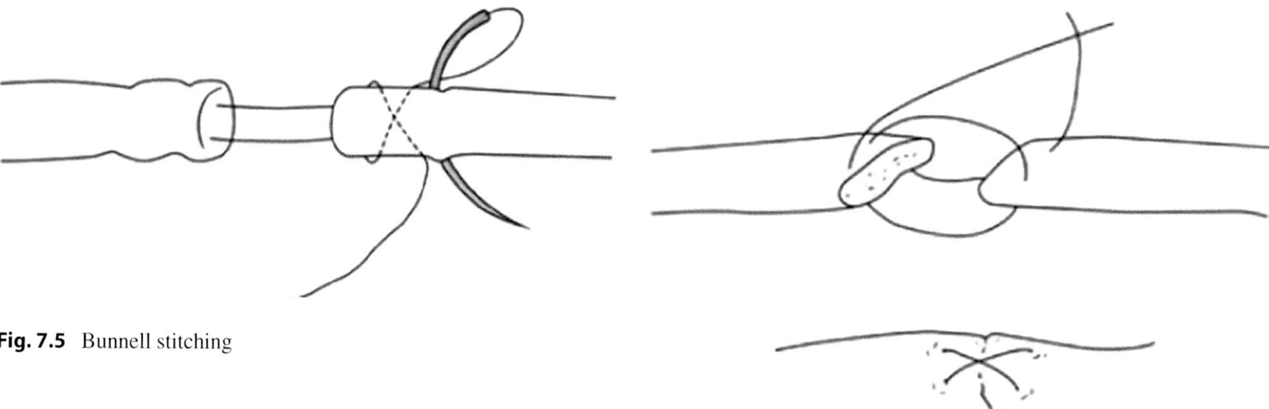

Fig. 7.5 Bunnell stitching

Fig. 7.7 Figure-of-8 stitching

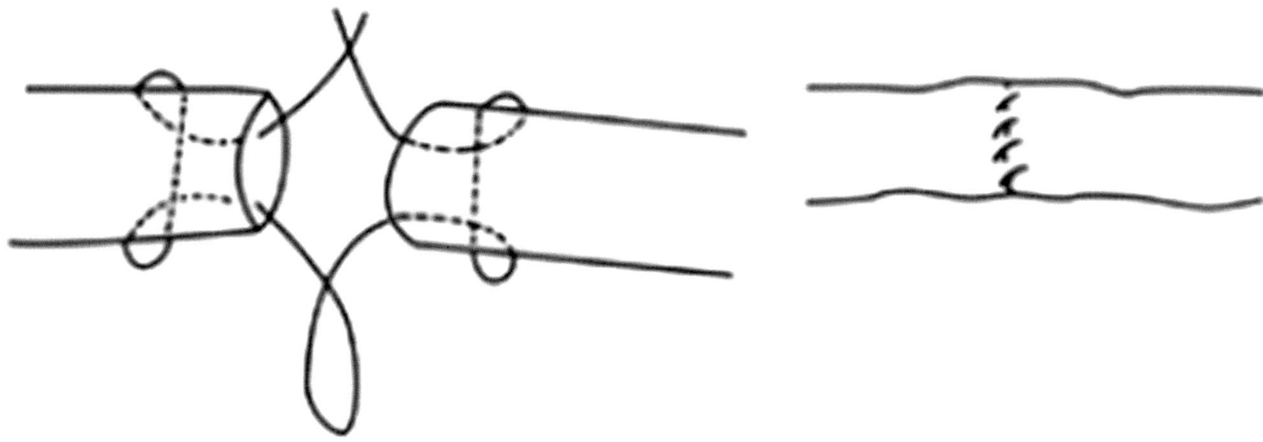

Fig. 7.6 Kessler stitching

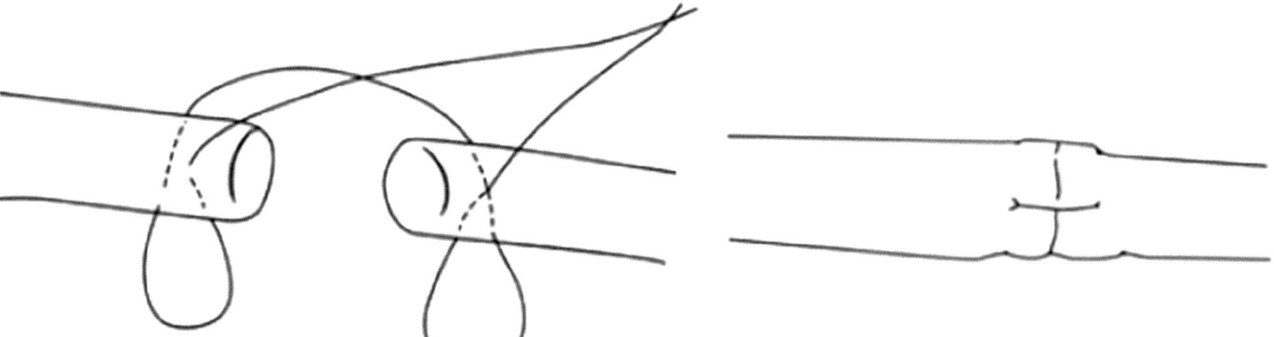

Fig. 7.8 Double cross stitching

The choice of tendon suture techniques can be determined according to the severity of tendon injury and the technique and conditions of the surgeon. In recent years, microsurgical stitchings have been used, aiming to minimize the impact on blood supply of the tendon to promote tendon healing and reduce adhesion.

Other tendon suture techniques are: fish mouth stitching (Fig. 7.11), double Tsuge stitching (Fig. 7.12), Tsuge buried loop stitching (Fig. 7.13), modified double loop stitching (Fig. 7.14), multiple intra-tendon stitching (M-Tang technique, Fig. 7.15), semi-knot locking stitching (Fig. 7.16), Strickland stitching, MGH stitching (Fig. 7.17),

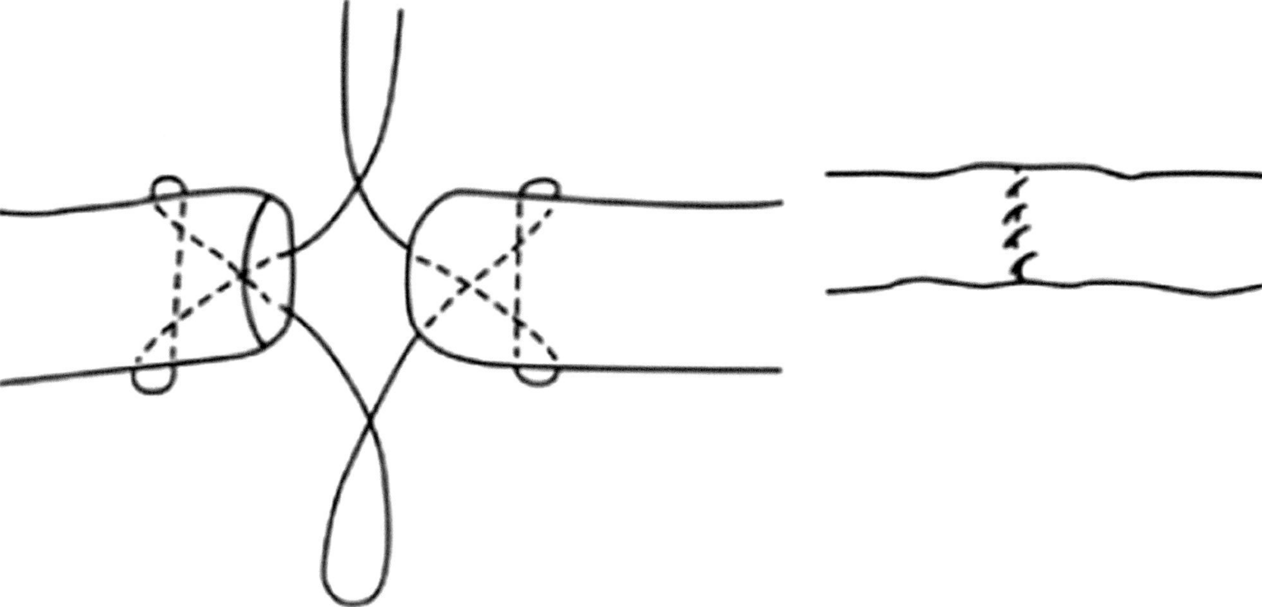

Fig. 7.9 Kleinert stitching

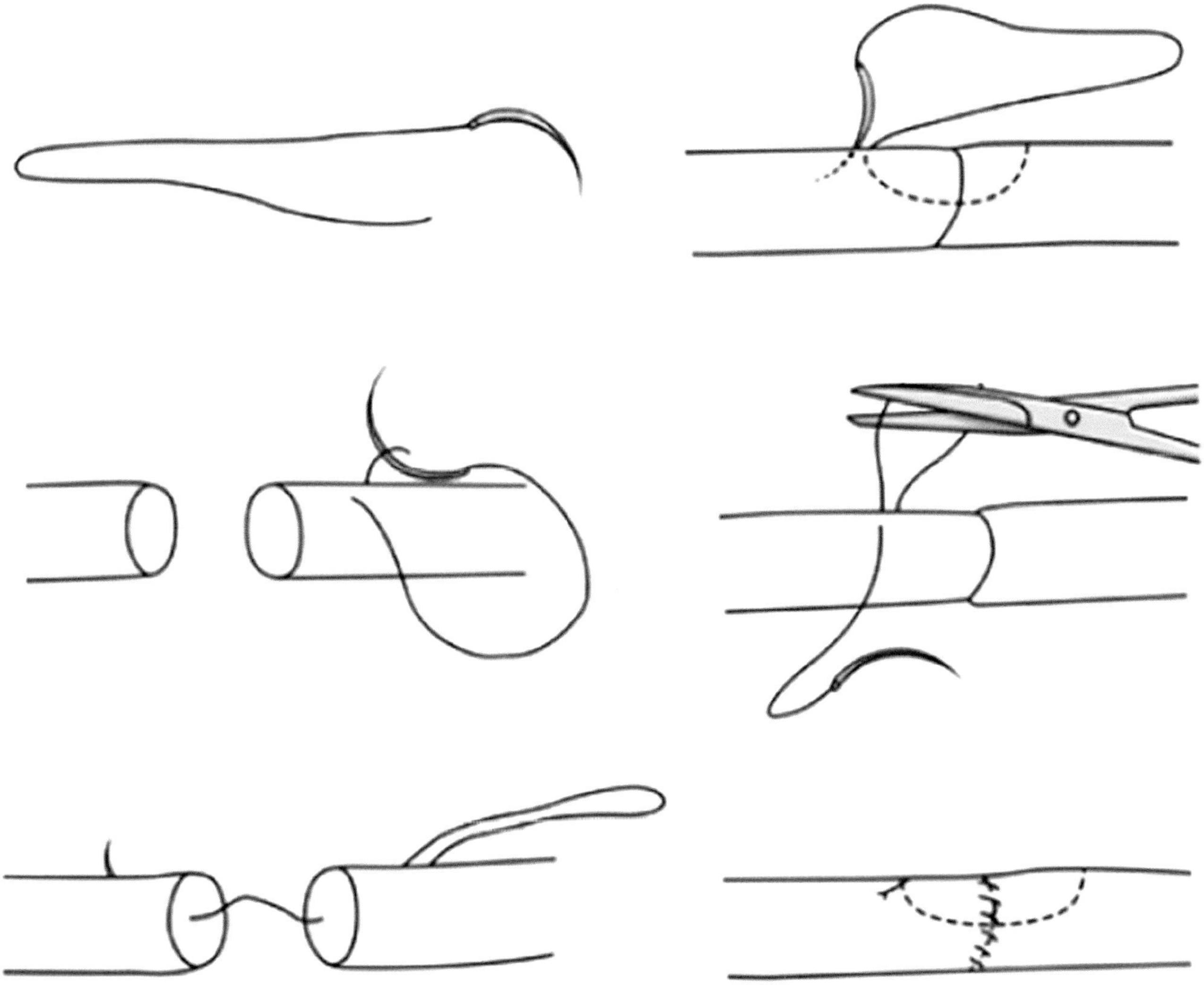

Fig. 7.10 Tsuge loop stitching

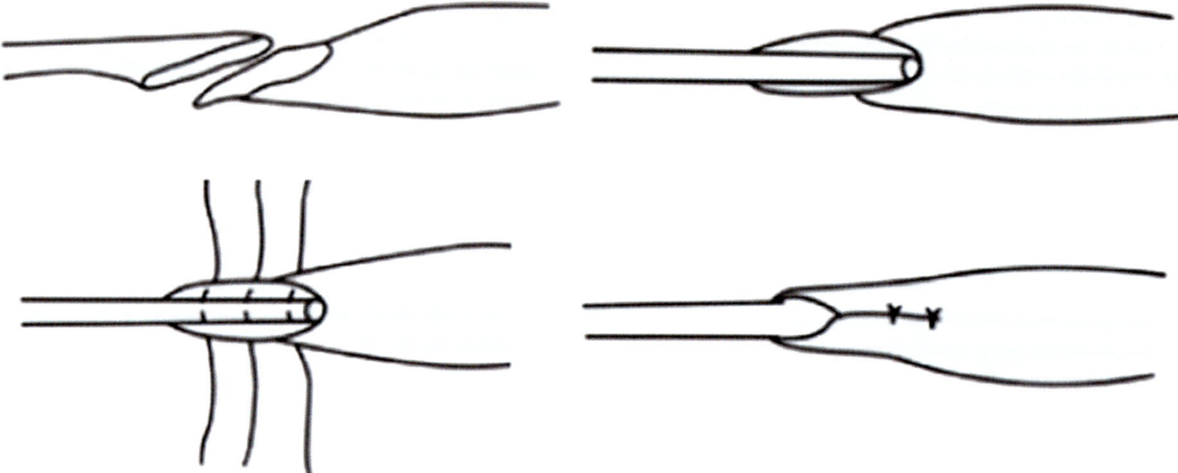

Fig. 7.11 Fish mouth stitching

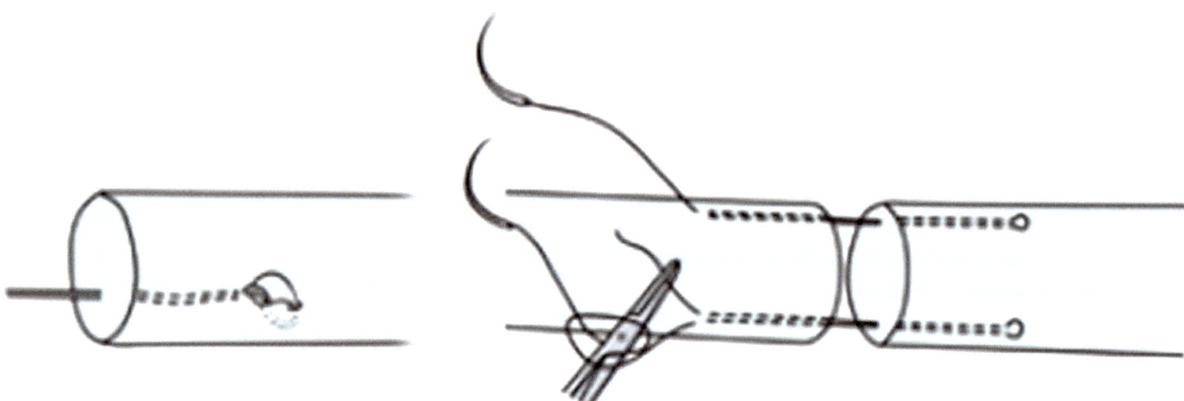

Fig. 7.12 Double Tsuge stitching

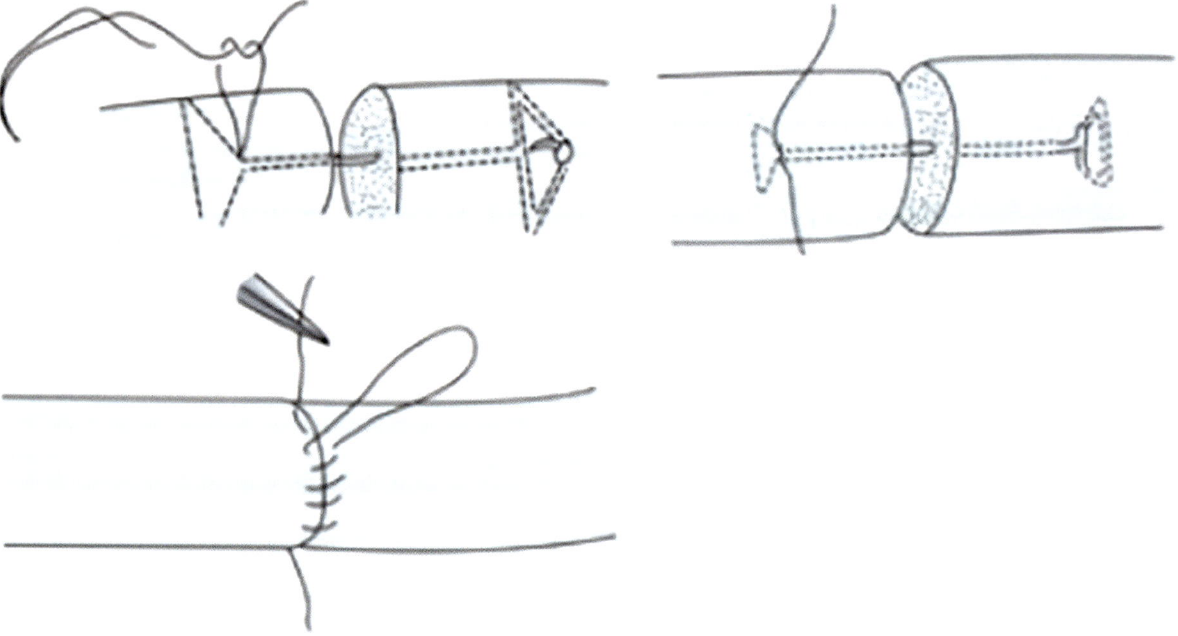

Fig. 7.13 Tsuge buried loop stitching

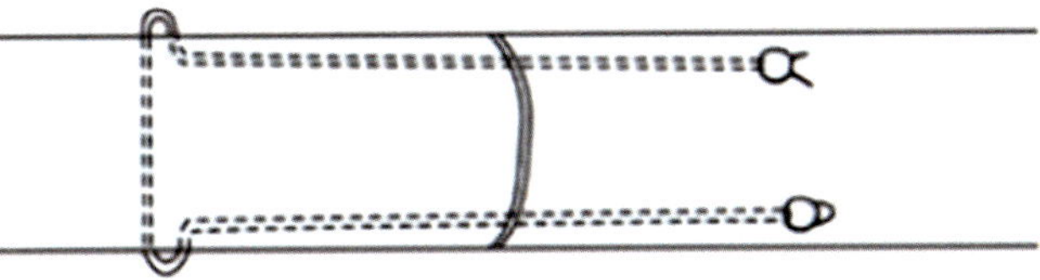

Fig. 7.14 Modified double loop stitching

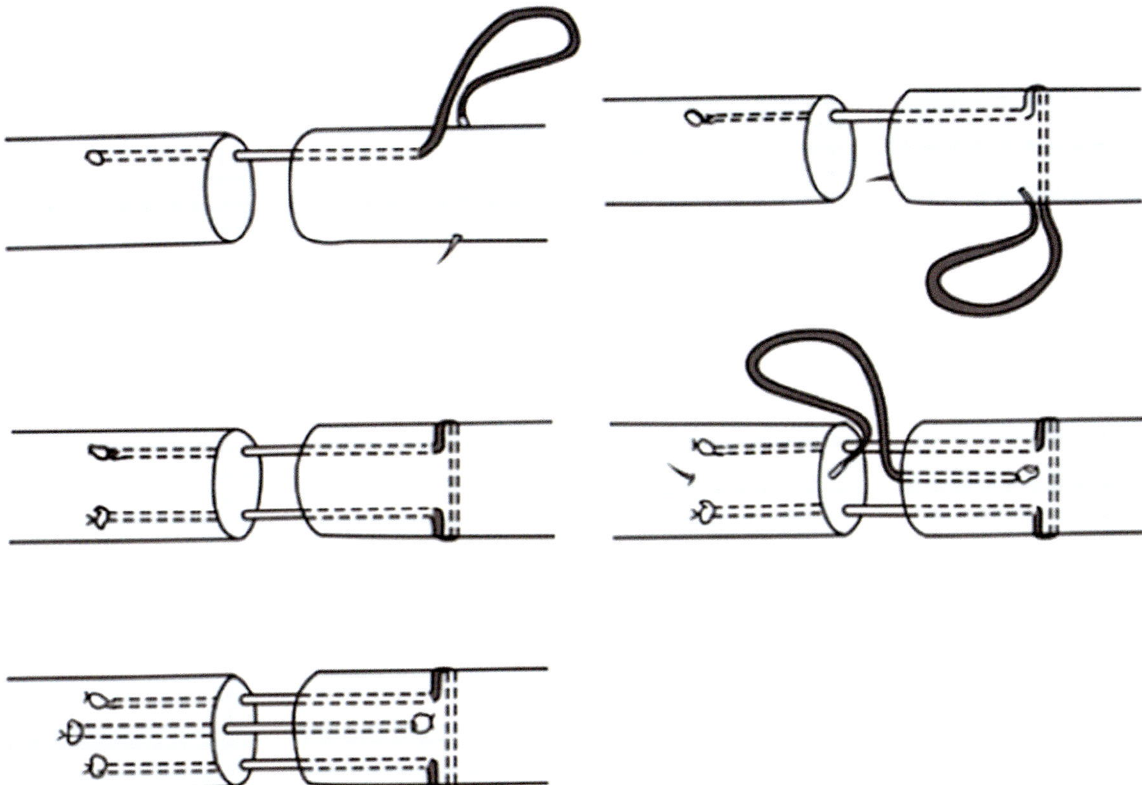

Fig. 7.15 Multiple intra-tendon stitching (M-Tang technique)

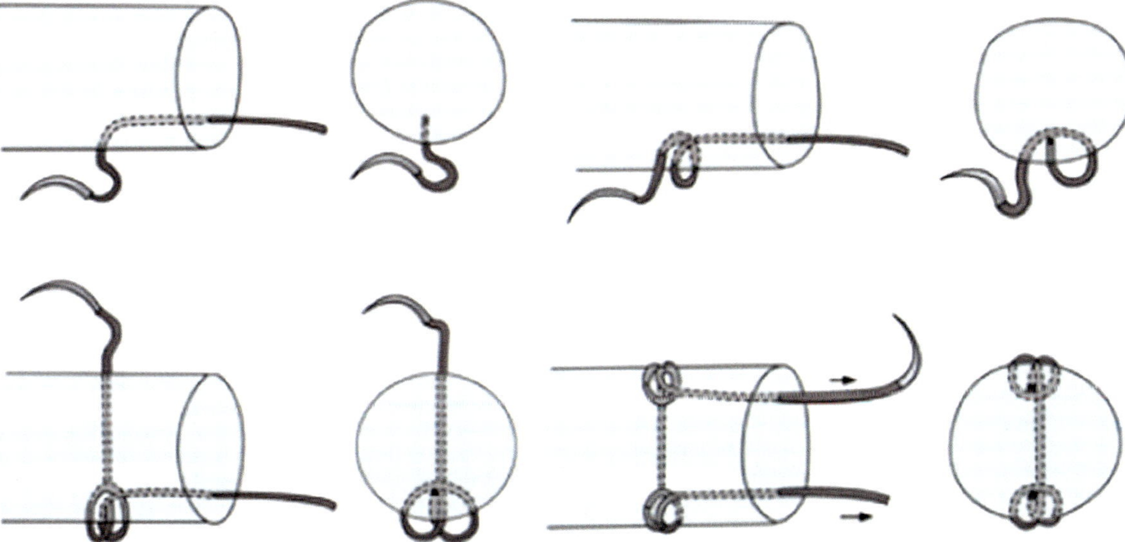

Fig. 7.16 Semi-knot locking stitching

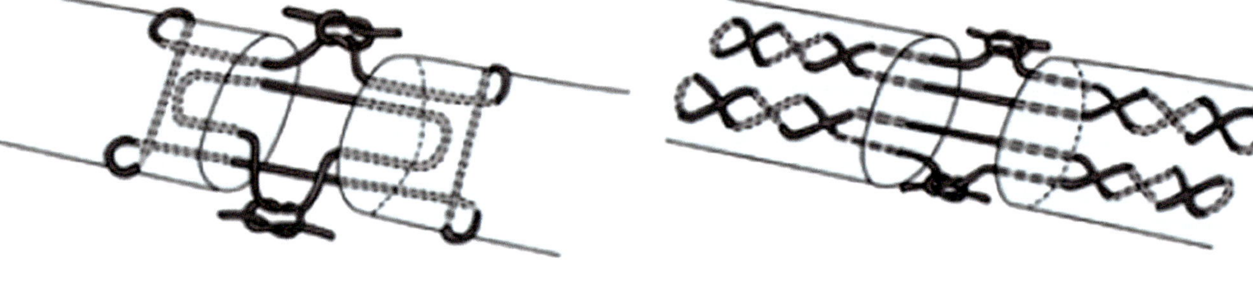

Fig. 7.17 Strickland stitching, MGH stitching

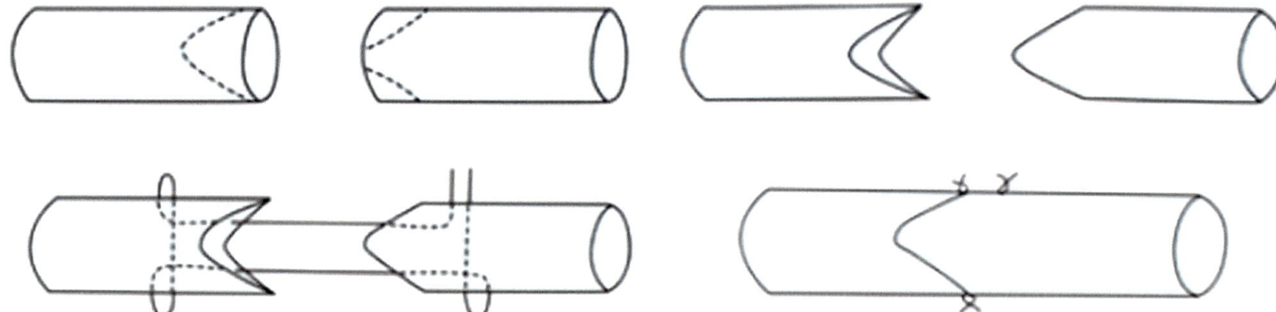

Fig. 7.18 Angular technique of interlocking

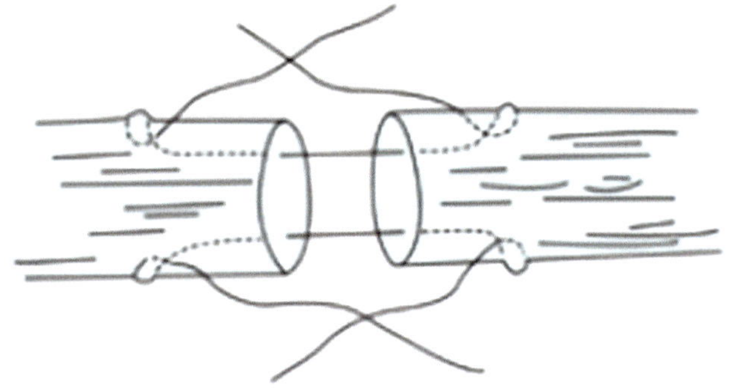

Fig. 7.19 Wilms stitching

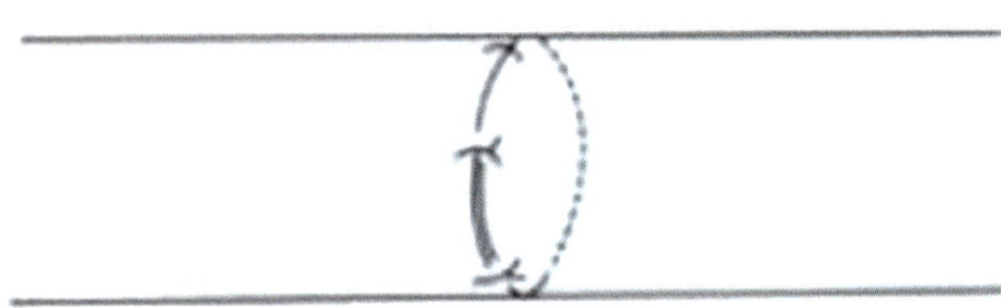

Fig. 7.20 Verden stitching

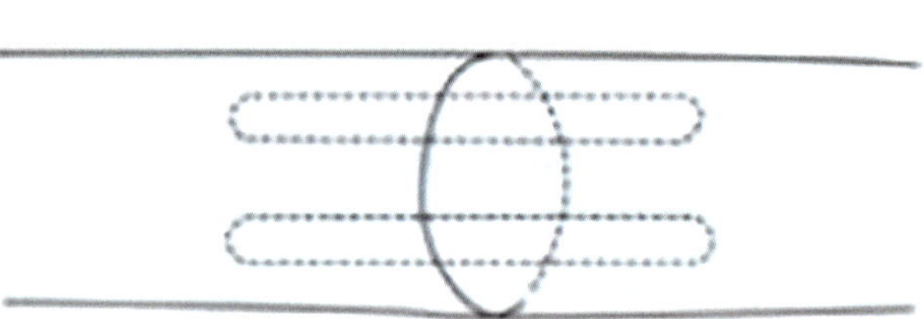

Fig. 7.21 Tajima stitching

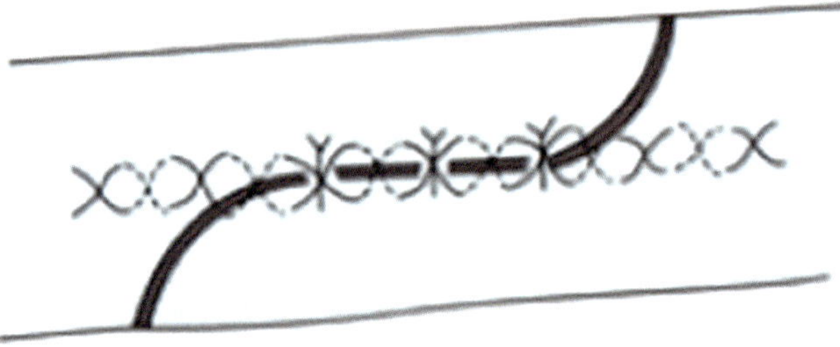

Fig. 7.22 D.Beden stitching

angular technique of interlocking (Fig. 7.18), Wilms stitching (Fig. 7.19), Verden stitching (Fig. 7.20), Tajima stitching (Fig. 7.21), D.Beden stitching (Fig. 7.22), Robertson stitching (Fig. 7.23), Running stitching (continuous peripheral, Fig. 7.24), Cross-stitch (Silfverskiold peripheral suturing, Fig. 7.25), Halsted stitching (peripheral suturing, Fig. 7.26), new peripheral technique (Fig. 7.27), central axis long distance buried stitching (steel wire, Fig. 7.28), central axis long distance buried stitching (Mersilk, Fig. 7.29).

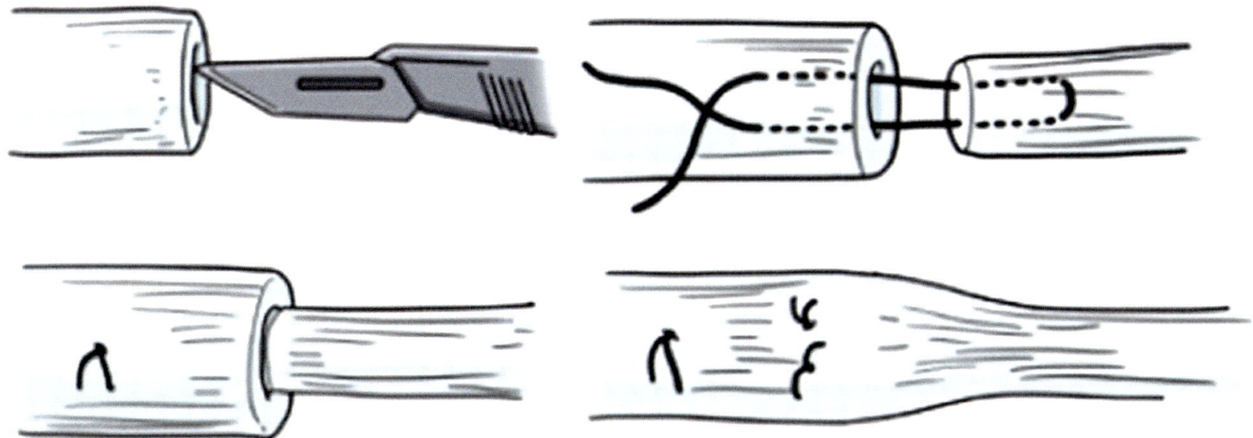

Fig. 7.23 Robertson stitching

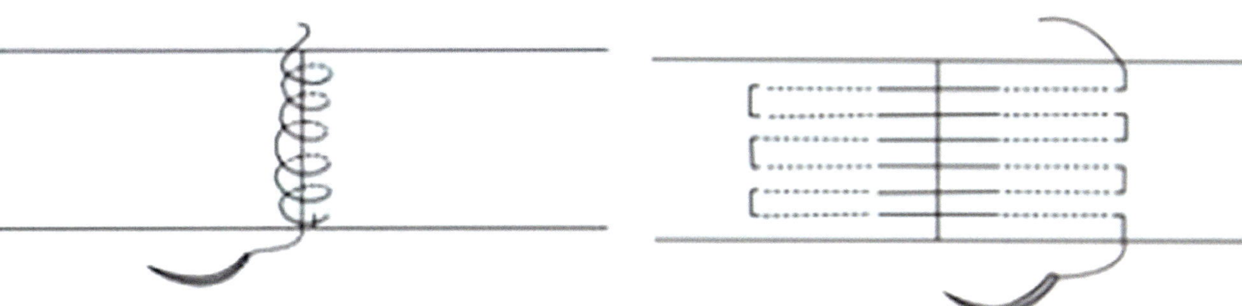

Fig. 7.24 Running stitching (continuous peripheral)

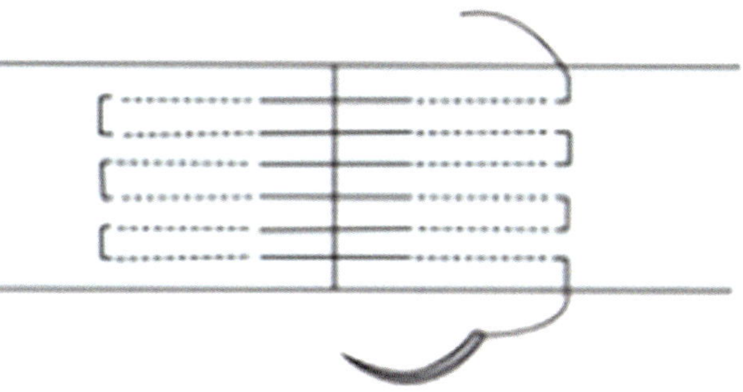

Fig. 7.26 Halsted stitching (peripheral suturing)

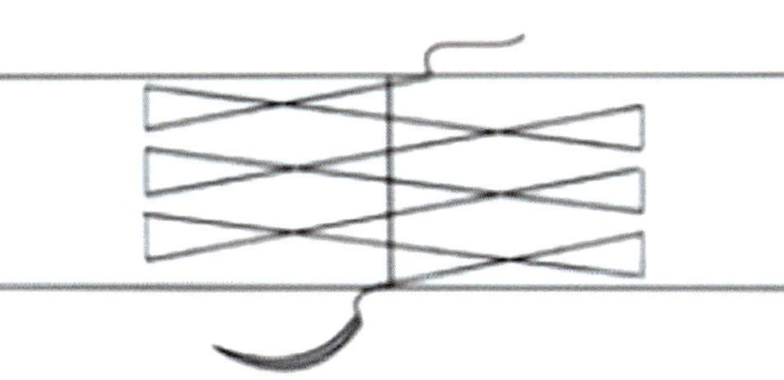

Fig. 7.25 Cross-stitch (Silfverskiold peripheral suturing)

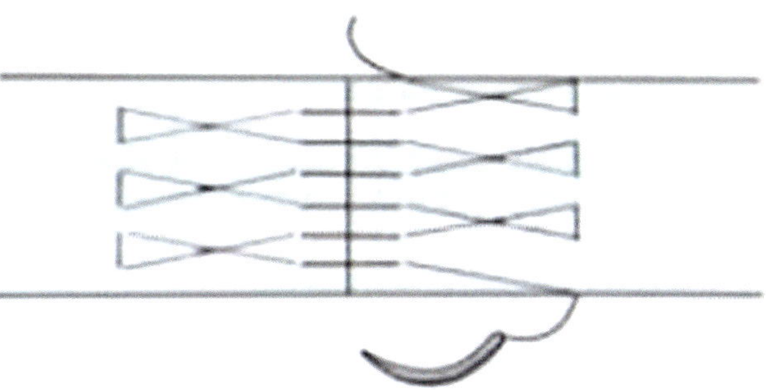

Fig. 7.27 New peripheral technique

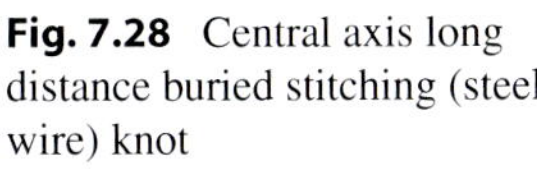

Fig. 7.28 Central axis long distance buried stitching (steel wire) knot

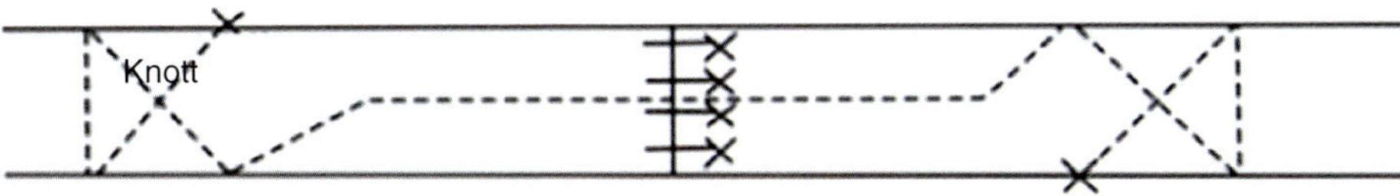

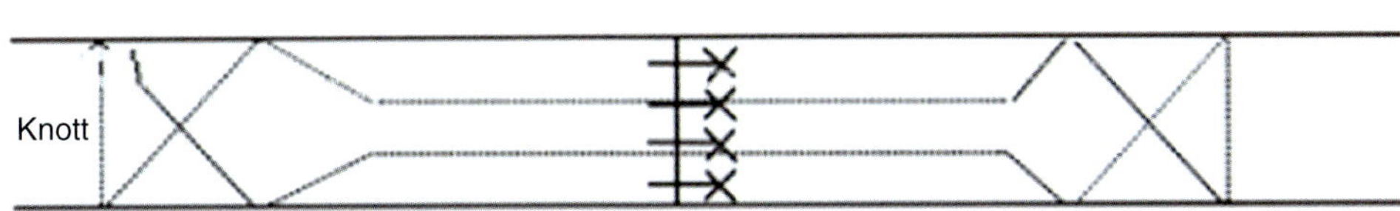

Fig. 7.29 Central axis long distance buried stitching (Mersilk)

7.6 Basic Tendon Suture Techniques for Hand Surgery

7.6.1 Bunnell Stitching

1. First clamp the tendon rupture end using hemostatic forceps, and pull it tight. At 1.5 cm from the rupture end, use the straight needle to cross the 3-0 polypropylene (PROLENE) bidirectional suture across the tendon (Fig. 7.30a).
2. Approximately 1 mm above the entry point, pass the two straight needles obliquely at 6 mm site (Fig. 7.30b).
3. Cut off the tendon rupture end with a blade approximately 5 mm to the exit point (Fig. 7.30c).
4. Insert the straight needle obliquely approximately 1 mm above the exit point, and pass through the tendon rupture end (Fig. 7.30d).
5. Tighten the suture passing through the tendon rupture end (Fig. 7.30e).

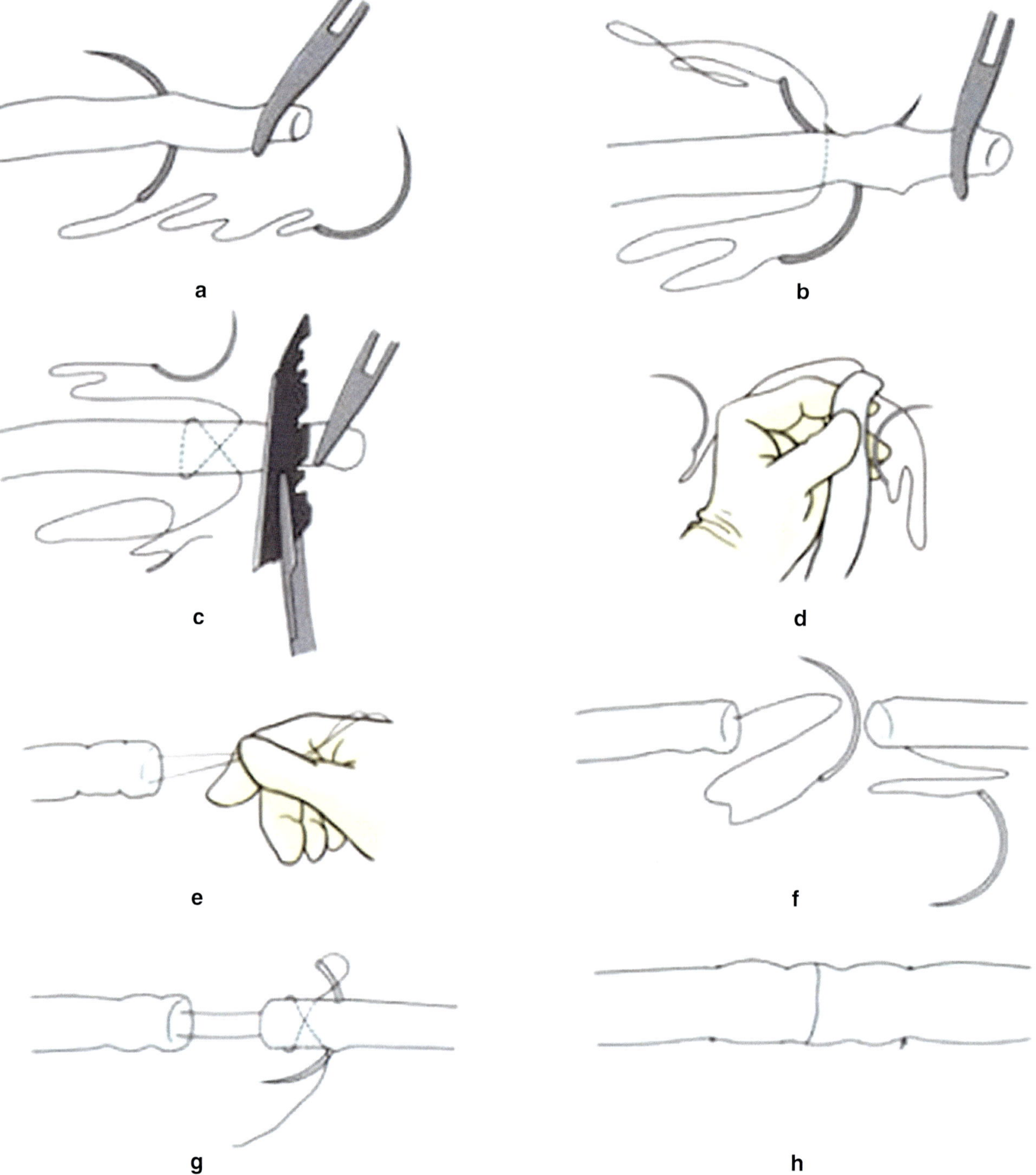

Fig. 7.30 Bunnell stitching

6. After trimming the other rupture end with a blade, pass the two straight needles obliquely from the rupture end to both sides 5 mm away from the rupture end (Fig. 7.30f).
7. Cross the two straight needles obliquely at 1 mm at the exit point and pass them out at 6 mm, and then pass the straight needles transversely 1 mm above the exit point (Fig. 7.30g).
8. Tighten the knot (Fig. 7.30h).

Comments:

1. The stitching is more reliable, unlike the simple tendon suture technique which is prone to split;
2. Less rough surface at the anastomotic site;
3. The technique is complicated and more invasive;
4. At present, it is used for the repair of flexor and extensor tendons in the forearm area, and is rarely used in repair for the tendons of fingers, palms, and wrists.

7.6.2 Modified Kessler Stitching

1. Fix both tendon ends with needles. Use a 3-0 polypropylene bidirectional suture (PROLENE), and firstly cross one end of the tendon at 8–10 mm to the end, then insert the double straight needle into the tendon slightly obliquely at 2–3 mm above the exit point, and pass through the tendon cross section after being parallel to the tendon.
2. Perform the procedure above on the other end of the tendon.
3. Bring the two rupture ends of the tendon together, tighten the suture and knot.
4. After core suturing of the tendon, make external continuous peripheral suturing around the anastomotic site at the rupture end with 5-0 or 6-0 monofilament (Fig. 7.31a–e).

Comments:

1. The operation is simpler, less invasive, and the blood supply in the tendon is less affected;
2. It is beneficial to early functional exercise, reducing postoperative tendon rupture and adhesion;
3. Simple Kessler stitching is prone to tear, but after continuous peripheral suturing around the anastomotic site at the rupture end, the tensile strength can be improved;
4. It can be used to repair flexor and extensor tendons in various zones.

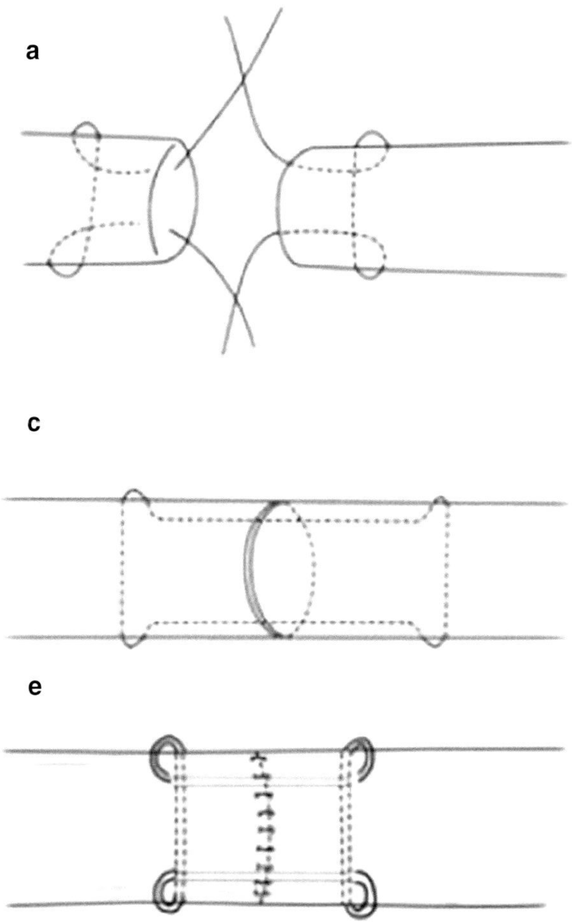

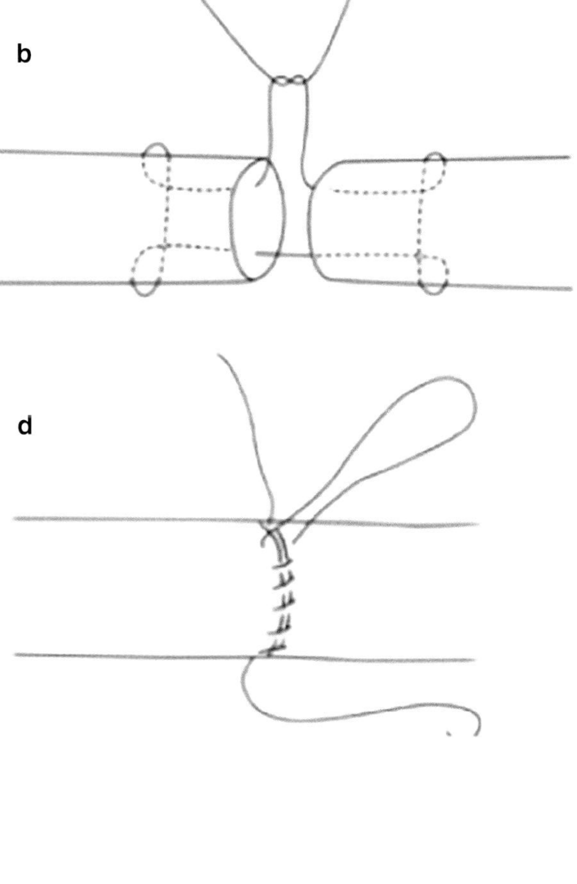

Fig. 7.31 Modified Kessler stitching

7.6.3 Tsuge Loop Stitching

Comments:

1. Using a special looped suture with needle is easy to operate and can suture in a small incision (Fig. 7.32);
2. There is less damage and the blood supply in the tendon is impacted less, and the tendon heals quickly;
3. Good and reliable matching of both rupture ends, with less and limited postoperative adhesion;
4. It can be used to repair flexor and extensor tendons in various zones.

7.6.4 Figure-of-8 Stitching and Double Cross Stitching

Comments:

1. Easy to operate (Fig. 7.33), and time saving, but with poor tensile strength;
2. Applicable only in emergency suturing.

7.6.5 Extensor Tendon Repair Technique

After core suturing of the tendon, make continuous peripheral suturing around the anastomotic site at the ruptured end (Fig. 7.34).

7.6.6 Fish Mouth Stitching

Comments:

1. It can be used for repairing the ruptured flexor tendons in forearm or palm;
2. It can be used in repairing with tendon transfer;
3. It is more applicable in suturing two ruptured ends in different sizes (Fig. 7.35).

7.6.7 Weaving Stitching (Fig. 7.36)

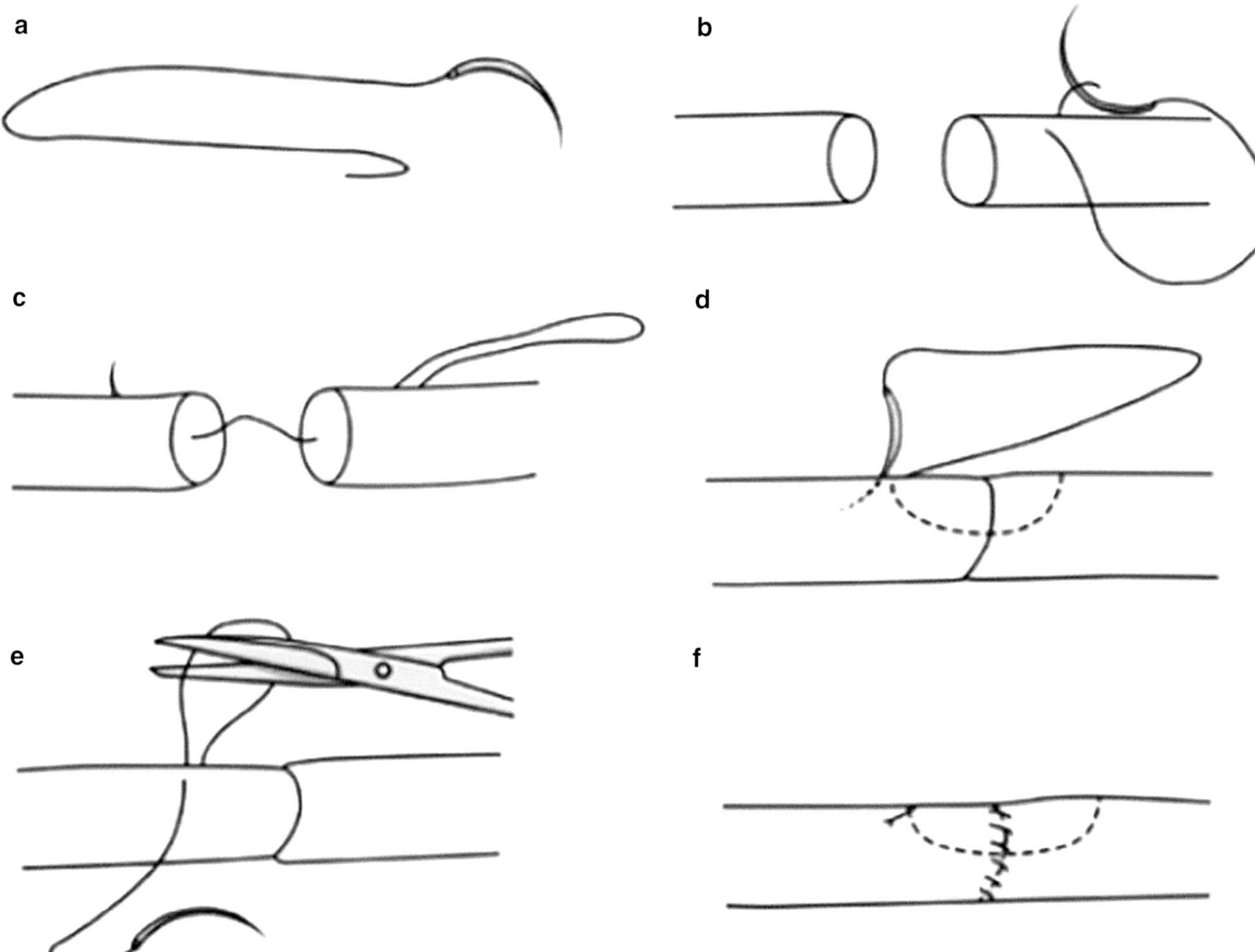

Fig. 7.32 Tsuge loop stitching

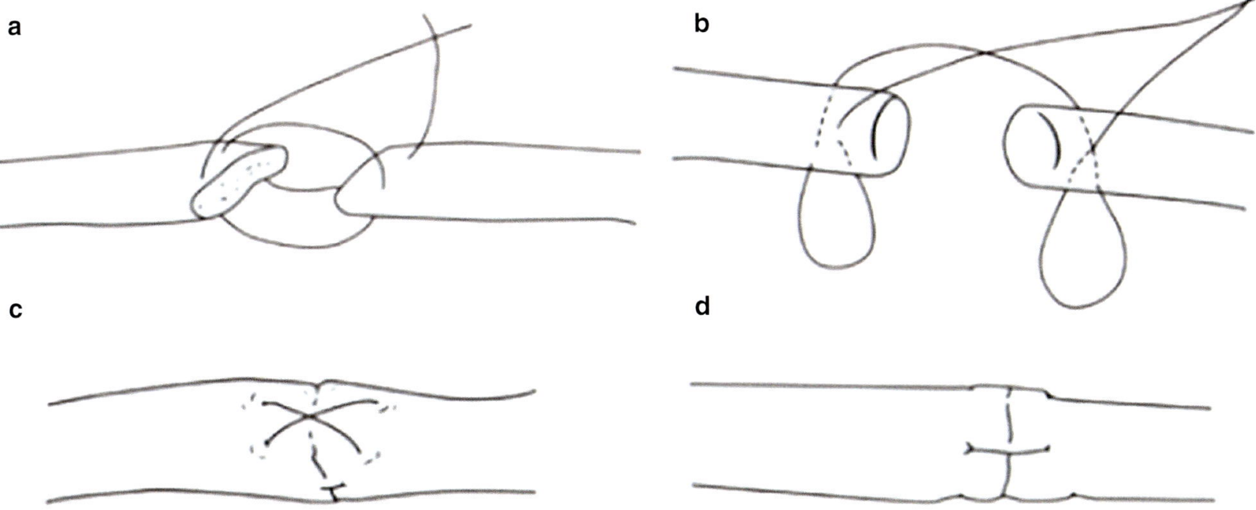

Fig. 7.33 Figure-of-8 stitching and double cross stitching

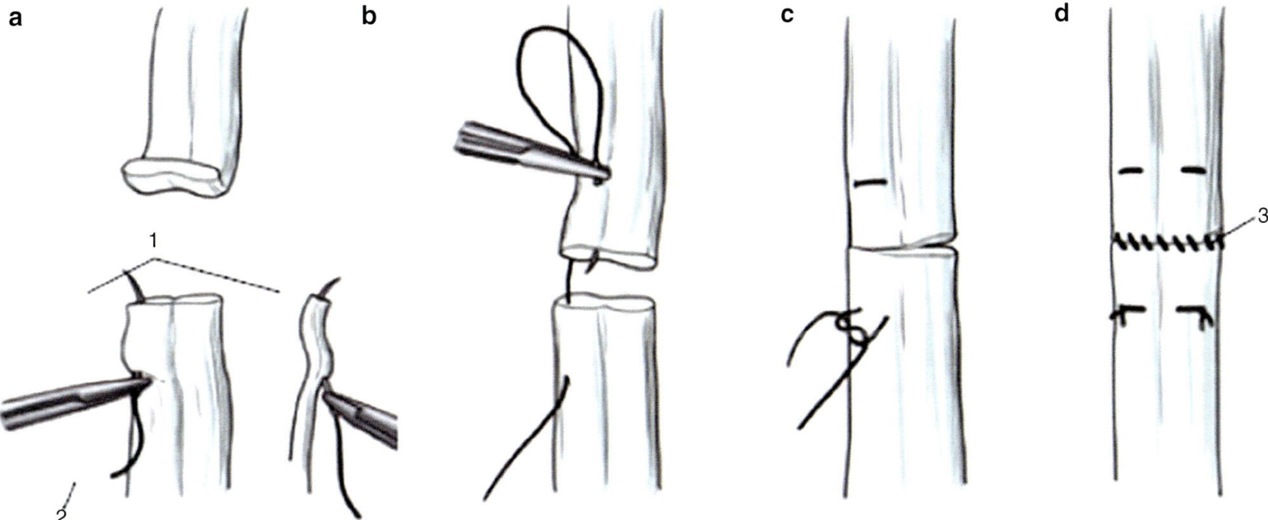

Fig. 7.34 Extensor tendon repair technique

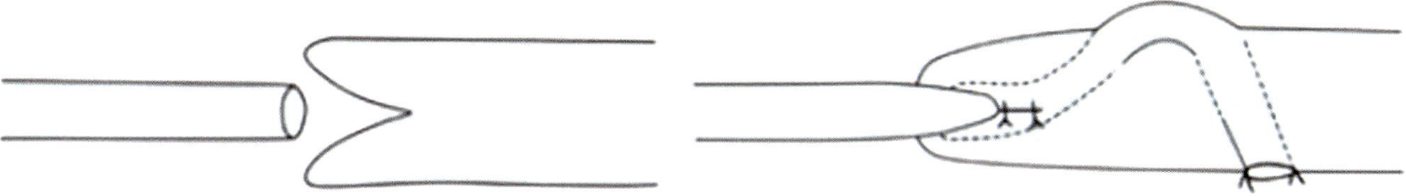

Fig. 7.35 Fish mouth stitching

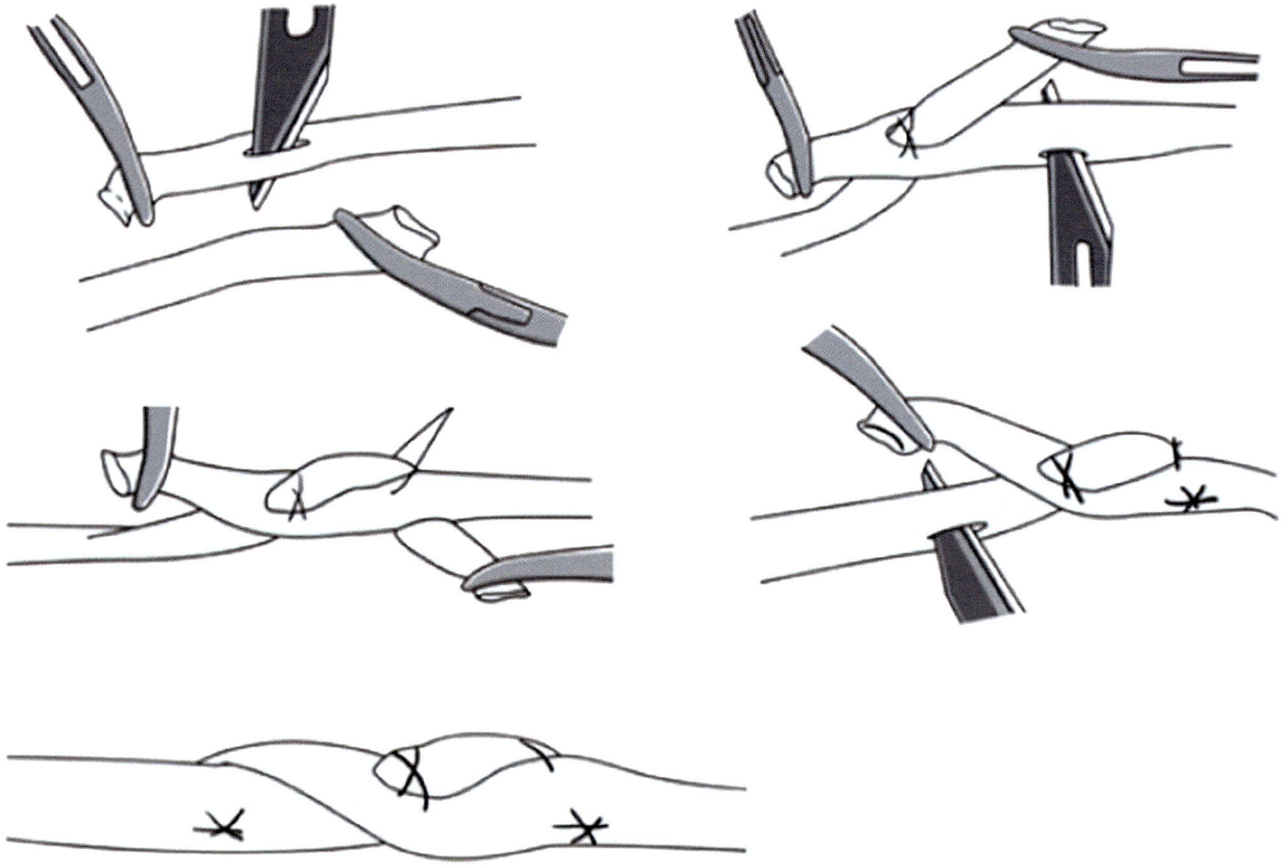

Fig. 7.36 Weaving stitching

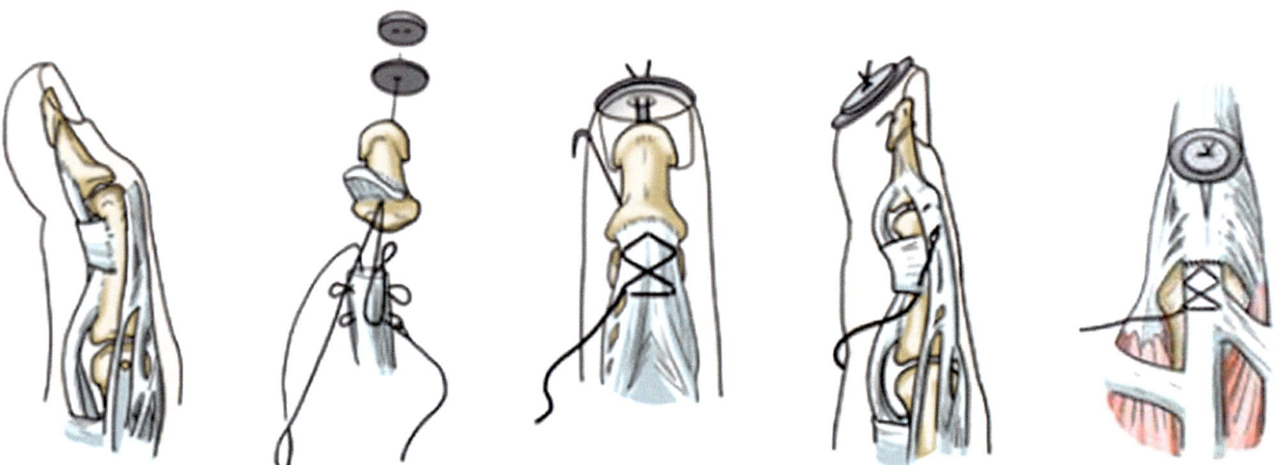

Fig. 7.37 Repair of extensor tendon insertion rupture

7.7 Common Repair Techniques for Tendon Rupture

7.7.1 Repair of Extensor Tendon Insertion Rupture (Fig. 7.37)

7.7.2 Repair of Middle Phalanx Level Extensor Tendon Rupture (Fig. 7.38)

7.7.3 Repair of Proximal Interphalangeal Joint Level Extensor Tendon Rupture (Fig. 7.39)

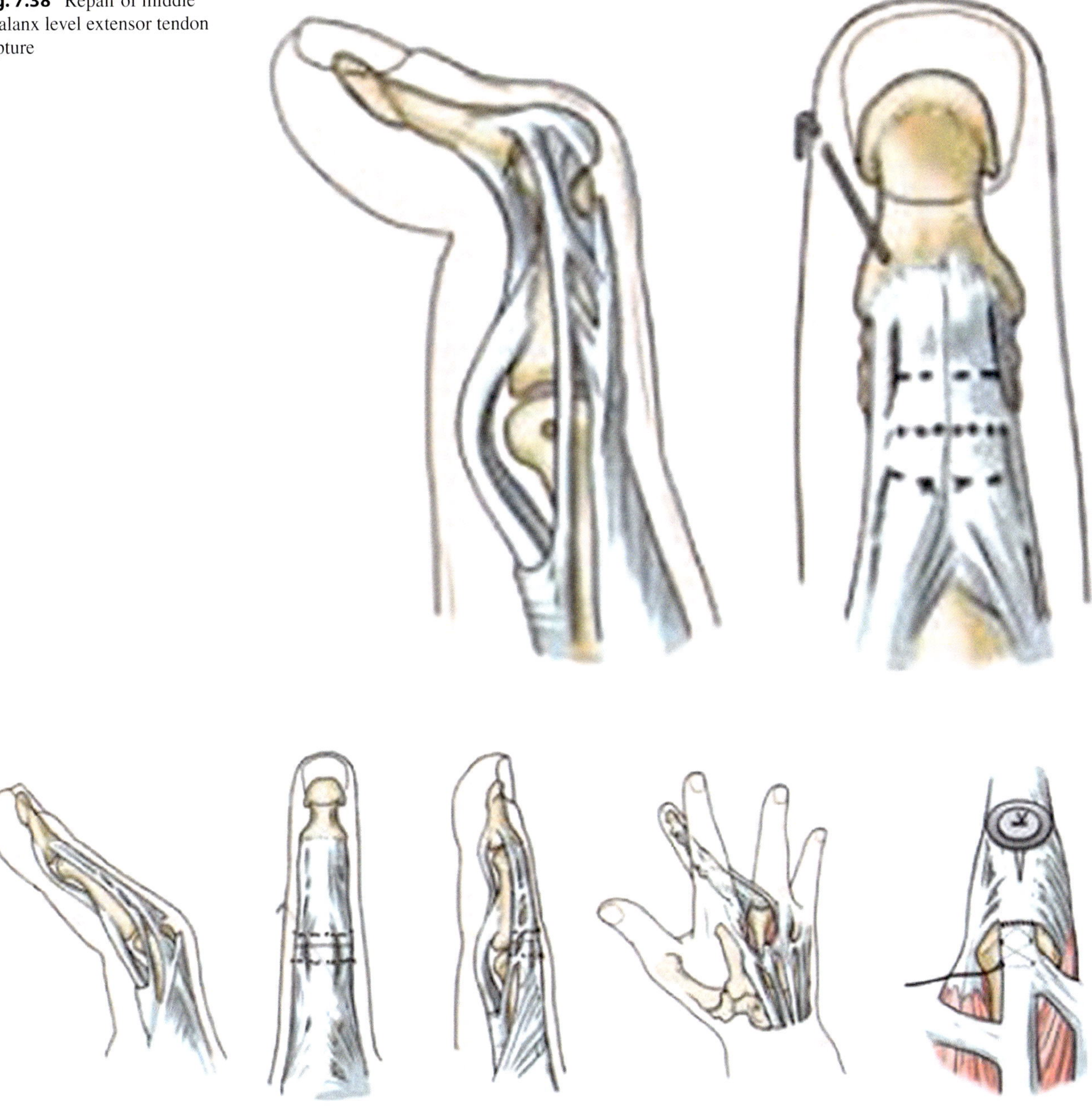

Fig. 7.38 Repair of middle phalanx level extensor tendon rupture

Fig. 7.39 Repair of proximal interphalangeal joint level extensor tendon rupture

7.7.4 Repair of Metacarpophalangeal Level Extensor Tendon Rupture (Fig. 7.40)

7.7.5 Repair of Flexor Tendon Insertion (Zone I Dp1) Rupture (Fig. 7.41)

7.7.6 Repair of Middle Phalanx Level Flexor Tendon Insertion (Zone II Dp2) Rupture (Fig. 7.42)

7.7.7 Repair of Proximal Phalanx Level Flexor Tendon Insertion (Zone II Dp2) Rupture (Fig. 7.43)

7.7.8 Repair of Palm Level Flexor Tendon Insertion (Zone III Dp3) Rupture (Fig. 7.44)

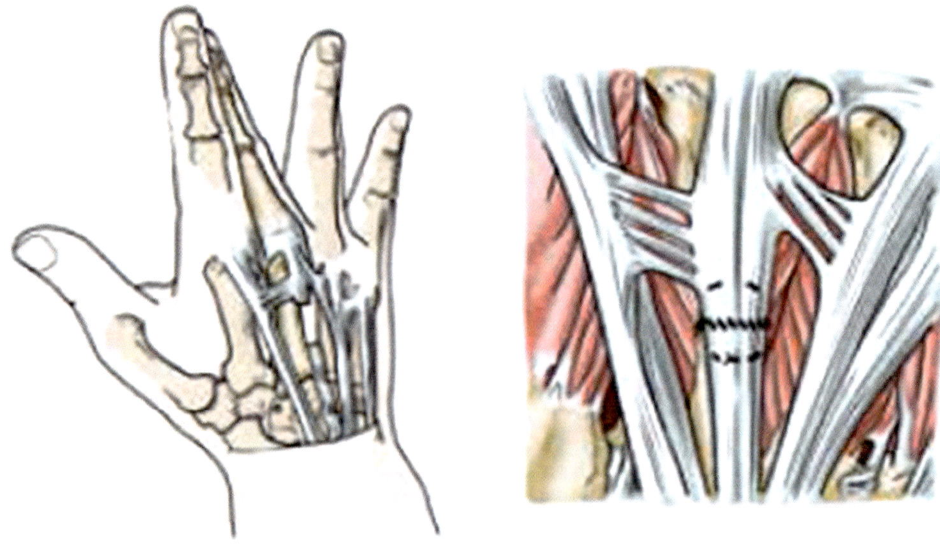

Fig. 7.40 Repair of metacarpophalangeal level extensor tendon rupture

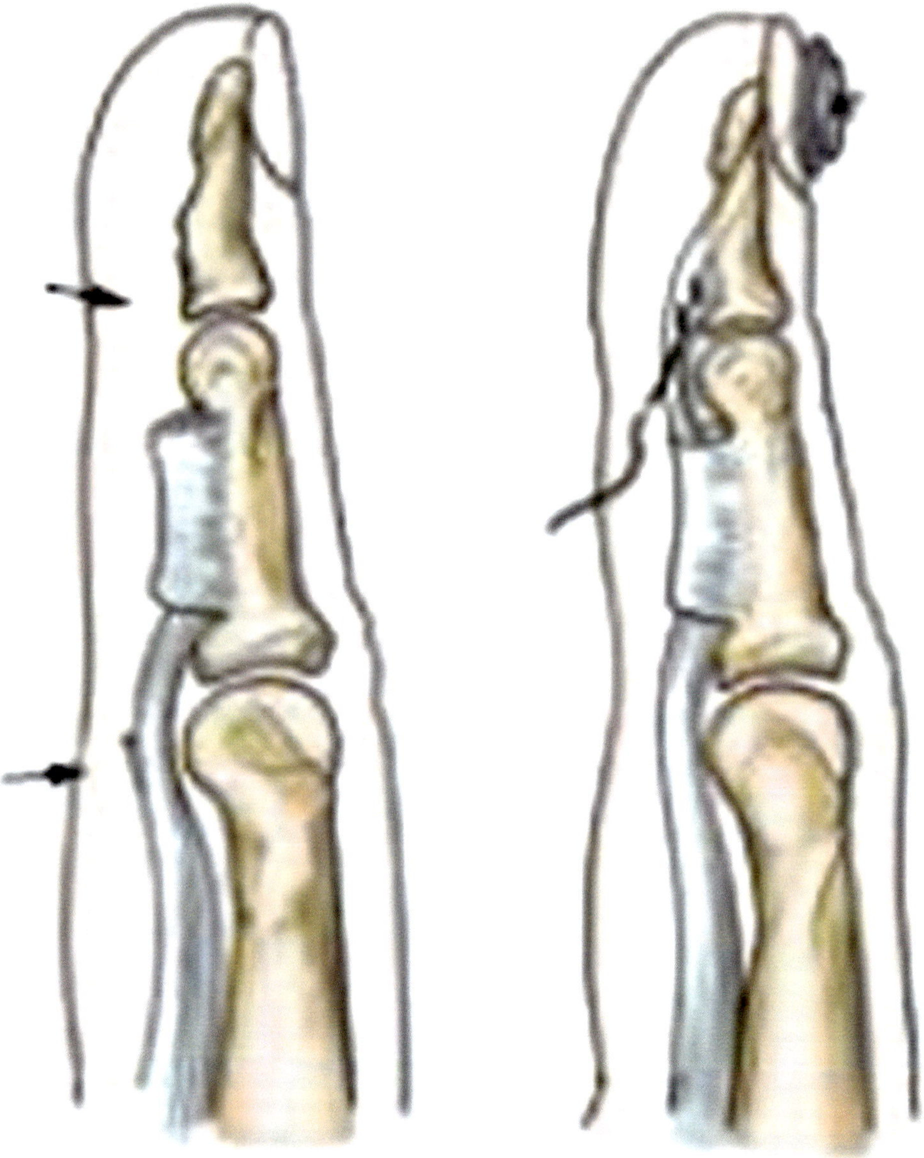

Fig. 7.41 Repair of flexor tendon insertion (zone I Dp1) rupture

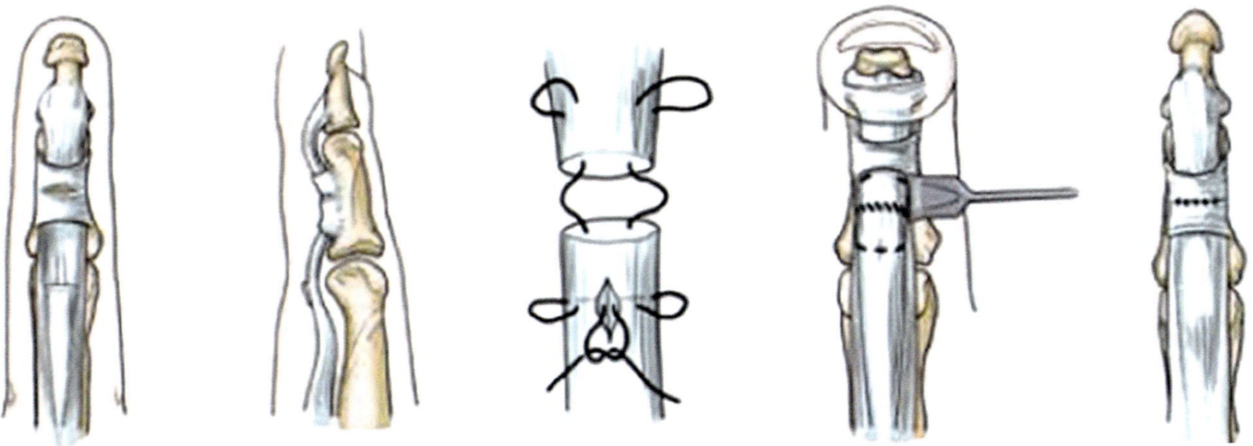

Fig. 7.42 Repair of middle phalanx plane flexor tendon insertion (zone II Dp2) rupture

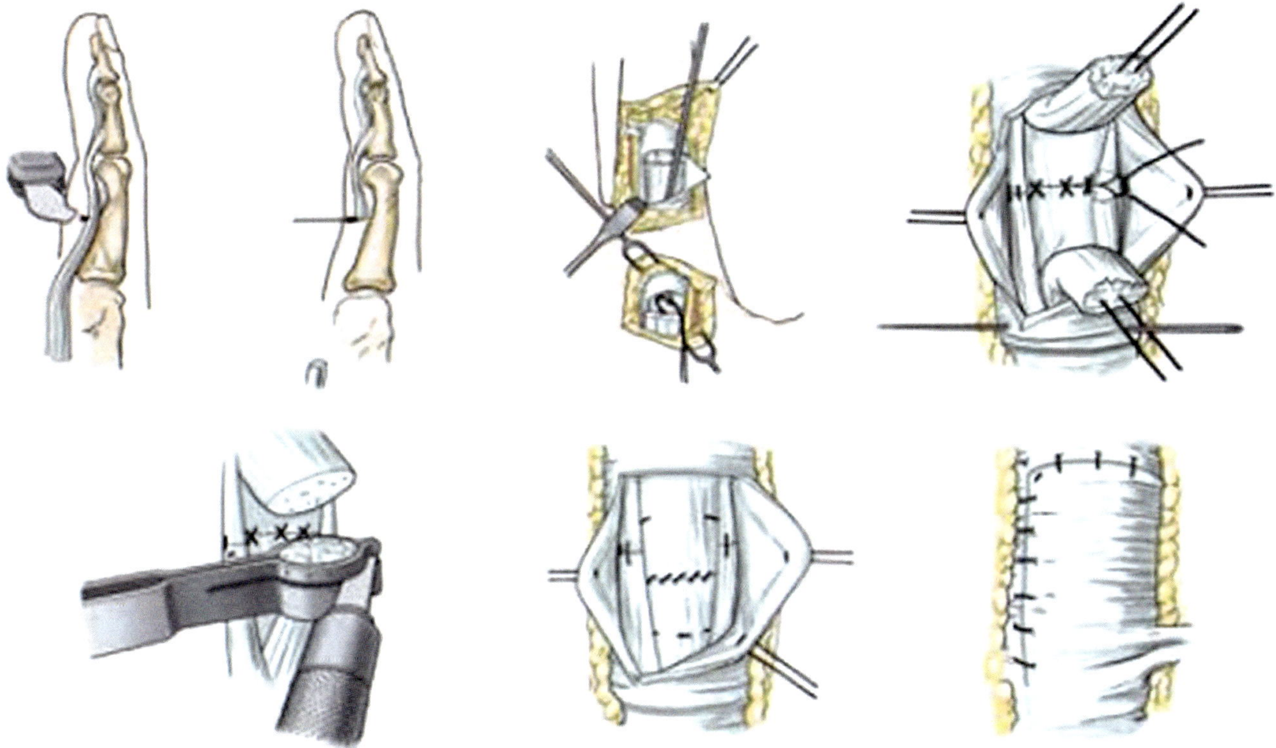

Fig. 7.43 Repair of proximal phalanx level flexor tendon insertion (zone II Dp2) rupture

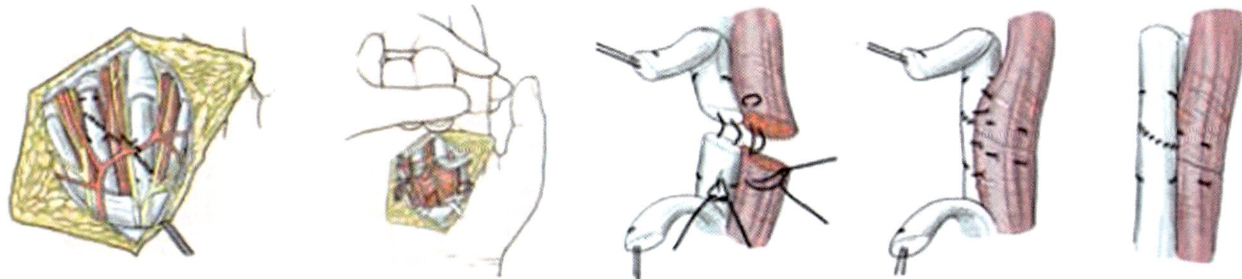

Fig. 7.44 Repair of palm level flexor tendon insertion (zone III Dp3) rupture

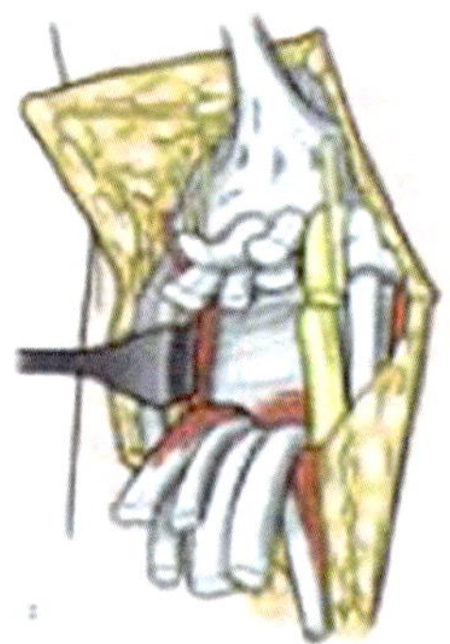
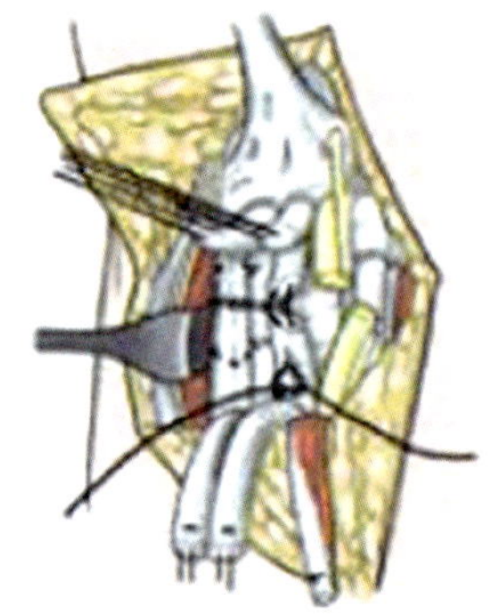
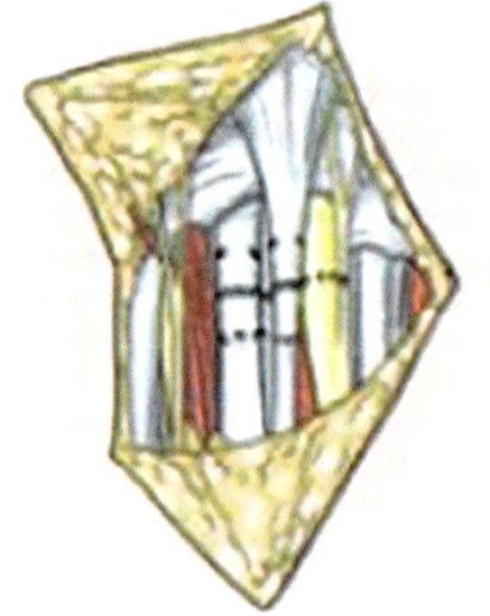
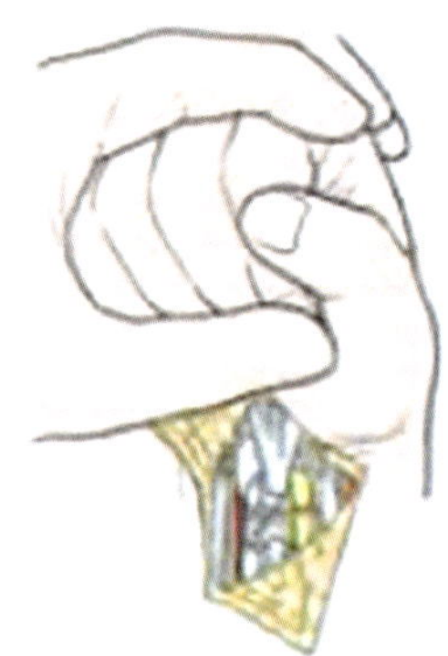

Fig. 7.45 Repair of wrist level flexor tendon insertion (zone IV Dp4) rupture

7.7.9 Repair of Wrist Level Flexor Tendon Insertion (Zone IV Dp4) Rupture (Fig. 7.45)

7.8 Early Rehabilitation after Tendon Repair

A healed tendon does not mean a functional tendon. If we need a tendon function well, the tendon needs to be able to slide in the body without resistance. Tendon adhesion is inevitable during tendon healing, which prevents the tendon from sliding. Rehabilitation training is to release the scar adhesion band with hand activities, restore the sliding property of the tendon, and transmit the muscle contraction force. The time to start rehabilitation exercise should be appropriate. After starting the rehabilitation exercise, patients should follow the medical order, and improve step by step. If rehabilitation exercise starts too early or too aggressive, as the tendon rupture ends have not been healed, the probability of tendon rupture increases. If it starts too late or too conservatively, the tendon adhesion scar band will turn harder and larger, making it hard to be released.

After suturing, tendon should be fixed for 3 to 4 weeks until it is healed. Then, remove the fixation to allow exercise for function restoration, accompanied with physical therapy. In the recent two decades, it is believed that early activity after tendon suture is beneficial to reduce adhesion and help to functional restoration. It is recommended to fix the affected finger in the flexion position with a rubber band after repairing the flexor tendon rupture, using active finger extension and passive flexion of the fingers with protective passive exercise early after the surgery. But it should be performed under the guidance of experienced physicians; otherwise, it may cause tendon rupture. Therefore, recent studies have shown that the combination of using tendon suture with good tensile strength and tendon stitching during the surgery, and the combination with active and passive postoperative exercise could improve the repair effect and reduce the risk of rupture [19–21].

7.9 Summary of Hand Surgery Tendon Repair

Try to repair hand tendon rupture at one stage. Commonly used repair techniques include modified Kessler stitching, Bunnell stitching, Tsuge loop stitching, etc. The surgery requires non-invasive repair; the suturing materials should have good tensile strength, less damage to the tendon, and can ensure active postoperative activities, such as monofilament non-absorbable polypropylene suture (PROLENE), which is smooth, has less damage, and less tissue reaction. Multifilament braided non-absorbable polyester suture (ETHIBOND), which has the characteristics of firm knotting and less tissue reaction. Both kinds are suitable for tendon suture; early postoperative exercise is necessary with combination of active and passive exercise, or mainly in active exercises, so as to maximize the restoration of hand joint function. The main issues for tendon repair: one is to prevent tendon adhesion, and the other is to prevent tendon rupture.

Search Terms
Hand surgery, Tendon injury, Suturing and repair

References

1. Newmeyer WL 3rd. Sterling Bunnell, MD: the founding father. J Hand Surg Am. 2003;28(1):161–4.
2. Verdan CE. Primary repair of flexor tendons. J Bone Joint Surg Am. 1960;42A:647–57.

3. Kleinert HE, Sister SA. Emergency hand operations. AORN J. 1965;3(5):53–66.
4. Belusa M, Schmickaly J. Primary flexor tendon suture in the "no man's land" of the hand. Zentralbl Chir. 1984;109(22):1441–50. German
5. Savage R. Strength of various suture techniques. J Hand Surg Br. 1992;17(6):705.
6. Silfverskiöld KL, May EJ. Flexor tendon repair in zone II with a new suture technique and an early mobilization program combining passive and active flexion. J Hand Surg Am. 1994;19(1):53–60.
7. Silfverskiöld KL, May EJ. Early active mobilization after tendon transfers using mesh reinforced suture techniques. Hand Surg Br. 1995;20(3):291–300.
8. Tang JB, Shi D. Subdivisions of "no man's land" of the digital flexor tendons and different management of tendon injuries in subdivisions. Chin J Surg. 1991;29(10):608–11.
9. Tang JB, Shi D, Gu YQ, Chen JC, Zhou B. Double and multiple looped suture tendon repair. J Hand Surg Br. 1994;19(6):699–703.
10. Elliot D, Barbieri CH, Evans RB, Mass D, Tang JB. IFSSH flexor tendon committee report 2007. J Hand Surg Eur Vol. 2007;32(3):346–56.
11. Verdan CE. Primary repair of flexor tendons. J Bone Joint Surg Am. 1960;42:647–57.
12. Verdan C. Basic principles in surgery of the hand. Surg Clin North Am. 1967;47(2):355–77.
13. Matthews P, Richards H. The repair potential of digital flexor tendons. An experimental study. J Bone Joint Surg Br. 1974;56(4):618–25.
14. From Dr. Sterling Bunnell, Secaucus, New Jersey. Cal State J Med. 1918;16(4):218–9.
15. Wang B, Tang JB. Increased suture embedment in tendons: an effective method to improve repair strength. J Hand Surg Br. 2002;27(4):333–6.
16. Cao Y, Xie RG, Tang JB. Dorsal-enhanced sutures improve tension resistance of tendon repair. J Hand Surg Br. 2002;27(2):161–4.
17. Tang JB, Chang J, Elliot D, Lalonde DH, Sandow M, Vögelin E. IFSSH flexor tendon committee report 2014: from the IFSSH flexor tendon committee. J Hand Surg Eur. 2014;39(1):107–15.
18. Wu YF, Tang JB. Recent developments in flexor tendon repair techniques and factors influencing strength of the tendon repair. J Hand Surg Eur. 2014;39(1):6–19.
19. Tang JB. Flexor tendon injuries. Clin Plast Surg. 2019;46(3):295–306.
20. Mehling IM, Arsalan-Werner A, Sauerbier M. Evidence-based flexor tendon repair. Clin Plast Surg. 2014;41(3):513–23.
21. Hundozi H, Murtezani A, Hysenaj V, Hysenaj V, Mustafa A. Rehabilitation after surgery repair of flexor tendon injuries of the hand with Kleinert early passive mobilization protocol. Med Arch. 2013;67(2):115–9.

8 Achilles Tendon Rupture Suture Techniques

Hua Chen and Hongzhe Qi

Abstract

It is always a controversial topic whether closed complete Achilles tendon rupture is repaired surgically. Some scholars believe that conservative treatment can reduce the risk of surgical incision infection; other scholars insist on recommending surgical treatment, and think that accurate suturing of ruptured Achilles tendon can increase the plantar flexion strength of Achilles tendon after surgery, and the optimization of surgical protocol can reduce the occurrence of surgical complications. The suggestions from Orthopedics Department of Chinese PLA General Hospital (301 Hospital) on closed Achilles tendon rupture are that young people need to recover motor function and should receive active surgical treatment; however, for the elderly with few activities, most of them suffer from diabetes, hypertension and other comorbidities, so conservative treatment is recommended. For the acute Achilles tendon rupture, the rupture ends are in horsetail shape, the defect of proximal retraction end is about 3 cm. With the plantar flexion of the ankle joint, the Achilles tendon rupture ends can touch each other and end-to-end suture could be made, such as the Krackow technique, Bunnell technique, and end-to-end modified Kessler suture augmented with interrupted suturing; the special device invented by our hospital is also particularly recommended, which realizes channel-assisted minimally invasive repair of acute Achilles tendon rupture, effectively avoids sural nerve injury and provides sufficient effective mechanical support, the surgery time is only 15–20 min, and the incision is only 1.5–2 cm. Subacute injury, Achilles tendon ruptured for more than 10 days, Achilles tendon contracture often reaches 3–6 cm, rupture ends degenerated with non-severe necrosis, and plantar flexion of the ankle joint alone cannot achieve end-to-end contact of the Achilles tendon rupture ends. Abraham V-Y suture technique is recommended. Old injury, Achilles tendon ruptured for more than 3 weeks; at this time, Achilles tendon contracture always exceeds 6 cm. It is recommended to use the Lindholm technique (gastrocnemius aponeurosis turndown flap) to repair the defect of the Achilles tendon rupture ends. If the strength of the Achilles tendon after suturing and repair is found to be insufficient during the surgery, the following methods can be used to strengthen the Achilles tendon, such as White Krynick technique, Rugg and Bogoe technique, simple plantaris reinforcement, use of peroneal brevis and artificial materials to repair, fascia lata transplantation, and other suturing techniques. However, for Achilles tendon rupture with defects of the calcaneus and skin, suggestions are as follows: ① Transposition of the pedicled tendon to repair Achilles tendon defects; ②Transposition of vascularized tissue flap to repair Achilles tendon defect; ③Free transplantation of vascularized composite tissue flap to repair Achilles tendon defect. For selection of sutures, it is recommended to use nonabsorbable 2# ETHIBOND (Polyester, ETHICON) for Achilles tendon suturing, absorbable 2-0, 3-0 VICRYL® Plus Control Release Suture (Polyglactin 910, ETHICON) for interrupted reinforced suturing, absorbable 0# VICRYL® Plus Control Release Suture (Polyglactin 910, ETHICON) for deep fascia suturing, absorbable 3-0 VICRYL® Plus Control Release Suture (Polyglactin 910, ETHICON) for subcutaneous suturing, and nonabsorbable 3-0, 4-0 PROLENE Suture (Polypropylene, ETHICON) for skin suturing.

Keywords

Achilles tendon rupture · Suture repair · Minimally invasive · Functional exercise

H. Chen (✉)
Department of Orthopedics, The First Medical Center of PLA General Hospital, Beijing, China

H. Qi
PLA Strategic Support Force Characteristic Medical Center, Beijing, China

P. Tang et al. (eds.), *Tutorials in Suturing Techniques for Orthopedics*, https://doi.org/10.1007/978-981-33-6330-4_8

8.1 Overview

The incidence of Achilles tendon rupture is 18/100,000, and there is an increasing trend, especially with the development of national sports. Achilles tendon rupture of many sports stars has made this sports injury a household name. Most of the onsets are related to excessive strain. The ankle is injured by sudden force in the hyperextension position, and the rupture usually occurs 4–6 cm above the insertion of the Achilles tendon.

Surgical incision and suture is the current standard surgical procedure for repairing Achilles tendon rupture, and it has good clinical results. However, the incidence of complications such as wound infection, wound dehiscence, and even Achilles tendon exposure (Fig. 8.1) is high. The attempt of percutaneous minimally invasive repair of Achilles tendon and the follow-up results have brought new hope to patients with small injury, and low re-rupture rate. Most importantly, the incidence of wound complications is greatly reduced, which is close to conservative treatment. However, iatrogenic sural nerve injury and concerns about suture strength are the biggest challenges. Domestic hospitals have explored and tried minimally invasive repair techniques, and many new techniques have been produced.

In addition, the series of problems caused by the use of local hormones and local injection therapy to treat Achilles tendonitis has gradually attracted the attention of surgeons. After local use of hormones, it causes inflammatory damage to small blood vessels around the Achilles tendon, increases vascular permeability, triggers intravascular coagulation, affects blood circulation around the Achilles tendon, and causes degenerative disease of the Achilles tendon, with increased fragility, weakened elasticity, and load reduced. Therefore, after local use of hormones, tendon load is impaired, and Achilles tendon rupture is prone to occur. For inflammation around the Achilles tendon that could be treated by general physical therapy, try not to use invasive treatment (local injection therapy). Even for the pain point injection, the indications and drug concentration should be strictly controlled, and weight-bearing activities should be avoided after treatment. Special care should be taken for its surgical treatment; otherwise, it is prone to have skin incision issues, Achilles tendon exposure, prolonged hospital stay, and increased treatment cost; for such patients, minimally invasive treatment has brought much greater benefits.

8.2 Anatomy of Achilles Tendon Injury

The Achilles tendon is the most robust and largest tendon in the human body. It is about 15.0 cm long. It starts from the middle 1/3 of the calf and ends at the calcaneal tubercle. The Achilles tendon gradually narrows and thickens from top to bottom, and the narrowest part is 4–6 cm above the calcaneal tubercle. The insertion is under the skin, above which in front of the Achilles tendon located the retrocalcaneal bursa, and behind the Achilles tendon, the subcutaneous bursa (Fig. 8.2).

There is no tendon sheath around the Achilles tendon, only loose mesh tissue (peritendinous tissue); the peritendinous tissue connects the tendon with its surrounding fascia. The blood vessels inside supply nutrition to the Achilles tendon. There are 7–8 lubricating layers on the back of the Achilles tendon, there are independent nutritional blood vessels between each layer, and there are blood vessels passing between layers; when the ankle joint is active, there may be movement between layers (Fig. 8.3).

The nutrition artery distribution of the Achilles tendon shows that the lower part of the area has relatively less blood supply. The number of blood vessels in the Achilles tendon

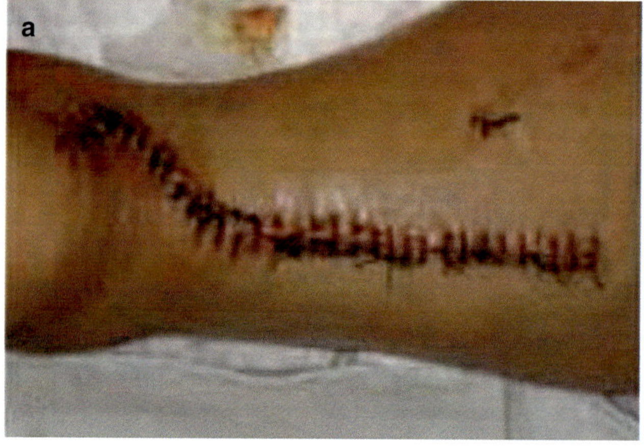

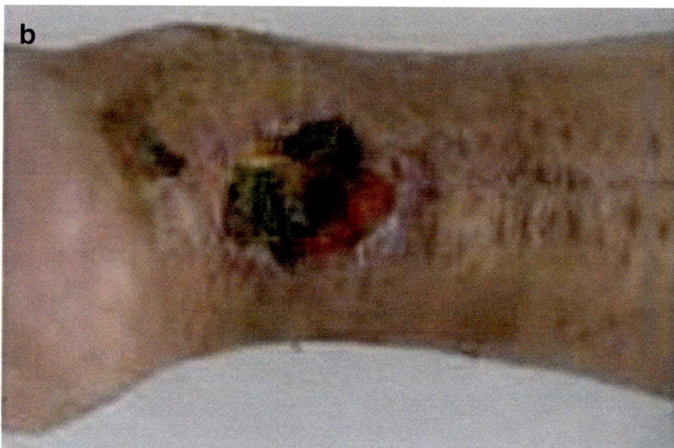

Fig. 8.1 Open repair of acute Achilles tendon rupture. (**a**) The incision is about 15 cm long. There are many patients with incision healing issues (including superficial infection or deep infection), and the incidence of clinical incision issues is as high as 34.1%. (**b**) This patient had incision skin necrosis and Achilles tendon exposure

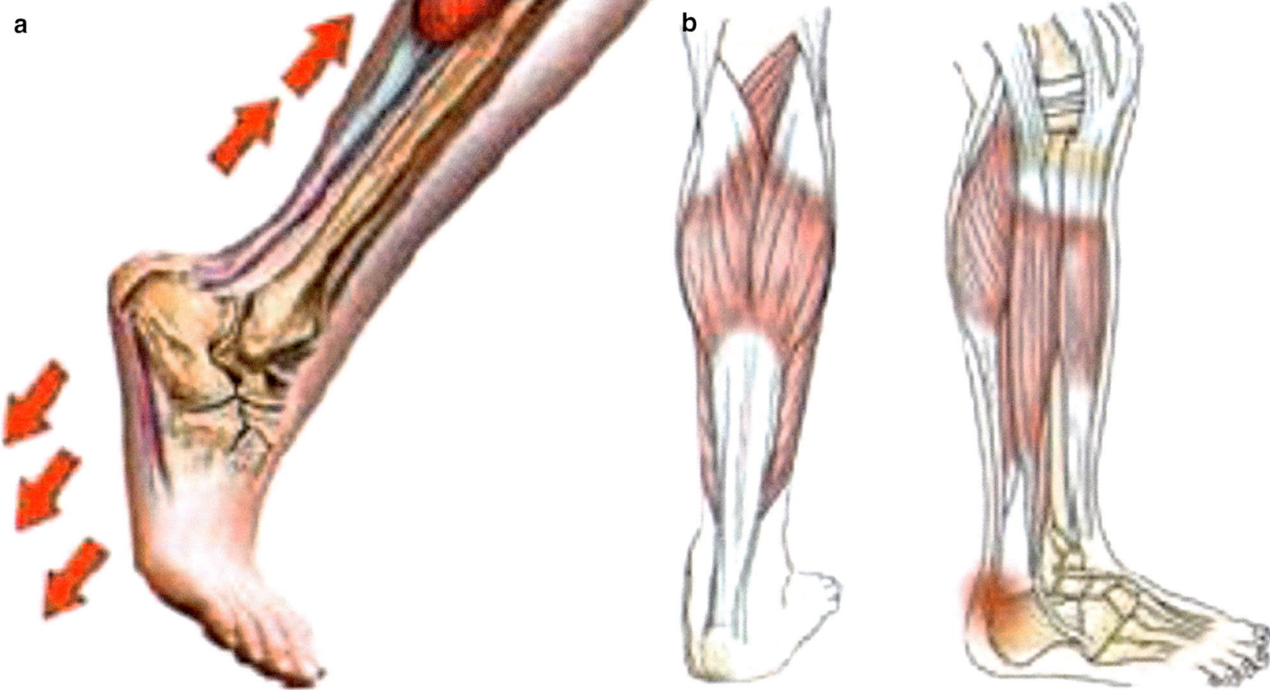

Fig. 8.2 Achilles tendon. (**a**) The function of the Achilles tendon; (**b**) The rupture site of the Achilles tendon is 4–6 cm above the insertion of the Achilles tendon

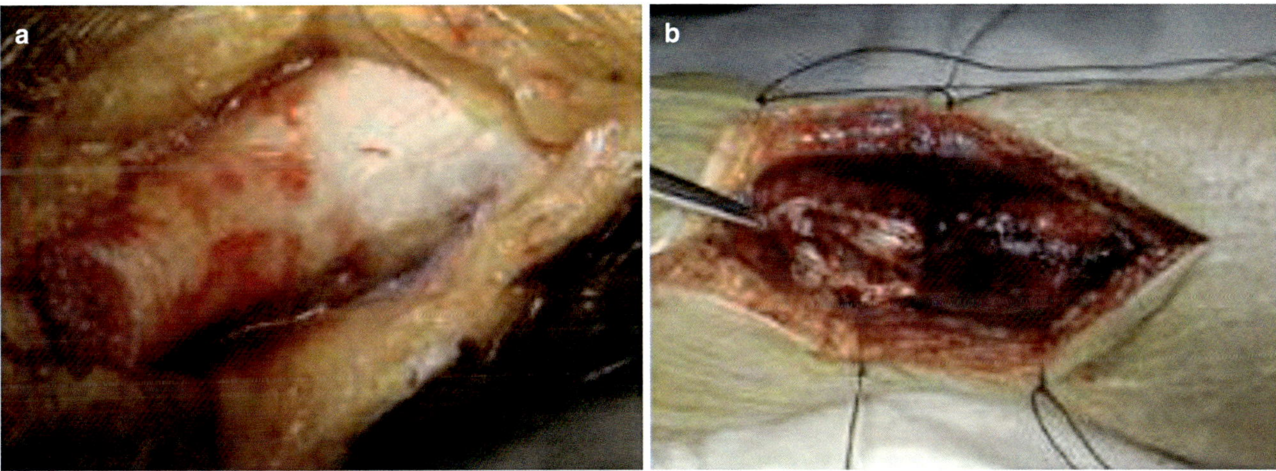

Fig. 8.3 Source of blood supply. (**a**) The peritendinous tissue around the Achilles tendon is transparent, and the Achilles tendon can be seen clearly. There are longitudinal blood vessels inside the peritendinous tissue, which is different from the tendon sheath of hand tendon; (**b**) After the Achilles tendon is ruptured, the peritendinous tissue is injured with congestion and swelling, like "snot" (must be protected and repaired during the surgery, and should not be resected)

gradually decreases with age. The blood supply of the Achilles tendon comes from two main arterial sources, namely the tibial artery and the peroneal artery. The deep and superficial branches of the medial Achilles tendon artery and the deep longitudinal branch of the Achilles tendon artery come from the tibial artery. The former nourishes the Achilles tendon from the medial side, from top to bottom; the latter runs through the entire Achilles tendon and is the most important nutritional artery for the Achilles tendon. The outer upper and lower arteries of the Achilles tendon come from the peroneal artery, and nourish the Achilles tendon from the lateral side. The abovementioned arteries form an arterial network between the outer and inner membranes of the Achilles tendon. Stein et al. also confirmed by radionuclide scans that there are fewer blood vessels visualized in the part 4–6 cm above the insertion of the Achilles tendon.

A. The blood supply of the Achilles tendon comes from the attachment point of the tendon, peritendinous tissue, and gastrocnemius; B. Intravascular injection of barium sulfate, the calf X-ray shows that there are abundant vessels for blood supply to the Achilles tendon after removing the gastrocnemius muscle [1].

8.3 Classification of Achilles Tendon Injury

Achilles tendon injuries are basically divided into two categories, open injuries and closed injuries. Open ruptures are mostly sharp cutting injuries, and some patients may have missed diagnosis. Closed Achilles tendon rupture refers to the complete disrupture of the anatomical continuity of the Achilles tendon. Some patients have scattered incomplete disconnection of the tendon bundles before the complete rupture, and in the event of sudden violence, complete rupture occurs; in addition, the chronically long-term stretching strain of the Achilles tendon causes Achilles tendonitis, peritendinitis, Achilles tendon tissue becoming brittle, peritendinitis affecting the microcirculation of the Achilles tendon, and then affects the blood supply of the Achilles tendon.

The General PLA Hospital (301 Hospital) recommends that Achilles tendon injuries should be divided into three types according to the characteristics of pathological changes after the Achilles tendon injury and the time of injury: ① 10 days after injury (acute injury); ② 10–20 days (subacute injury); ③ after 20 days (old injury). Acute injury: within 1 week after the injury, no more than 10 days at most, the Achilles tendon fibers are bright white during surgical incision, with good flexibility, no edema or very light edema, and the tissue holds the suture very well during suturing, simple plantar flexion of the ankle joint can make the Achilles tendon rupture ends contact. Subacute injury: 10–20 days after injury, the peritendinous tissue is swollen, the granulation scar is brittle, the Achilles tendon fibrous tissue becomes brittle, holds the suture poorly, the suture firmness is reduced, and plantar flexion of the ankle cannot make the Achilles tendon rupture ends contact. Old injury: after 20 days of injury, the Achilles tendon fiber swelling subsides, the scar is slightly aging, the holding strength to the suture is enhanced, but the Achilles tendon is often shortened by more than 6 cm, with plantar flexion of the ankle joint and V-Y lengthening of Achilles tendon cannot make the Achilles tendon rupture ends contact.

Myerson classifies Achilles tendon injuries according to the size of the defect at the Achilles tendon rupture site: Type I, the defect length is less than 2 cm, and the end-to-end suturing could be made after plantar flexion of the ankle joint; Type II, the defect length is 2–5 cm, use triceps tendon-belly junction V-Y advancement repair, or combined with tendon transfer for strengthening; Type III, defect length > 5 cm, use tendon transfer bridging Achilles tendon defect, or combined with triceps tendon V-Y advancement. For Myerson Type III Achilles tendon rupture, because the Achilles tendon defect is large, after the traditional surgical repairing, most of the part is filled with advanced scar tissue. After the operation, there might be Achilles tendon lengthening, triceps surae weakness, decreased pedal strength, difficult dorsiflexion of the ankle joint, skin adhesion, and other complications.

8.4 Evaluation of Achilles Tendon Injury

8.4.1 Clinical Evaluation

- Medical history: Direct Achilles tendon cutting or hitting by a sharp or blunt instrument or feeling of being kicked at the back after running and jumping or other vigorous exercises.
- Symptoms: Local swelling and pain in the Achilles tendon, plantar flexion or less pedal strength, difficulty in standing or walking.
- Physical examination: Touching Achilles tendon reveals its continuity interrupted with depression (Fig. 8.4), the toe

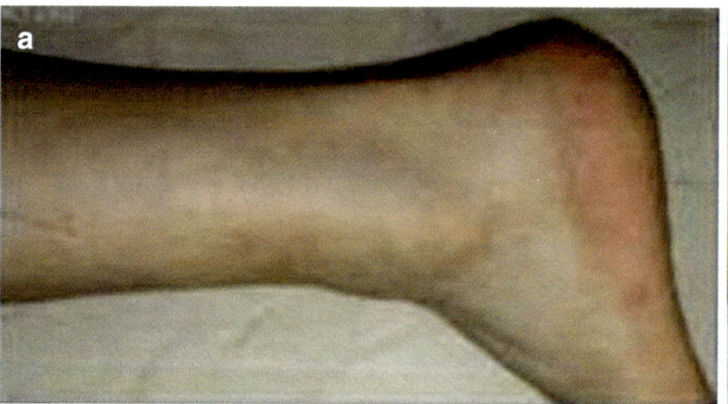

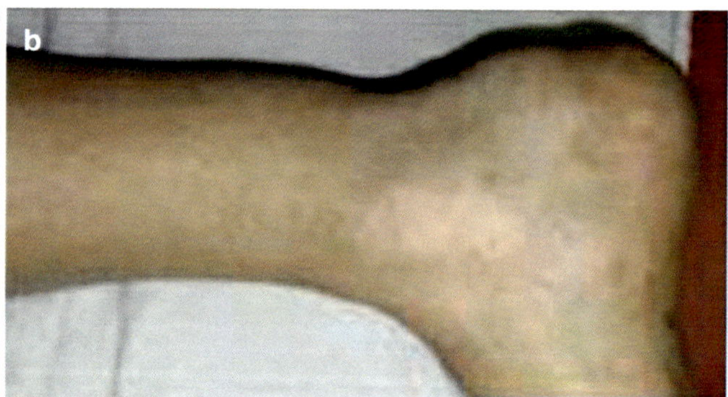

Fig. 8.4 Lateral view of Achilles tendon. (**a**) The normal Achilles tendon is locally continuous and full with elasticity and tension when being touched; (**b**) The Achilles tendon is completely ruptured, with local depression, feels empty, tension-free and nonelastic when being touched

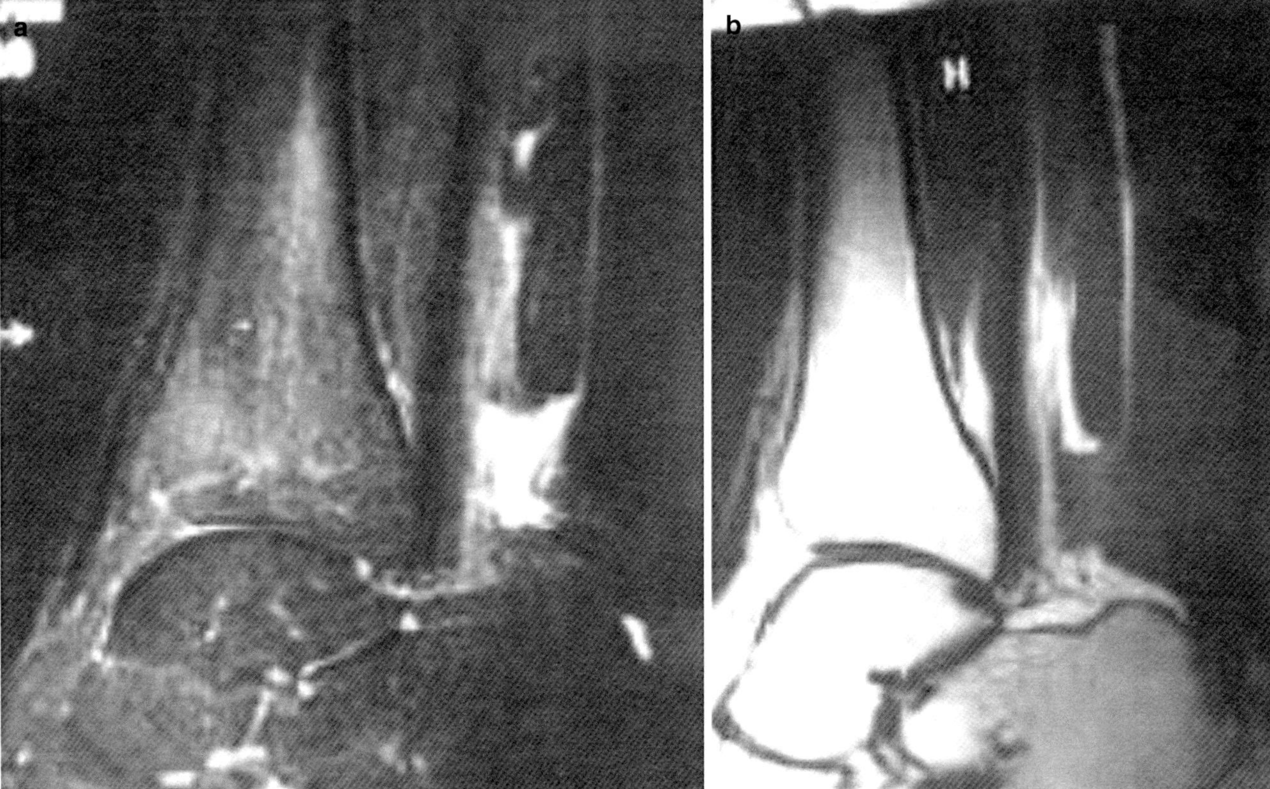

Fig. 8.5 MRI shows complete rupture of the Achilles tendon. (**a**) T2 weighted; (**b**) T1 weighted

flexion strength is significantly weakened, calf raises cannot be made (heel-raising test positive), and the Thompson sign is positive (have the patient knelt on the bedside, and there is plantar flexion movement when appropriately pinching the gastrocnemius muscle; absence of plantar flexion movement indicates Achilles tendon rupture).

- According to the patient's medical history, symptoms, signs, and imaging examinations, the diagnosis of Achilles tendon rupture is generally not difficult, but it could be easily ignored by young doctors and cause missed diagnosis.
- The reasons for the missed diagnosis are: ① The open injury is only considered to be a skin and soft tissue laceration, and detailed examination is not performed; ② After the Achilles tendon rupture, the plantar flexion does not completely disappear, because the posterior tibialis, peroneus longus and brevis, and digital flexor could still bend ankle and toe; ③ After the Achilles tendon rupture, some patients could still stand and limp.

8.4.2 Imaging Evaluation

- X-ray examination shows local soft tissue swelling and a positive Kager sign in front of the Achilles tendon; it clearly shows the small bone block attached to the avulsion of the Achilles tendon insertion.
- B-ultrasonography or MRI: is the most reliable imaging evidence for diagnosing Achilles tendon rupture, which can directly show the interrupted continuity of the Achilles tendon (Fig. 8.5).

8.5 Treatment of Achilles Tendon Injury

8.5.1 Treatment Principles

Whether the closed Achilles tendon rupture should be repaired and sutured surgically has always been a subject for debate. Some scholars believe that the repair technique of Achilles tendon rupture is scar healing, by choosing conservative treatment, as long as the ankle joint is maintained in plantar flexion, the ruptured Achilles tendon eventually can heal, whereas surgical incision has the risk of incision infection; other scholars insist to recommend surgical treatment, believing that precise suturing of the ruptured Achilles tendon after surgical treatment greatly increases the strength of the plantar flexion of the Achilles tendon after surgery, and the optimization of the surgical plan can greatly reduce the incidence of surgical complications.

In 2005, the *JBJS* journal published a paper of Meta-analysis on randomized and controlled clinical studies on the treatment of Achilles tendon rupture, involving 12 studies and 800 patients. In the study, three scholars analyzed the data and used 10 criteria for independent evaluation. They found the incidence of re-rupture of Achilles tendon was 12.6% in the conservative treatment group and only 3.5% in the surgical treatment group; the incidence of wound infection was 4% in the surgical treatment group and 0 in the conservative treatment group. The re-rupture rate of percutaneous minimally invasive suture of Achilles tendon was close to that of the surgical group, while the incidence of infection was only 2.4% [2].

The Orthopedics Department of General PLA Hospital (301 Hospital) recommends on closed Achilles tendon rupture is that young people need sports, and the firmness of the Achilles tendon is very important to the degree of sports, and surgical treatment is recommended; while the elderly have little activities, most of them have diabetes, hypertension, and other comorbidities, and conservative treatment is recommended.

1. **Nonsurgical treatment**

- Mostly use Achilles tendon boots, plasters, or braces to fix the foot in the plantar flexion position for 8–12 weeks.

2. **Choice of open suturing and repair techniques (recommended by Orthopedics Department of 301 Hospital):**
   (a) For the acute Achilles tendon rupture, the rupture ends are messy and in horsetail shape, the defect of the proximal retraction end is about 3 cm. With the plantar flexion of the ankle joint, the Achilles tendon rupture ends can touch each other and end-to-end suture could be made, such as Krackow technique, Bunnell technique, and end-to-end modified Kessler suture augmented with interrupted suturing; the special device invented by our hospital is also particularly recommended, which realizes channel-assisted minimally invasive repair of acute Achilles tendon rupture, effectively avoids sural nerve injury, and provides sufficient effective mechanical support, the surgery time is only 15–20 min, and the incision is only 1.5–2 cm.
   (b) Subacute injury, Achilles tendon ruptured for more than 10 days; Achilles tendon contracture often reaches 3–6 cm, rupture ends degenerated with non-severe necrosis, and plantar flexion of the ankle joint alone cannot achieve end-to-end contact of the Achilles tendon rupture ends. Abraham V-Y suture technique is recommended.
   (c) Old injury, Achilles tendon ruptured for more than 3 weeks; at this time, Achilles tendon contracture always exceeds 6 cm. It is recommended to use the Lindholm technique (gastrocnemius aponeurosis turn-down flap) to repair the defect of the Achilles tendon rupture ends. If the strength of the Achilles tendon after suturing and repair is found to be insufficient during the surgery, the following methods can be used to strengthen the Achilles tendon, such as White Krynick technique, Rugg and Bogoe technique, simple plantaris reinforcement, use of peroneal brevis and artificial materials to repair, fascia lata transplantation and other suturing techniques.
   (d) Achilles tendon injuries caused by traffic accidents are often accompanied by defects of the calcaneus and skin. It is difficult to succeed by local skin tension-reduced suture/free skin grafts. At present, mostly used are: ① Transposition of the pedicled tendon to repair Achilles tendon defects; ② Transposition of vascularized tissue flap to repair Achilles tendon defect; ③ Free transplantation of vascularized composite tissue flap to repair Achilles tendon defect.

8.5.2 Krackow Lockstitch Suture for Open Repair of Acute Achilles Tendon Rupture

The patient is in the prone position, with local anesthesia or continuous epidural or sciatic nerve block anesthesia, and a pneumatic tourniquet is tied to the middle and upper thigh.

Routine iodine and alcohol disinfect the skin of the affected limb, spread sterile drape sheets, and stick sterile membrane. Drive the blood with the blood-driving band, and apply the tourniquet.

A longitudinal incision is made on the medial side of the Achilles tendon, with a length of 10–15 cm (the incision is 1 cm away from the Achilles tendon, that is, the incision is far away from the center to prevent the shoe from rubbing against the Achilles tendon and causing local irritation of the Achilles tendon). The Achilles tendon is exposed through three main incisions, the posterior median approach, the lateral approach, and the medial approach. The median approach is better for the exposure of the Achilles tendon, but after the long-term incision scar healing, the friction between the scar and the shoe could cause pain. In addition, the incision suturing has the highest tension, which affects the healing of the incision and could easily cause the exposure of the Achilles tendon; the lateral approach could easily damage the heel branch of the sural nerve, resulting in loss of skin sensation on the heel, long-term skin innervation malnutrition, and other issues; the Achilles tendon medial longitudinal approach is relatively safe, it could avoid the damage to the posterior cutaneous nerve of the calf, reduce the high skin necrosis and incision infection rate caused by middle posterior straight incision.

Incise the skin, subcutaneous tissue, and deep fascia, protect the deep fascia and connect it to the subcutaneous tissue (suture the skin and deep fascia with silk and fix it on the peripheral skin), that is to say, no dissection of the subcutaneous tissue, protect the peritendinous tissue and fully expose the ruptured Achilles tendon (Fig. 8.6a, b). The sharp incision should be made to the deep fascia (epitendineum) to avoid destruction of the subcutaneous nutrient vascular network and fat liquefaction caused by blunt dissection, thereby reducing incision skin necrosis, infection, and adhesion; protect the peritendinous tissue, and avoid damage to the vascular bundle that enters the Achilles tendon from the ventral side (Fig. 8.7a, b); suturing: suture the Achilles tendon rupture ends with nonabsorbable 2# ETHIBOND® Suture (Polyester, Ethicon Inc.) Krakcow, and use Absorbable 2-0 antibacterial PDS®Plus Suture (polydioxanone, Ethicon Inc.) for interrupted suturing to strengthen the rupture ends (Fig. 8.6c). Strengthening suturing buries the knot in the rupture end, and the interrupted suturing of the epitendineum makes the knot in the subcutaneous tissue, which can reduce the knot irritation. After the repair, the Achilles tendon should have enough strength and the tension should not be too high, so as not to block the blood supply of the rupture ends or affect the healing; suture the peritendinous tissue and completely wrap the Achilles tendon to reduce the postoperative adhesion of the Achilles tendon (Fig. 8.6d); postoperative plaster support is fixed in knee flexion and plantar flexion position to reduce the tension at the anastomotic site. Leave the negative pressure drainage tube, the distal end of outlet, drainage tube at high position are placed at the lowest part of the wound; if a rubber strip is used for drainage, the outlet is located at the lowest position of the drainage, opposite to the negative pressure drainage tube. For tight closing of the deep fascia, the effective method is figure-of-8 suturing stitch by stitch without knotting, after the suturing is completed, knot to close the deep fascia, and put the knots under the skin (Fig. 8.6e); for suturing subcutaneous tissue, leave the knot in the deep tissue; suture the skin to ensure the tight closure of the incision.

Use long leg plaster or brace (Fig. 8.6f, g, h) to fix the knee joint at the knee flexion 10 15°, plantar flexion of the ankle joint 30° position (this position can relax the gastrocnemius muscle, and the tension at the anastomotic site of Achilles tendon rupture is the lowest, creating conditions for the Achilles tendon to heal under tension-free conditions).

8.5.3 Percutaneous Minimally Invasive Suture and Repair of Acute Achilles Tendon Rupture

In 1977, Dr. Ma and Griffith first used and reported this method, but the sural nerve injury rate reached 13% [3]. Therefore, some doctors used absorbable suture or modified surgical incisions to invent auxiliary suturing surgical instruments, such as Mayo needle (BL059N), French Achillon Achilles device, etc., in an attempt to reduce the risk of sural nerve injury.

One of the most promising tools is the Achillon device, invented by a Swiss orthopedic surgeon. The "box" suturing technique is used. In clinical practice, we found that the suture could easily cut the Achilles tendon, and the mechanical strength of the early suturing is questioned; the latest research shows that it cannot provide sufficient initial mechanical strength, which is only 1/10 of the Krackow technique. Therefore, it must be fixed and protected by plaster or brace after the surgery; in addition, the risk of sural nerve injury is extremely high in the cadaver operation study, and it is found that the incidence of direct suturing puncture injury and nerve suturing is as high as 25.6%. In 2007, China introduced the Achillon device. At present, due to its unreliable suturing, sural nerve damage, and other issues, it has not been well promoted.

1. **Development and design of channel-assisted suturing system**

In order to avoid the iatrogenic injury of the sural nerve and the concern about the mechanical strength of the suture, since 2010, the Achilles tendon minimally invasive research group of 301 Hospital has explored the minimally invasive suture of the Achilles tendon.

In 2010, the research team tried to modify the Bunnell method (one of the most reliable methods for open repair and suturing of the Achilles tendon, Fig. 8.8a) during the open repair of the Achilles tendon, and invent a new suturing technique (Fig. 8.8b), that is, the oblique needle passing is changed to a horizontal needle passing; the knot is changed from inside the tendon to outside the tendon. Preliminary mechanical studies have shown that this method can meet the mechanical requirements for Achilles tendon suturing and repair and has better clinical efficacy.

In 2012, for this modified Bunnell suture technique, a channel-assisted minimally invasive repair (CAMIR) system was designed and developed. In 2015, the national invention patent authorization was obtained. This system (Fig. 8.9) realizes the percutaneous minimally invasive suture of the Achilles tendon with five innovative technologies and avoids iatrogenic injury of the sural nerve.

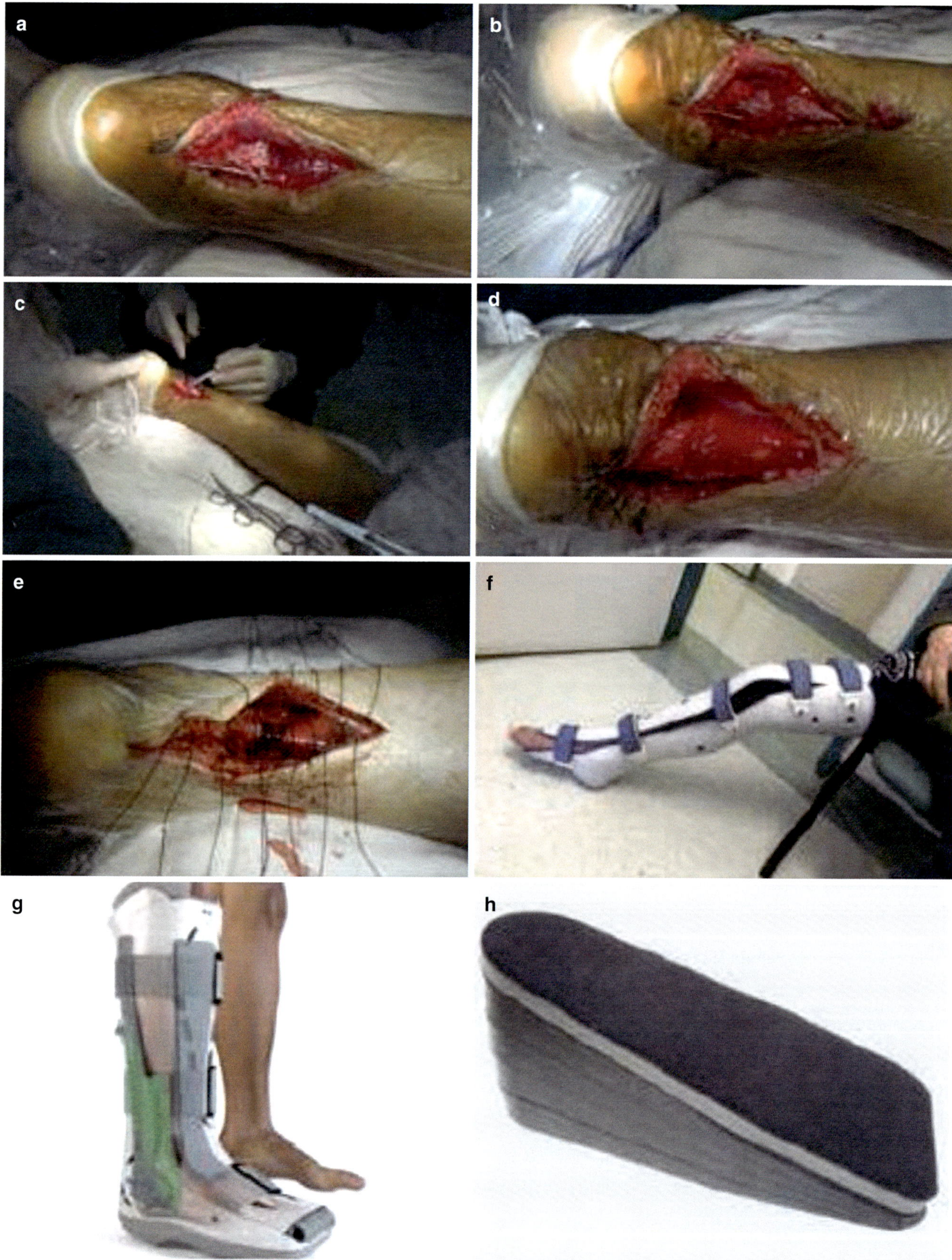

Fig. 8.6 Open repair of acute Achilles tendon rupture with Krackow lockstitch

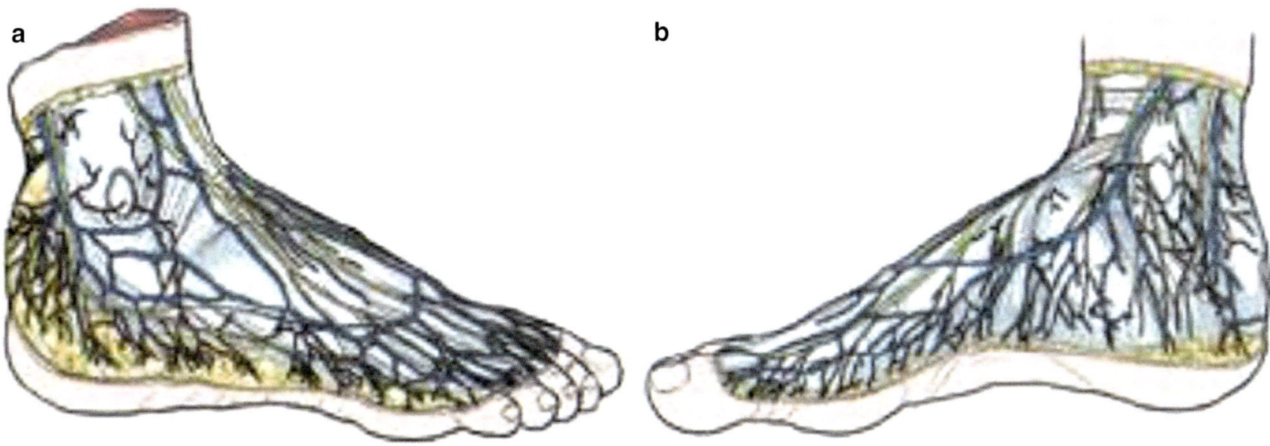

Fig. 8.7 Achilles tendon peripheral surface anatomy. (**a**) Lateral view; (**b**) Medial view

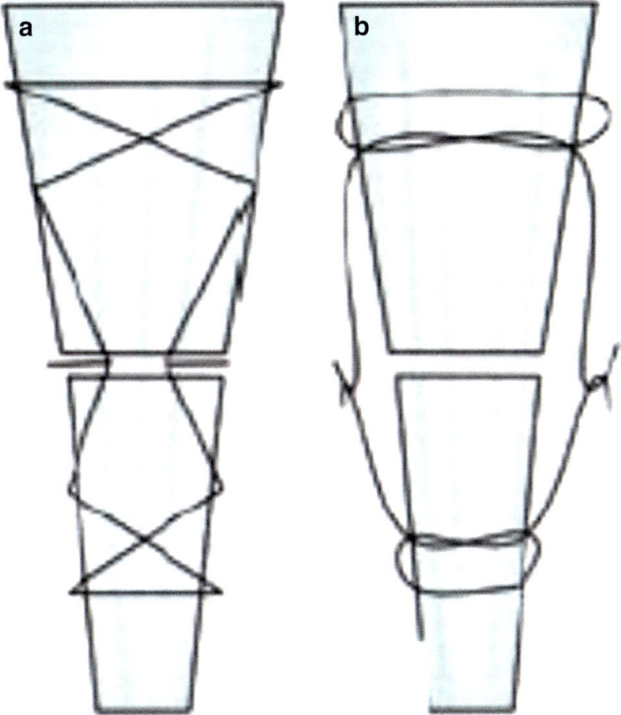

Fig. 8.8 Bunnel suture technique (**a**) Classic suture technique; (**b**) Modified Bunnel suture technique

(a) Technique 1 enables relative movement between the stapler and the Achilles tendon: under normal circumstances, the open exposure of the Achilles tendon needs to pass through the skin, subcutaneous tissue, and deep fascia. The deep fascia wraps around the Achilles tendon and forms a fibrous channel. The Achilles tendon moves in this channel and completes the plantar flexion and dorsal extension of the ankle joint. The Achilles tendon skin has a certain degree of mobility. Therefore, a longitudinal incision must be made in the deep fascia to realize the relative sliding between the stapler and the Achilles tendon. A 30° transverse blade at the side of the sleeve-core end specially designed for this system could complete the incision after passing through the deep fascia.

(b) Technique 2: Create a safe suture channel to avoid sural nerve injury: sharply incise the skin 5 mm at the insertion point of the channel, insert a hemostatic forceps to bluntly release the tissues to the deep fascia, especially the sural nerve; then insert the specially designed sleeve core, penetrate deep fascia and enter into the sheath of Achilles tendon; insert the contralateral channel in the same way; adjust the blade of sleeve core to be parallel to the direction of Achilles tendon, push the stapler up and down to cut deep fascia for 1 cm; follow the sleeve core to screw in the sleeve to establish the suturing channel.

(c) Technique 3: Horizontal needle passing prevents suture cross-cutting: Specially designed neutral and eccentric position suture guide avoids cutting between the horizontal needle sutures or causing suture breakage.

(d) Technique 4: The suture in the Achilles tendon sheath is pulled out from the incision site without increasing the incision: The uniquely designed inner-arm holding suture pulls the suture out from the incision site from the tendon sheath.

(e) Technique 5: The reconstruction sleeve distal to the Achilles tendon insertion realizes the reconstruction of the Achilles tendon insertion: For injuries close to the Achilles tendon insertion rupture, the specially designed stapler arm can percutaneously establish a channel between the deep fascia and the calcaneus. Insert the sleeve, insert the suture in the calcaneal drill bone canal, and pull out the suture by the stapler.

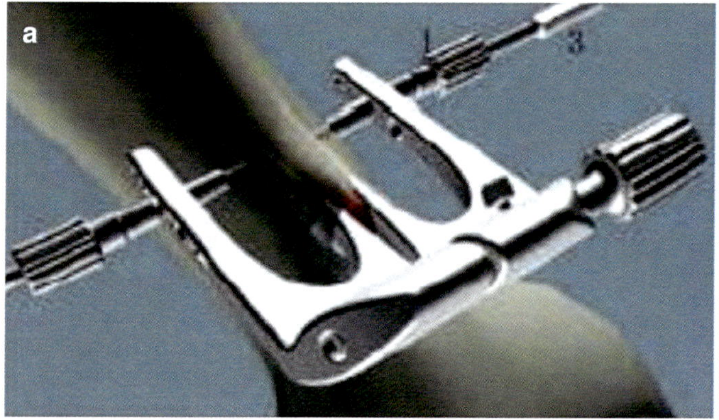

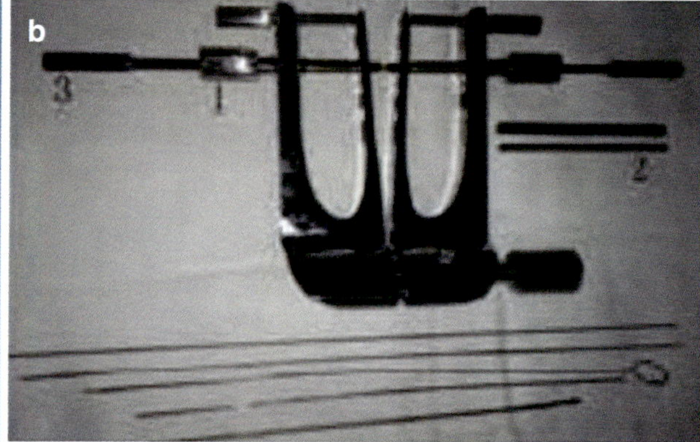

Fig. 8.9 Achilles tendon channel-assisted minimally invasive repair system (CAMIR) invented by this research group. (**a**) Processing design drawing of ProE software; (**b**) Physical picture. 1. Specially designed auxiliary channel, passing through the skin, subcutaneous tissue, Achilles tendon sheath, the sural nerve located outside the channel; 2. Central and eccentric guiders guide the suturing to avoid suture cutting caused by suture crossing; 3. Specially designed Trocar, a 30° transverse blade on the tip side can cut the tendon sheath after passing through the deep fascia, so that the channel and the stapler can move on the surface of the Achilles tendon, similar to sewing machine suturing

2. **Channel-assisted minimally invasive repair (CAMIR) of acute Achilles tendon rupture**

The patient is placed in the prone position, using sciatic nerve/lumbar plexus block anesthesia, tourniquet placed on the middle and upper thigh, blood being driven for the lower limb, the tourniquet pressure is 320 mmHg (1 mmHg = 0.133 kPa).

After successful anesthesia, 1 g of cefmetazole sodium is injected intravenously for preventing infection. First, touch the rupture ends of the Achilles tendon, and make a 1.5-cm transverse incision on its surface perpendicular to the direction of the Achilles tendon. Incise the skin, subcutaneous tissue, and Achilles tendon fascia sheath to expose the Achilles tendon rupture ends. Use Kocher forceps to hold the proximal end of the ruptured Achilles tendon, pull it out from the incision, insert the CAMIR inner arm into the Achilles tendon fascia sheath, and clamp the Achilles tendon. Make a forceps incision with a length of 5 mm on the skin along the guide hole of the lateral arm. Use hemostatic forceps to push the sural nerve that may run through the incision (Fig. 8.10a), and insert the sleeve and 1.5-cm-long double-sided sharp cone through the guide hole of the lateral arm (Fig. 8.10b), pierce the Achilles tendon fascia sheath bluntly, push CAMIR toward the distal and proximal directions of the Achilles tendon rupture ends (Fig. 8.10c), use the side blade at the sharp cone end to cut the fascial sheath for 1.0–1.5 cm, and screw the sleeve along the sharp cone, so that the sleeve enters the inner arm of the stapler to establish the suturing channel (Fig. 8.10d). Pass the needle along the central or eccentric guider to complete the modified Bunnel suture technique grasping the proximal end of the ruptured Achilles tendon (Fig. 8.10e), pull out the CAMIR inner arm from the incision, and pull out the suture that holds the proximal end of the ruptured Achilles tendon from the incision (No. 2 Ethicon suture) (Fig. 8.10f, g). In the same way, use the suture to grasp the distal end of the ruptured Achilles tendon (Fig. 8.10h), pull out the suture, tighten the suture, knot, and complete the suturing fixation of the Achilles tendon (Fig. 8.10i). Use the Absorbable 3-0 VICRYL® Plus Control Release Suture (Polyglactin 910, Ethicon Inc.) to strengthen interrupted suturing of the Achilles tendon rupture ends, and suture the surrounding tissue of Achilles tendon.

Close the incision layer by layer, compress with the elastic bandage, and release the tourniquet. Postoperative treatment and rehabilitation are the same as the open repair.

8.5.4 Repair of Subacute Achilles Tendon Rupture with Abraham V-Y Plasty

The patient is placed in the prone position, a tourniquet is placed on the proximal thigh, and a straight incision of about 15 cm in length is made at the medial side of the Achilles tendon attachment to the middle part. Pay attention to protect the sural nerve and superficial peroneal nerve.

Open the Achilles tendon membrane, explore the injury, and completely remove scar tissue of the rupture ends. Make the knee joint at 30° flexion and the ankle at 20° plantar flexion to measure the length of the tendon defect. If the defect length is 3–6 cm, perform the Abraham V-Y technique. (Fig. 8.11). Make an inverted "V"-shaped incision about 1 cm distal to the junction of the muscle-tendon of triceps surae. The length of the two incisions that make up the "V"-shaped incision is at least 1.5 times longer than the defect. After opening all the tendon sheath, advance down-

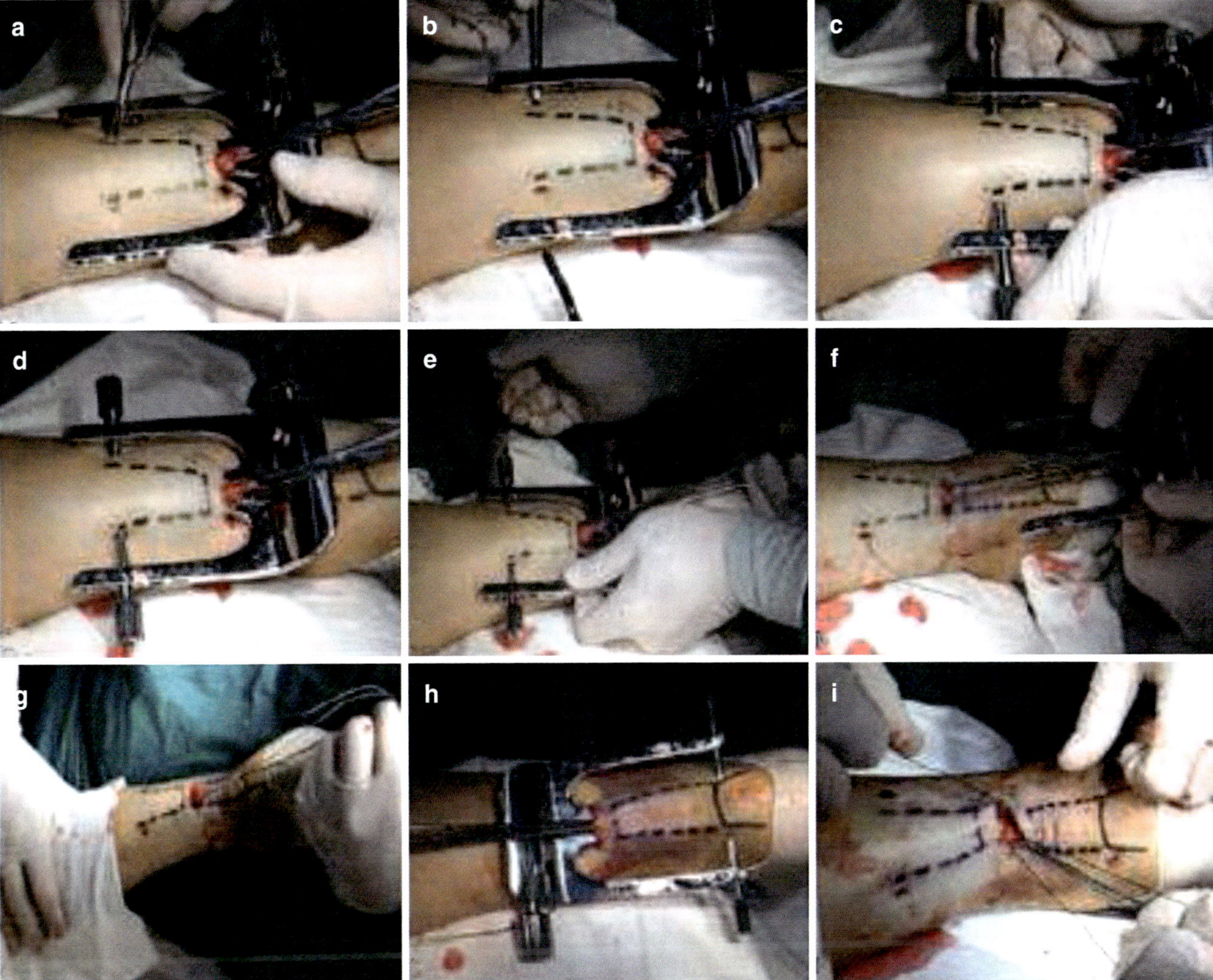

Fig. 8.10 CAMIR of acute Achilles tendon rupture

ward to complete the end-to-end anastomosis. Make end-to-end suturing of the Achilles tendon rupture ends with Nonabsorbable 2# ETHIBOND® Suture (Polyester, Ethicon Inc.) with modified Kessler technique, and suture the inverted "V-Y"-shaped incision with Absorbable 2-0 VICRYL® Plus Control Release Suture (Polyglactin 910, Ethicon Inc.), repair the Achilles tendon membrane and suture the wound.

Postoperative treatment and rehabilitation are the same as open repair.

8.5.5 Lindholm Technique to Repair Old Achilles Tendon Rupture

The patient is in a prone position and makes a posterior curved incision from the middle of the calf to the calcaneus. Open the deep fascia in the midline direction to expose the rupture ends of the Achilles tendon.

Debridement first, trim the rupture ends, use thick silk or thin stainless steel wire for mattress suture, or use thin silk for interrupted suture. Take a piece of gastrocnemius aponeurosis and Achilles tendon flap with a length of 7–8 cm and a width of about 1 cm from both sides of the proximal rupture end of the Achilles tendon, flip to the distal end, leave the base part at the proximal rupture end of the Achilles tendon, and suture them to the distal Achilles tendon end. Suture the edges of the tendon strips, and suture the two tendon strips to each other to completely cover the rupture part of the Achilles tendon. When the tension is large and there is a gap, the gastrocnemius tendon flap can be used to have direct anastomosis with the distal end, make reinforcement suturing at the proximal end. If there is a plantar tendon, use this tendon for reinforcement. Suture the defect of the aponeurosis to close the gap left by the tendon flip. Suture the tendon sheath and surrounding tissue and skin (Fig. 8.12).

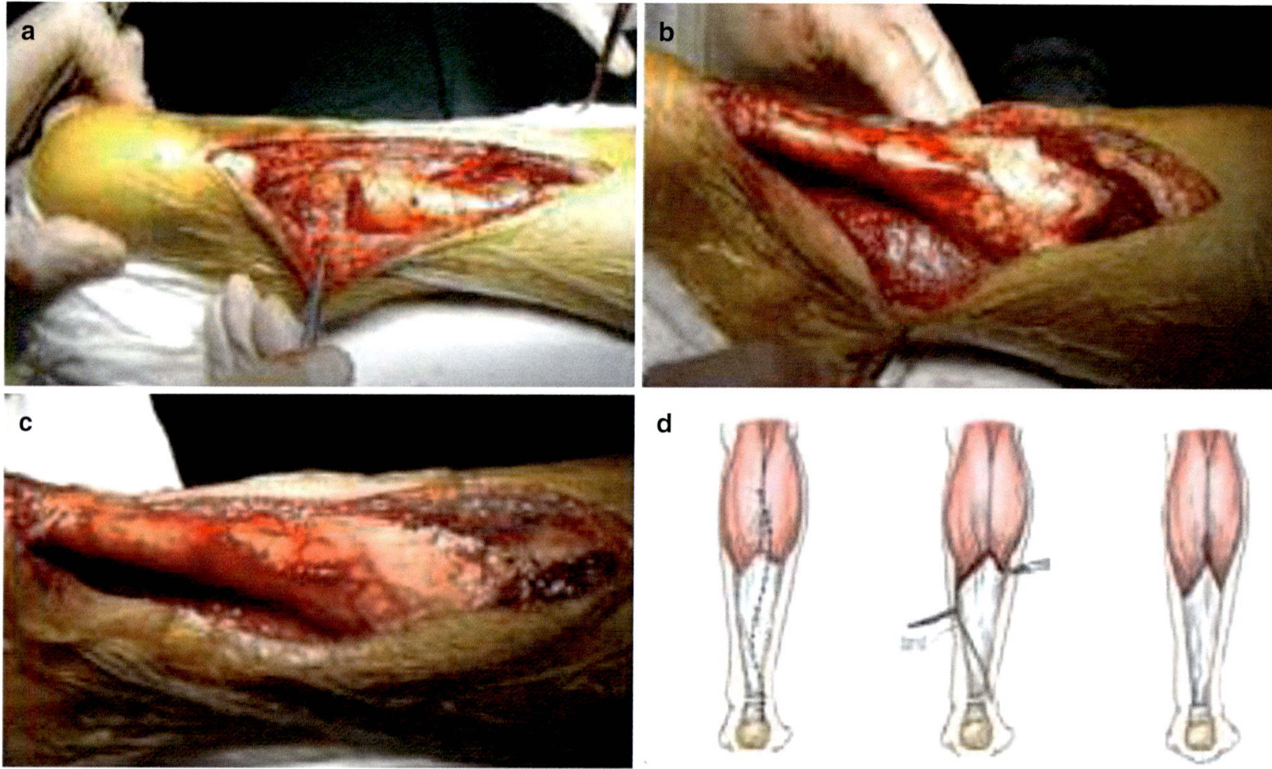

Fig. 8.11 Abraham V-Y advancement and repair of subacute Achilles tendon rupture

8.6 Complications and Prognosis of Achilles Tendon Injury

During the diagnosis and treatment process of Achilles tendon injury, problems such as missed diagnosis, wound infection and necrosis, Achilles tendon re-rupture, joint stiffness, Achilles tendon adhesion, sural nerve, and incision problems may occur.

8.6.1 Misdiagnosis or Missed Diagnosis of Achilles Tendon Rupture

Open Achilles tendon injury, because of the superficial position of the Achilles tendon, it could be found by careful inspection of the wound during debridement. It is unlikely to be misdiagnosed. The main reason for misdiagnosis or missed diagnosis is over-negligence and lack of responsibility.

For closed Achilles tendon rupture, according to medical history; chief complaints of local "feeling of being hit" and sounds, followed by local swelling, pain, and weakness in heel raising; a transverse groove could be palpated at the Achilles tendon rupture, with tenderness; positive Thompson sign, could confirm the diagnosis. However, it must be clear that even without these signs, Achilles tendon rupture cannot be completely ruled out. For Achilles tendon rupture, the above signs may not appear, comprehensive judgment is needed. Doppler ultrasound or MRI examination are needed to help judge.

1. Regarding the palpable transverse groove at the Achilles tendon rupture, this sign only appears in patients with complete rupture of the Achilles tendon with retracted rupture ends; in the case of incomplete rupture, intact tendon sheath, or old rupture ends filled with scar tissue, the sign "transverse groove" is not obvious.
2. A positive Thompson sign is tenable for the diagnosis of Achilles tendon rupture, but a negative Thompson sign does not completely rule out the Achilles tendon rupture. Because the muscle strength of plantar flexion of the ankle joint is not limited to the triceps surae and the Achilles tendon of its continuation, the deep tibialis posterior muscle, peroneus longus and brevis, plantar flexor and plantaris muscles are also involved in the plantar flexion of the ankle joint. So, for simple Achilles tendon rupture, the plantar flexion function of the ankle joint is not completely lost, only manifestations are the weakness of plantar flexion of the ankle joint and the limited range of plantar flexion. At this time, the Thompson sign is false-negative; especially for incomplete Achilles tendon rupture, the Thompson sign is also false-negative.

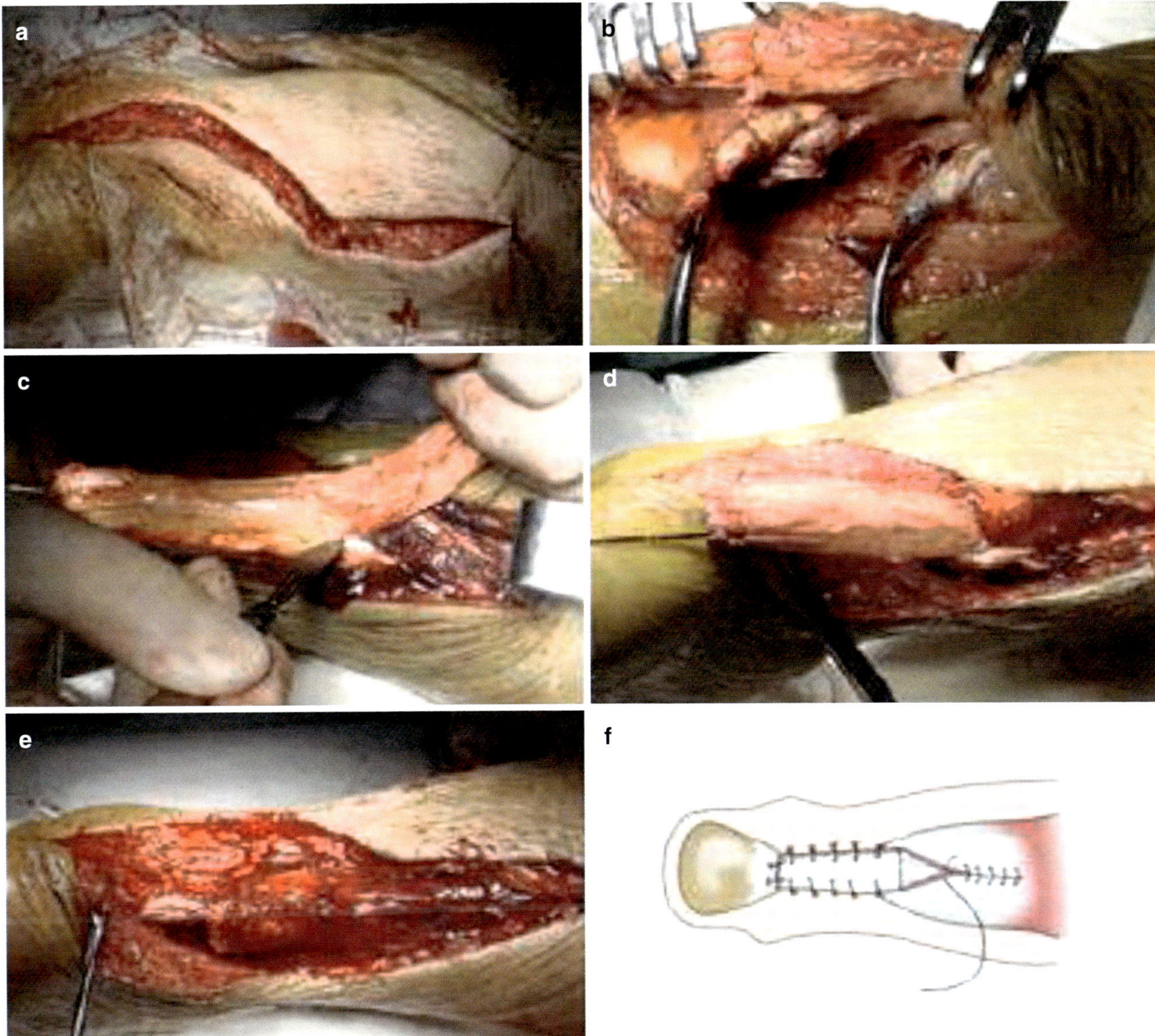

Fig. 8.12 Lindholm technique to repair old Achilles tendon rupture

3. Inadequate understanding of the plantar tendon. The plantaris muscle is located between the gastrocnemius muscle and the soleus muscle. It starts from the posterior upper bony surface of the lateral femoral condyle and the knee joint capsule, and ends at the calcaneus on the medial edge of the Achilles tendon. The muscle belly is in the shape of a small fusiform, generally no more than 7 cm, and goes down into a small tendon. When the Achilles tendon is completely ruptured and the plantaris muscle is intact, the plantar tendon could be palpated and misjudged as the medial half of the Achilles tendon, thereby mistakenly judging that the Achilles tendon is partially ruptured.
4. The one-foot standing heel-raising test is used to preliminarily judge Achilles tendon rupture. But in clinical practice, it is found that this test is reliable, but because of pain aggravation, patients often cannot cooperate.

8.6.2 Incision Issues

The postoperative infection rate of acute Achilles tendon rupture is 7.15%. This is because the Achilles tendon is superficial, covered only by skin and a thin layer of subcutaneous tissue. Avoid the posterior midline incision on the Achilles tendon surface, make a sharp dissection, pay attention to repairing the peritendinous tissue surrounding the Achilles tendon, and make thorough hemostasis before closing the incision. For old injury, it is even higher, reaching 27.78%, which may be related to untimely treatment after injury, poor blood supply; block treatment history; excessive local tension and other factors. The longitudinal incision on the medial side of the Achilles tendon has less damage to the blood supply around the tendon. It not only avoids the pain caused by friction between the scar and shoes but also there is little tension on the incision. There should be attention during the surgery:

1. When repairing the Achilles tendon, try to keep the ankle at plantar flexion position as much as possible (at this time, the Achilles tendon is relaxed, do not overlap and shorten, as long as the continuity of the Achilles tendon is restored, a certain tension is maintained after suturing the Achilles tendon, bilateral Thompson tests are roughly the same after suturing, indicating that the tightness is appropriate).
2. The strength of the Achilles tendon suture can independently maintain the ankle joint in the neutral position.
3. The tendon sheath of the Achilles tendon must be completely repaired, and the deep fascia is well aligned. The deep fascia can resist the tension of the Achilles tendon's backward bowstring and reduce the tension on the skin, so that the skin can be sutured without tension to avoid edge necrosis.
4. Unless the tendon sheath suture is not satisfactory, try not to implant the anti-adhesion membrane, so as to avoid increasing the difficulty of suturing.
5. After the surgery, the ankle joint is fixed in plantar flexion; use Kessler suture technique to anastomoses the Achilles tendon rupture ends and repair the aponeurosis, and reduce the interference to the blood circulation inside and outside the tendon.

8.6.3 Postoperative Adhesion

During the surgery, minimally invasive operation is prioritized to protect and restore the blood circulation of the rupture ends. Our experience is:

1. The blood supply of the Achilles tendon mainly comes from the junction of the tendon and muscle belly, the tendon-bone junction, and peritendinous tissue. When the incision is made on the medial side of the Achilles tendon, the skin, subcutaneous tissue, and deep fascia should be incised in sequence, avoid stripping the three parts. Retract to both sides at the same time, sharp dissection exposes the Achilles tendon, avoid violent operation to reduce the damage of the Achilles tendon blood supply.
2. There is a semicircular avascular area 10–18 mm proximal to the Achilles tendon insertion, accounting for 1/2 to 2/3 of the ventral Achilles tendon. Therefore, the operation in this area should be minimized during the surgery.
3. Traditionally, Achilles tendons are sutured with silk. Silk is prone to cause tissue reactions and adhesions. Although Steel Suture has light tissue reactions and high tensile strength, they could easily cut the tendon and need to be removed by a second operation. We recommend Nonabsorbable 2# ETHIBOND® Suture (Polyester, Ethicon Inc.), and then use Absorbable 2-0 VICRYL® Plus Control Release Suture (Polyglactin 910, Ethicon Inc.) for strengthening interrupted suturing, Absorbable 3-0 VICRYL® Plus Control Release Suture (Polyglactin 910, Ethicon Inc.) to close the peritendinous tissue; try to trim the fascia and Achilles tendon smoothly as much as possible, and repair the deep fascia around the Achilles tendon to reduce postoperative adhesions.
4. Fully remove the ischemic necrosis tissue at the Achilles tendon rupture ends, remove the scar tissue from the rupture ends for the relatively old injury, and irrigate the surgical field with normal saline before obtaining the gastrocnemius fascia flap.
5. Tension adjustment during Achilles tendon anastomosis is the most critical issue in Achilles tendon repair surgery. The tension during Achilles tendon anastomosis should be the same as that of the contralateral Achilles tendon. Excessive tension will lead to difficulty in dorsiflexion of the ankle joint, and too little tension will produce weak plantar flexion. Our suggestion is to check the Achilles tendon tension in the resting position of the healthy side Achilles tendon before the surgery (knee flexion 20°, plantar flexion of the ankle joint 30°), and suture Achilles tendon under appropriate tension, and better results could be obtained.
6. Surgery timing, in general, 3 weeks after the rupture of the Achilles tendon, the elasticity of the tendon sheath is lost, the inner diameter is reduced, the tendon is retracted for too long, difficult to pull together, and the repairing difficulty increases significantly. Studies have reported that the average plantar flexion force of patients who receive surgeries within 1 week after rupture was 91% of the healthy side, while the plantarflexion force of those who receive surgeries 1 week later was only 74% of the healthy side. We suggest that once the diagnosis is clear, the relevant examinations should be completed and the surgery should be performed as soon as possible.

8.7 Rehabilitation of Achilles Tendon Injury

It is necessary to follow the pathophysiological mechanism of Achilles tendon healing, not only to prevent excessive load on the unhealed tissue but also to prevent the negative impact of immobilization and disuse on the healed tissue.

1. 1–4 weeks after surgery (28 days in total): Long leg plaster support for fixation, with crutches, is necessary.
2. 5–6 weeks after surgery (2 weeks in total): Change to short leg plaster support (cut and shorten the long leg plaster support to 3 cm below the capitula fibula, and start to move the knee joint). Remove the plaster support every day, soak the Achilles tendon area in warm water, massage the Achilles tendon, and appropriately increase the ankle dorsiflexion and plantarflexion activities. Conduct foot rolling bottle training, toe grasping towel training (maintain the ankle joint in plantar flexion).
3. 7–14 weeks after surgery (8 weeks in total): Remove the short leg plaster posterior support, walk in Achilles boots, and pad a 2.5 to 3 cm high heel pad composed of ten layers of thin plates between the heel and the shoe sole when walking. During this period, it is necessary to prevent the stretch of the Achilles tendon from falling or kicking suddenly. Both feet heel raising exercises in seat position.
4. 15–19 weeks after surgery (5 weeks in total): Walk on the whole soles of the feet, exercise ankle joint function, and make the range of motion of the ankle joint completely normal. Start to practice triceps surae strength. At the beginning, exercise the heel raising of both feet, gradually increase the load on the affected limb, and finally transition to single foot heel raising. At this point, people who are engaged in easier work can start working. During this period, it is still necessary to prevent the stretch of the Achilles tendon caused by falling or kicking suddenly.
5. 20–24 weeks after surgery (5 weeks in total): Continue to exercise single foot heel raising, correct residual plantar flexion of the ankle joint or dorsiflexion dysfunction, start jogging with the whole soles of the feet, and gradually restore the flexibility of the ankle joint and triceps surae muscle strength and dimension. At this point, athletes can start to participate in light training, and those engaged in moderate physical labor can participate in the work.
6. Twenty-four weeks after surgery, athletes can participate in formal training, and the general population can participate in heavy physical labor.

8.8 Author's Comments

Achilles tendon rupture is a common injury, which has been increasing year by year with the increase of sports activity. Elderly patients and patients with low sports needs can be treated conservatively, but for young patients with sports needs, surgical repair is undoubtedly the best choice. However, during clinical treatment, there are many complications of surgical open repair, which severely affect the physical and mental health of patients. In 1977, Ma and Griffith's percutaneous suture technique provided clinicians with a new idea [3]. Is it possible to minimize the incision exposure of the clinical commonly used open suturing technique by percutaneous or minimally invasive or small incision technique, protect the sural nerve in the incision at the same time, and finally realize the suturing and repair of the Achilles tendon? With this idea, many surgeons thought and put forward new challenges for clinical surgeons.

Under the leadership of Professor Tang Peifu, Orthopedics Department of 301 Hospital, some exploratory work has been carried out, the channel minimally invasive Achilles tendon anastomosis system was invented, which avoids the sural nerve from damage. It modifies the Bunnell suture technique, a classic surgical procedure of open suturing, realizes the small incision minimally invasive Achilles tendon rupture end anastomosis. The surgery time is only 15–20 min, and the surgical incision is only 1.5–2 cm. It is currently used to repair horsetail avulsion, Achilles tendon insertion reconstruction, old Achilles tendon rupture (defect), and other Achilles tendon injuries. Surgical trauma is greatly reduced, and the patient recovery is faster and the incidence of complications is significantly lower compared with open repair techniques. For this reason, it has received funding from the Capital Special Fund and two-episode exclusive interview "Approach to Science" column of CCTV 10, which brings a good response from the society. Compared with foreign minimally invasive devices (such as the Achillon device, invented by Assal in Switzerland; PARS device, invented by Robert in the United States), it has obvious advantages; it is believed that this technique will be comprehensively popularized in China, offering benefit to patients with Achilles tendon rupture.

Search Terms

Achilles tendon rupture, suture and repair, minimally invasive, functional exercise

References

1. Carr AJ, Norris SH. The blood supply of the calcaneal tendon. J Bone Joint Surg (Br). 1989;71(1):100–1.
2. Khan RJ, Fick D, Keogh A, et al. Treatment of acute achilles tendon ruptures. A meta-analysis of randomized, controlled trials. J Bone Joint Surg Am. 2005;87:2202–10.
3. Ma GWC, Griffith TG. Percutaneous repair of acute closed ruptured Achilles tendon. A new technique ClinOrthop. 1977;128:247–55.

Suturing Techniques in the Repair and Reconstruction of Peri-Articular Injuries of Upper Limbs

9

Zhongguo Fu, Danmou Xing, Jingming Dong, Jianhai Chen, Zhengren Peng, Dong Ren, Wei Feng, Yan Chen, Huan Wang, Junlin Zhou, Qi Yao, Chengyu Zhuang, and Xiaoming Wu

Abstract

Cartilage fractures around the elbow joint are a group of special types of intra-articular fractures. Due to the characteristics of its anatomical structure and limited space, it is much more difficult to fix those (1) fragments which are small and completely separated from articular surface, (2) subchondral bones, (3) small bone fragments, and (4) multiple bone fragments. The suture-assisted fixation technique effectively solves these problems. This article introduces in detail the application of suture-assisted fixation technique in various types of articular cartilage fractures of the elbow.

Keywords

Shoulder joint · Clinical anatomy · Repair of injuries Anatomical landmark · Fracture reduction · Fixation Proximal humeral fractures · Suture-assisted "parachute" principle · Shoulder fractures · Arthroplasty Replacement · Rotator cuff injury · Rotator cuff repair Shoulder joint instability · HAGHL injury · Ligamentous laxity · Ligament absence · Superior capsular reconstruction · Acromioclavicular joint · Acromioclavicular joint injury · Open reduction · Ligament reconstruction Acromioclavicular joint dislocation · Coracoclavicular ligament reconstruction Weaver–Dunn technique Artificial shoulder arthroplasty · Rotator cuff functions Greater and lesser tubercles · Suturing techniques Lateral collateral ligament of the elbow joint · Instability of posterolateral rotation · Repair · Reconstruction Distal triceps brachii tendon · Acute injury · Old injury Avulsion · Rupture · Reconstruction · Biceps tendon Acute injury · Injury · Recovery · Articular cartilage fracture of the elbow · Suture repair · Auxiliary fixation

Z. Fu (✉) · J. Chen
Peking University People's Hospital, Beijing, China

D. Xing · Z. Peng · D. Ren · W. Feng · Y. Chen · H. Wang
Wuhan No. 4 Hospital, Wuhan, China

J. Dong
Tianjin Hospital, Tianjin, China

J. Zhou
Beijing Chao-Yang Hospital, Capital Medical University, Beijing, China

Q. Yao
Beijing Shijitan Hospital, Capital Medical University, Beijing, China

C. Zhuang
Ruijin Hospital, Shanghai JiaoTong University School of Medicine, Shanghai, China

X. Wu
Shanghai General Hospital, Shanghai, China
e-mail: drwxm@263.net

9.1 Clinical Anatomy of Shoulder Joint and Principles for Repair of Injuries

Zhou Junlin

Abstract Shoulder joint is one of the most important joints of human body and its function has a great impact on life. Further knowledge of the anatomy of the shoulder joint will enable us to improve our understanding of shoulder joint operation as well as the techniques for intraoperative reduction and fixation. This chapter provides an elaboration on the clinical anatomy of the shoulder joint and the principles for repair of its injuries by individual parts.

9.1.1 Clinical Anatomy of Shoulder Joint

Shoulder joint is one of which the range of motion is the largest. In terms of bone structure, the shoulder joint, also known as the glenohumeral joint, is composed of the humeral head and the scapular glenoid. In addition to its bone structure, the glenohumeral joint is also surrounded by coracohu-

P. Tang et al. (eds.), *Tutorials in Suturing Techniques for Orthopedics*, https://doi.org/10.1007/978-981-33-6330-4_9

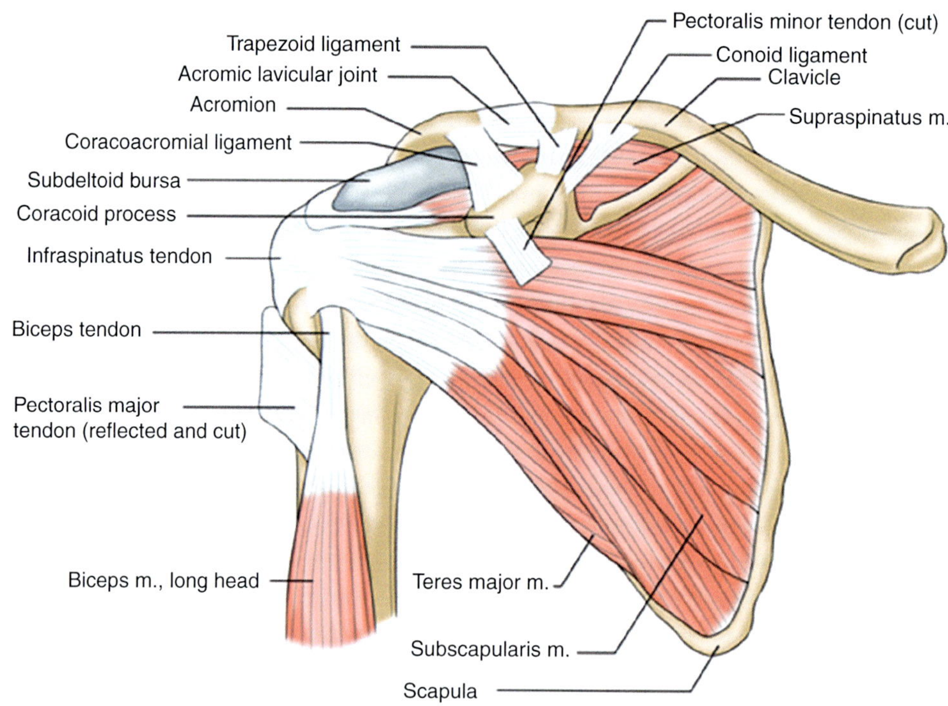

Fig. 9.1 Front view of shoulder joint

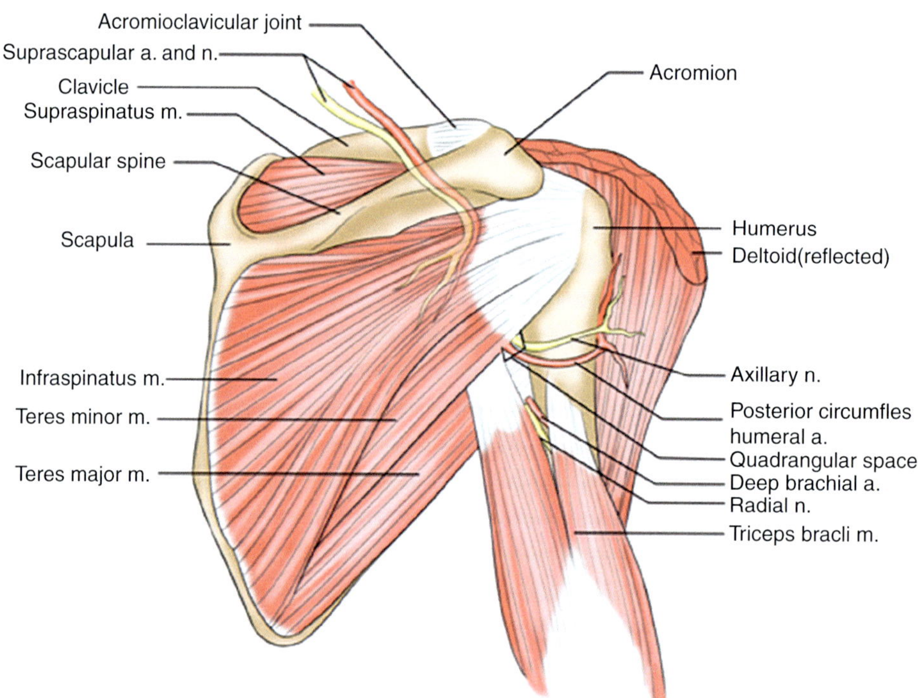

Fig. 9.2 Back view of shoulder joint

meral ligament, glenohumeral ligament, coracoacromial ligament, supraspinatus, infraspinatus, teres minor, teres major, subscapularis, deltoid, trapezius, latissimus dorsi, serratus anterior, etc. (Figs. 9.1 and 9.2). These structures increase stability of the shoulder joint while restricting its activity to a certain extent [1–3].

The shoulder joint is a typical multi-axial ball and socket joint, including the humeral head similar to a ball and the shallow and small glenoid. The surface of the shoulder joint is covered with hyaline cartilage, usually 2–7 mm thick [4–6]. The articular cartilage not only increases the smoothness of the articular surface, but also reduces the friction of the articular surface during the movement of the joint. The shoulder capsule is composed of fibrous connective tissues. The proximal end of the articular capsule fiber inserts at the glenoid labrum and the distal end at the anatomical neck of the humerus. It reaches as far as the surgical neck of the humerus on the medial side, and its proximal and distal ends fuse with the periosteum to enclose and seal the joint. The synovial layer of the joint capsule can bulge to form a synovial sheath or synovial capsule, facilitating tendon movement. The synovial sheath is formed in the groove between the greater and lesser tubercles of the shoulder joint capsule, and surrounds the long head of the biceps tendon (LHBT) which originates from the supraglenoid tubercle of scapula and meets the short head in the middle of humerus through the intertubercular groove to form the venter of biceps brachii. The biceps brachii descends to the lower end of the humerus and, in the end, the tendon stops at the radial tuberosity and the aponeurosis of the forearm. The thickness of the shoulder joint capsule varies in different parts, which is very thin where ligament reinforcement is absent. The inferior wall of the joint capsule is, relatively, the thinnest and, therefore, the humeral head often slips off the lower part in a dislocating shoulder joint and results in anterior inferior dislocation [7].

The joint capsule is thicker in the front for the coracohumeral ligament and the glenohumeral ligament. The shoulder joint cavity can also connect with the surrounding bursae, with the anterior part able to be connected with the subscapular bursa. The glenoid labrum of shoulder joint is the fibrocartilage tissue around the scapular glenoid, which deepens the articular surface and increases the stability of the joint. The glenoid fossa can still hold only 1/4–1/3 of the humeral head although its depth is deepened by the glenoid labrum. Such a form of the bone structure of shoulder joint reduces the stability of the joint, while increasing the range of motion. In case of repeatedly dislocation of the shoulder joint, the glenoid labrum will be torn off the glenoid edge and result in structural injury of the glenoid labrum. The number of cases of glenoid labrum degradation is also significant among elderly patients having suffered no dislocation before [8].

View of the bony-soft tissue ring-consisting of:
1. Superior strut-middle and lateral third of clavicle.
2. Inferior strut-junction of most lateral portion of the scapular body and medial portion of glenoid neck

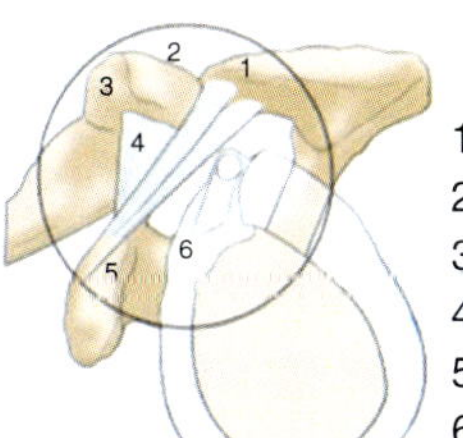

Fig. 9.3 Suspension complex of upper shoulder joint

Therefore, elderly patients or patients with shoulder dislocation experience some decrease in shoulder joint stability and are prone to joint injuries.

The main role of the shoulder joint is to suspend the upper limb and provide its movement [1, 2, 4, 9]. The suspension of the strength of the upper limb is also shared by muscles around the shoulder joint, the major and minor tubercles of the shoulder, the acromion and other bony structures, in addition to the shoulder capsule ligament. The superior shoulder suspensory complex (SSSC), of which the role is to maintain the stability of the upper limb, is a circular structure composed of distal clavicle, acromioclavicular joint and ligament, acromion, glenoid, scapular neck, coracoid process, and coracoclavicular ligament (Fig. 9.3). These structures not only share the weight on the shoulder joint, but also limit the movement of the ball and socket joint, so as to stabilize the shoulder joint. Therefore, the muscles and ligaments around the joint play an important role in the stability of the shoulder joint.

9.1.2 Clinical Structure of Shoulder Joint and Principles for Repair of Injuries

With a wide range of motion, the shoulder joint is one of the most flexible joints of the whole body and can move in three axial planes, that is, the flexion and extension on the coronal axis, the retraction and extension on the sagittal axis as well as the medial and lateral rotation and circumduction on the vertical axis. An arm abduction over 40°~60° and further elevation to 180° is often accompanied by movement of the sternoclavicular joint (SCJ) and the acromioclavicular joint (ACJ) as well as rotation of the scapula. Flexibility of the shoulder joint also results in its proneness to injuries. With the development of new artificial substitutes, the treatment of shoulder joint injuries is constantly improving. Whichever repair or replacement, humeral head replacement, total joint replacement including the glenoid, or even reverse shoulder joint replacement, cautious repair of tissues around the shoulder joint is very important to the prognosis of patients. Our discussion of the composition of shoulder joint will be based on its division into bony structures, surrounding muscles, innervating nerves and important peripheral blood vessels, etc. Our presentation on the principles for the repair of should joint injuries synchronizes with the analysis of different structures.

1. *Bony Structures of the Shoulder Joint*

   Bones making up the shoulder joint include: the clavicle, the scapula, and the proximal humerus.

   The clavicle is the limb girdle, a long S-shaped bone located transversely in the upper anterior part of the thorax, with its full length able to be touched on the body surface. The medial end, which is big and thick, is the sternal end, with articular surface connected with the sternal stem. The lateral end, which is flat, is the acromial end, with facet joint connected with the acromion of scapula. The medial 2/3, in a triangular shape, is convex forward; and the lateral 1/3, in a flat shape, is convex backward. Fractures are most likely to occur where its shape changes. The clavicle, which is in a superficial position, is smooth on the top and rough on the bottom. It looks like a long bone, but has no marrow cavity. The clavicle is the only upper limb bone directly connected with the trunk. It supports the scapula like a lever, and keeps the upper limb away from the chest wall to ensure flexible movement of the upper limb and transmit the stress from the upper limb to the trunk.

The clavicle mainly works to keep the upper limb away from the trunk and increase its range of motion. The fibrocartilage disc is located in the middle of SCJ, which enables 35° anteroposterior motion, 30°–35° upward and downward motion and 44°–50° rotational motion. The upward and downward motion of SCJ mainly occurs between the fibrocartilage disc and the clavicle. The anteroposterior and rotational motions occur between the fibrocartilage disc and the sternum. However, when the distal end of the clavicle is under a downward force, the clavicle can move upward with the rib as the fulcrum. SCJ is strengthened by the anterior and posterior sternoclavicular ligaments (SCL) around it. The posterior sternoclavicular ligament (PSCL) is stronger and can prevent the clavicle from moving upward. The space between the two clavicles is strengthened by the interclavicular ligament (ICL), which can prevent the clavicle from moving outward. ICL consists of the anterior ligament and the posterior ligament, which prevent the clavicle from moving laterally or medially. The involutory surface of the acromioclavicular joint (ACJ) is small, and the ACJ capsule is very weak, making ACJ prone to dislocation. The coracoid is connected with the clavicle by coracoclavicular ligament (CCL), which consists of the medial conical ligament and lateral trapezoid ligament. In case of an injury, it is important to pay attention to CCL and, if necessary, repair it as it is the main structure for static stability to ensure suspension of the scapula and even the upper limb. The range of motion of ACJ is 5°–8°. At both ends of the clavicle is synovial joint, which substantially increases the range of motion of the clavicle. The motion of SCJ and ACJ inevitably coincides with the motion of scapula.

Early surgical indications of a clavicle fracture include open fracture, skin or pleura about to be punctured by the fracture end, or accompanying neurovascular bundle injury. Relative surgical indications include accompanying ipsilateral upper limb injury, spinal cord injury, or multiple traumas. A surgical therapy is necessary for the "floating shoulder (FS)" with severe displacement or ipsilateral instability of scapular neck and clavicle fracture, and it may also be considered for a case of simple clavicle fracture.

The scapula is a triangular flat bone attached to the back outside of the thorax, between the second and the seventh ribs. It can be divided into two sides, three edges and three angles. The ventral or costal side, a large shallow fossa called subscapular fossa opposite to the thorax, is where the subscapular muscle starts. The transverse ridge on the dorsal side is called scapular spine. The shallow fossae above and below the scapular spine, from which supraspinatus and infraspinatus originate, are called supraspinatus fossa and infraspinatus fossa, respectively. Acromion, the flat protrusion extending laterally from scapular spine, is connected to the lateral end of the clavicle. It is one of the bony structures of ACJ. The upper edge of the scapula is short and thin, with a scapular notch on the lateral side, where there is the suprascapular transverse ligament. More laterally is the finger-like protrusion called coracoid, where CCL starts. A complete fracture of the coracoid will affect the function of CCL and, therefore, repair of the fractured coracoid is recommended. The acromion is connected with the coracoid by CAL to form the coracoacromial arch, which makes up the second shoulder joint with the supraspinatus and the humeral head. The thin and sharp medial edge of the scapula is also called the vertebral border for its adjacency to the spine. The lateral edge is also called the axillary border for its adjacency to the axillary. The superior border meets the vertebral border at the superior angle of the scapula, which is parallel to the second rib, while the vertebral border meets the axillary border at the inferior angle, which is parallel to the seventh rib or the seventh intercostal space and is a landmark for counting the ribs. The thickest lateral angle is the junction between the axillary border and the superior border, where pear-shaped shallow fossa, called glenoid, faces outward. Connected to the humeral head, the glenoid is surrounded by the glenoid labrum for increased its depth. A rough protrusion is located above and below the glenoid, which is called the supraglenoid tubercle and the infraglenoid tubercle, respectively. The long head tendon of the biceps brachii (BB) originates from supraglenoid tubercle, while the infraglenoid tubercle is one of the starting points of the triceps brachii (TB). The scapular spine, the acromion, the inferior angle of scapula (IAS), the medial margin and the coracoid, palpable on the surface of the body, are all bony landmarks during surgical operation or physical examination. Scapular fractures are often seen in injury due to direct violence, which can be divided into body fracture, scapular neck fracture, scapular spine fracture, scapular glenoid fracture, coracoid process fracture, and acromial fracture, among which fracture of the scapular body is the most common. Surgical repair is recommended when a scapular fracture involves the glenoid together with a dislocation of the fracture.

In most cases, fracture of the scapular body can be treated conservatively by immobilizing the shoulder joint until the pain disappears. A surgical therapy will not be applied unless the fracture block is obviously displaced and the motion of the scapula or the glenohumeral joint (GHJ) is affected. In case of a scapular process fracture, the non-union rate of displaced scapular spine fracture is high, and malunion may lead to restricted function of the shoulder joint. Therefore, displaced scapular spine fracture needs surgical treatment. If coracoid fracture is accompanied by ACJ dislocation, the coracoid fracture block will dislocate with the lateral end of the clavicle. A surgical therapy may be applied under such an unstable circumstance. Scapular neck fracture will cause decline in the function of the rotator cuff and, possibly, shoulder joint instability as well.

Humerus, the largest tubular bone in the upper limb, consists of the humeral body as well as the upper and lower ends. The upper end includes a hemispherical humeral head which faces toward the upper posterior medial side and connects with the glenoid of the scapula. The shallow annular groove around the head is called anatomical neck. The protuberances on the lateral and anterior sides of humeral head are called greater tubercle and lesser tubercle, which extend downward into the greater tubercle ridge and the lesser tubercle ridge, respectively. The longitudinal groove between the two tubercles is called intertubercular groove. The thinner junction of the upper end with the body, where it is prone to fracture, is called surgical neck, where the cancellous bone of humeral head and cortical bone of humeral shaft share border. Humeral head has a 130° to 135° neck-shaft angle and a 15° caster angle with humeral shaft.

A surgical therapy is recommended for a dislocation of the fracture block of greater tubercle and lesser tubercle over 6 mm. For a Type A fracture of the proximal humerus, a surgical therapy may be applied in case of a relatively high requirement for the shoulder joint function. In a Type B fracture, the instable surgical neck of a Type B2 fracture, if accompanied by rotation and displacement of the humeral head fracture block, may be subject to a surgical reduction. A surgical reduction is recommended for a Type B3 fracture as most of the closed reduction can hardly maintain the stability of fractured end. Generally, a surgical therapy is recommended for cases of Type C fracture.

2. *Muscle Structure of the Shoulder Joint*

This mainly includes the shoulder cuff, the teres major, and the deltoid.

Shoulder cuff, also known as the rotator cuff (Fig. 9.4), is a group of tendon complex around the humeral head. The anterior part of the humeral head is the subscapular tendon, the top is the supraspinatus tendon (SST), and the posterior part is infraspinatus tendon (IST) and teres minor tendon [2, 3, 6]. Contraction of these tendons causes inward and outward rotation and raising of the shoulder joint. More importantly, however, they stabilize humeral head on the scapular glenoid, playing a pivotal role in maintaining the stability of the shoulder joint and its motion. The supraspinatus originates from 2/3 of the bone surface in the medial part of the supraspinatus fossa and its surface fascia, moves forward as a short and flat tendon, and inserts at the superior part of greater tubercle. The infraspinatus, a broad bipennate muscle with visible yellow fat line in the middle, originates from the infraspinatus fossa and its surface fascia, and inserts at greater tubercle below the insertion of the supraspinatus. The teres minor originates from the back of 1/3 of the outer edge of scapula and inserts at greater tubercle below the insertion of the infraspinatus. The supraspinatus is mainly as an abductor muscle of the shoulder. When the shoulder abduces to an angle below 30°, it pulls the humeral head inward and downward to the glenoid to stabilize the shoulder joint, assisting the deltoid muscle to complete abduction of the shoulder. Infraspinatus and teres minor are the major extortors of the shoulder which can stabilize the shoulder joint during the motion of the shoulder. Supraspinatus and infraspinatus are innervated by the suprascapular nerve, and teres minor is innervated by the axillary nerve. The suprascapular artery accompanying subscapular nerve is involved in the formation of the scapular artery network to nourish the muscle group. The subscapular muscle originates from nearly all the costal surface of the scapula, passes the anterior part of the shoulder joint, and inserts at lesser tubercle. A bursa is located between the muscle and the scapular neck, which is mostly connected with the shoulder joint cavity. It is

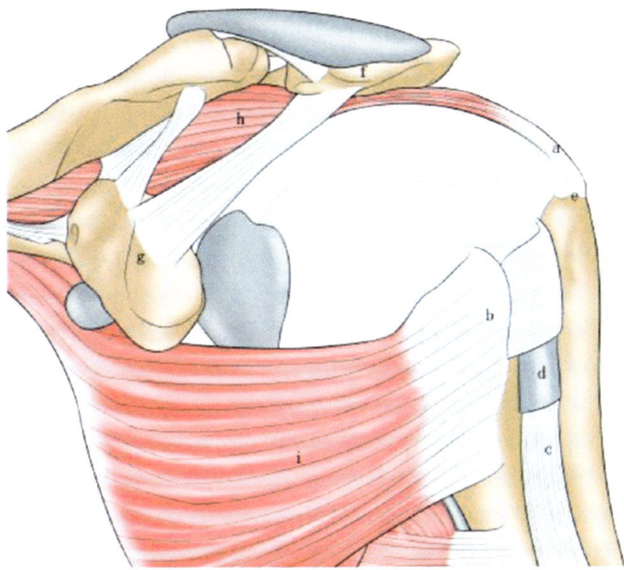

Fig. 9.4 Structure of rotator cuff. (**a**) Supraspinatus tendon; (**b**) Subscapular tendon; (**c**) Long head tendon of BB; (**d**) Long head of biceps tendon sheath; (**e**) Greater tubercle of humerus; (**f**) Acromion; (**g**) Coracoid; (**h**) Supraspinatus; (**i**) Subscapular muscle

innervated by the superior and inferior subscapular nerves and nourished by branches of the subscapular artery. The subscapular muscle mainly works to enable adduction and inward rotation of the shoulder joint. These four muscles constitute the rotator cuff and an important dynamic stability structure of the shoulder joint. Arthroscopy may be applied in case of an injury which affects movement of shoulder joint.

Teres major originates from the back of the IAS and inserts at the ridge of lesser tubercle. As it carries forward, the long head of TB runs from between the teres major and the teres minor. The latissimus dorsi surrounds the insertion of the teres major from the back to the front. Innervated by the subscapular nerve, the teres major enables adduction, inward rotation, and dorsal extension of the shoulder joint.

The deltoid originates from 1/3 of the clavicle and full length of the acromion and the scapular ridge. It originates from the insertion of the trapezius muscle and inserts at the tuberosity of the deltoid on the lateral side of the humeral shaft. The deltoid is so called because the fibers are distributed in the front, external, and back sides of the shoulder joint. The fibers in the middle are mainly for abduction, the anterior fibers for flexion and inward rotation, and the posterior fibers for dorsal extension and outward rotation of the shoulder joint. The lower part of the anterior and posterior fibers can adduce the shoulder joint to some extent when the shoulder joint is in a neutral position [9]. The deltoid is innervated by the axillary nerve, which moves upward and forward after separating from the posterior bundle to bypass the surgical neck of the humerus and access branches, and innervate the deltoid. Therefore, the position of the axillary nerve is lower in the posterior fibers of the deltoid than in the anterior fibers. Therefore, the axillary nerve should be specially protected if the deltoid is split longitudinally from 1/3 the anterior middle. Arterial supply is provided by the posterior humeral circumflex artery (PHCA). The borders of the fibers of the deltoid are visible to the naked eye and can be divided into three separate parts for the innervation by different branches of the axillary nerve along the way, which are relatively independent in function. Knowing this point will help understand the various functions of the deltoid and the fact that longitudinal deltoid splitting is often used in some operative approaches.

3. *Cutaneous Sensory Nerves of the Shoulder Joint*

The cutaneous sensation in the superior part of precordium is innervated by supraclavicular nerve, which is the branch of C1 and C4 of the cervical plexus. The skin of the thoracic region is innervated by the intercostal nerve (ICN), while the level of the sternal stem is innervated by T2. The dorsal skin is innervated by ICN, and the upper lateral arm innervated by the axillary nerve. The axillary base and the medial arm are innervated by the intercostobrachial nerve (ICBN) from T2 or T2, T3. The lower part of the medial arm is innervated by the medial brachial cutaneous nerve from the medial fasciculus (Fig. 9.5).

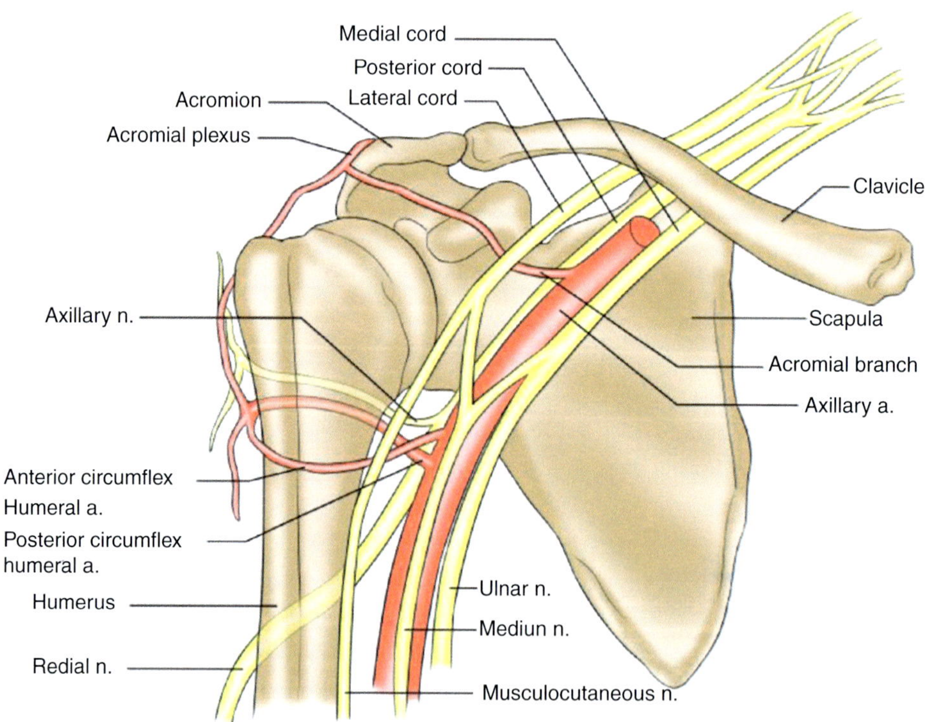

Fig. 9.5 Distribution of important nerves and blood vessels around shoulder joint

4. *Important Blood Vessels Around the Shoulder Joint*

Important arteries include axillary artery, etc. The axillary artery goes on from the subclavicular artery at the lateral border of the first rib and then moves forward through the depth of the axilla to the lower border of the latissimus dorsi, with branches as follows: the superior thoracic artery, which is located in the space between the first and the second ribs; the thoracoacromial artery, which is divided into several branches distributed in the pectoralis major, the pectoralis minor, the deltoid, and the shoulder joint. The lateral thoracic artery runs in company with the long thoracic nerve and is distributed in the serratus anterior, the pectoralis major, the pectoralis minor, and the breast. The subscapular artery is composed of the thoracodorsal artery and the circumflex scapular artery. The former extends to the latissimus dorsi and the serratus anterior, while the latter passes through the trilateral foramen to the muscles near the infraspinatus fossa to mold to the suprascapular artery. The posterior humeral circumflex artery accompanies the axillary nerve, runs through the quadrilateral foramen, winds through the surgical neck of the humerus to the deltoid and the shoulder joint, etc., to mold to the anterior humeral circumflex artery. The anterior humeral circumflex artery, to the shoulder joint and adjacent muscles.

Important veins around the shoulder joint include axillary vein, etc. [2, 3, 10] Deep veins of the upper limb, usually two, are accompanied by the artery of the same name. Venous blood in the upper limb is mainly drained by the superficial vein, so the deep veins are thinner. Two brachial veins meet at the lower border of teres major and make up the axillary vein, which is located in the anteromedial part of the axillary artery and changes to be the subclavian vein at the lateral edge of the first rib. The axillary vein collects all the blood from the superficial veins and the deep veins of the upper limb. Superficial shoulder veins are mainly upper ends of the cephalic vein, which is located between the deltoid and the pectoralis major and passes through the clavipectoral fascia into the axillary vein. The cephalic vein originates from the radial side of the dorsal venous network of hand, moves up along the radial side of the lower forearm, the superior part of the forearm, the anterior side of the elbow and the lateral groove of BB, and then passes through the groove between the deltoid and the pectoralis major to the subclavian fossa, and then through the deep fascia into the axillary vein or the subclavian vein. It communicates with the basilic vein through the median cubital vein at the cubital fossa. The cephalic vein collects venous blood from superficial structures of the hand and the radial side of the forearm. The basilic vein originates from the ulnar side of the dorsal venous network of hand, moves up along the ulnar side of the forearm, turns to the front side of the elbow, embraces the median cubital vein at the elbow fossa, passes the medial groove of the BB to the midpoint plane of the arm, and runs through the deep fascia and into the brachial vein, or goes up in company with the brachial vein into the axillary vein. The basilic vein collects venous blood from the superficial structure of the ulnar side of the hand and the forearm.

Conclusively, the bony structure of the shoulder joint consists of the clavicle, the scapula, and the humerus, and the muscles include the rotator cuff, the teres major, and the deltoid, with important nerves and blood vessels around. Therefore, anatomical knowledge and insights into the shoulder joint will help improve understanding of the shoulder joint surgery and the repair skills. The general principle of shoulder joint repair is to restore the function of the shoulder joint as much as possible to minimize the impact of the injury.

9.2 Learn to Use Anatomical Landmarks in Reduction and Repair

Zhou Junlin

Abstract Many anatomical landmarks of the shoulder joint are available. It is the key to an operation on the shoulder joint how to make good use of each individual anatomical landmark. With a focus on different surgical approaches and various internal fixations, this section investigates the methods for repairing or reconstructing the shoulder joint as much as possible and restoring its function.

9.2.1 Anatomical Landmarks of the Shoulder Joint

There are many anatomical landmarks of the shoulder joint. The bony landmarks include the greater tubercle, the lesser tubercle, the intertubercular groove, the anatomical neck, the surgical neck, the acromion, the coracoid, the distal clavicle, the scapular spine and the lateral border of scapula, etc. (Fig. 9.6). Muscular landmarks include the long head tendon of the biceps brachii, the rotator cuff, the teres major, the deltoid and the latissimus dorsi, etc., together with other soft tissue landmarks such as the cephalic vein, the brachial plexus, the axillary arteries and veins, the trilateral foramen, the quadrilateral foramen and the axillary nerve, etc. It is of critical importance to know these anatomical landmarks in the repair of a shoulder joint injury [11–13] as the shoulder joint can be exposed, reset, and fixed or reconstructed based on these anatomical landmarks during the surgical operation.

First of all, it is of critical importance to correctly distinguish between anatomical neck fracture and surgical neck

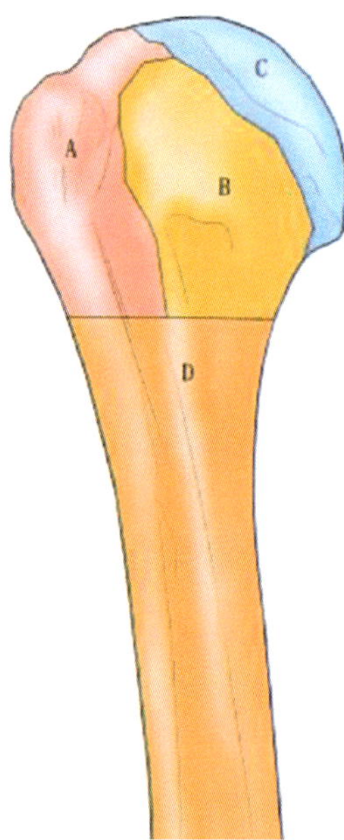

Fig. 9.6 Bony landmarks of proximal humerus. (**a**) Greater tubercle; (**b**) Lesser tubercle; (**c**) Humeral head; (**d**) Humeral shaft

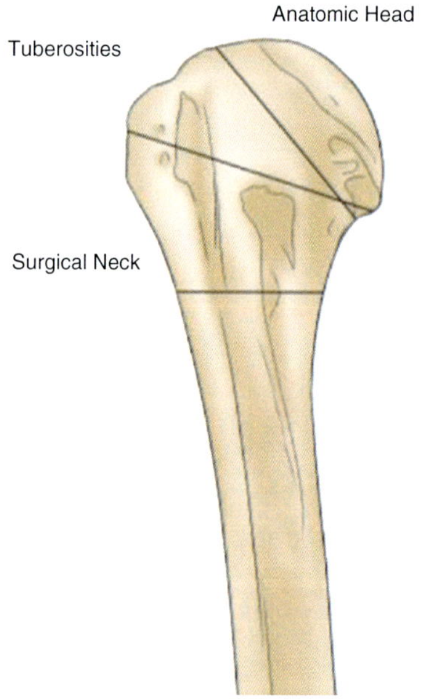

Fig. 9.7 Surgical neck and anatomical neck of humerus

fracture (Fig. 9.7) [6, 14, 15], because the main blood supply of the humeral head fracture block is usually damaged after the fracture of anatomical neck of the humerus, which makes avascular necrosis of the humeral head very likely to occur. Fracture of the surgical neck of the humerus, by contrast, is better, because the blood supply to the humeral head is usually preserved well. The lateral ascending branch of the anterior humeral circumflex artery is located in the intertubercular groove, often a few millimeters posterolateral to the long head of the biceps brachii tendon and moving upward with it in parallel. In dissecting and separating the long head tendon of the biceps brachii, therefore, attention should be paid to the lateral ascending branch of the anterior humeral circumflex artery, so as to prevent damage on it and, consequently, any impact on blood supply to the humeral head.

The anatomical position of the long head tendon of the biceps brachii is very important (Fig. 9.8) for fracture classification and prognosis of the patient, even as well as the selection of surgical approach and the placement of internal fixation [9, 10, 16]. Therefore, the first thing is to find the long head tendon of the biceps brachii in an open reduction and internal fixation surgery. The blood supply on the medial side of the shoulder joint capsule also plays an important role. It has a positive effect on the prognosis of the fracture if there is a substantial, complete fracture block in the medial humeral head. The long head tendon of the biceps brachii is important for identifying the ascending branch of the lateral circumflex humeral artery and reducing the greater and the lesser tubercles. If the fracture cannot be reduced by a closed approach, it may be due to the embedment of the long head tendon of the biceps brachii between the fracture blocks. Equally important are other soft tissues as anatomical landmarks. The acromion, the coracoacromial ligament, and the coracoid, for instance, make up the coracoacromial arch to restrict movement of the humeral head below it, with the rotator cuff sliding under the coracoacromial arch. The injury, if any, may affect the function of the shoulder joint.

9.2.2 Surgical Approaches for Shoulder Joint

Common surgical approaches for the shoulder joint include: the deltoid-pectoralis major groove approach and the lateral deltoid approach. The choice of these two surgical approaches is also made according to the anatomical landmarks of the shoulder joint. The following is an elaboration on these two approaches.

Deltoid-pectoralis major groove approach (Fig. 9.9): The incision originates from between the coracoid and the clavicle and extends obliquely to the deltoid attachment. The incision of the surgical approach originates from the coracoid and extends to the tuberosity of the deltoid of the humerus. Find the cephalic vein at the proximal end and pull it aside for exposure of the deltoid–pectoralis major interface. Cut open the clavipectoral fascia on the lateral side of the conjoint tendon, and leave the coracoacromial ligament at the proximal end. Cut 1–2 cm open from the upper edge of the insertion of the pectoralis major to the distal end. Locate the fracture block, and remove the hematoma. The long head

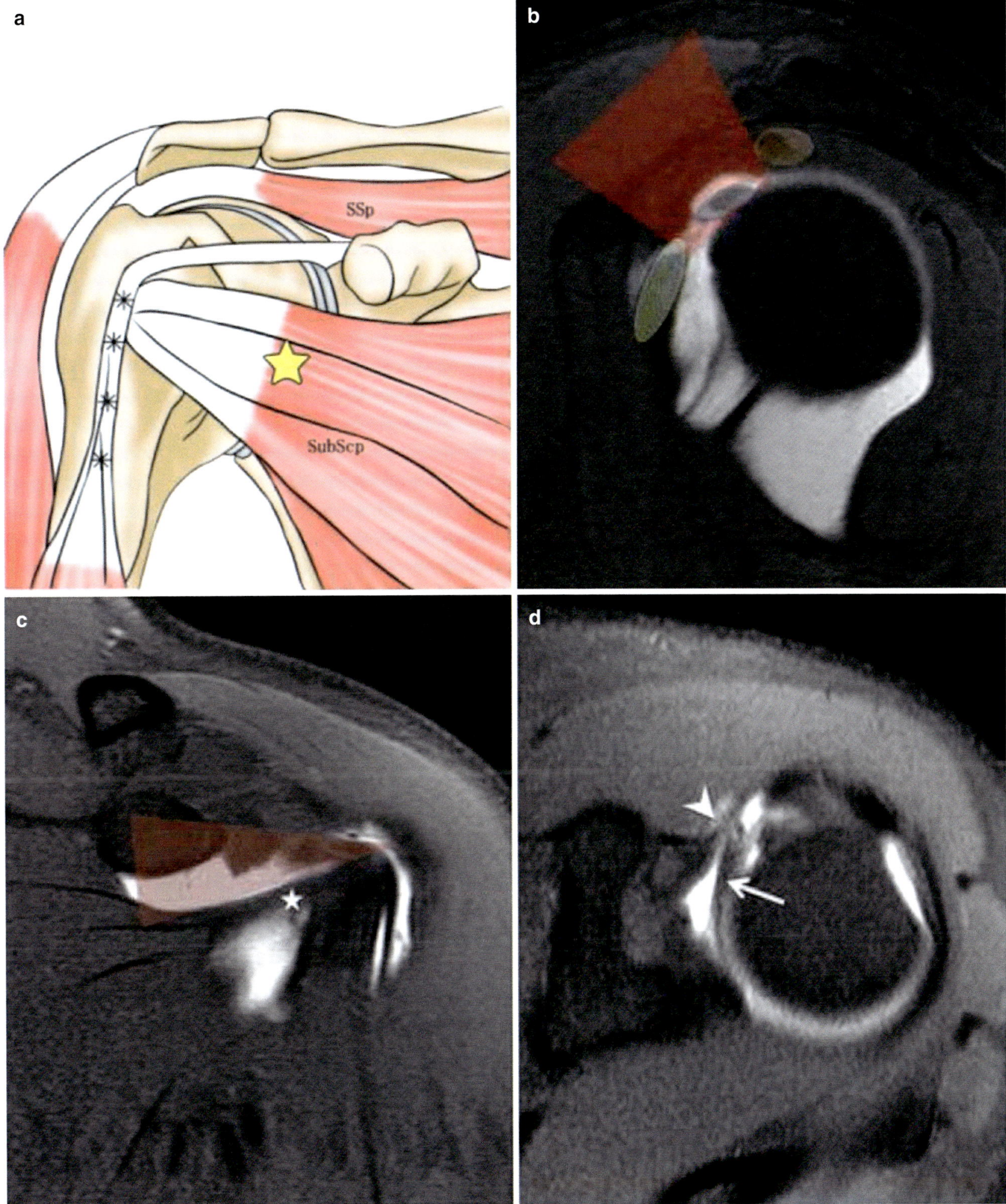

Fig. 9.8 Anatomical position of the long head tendon of biceps brachii. (**a**) Simple image; (**b**) MRI oblique sagittal; (**c**) MRI oblique coronal; (**d**) MRI axial

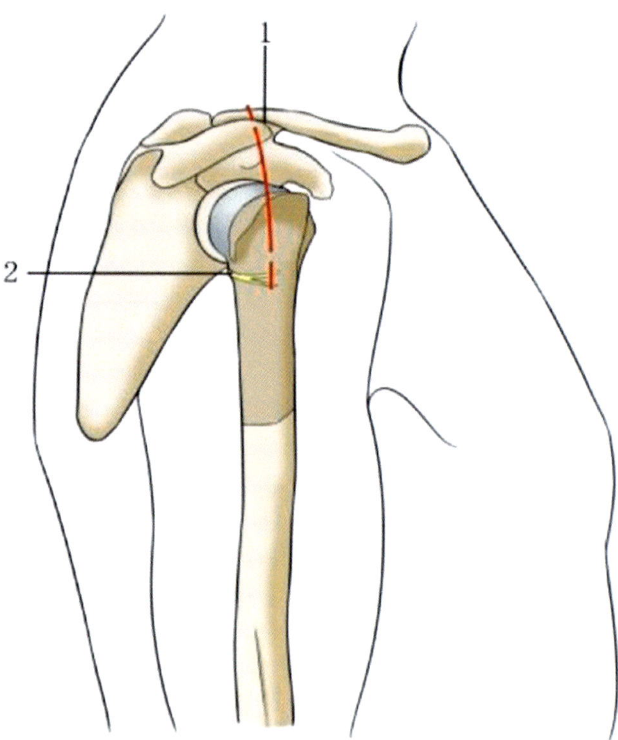

Fig. 9.9 Lateral deltoid approach. 1. Acromioclavicular joint, 2. Axillary nerve. The incision of this approach originates from not more than 5 cm below the distal end of the anterolateral angle of the acromion

tendon of the biceps brachii, an important landmark for identifying the greater and the lesser tubercles as well as the attached rotator cuff tissue, can be found in the depth of the pectoralis major. Exposure of the space below the deltoid via abduction of the shoulder joint can enable operation on proximal fracture. Application of a long plate for distal extension of the fracture needs separation of the anterior 1/2 of the distal insertion of the deltoid. The retractor should be placed carefully behind the proximal fracture block, so as to prevent damage on the axillary nerve. Reduce the fracture under the premise of protected blood supply of the fracture block. When a steel plate is used, the plate should be placed on the lateral side of the intertubercular groove, so as to prevent damage on the ascending branch of the anterior humeral circumflex artery.

Lateral deltoid approach (Fig. 9.9): The incision of this approach originates from not more than 5 cm below the distal end of the anterolateral angle of the acromion (marked with "safe suture" to prevent damaging the axillary nerve), passes through the lateral deltoid approach, follows the separation between the anterior and central deltoid to the subdeltoid bursa. The anterior part of the deltoid and the anterior border of the trapezius muscle can be separated sharply at the lateral end of the clavicle and the acromion in case of a need for extension of the incision, which needs to be sutured to the original insertion when it is being closed. Through inward and outward rotation of the upper arm, we can detect the greater and the lesser tubercles or the rotator cuff as well as reduction and fixation of fracture block. Split the deltoid longitudinally at the anterior angle of the acromion, that is, the intersection at 1/3 of the anterior and central deltoid as it is a natural dividing line of the deltoid where it bleeds less. The longitudinal split may reach upward the deltoid and start from the acromion. If necessary, the starting point of the deltoid may be stripped toward the anterior or below the posterior periosteum. It may reach downward to 3.8 cm below the acromion, where a stich can be made transversely across the extension line of the incision with Non-Absorbable ETHIBOND® Suture (Polyester, Ethicon Inc.) to prevent the deltoid from further splitting downward, and thus damaging the axillary nerve. It is generally believed that the axillary nerve is located 4 cm below 1/3 of the anterior and central deltoid and that the damage on this nerve may lead to denervation of anterior fibers of the deltoid.

For proximal humeral fractures, reduction and repair are carried out in ways that vary with different surgical methods. The following is about how to fulfill exposure, reduction, and fixation of the fracture based on anatomical landmarks by individual different surgical methods.

Open reduction and internal fixation with steel plate for proximal humeral fracture: Position and preoperative preparation: In beach chair position, with the trunk placed on the edge of the bed, a cushion placed behind to make the patient tilt slightly to the opposite side, and a radiolucent upper limb or shoulder support placed along the side of the bed. The whole upper limb must be able to move or operate freely during the operation. C-arm assisted fluoroscopy is to be performed from multiple angles, including the axillary position as well as the anteroposterior (AP) position, with attention to be paid to rotating the upper arm and observing the length of the screw from multiple angles in case of an AP position. Mark the bony landmarks of the clavicle, the acromion, the scapular spine, and the coracoid with a pen in surface projection of the incision. Open the skin and the subcutaneous tissue, and perform conventional open reduction of proximal humerus and internal fixation or humeral head replacement via the deltoid-pectoralis major sulcus approach. For fracture of the greater tuberosity with backward displacement, sometimes, the fixation might be difficult through the deltoid-pectoralis major approach alone, which can be addressed by combining the conventional deltoid-pectoralis major groove approach with the deltoid splitting approach. Separate the deltoid from the pectoralis major at the distal end of the incision, where it is easy to find the cephalic vein. Bluntly separate the lateral side of the cephalic vein from the deltoid fibers. Pull the cephalic vein and the small deltoid fibers to the medial side for protection, and bluntly separate the deltoid-pectoralis major sulcus from the sternoclavicular fascia to expose the proximal humerus. At the distal end of the incision, release the anterior 1/3 of the deltoid insertion laterally along the humerus surface. In the middle of the incision, release the superior part of the insertion of the pectoralis major at the ridge of the greater tuberosity of the humerus, so as to facilitate exposure, reduction, and fixation of the fracture block. Always bear in mind during the operation to avoid damaging the axillary nerve or the musculocutaneous nerve. Abduction of the upper limb during the operation can relax the deltoid, and help expose the incision. Fracture reduction and fixation techniques: Different techniques are available for reduction of fractures of different Neer types. 2-part fracture of the surgical neck of humerus can be reduced by pulling the affected limb. In case of any impaction at the fracture end, a blunt periosteum elevator can be inserted into the gap between the fracture ends during the traction, which may be used as a lever for prying and reducing the fracture. Pay attention to confirming the alignment of rotation upon reduction of the proximal humeral fracture through the surgical neck. Landmarks for the reduction include the alignment of fracture lines and intertubercular groove. The retroversion angle of the humeral head should also be checked, at the time of which the elbow may be bent 90°. Observe the included angle between the axis of the humeral head and that of the humeral condyle, which should be 30°. 3-part fracture of the proximal humerus, suture the insertion of the subscapularis muscle and the supraspinatus tendon with thick non-absorbable sutures, pull forward to expose the posterior infraspinatus tendon insertion and suture, similarly, the insertion of the subscapular muscle and the supraspinatus tendon with thick Non-Absorbable 2# ETHIBOND® Suture (Polyester, Ethicon Inc.). Carry out the reduction under direct vision, and pay attention to observing whether the fracture line is aligned and whether any terrace is left. For 2-part fractures, a threaded guide pin may be inserted into the proximal bone block as a lever, or a non-locking screw may be used to reduce the position relationship with the humeral shaft through the plate. Pay attention to detecting rotation displacement upon reduction, which can be marked by the alignment of the fracture lines and the intertubercular groove.

In case of a patient with osteoporosis, the retained suture should be pulled and tied tight to enhance the fixation.

For 3-part fracture of the proximal humerus, the 3-part fracture can be converted into a 2-part fracture. The use of a reduction forceps may lead to further crushed bone block, increased reduction difficulty, and impact on the stability after reduction. Sew Non-Absorbable 2# ETHIBOND® Suture (Polyester, Ethicon Inc.) at the insertion of the subscapularis muscle, the supraspinatus and the infraspinatus tendon, respectively, fasten the suture, and reduce the fracture to transform the 3-part fracture to a 2-part fracture. After the fracture is changed into a two-part one, a threaded guide pin can be used as a lever to reduce the metaphysis and humeral shaft, or a steel plate is used to reduce the humeral shaft and the metaphysis with non-locking screws. It should be noted that the direction to place the screw is subject to the fracture displacement, and the holes should be drilled perpendicular to the displaced humeral shaft. After reduction, use a Kirschner wire for temporary fixation after reduction, and it should be noted that the Kirschner wire should be placed from the front, so as to avoid affecting the placement of the lateral steel plate. After fracture reduction and temporary fixation, check the retroversion of the humerus head and, more importantly, the recovery of the neck-shaft angle of the humerus, that is, a 135° angle between the axis of humeral neck and the long axis of the humerus.

4-part fractures of the proximal humerus: For a case of 4-part fracture of proximal humerus, reduce the humeral head bone block first after pulling aside the bone block of the greater and the lesser tubercles. Put something under the armpit or use the fist as the fulcrum, drag the affected limb at the same time, and reduce the everted humeral head by using the lever principle. Or, use a blunt-headed periosteum elevator to assist in the reduction of the humeral head fracture block. Fix the humeral head and shaft temporarily with Kirschner wire. Tighten the retained suture afterwards, and reduce the bone block of the greater and the lesser tubercles. In addition to checking the cervical trunk angle, axillary or lateral fluoroscopy also needs to be performed to check whether there is a forward or backward angle between the humeral shaft epiphysis and the humeral shaft.

The steel plate should be placed along the axis of the humerus, with the maximum height of the plate 5–8 mm below the top of the greater tubercle, and the medial margin of the plate 2–4 mm behind the intertubercular groove. The height of the plate through fluoroscopy should not protrude upward, that is, the Kirschner wire positioned at the top of the plate should not exceed the highest point of the humeral head; otherwise, subacromial impingement syndrome (SAIS) will occur after the operation. Insert the locking screw, and fix the length of the screw to the subchondral bone of the articular surface of the humeral head, where the pull-out resistance is the strongest. For patients with unstable medial support and osteoporosis, it is recommended to have 1–2 humeral calcar screws applied, so as to obtain sufficient medial support. Generally, five screws are screwed into the humeral head. The number of screws depends on the osteoporosis of the humeral head. More screws can be used appropriately in case of osteoporosis. In order to stabilize the position of the greater and the lesser tubercles, suturing can be made at the tendon-bone junction of the insertion of the supraspinatus, the infraspinatus and the subscapularis muscle, pulling the sutures through the suture hole around the plate, and tie them tight for the tension band effect, and further stabilize the rotator cuff structure.

During the operation, the shoulder joint may be abducted, and the deltoid muscle relaxed for better exposure of the fracture. Suture and fix the insertion of the rotational axis to improve reduction and fixation of the fracture block. Forward inclination of fracture of the surgical neck of humerus is likely to be angulated. Correct the deformity due to angulation by lifting the distal end of the upper arm and pushing the fracture site downward toward the ground. In the reduction and fixation of proximal humerus fractures, the medial cortex is an important supporting structure. For proximal humeral fractures with incomplete or defective medial cortex, bone grafting, fixation of medial bone block with screws or use of mini-plates as backup may be applied to maintain stability of the medial column. It is recommended that the bone calcar screws be inserted. Screws may be implanted outside the steel plate as bone calcar screws if holes for such screws are unavailable.

The steel plate should not be placed much too forward; otherwise, it will be excessively close to the intertubercular groove and affect the long head tendon of the biceps brachii and the ascending branch of anterior humeral circumflex artery which moves along in the intertubercular groove, thus affecting the blood supply of the humeral head. To prevent displacement of the fracture block after the operation, the tip of the screw should be as close to the subchondral bone as possible. However, a distance of approximately 5 mm must be kept with the articular surface, so as to prevent the screw from sliding out. Rotate the upper arm inward as much as possible after screw implantation due to the 30° retroversion angle of the humeral head. Most of the articular surface of the humeral head can be observed through fluoroscopy in the anteroposterior position.

In the application of intramedullary nail fixation: Before placement of the intramedullary nail, the needle entry point will be under the acromion if the proximal end of the fracture is in an abduction position, when the threaded guide pin can be inserted as a lever for prying and reducing the fracture.

For humeral head replacement, the deltoid-pectoralis major intermuscular groove approach can be used [3, 15]. Firstly, identify the long head tendon of the biceps brachii, and find the greater and the lesser tubercles on the lateral side within the tendon. Mark them with non-absorbable sutures, drag them to the medial and the lateral sides to expose the humeral head and the glenoid. Remove the comminuted humeral head. Be careful not to damage the blood vessels and nerves in the axillary region if the humeral head is located under the coracoid. Drag the greater tubercle and the humeral shaft to the lateral side, so that it is easier to take out the humeral head if the humeral head bone block falls into the back of the joint. For a case of old fracture, the humeral head may be trapped in the scar. Crush the humeral head first, and remove it little by little. Sew the reserved Non-Absorbable 2# ETHIBOND® Suture (Polyester, Ethicon Inc.) where the tendon attaches to the bone at the greater and the lesser tubercular bone block. Trim the proximal humerus, and then expand the cavity slightly with an intramedullary file. Drill in the cortex of the proximal humerus, and insert steel wire or non-absorbable suture into the bone foramen, so as to facilitate fixing the greater and the lesser tubercles. Inject bone cement into the medullary cavity of the proximal humerus, and insert appropriate prosthesis.

Pay attention to the retroversion of the humeral head, which is usually 25° to 40° backward, during the operation. Place the forearm in neutral position, take the internal and external condyles of the distal humerus with the thumb and the index finger as the reference on the horizontal plane. Tilt the prosthesis 25° to 40° backward. The wing of the prosthesis should be aligned to the posterior part of the intertubercular groove. Try the reduction of the prosthesis, and carry out inward and outward rotational activities. Stability of the joint when the inward and outward rotation reaches 50° indicates appropriate backward inclination angle. Should posterior fracture dislocation occur, the backward inclination should be reduced by 5° to 10° while it should be increased by 5° to 10° in case of anterior fracture dislocation. The principle is that the backward inclination should not be $<20°$ or $>40°$.

Selection of prosthesis stem depth: Much too deep prosthesis stem will lead to reduced length of the humerus and shorter effective length of the deltoid. The space for placing the greater and the lesser tubercles must be allowed under the humeral head to maintain appropriate tension of the biceps tendon. For patients with osteoporosis, it should be noted that roomy proximal humeral medullary cavity will make it hard to achieve tight fit with the prosthesis. Therefore, bone cement is often used to fix the prosthesis. Note that the humerus should be drilled and preset with steel wire or non-absorbable suture before the injection of bone cement; otherwise, it will be very difficult to fulfill this operation after the bone cement is injected into the medullary cavity.

For fixation of the greater and the lesser tubercles, drill holes on these tubercles, and drag closer the tubercular bone blocks through the reserved suture. The suture at this site is used to resist the stress of the long axis of the humerus. Loop the sutures reserved in the tendon-bone junction of the greater and the lesser tubercles around the prosthesis stem in the medial side to complete the cerclage, and the suture at this site is used to resist the separation stress of the greater and the lesser tubercles. Insert the steel suture or Non-Absorbable ETHIBOND® Suture (Polyester, Ethicon Inc.) preset on the humeral shaft into the greater and the lesser tubercles, respectively, and tighten it up. Fix the greater and the lesser tubercles together with the humeral end and the prosthesis wing to make up a total movement unit restore the dynamic device of the shoulder joint. Take the graft of the humeral head, and implant it into the fracture space between the greater and the lesser tubercles and the humeral shaft, so as to obtain plenty greater tubercle of the humerus, which is helpful to the bony union of the greater and the lesser tubercles with the shaft and reduce bony absorption of the greater and the lesser tubercles. Desirable shoulder joint function will not be obtained unless bony union is achieved between the greater and the lesser tubercles and the humeral shaft. Take the cancellous bone in the humeral head, and implant it into the fracture space. The goal of joint replacement is to reconstruct a stable, painless, and effectively functional shoulder joint. Good reduction and firm fixation are the precondition for early functional exercise after the surgical operation.

Poor repair of the shoulder cuff injury will lead to postoperative pain and, therefore, the restoration of its integrity is of great importance. The shoulder cuff may be repaired and the healing may be enhanced by means of suturing (Fig. 9.10), so as to reduce postoperative pain and other complications. In the control of the retroversion angle of the prosthesis, the retroversion angle device of the shoulder prosthesis implanting system is used to control the angle at about 30°. The intertubercular groove can be used as a reference for prosthesis implantation. It is required that the wing of the prosthesis should be placed 1 cm behind the intertubercular groove. The greater and the lesser tubercles will not be reduced to the normal anatomical position unless the retroversion of the humeral head is kept within the appropriate range of angle. Poor reduction and insufficient healing of the greater and the lesser tubercles are important factors that affect the prognosis.

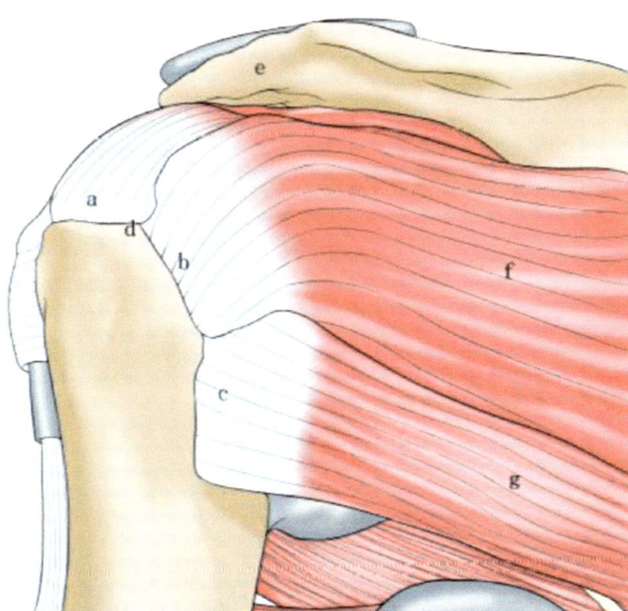

Fig. 9.10 Anatomy of rotator cuff. (**a**) supraspinatus tendon; (**b**) infraspinatus tendon; (**c**) teres minor; (**d**) greater tubercle; (**e**) acromion; (**f**) infraspinatus; (**g**) teres minor

For control of prosthesis height, the fracture will cause damage on bony landmarks. The lack of reference for the height of prosthesis to be placed increases the difficulty in prosthesis placement. The height of the prosthesis determines the tension of the soft tissue around the shoulder joint. Excessive height of the prosthesis will limit the movement of the shoulder joint on the one hand and result in excessive tension between the greater and the lesser tubercles and the bone shaft, which will, in turn, affect the bone healing between the greater and the lesser tubercles and the bone shaft. Insufficient height of the prosthesis will lead to decline in the tension of surrounding tissue and instability of the shoulder joint. The loss of the shoulder cuff function due to any cause will lead to the loss of inward tension of the humeral head. The shoulder joint will not be able to fulfill its normal functions if no fulcrum can be formed for lever movement during the motion of the shoulder joint. The special design of the reverse shoulder prosthesis can ensure that the shoulder joint obtains the fulcrum of the lever and complete the function of the shoulder joint even if the shoulder cuff loses its function.

In conclusion, many anatomical landmarks of shoulder joint are available. First of all, it is important to identify whether it is a case of anatomical neck fracture or surgical neck fracture. The anatomic site of the long head tendon of the biceps brachii is very important and should be determined first during the operation. Appropriate anatomic landmarks should be selected for the deltoid-pectoralis major sulcus approach and the lateral deltoid approach. For proximal humerus fractures, the fracture repair method varies with different surgical approaches; therefore, the anatomical landmarks to be followed are different. It is important, therefore, to identify appropriate anatomical landmarks according to different surgical methods and repair or reconstruct the shoulder joint as much as possible to restore its function.

9.3 Suture-Assisted Technique for Plate Nails and Intramedullary Nails in Internal Fixation of Proximal Humeral Fractures

Fu Zhongguo

Abstract Proximal humeral fractures account for 4%–5% of systemic fractures and are particularly common in the elderly with osteoporosis. A wide range of surgical solutions, including open reduction internal fixation (ORIF) with locking plates, internal fixation with intramedullary nails and joint replacement are available for the treatment of proximal humeral fractures. No consensus has been reached so far, however, on the gold standard for the treatment of proximal humeral fractures, and there are still some complications, including the loss of reduction, tubercular displacement, and malunion after the treatment. The use of the suture-assisted technique for reduction and fixation of the shoulder cuff and the tubercle bone block in the operation of proximal humerus fractures by means of internal fixation with steel plates or intramedullary nails not only helps fracture reduction in the operation, but also ensures the stability of fracture block fixation, so as to create better conditions for healing. In internal fixation of proximal humeral fractures, appropriate use of suture-assisted reduction and fixation will enable you to achieve a satisfactory process and effect of treatment.

9.3.1 Suture-Assisted Repair of Proximal Humeral Fractures with Steel Plates

In treating proximal humeral fractures, locking plate is a common internal fixation solution. Suture holes are available in commonly used anatomical plates for proximal humeral fractures and appropriate application of sutures to assist reduction and fixation will make the operation successful and achieve desirable results of treatment (Fig. 9.11). When the tubercle bone block and rotator cuff tissue are fixed with suture, the suture requires high-tensile strength and high tension (here, Non-Absorbable 2#, 5# ETHIBOND® Suture (Polyester, Ethicon Inc.) is recommended), and the suture site is the tendon-bone junction, because the tendon-bone junction has the best holding force, the knot can be tied with square knot. If necessary, assist metal band fixation, so as to ensure the fixation of fracture is stable, so as to create better healing conditions.

Bundle therapy is very popular for cases of proximal humeral fracture but the choice of right indications is very important. Even the application of a Kirschner wire with even stronger tension will result in a failure if the fracture is a type not suitable for the bundle therapy (Fig. 9.12).

The following is a case of suture-assisted reduction and fixation of complex proximal humerus fracture: Take a 2-part proximal humerus fracture under the Neer Classification System, for example. In spite of the fracture of the greater and the lesser tubercles of this type not more than 1 cm, sometimes there are too many fracture fragments, which not only cause many troubles for fixation (Figs. 9.13, 9.14 and 9.15) but even the reduction is a thorny problem (Fig. 9.16).

When the Kirschner wire cannot do with the reduction, reduction via suture traction is a technique worth trying. It is easy to handle and practical, with definite effect of reduction (Fig. 9.17). The position of suture fixation is usually above the insertion of the tendon, where the tendon is strong and tough, facilitating traction and fixation (Fig. 9.18).

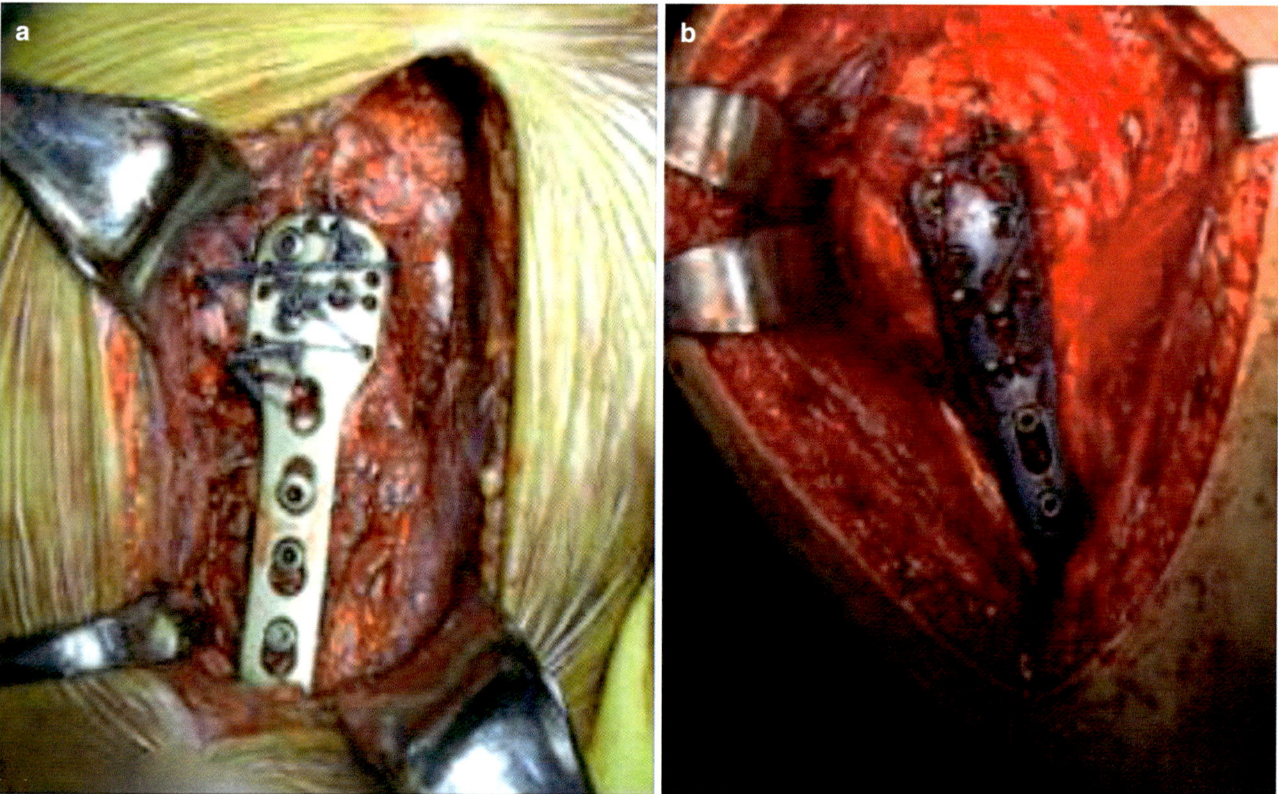

Fig. 9.11 Suture-assisted repair of proximal humerus fracture with steel plate. (**a**, **b**) Fixation by steel plate with suture

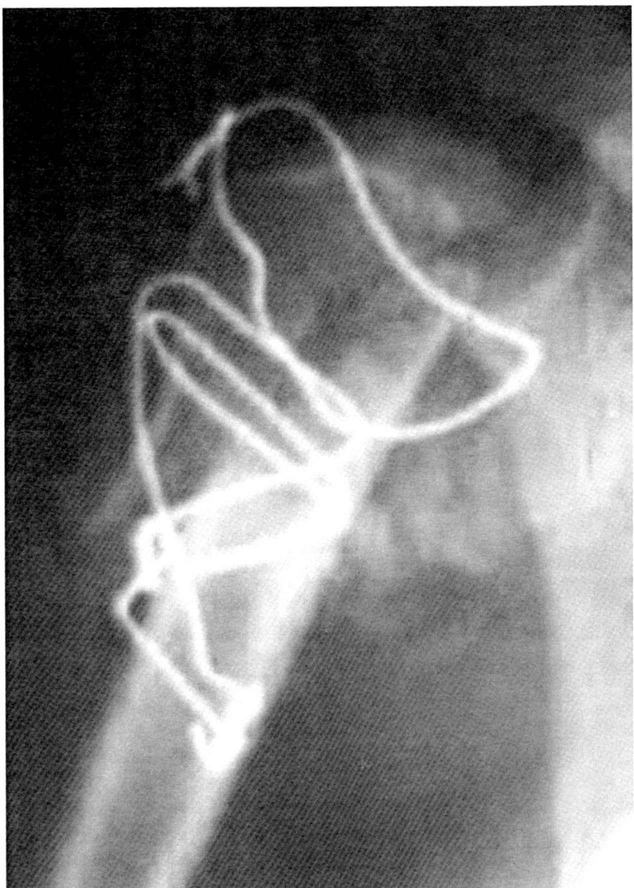

Fig. 9.12 Failure of the bundle and fixation of proximal humerus fracture

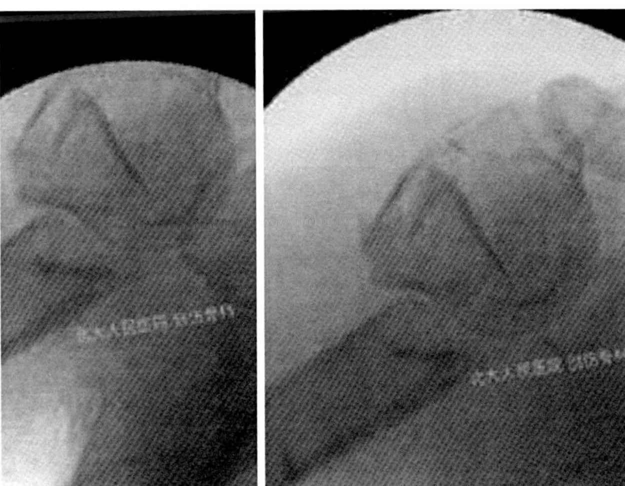

Fig. 9.13 X-ray film of 2-part proximal humerus fracture (Neer Classification System), showing the fracture in the surgical neck of the proximal humerus with evident displacement

Proximal humeral fractures often result in considerable loss of bones. In this case, implantation of an artificial humerus not only fills up the bone loss but also makes it easier to reduce the bone fragments (Fig. 9.19).

After the reduction with suture, put the primary fixation suture for the traction of the shoulder through the suture holes of the corresponding plate before the nails are fixed, so as to avoid the inconvenience in inserting the sutures afterwards. It may also be used as a reference for plate placement height (Fig. 9.20).

After suture-assisted reduction, the sutures can be led into the corresponding appropriate suture holes in the fixation plate, so as to enable long-acting fixation and protection of the shoulder cuff through internal fixation (Fig. 9.21), with desirable fixation effect able to be achieved after the operation (Fig. 9.22).

We need to pay attention to the followings during the course of repair:

1. Proper bone grafting not only fills up the bone loss, but also supports stability of the fracture (Fig. 9.23).
2. Take due care of "each and every" aspect of the shoulder cuff during suturing and, particularly, do not give up any bone fragments that may lead to connection of the shoulder cuff to the tubercles due to the fracture (Fig. 9.24). This requires careful preoperative assessment of the injury by the surgeon and meticulous detection during the operation to maximize the recovery of shoulder cuff function after the operation and achieve a satisfactory therapeutic effect.
3. Normal anatomical structure must be always followed during the course of reduction (Fig. 9.25a).
4. After the prefabrication of the traction suture for the shoulder cuff, fulfill upside and back-and-forth sliding contact in the tubercular zone with the fingers, so as to check whether there are any bone fragments associated with the rotator cuff missed during the reduction of the fracture. This is a very important step as, in clinical practice, missed bone blocks are often found during the X-ray examination after fixation with the plates and the nails, thus affecting the postoperative recovery of the functions.

The above is an elaboration on suture-assisted plate fixation technique for 2-part proximal humeral fracture (Neer Classification System). Sometimes, the fracture is relatively simple and can be repaired through a small incision. In such cases, the assistance of sutures also plays a very important role (Figs. 9.25b, 9.26 and 9.27).

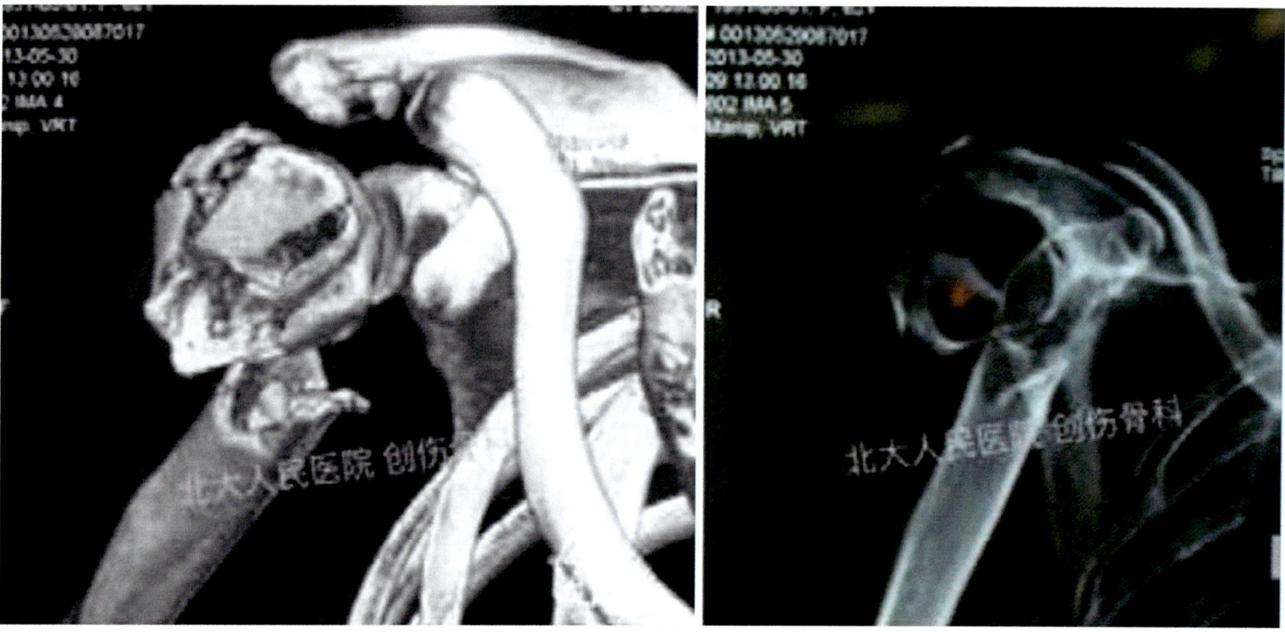

Fig. 9.14 3D CT reconstruction of a 2-part proximal humerus fracture (Neer Classification System), showing fracture of the greater and the lesser tubercles with displacement not obvious

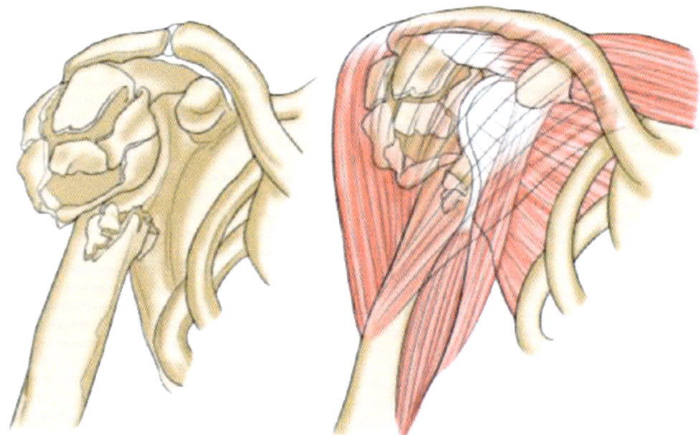

Fig. 9.15 Proximal humerus fracture

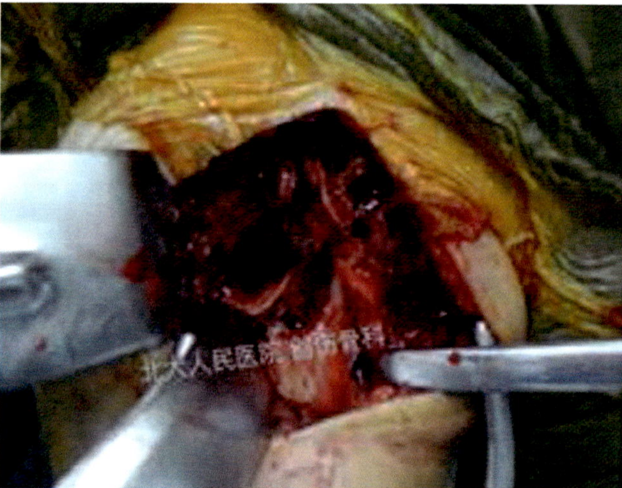

Fig. 9.16 Many fracture fragments are found during the operation, which leads to difficult reduction

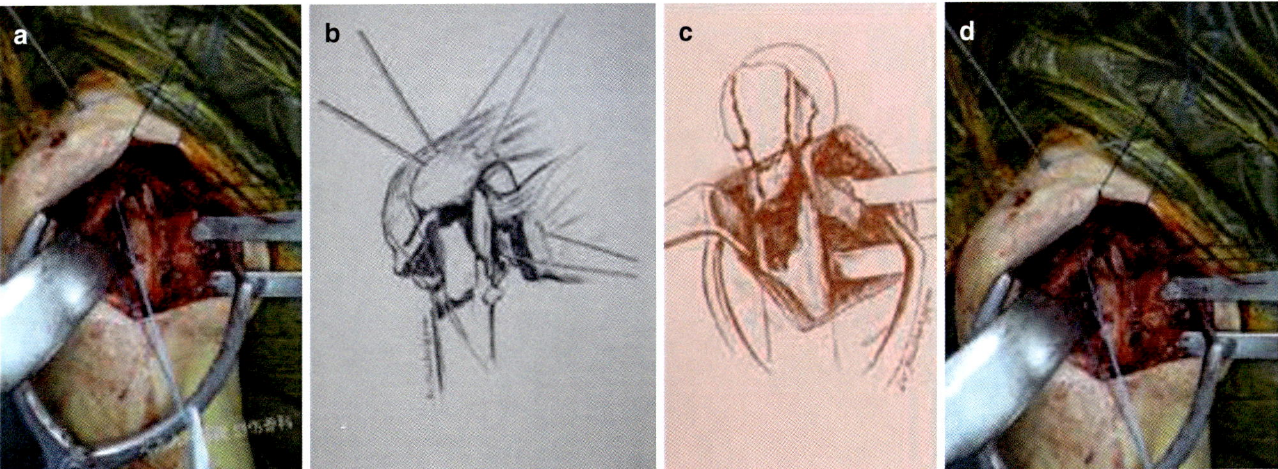

Fig. 9.17 Reduction via suture traction. (**a**) Reduction with Kirschner wire; (**b**) Operation of reduction with Kirschner wire; (**c**) Effect of reduction; (**d**) Application of the sutures and the Kirschner wire technique in fracture reduction

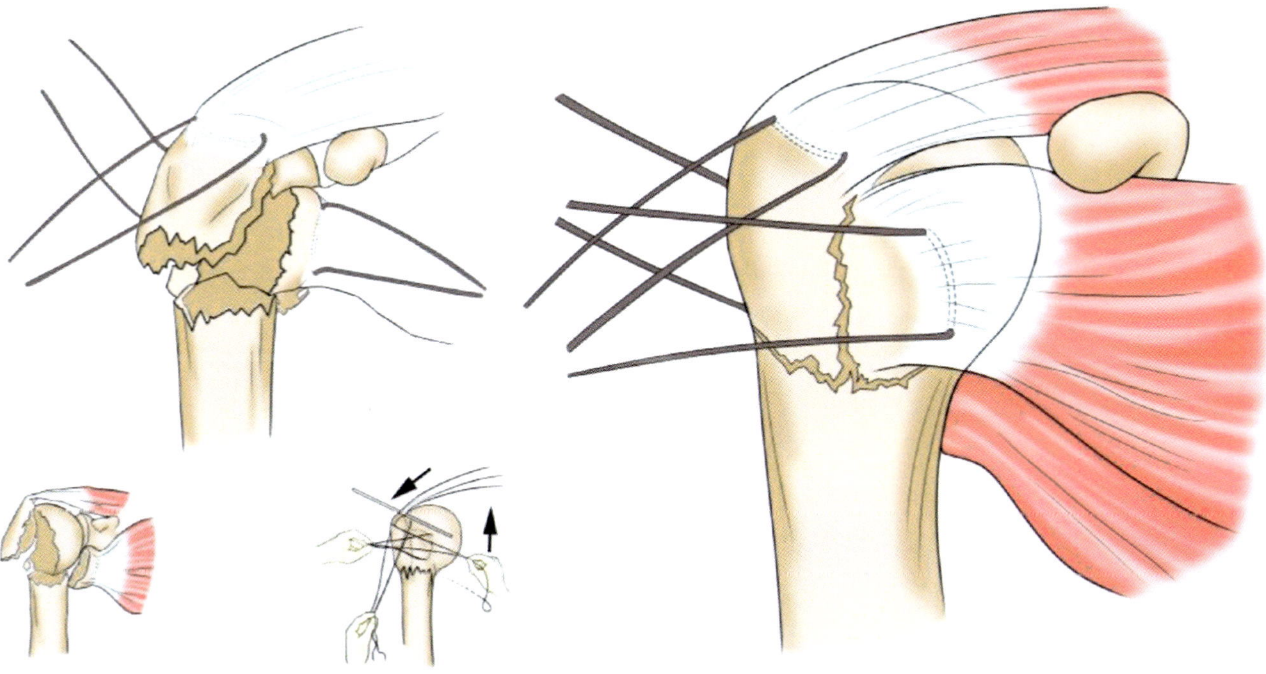

Fig. 9.18 Basic wiring locations

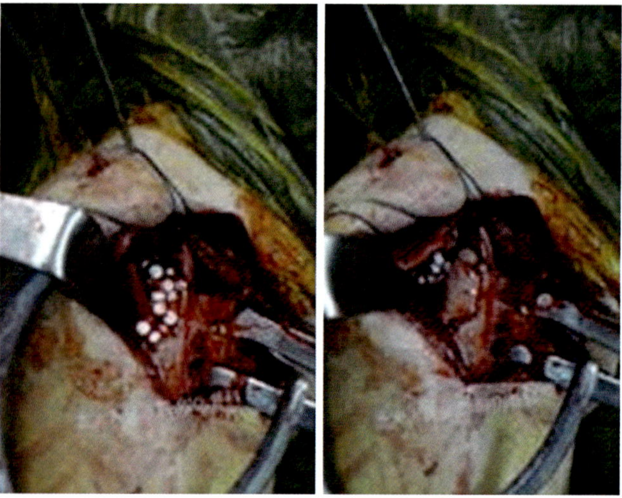

Fig. 9.19 Implantation of artificial bone

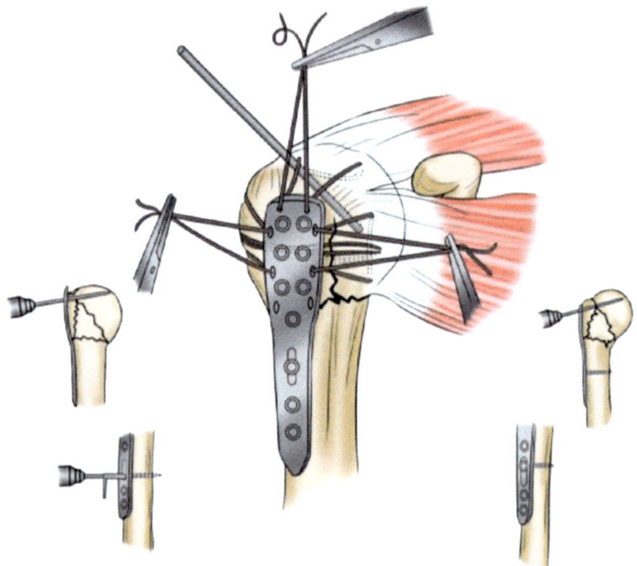

Fig. 9.21 Suture-assisted plate fixation

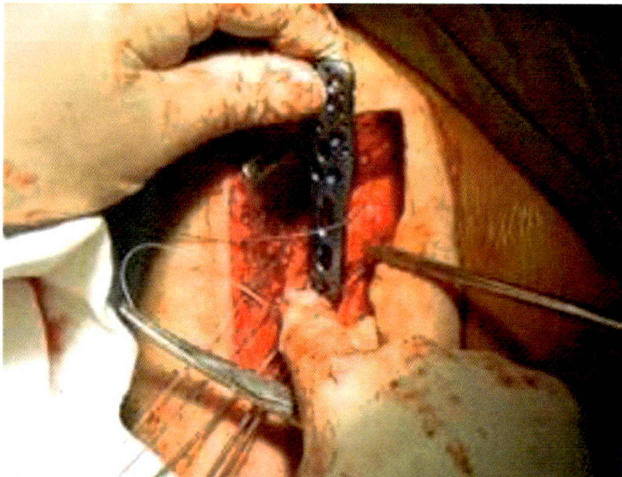

Fig. 9.20 Steel plate placing and pre-threading

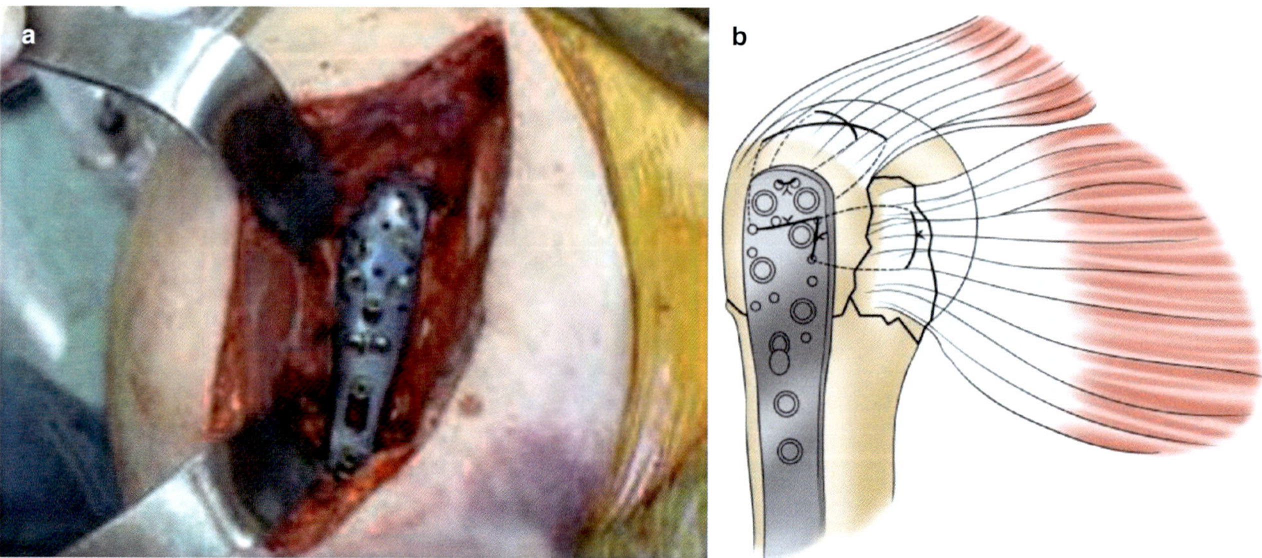

Fig. 9.22 Postoperative effect. (**a**) Effect of suture-assisted plate fixation; (**b**) Schematic diagram

Technical Summary for Different Bone Fractures

- This technique is also applicable for fractures at the lesser tubercle, but the suture needs to pass through the subscapular muscle tendon to increase fixation strength. Better fulfill this operation via the deltoid-pectoralis major approach.
- For 4-part fractures with eversion and impaction, suture not only between the greater and the lesser tubercles but also at each side of the humeral head and shaft under the apex of the fracture block of the humeral head, which helps to balance the strength of muscles of the shoulder joint to prevent deformity and retain the arm of force of the shoulder cuff.
- For 3-part fractures at the greater tubercle, the suture must pass through the entire lesser tubercle to maintain balance among all shoulder cuff tendons, so as to enable early start of the rehabilitation exercise.

A recent biomechanical study compared transosseous suturing, tension bands, and cancellous screws and found that the load at failure of transosseous suturing is significantly higher than that of the other two approaches, respectively.

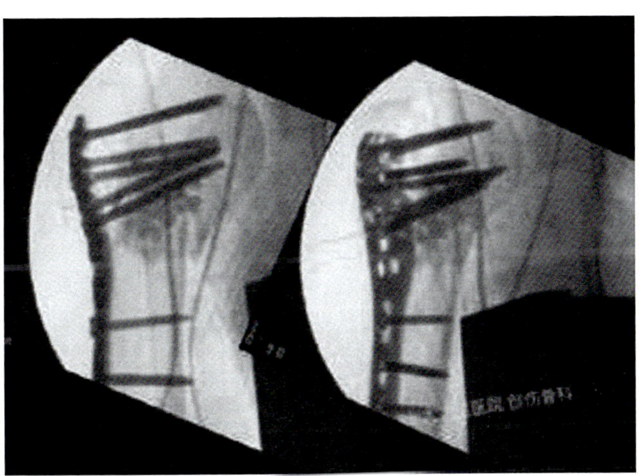

Fig. 9.23 Postoperative X-ray film

Precautions in the Repair of Proximal Humerus Fracture via Small Incision

- A likely trap in the reduction is that, due to the limitation of the incision or the blocking of the shoulder cuff, the anatomical reduction of the tubercular fracture is difficult, resulting in poorer fixation than expected and directly affecting postoperative functional recovery.
- Try to “take care of” the rotator cuff with sutures although it is a small-incision operation.
- Due care should be given to stable fixation of the greater and the lesser tubercles, which is closely related to postoperative functional recovery.

1. 4-Part Proximal Humeral Fracture (Neer Classification System)

   As shown in Fig. 9.28, a patient suffered a 4-part humeral fracture (Neer Classification System) due to an injury, and we chose to treat the case with the intramedullary nail therapy. Kirschner wire prying technique was applied to reduce the humeral head (Fig. 9.29), with relatively more difficulty in the reduction of the greater and the lesser tubercles. The author is used to considering the reduction and fixation of the greater and the lesser tubercles after intramedullary nailing for the proximal humeral fracture (Fig. 9.30).

   After intramedullary nailing, fulfill reduction and fixation of the greater and the lesser tubercles through suture assistance and traction (Non-Absorbable 2# ETHIBOND® Suture (Polyester, Ethicon Inc.) is recommended) (Figs. 9.31 and 9.32). Attention should be paid to the repair of the shoulder cuff, which plays an important role to ensure postoperative functional recovery (Fig. 9.33). Figure 9.34 indicates the effect of fixation by means of suture-assisted intramedullary nailing.

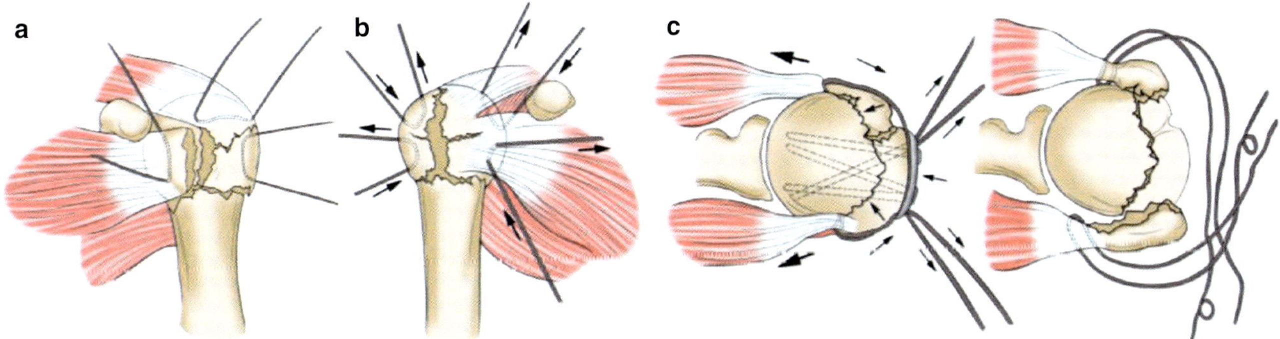

Fig. 9.24 Reduction of fracture block. (**a**, **b**) Reduction of shoulder cuff structure via suture traction; (**c**) Reduction and fixation of fracture and shoulder cuff structure with suture-assisted steel plate

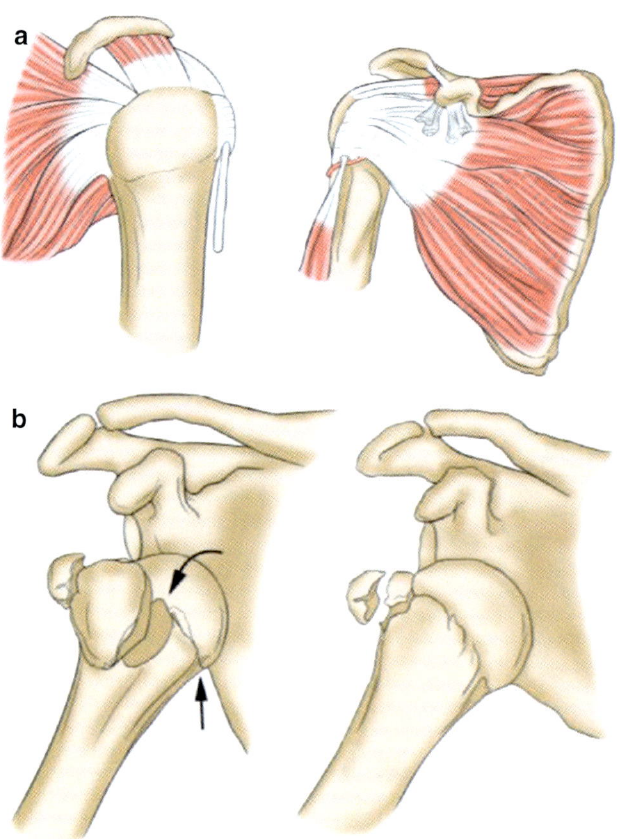

Fig. 9.25 (**a**) Anatomical structure of the insertion of normal shoulder cuff. (**b**) 2-Part fracture of the greater tubercle of proximal humerus (Neer Classification System)

2. 3-Part Proximal Humeral Fracture (Neer Classification System)

   For 3-part proximal humeral fractures (Neer Classification System) (Fig. 9.35), we may also choose the suture-assisted intramedullary nailing technique, and achieve very good effect of fixation. Fully assess the patient's injury before the operation with consideration of imaging examination data, execute examination and detection carefully during the operation, fulfill traction of the structure and tissues of the shoulder cuff with the sutures, and complete transfixion with sutures and fixation with intramedullary nails after reaching the anatomical site. As the greater and the lesser tubercles are not stable after the fixation with intramedullary nails and stabilization of the head and shaft structures in case of such fractures, the Nice knot may be used in the operation to achieve rigid fixation (Fig. 9.36).

In the application of intramedullary nailing for proximal humeral fractures, the role of sutures should not be ignored. Sutures play an indispensable part in the fixation and protection of the shoulder cuff under the "Parachute" principle. The author recommends application of single-thread sliding locking knot for the suture knotting technique, because only through sliding can the shoulder cuff and free bone block be stabilized and controlled. Nice knots may be used in case of a need for more rigid fixation of the free bone block.

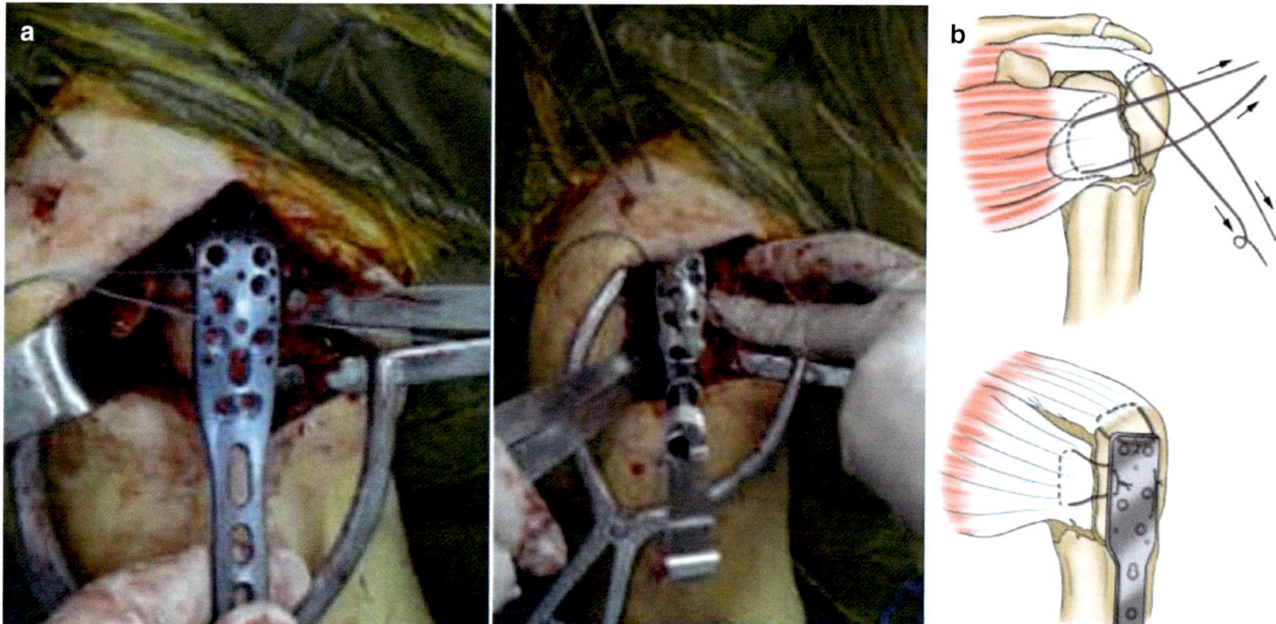

Fig. 9.26 Suture-assisted fixation with steel plate. (**a**) Fixation during the operation; (**b**) Schematic diagram

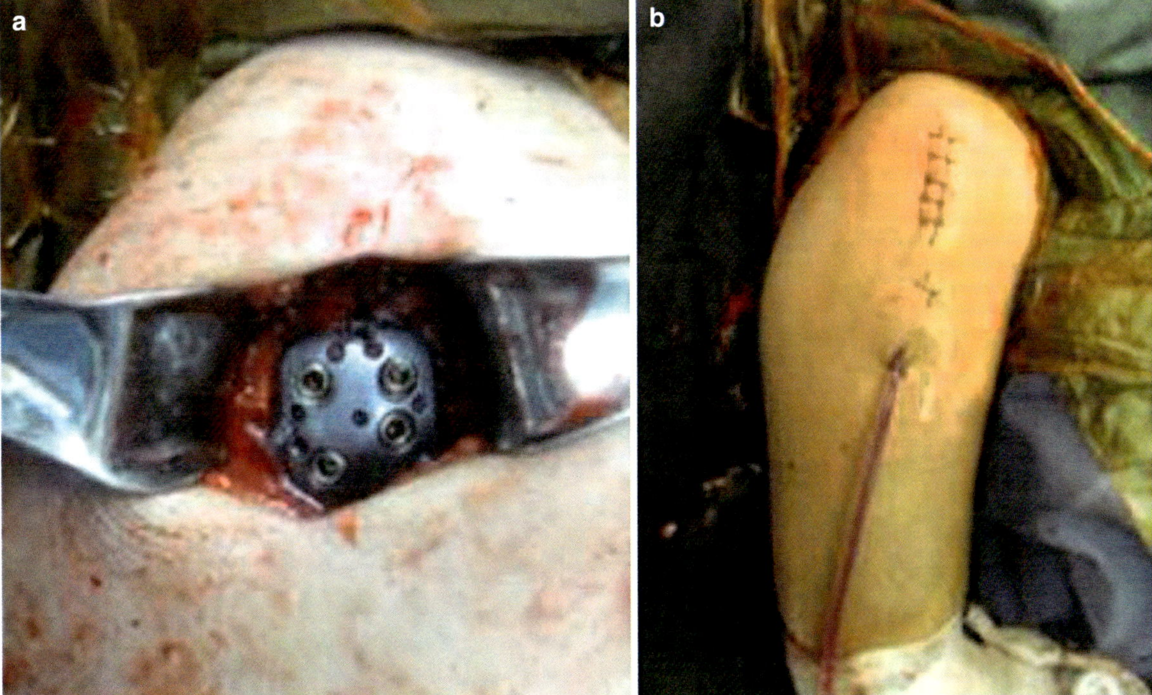

Fig. 9.27 Effect of suture-assisted fixation with steel plate. (**a**) Effect of fixation with steel plate; (**b**) Closing of the incision

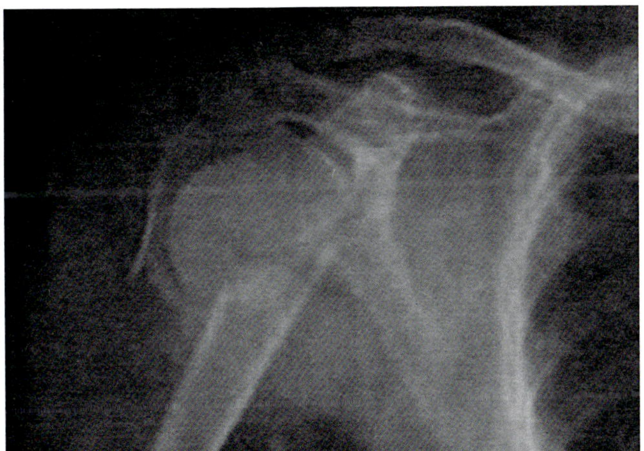

Fig. 9.28 4-part proximal humeral fracture (Neer Classification System)

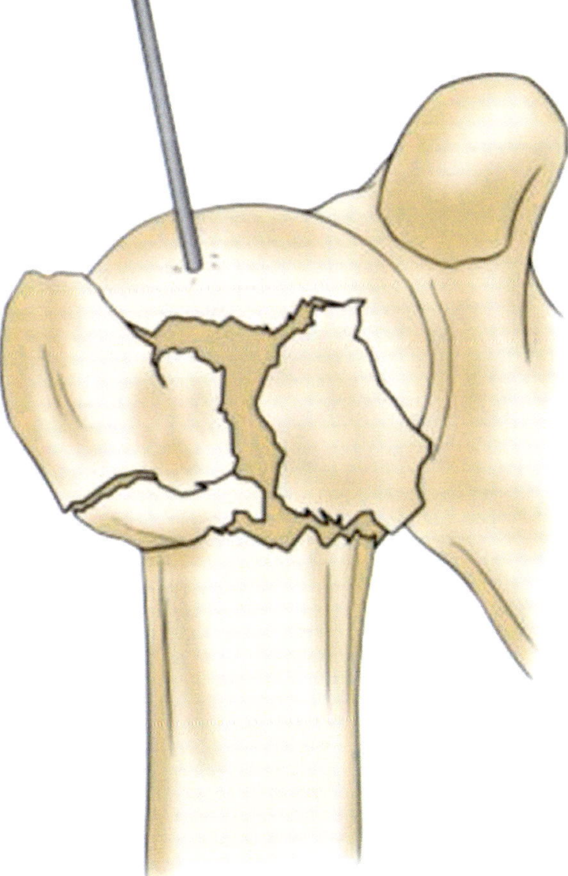

Fig. 9.29 Reduction of humeral head by prying with Kirschner wire

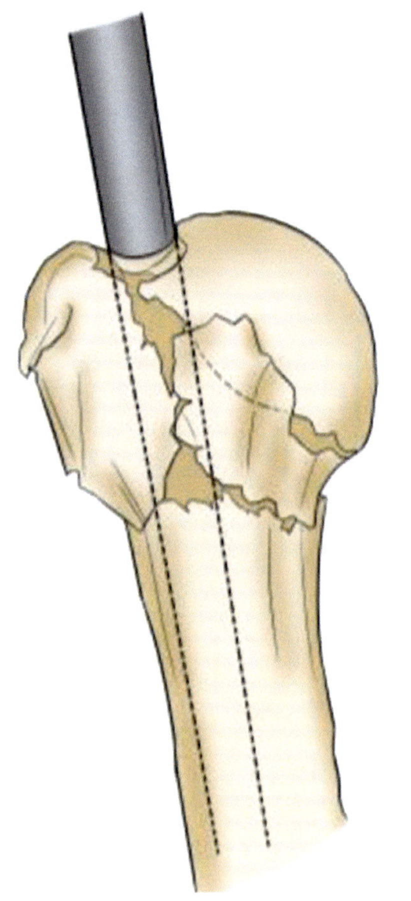

Fig. 9.30 Intramedullary nailing

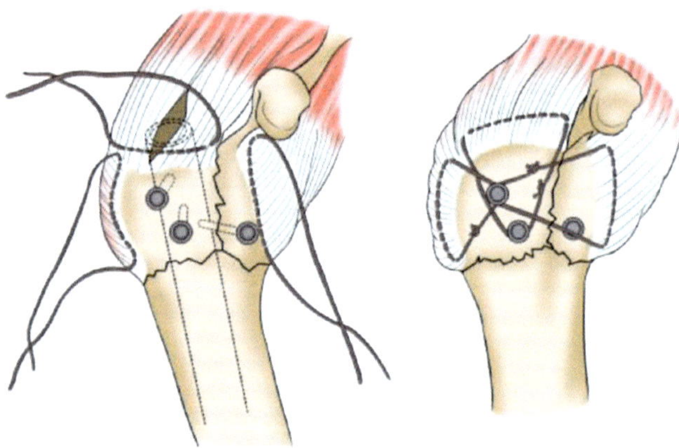

Fig. 9.31 Suture-assisted fixation of the greater and the lesser tubercles

9.4 Shoulder Prosthesis and Suturing Techniques

Dong Jingming

Abstract Proximal humeral fractures account for approximately 10% of fractures among the elderly. Non-surgical solutions, with satisfying outcome, are available to most of the cases. However, for more complex fractures, such as 3- or 4-part fractures under the Neer Classification System, fracture dislocation and humeral head fracture, shoulder replacement is often required. Conventionally, shoulder hemiarthroplasty is widely applied, but it is difficult to achieve perfect prosthesis height and proper prosthesis position due to high technical requirement, which is one of the most important factors affecting the postoperative efficacy. Currently, the indications of reverse shoulder replacement have been extended to complex proximal humeral fractures. Compared with shoulder hemiarthroplasty, it has less dependence on shoulder cuff repair and tubercular healing, and its popularity increases year by year. However, prior training still takes a long time. The postoperative effect will be more guaranteed only when a full understanding of the prosthesis principle has been acquired and when the operation is carried out by experienced surgeons specialized in upper limbs.

9.4.1 Overview

The incidence of proximal humeral fractures, as one of the brittle fractures among the elderly, is extremely high, ranking the third in osteoporotic fractures. Although the majority of proximal humeral fractures can be treated conservatively, surgical therapy is still the gold standard for cases such as the 3- and 4-part proximal humeral fractures with considerable displacement, fractures combined with glenohumeral joint dislocation, etc. The current mainstream surgical methods include internal fixation, such as open reduction with plate fixation and closed reduction with intramedullary nail fixation, and prosthesis replacement, such as shoulder hemiarthroplasty and reverse shoulder replacement.

For proximal humeral fractures, the incidence of avascular necrosis of the humeral head is extremely high if the residual of the medial wall attached to the humeral head is

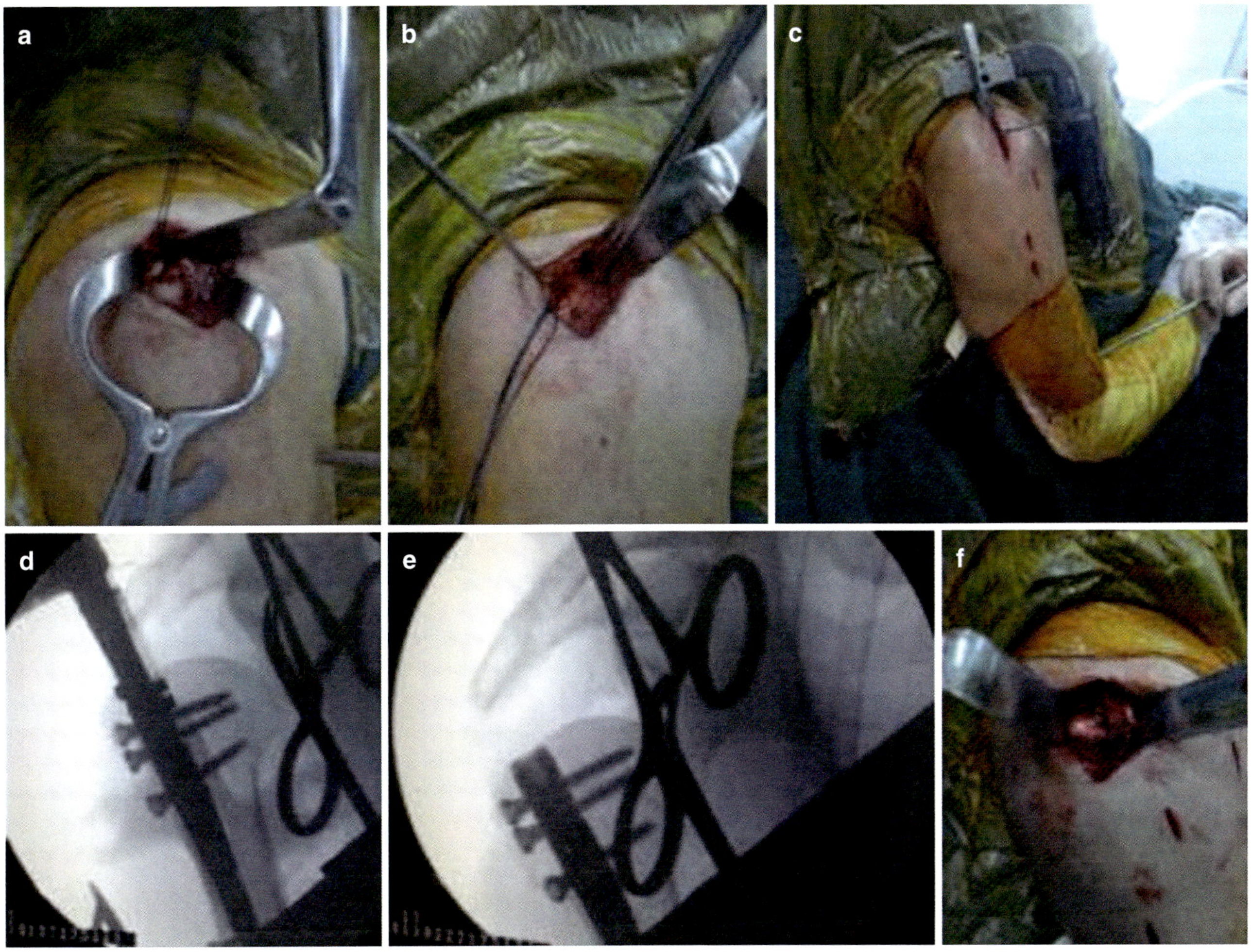

Fig. 9.32 Effect of suture-assisted fixation. (**a**, **b**) Exposure of the nail entry point through small incision; (**c**, **d**) Insertion of intramedullary nail into the medullary cavity of the humerus and fluoroscopy to complete proximal locking; (**e**, **f**) Effect and X-ray film of locking with intramedullary nails

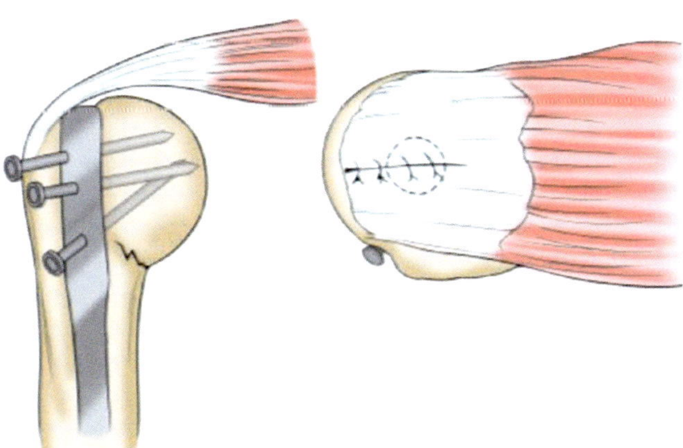

Fig. 9.33 Repair of shoulder cuff after fixation with intramedullary nails

less than 8 mm. Some scholars point out that the incidence of humeral head necrosis due to proximal humeral fracture can even reach 35%. Additionally, the internal fixation technology will be more complex, the operation will be more difficult, and the postoperative curative effect will be poorer than expected in case of much too comminuted proximal humerus, such as fracturing or compression of the humeral head, serious irreparable tubercular comminution, or even unstable glenohumeral joint. For the complex proximal humerus fractures among the elderly, more and more scholars use shoulder joint replacement and have achieved certain curative effect. Boileau et al. have reported that shoulder hemiarthroplasty is designed to replace the humeral head based on the anatomical structure [17]. It is still necessary to reduce the greater and the lesser tubercles and fix them firmly in their respective

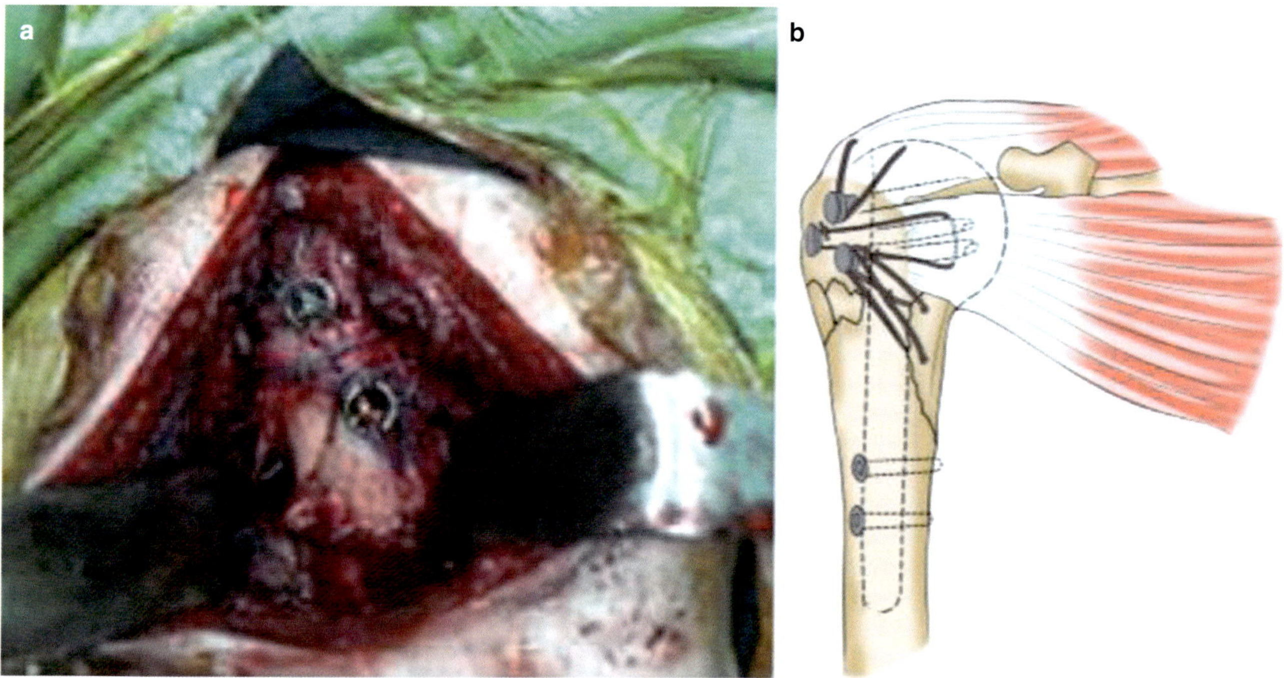

Fig. 9.34 Postoperative effect of suture-assisted fixation with intramedullary nails. (**a**) During the operation; (**b**) Schematic diagram

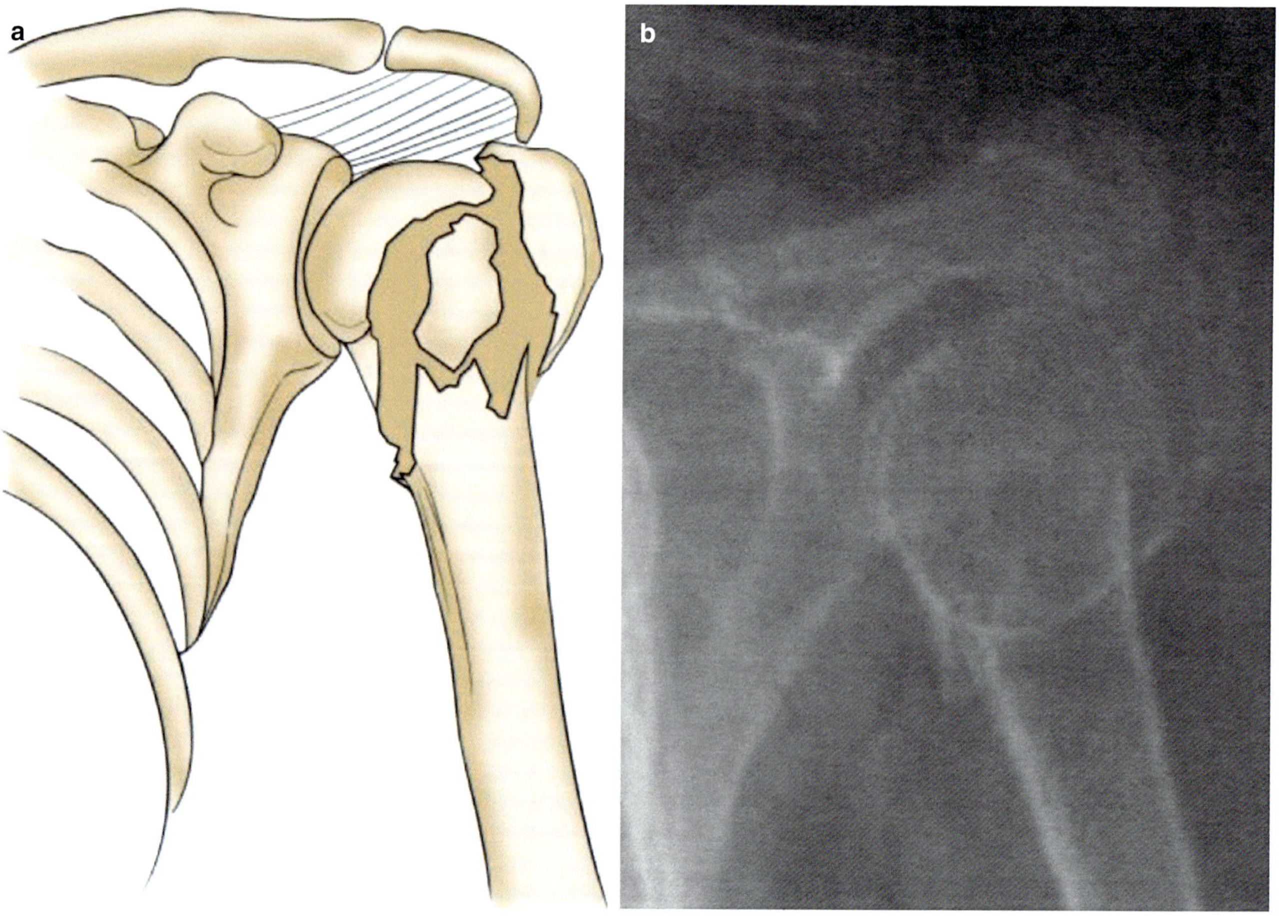

Fig. 9.35 3-part proximal humerus fractures (Neer Classification System). (**a**) X-ray fracture manifestation; (**b**) Schematic diagram of fracture

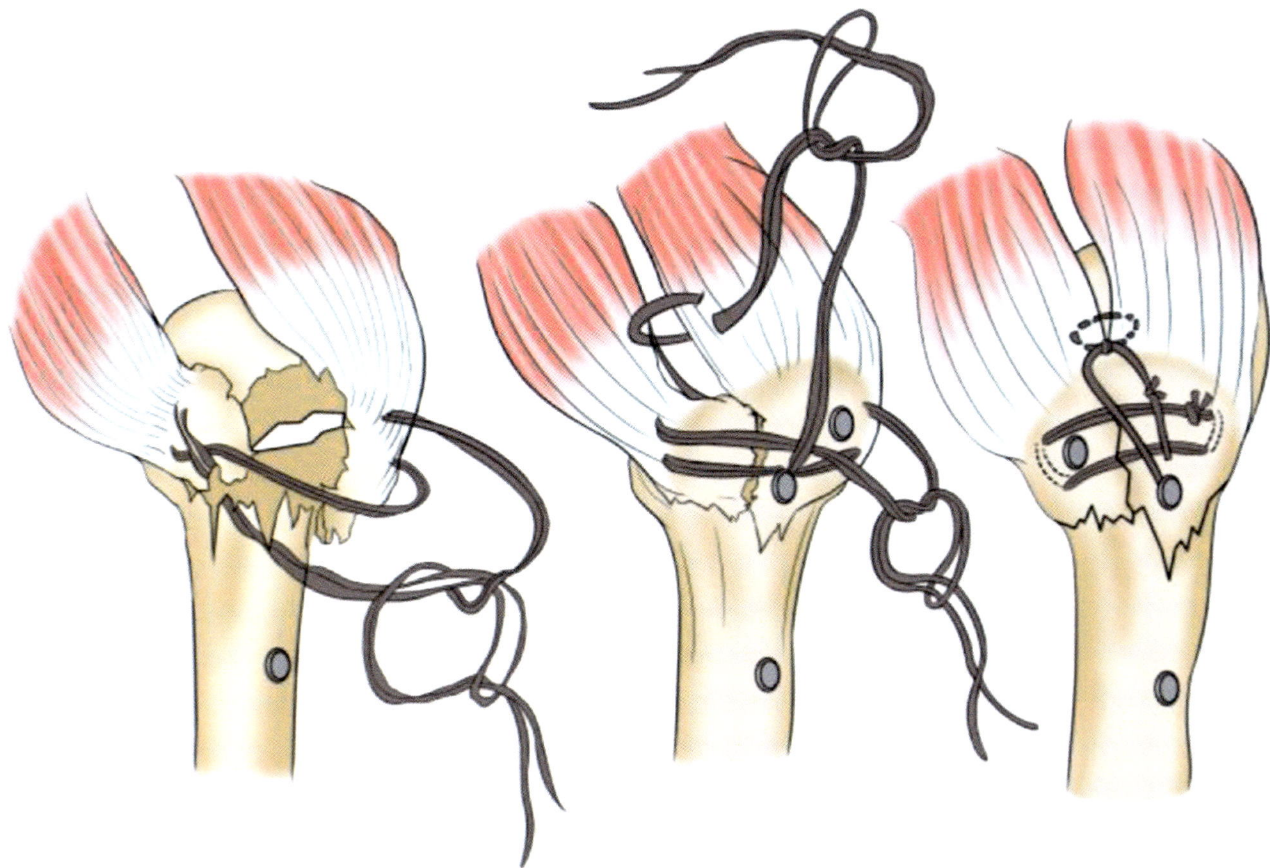

Fig. 9.36 Suture-assisted fixation of the greater and the lesser tubercles

anatomical sites during the operation. Only when the greater and the lesser tubercles are correctly positioned and healed can the shoulder cuff play its normal function. Therefore, the main complication of shoulder hemiarthroplasty is poor postoperative function, particularly abduction and lifting. That is why we would say that the recovery of the greater tubercle is the key to whether the patient can lift his or her shoulder joint or not after the shoulder hemiarthroplasty. However, shoulder hemiarthroplasty is evidently no longer appropriate in case of proximal humeral fractures with comminuted greater tubercle, or combined with severe supraspinatus tendon injury, which we often encounter in clinical practice. As a result, the reverse shoulder replacement receives more and more praises from scholars in the treatment of complex proximal humeral fractures among the elderly.

The development of reverse shoulder replacement provides more options for upper limb surgeons in treating complex proximal humeral fractures among the elderly. Results of early reports indicate that the average prognostic function might be superior to that of shoulder hemiarthroplasty in some patients and specific clinical studies. In addition, these results seem able to be achieved more quickly with less dependence on rehabilitation exercise. In patients over 70 years of age, particularly those with severe comminuted fractures, these factors may seriously affect the result of the shoulder hemiarthroplasty and internal fixation, but their impact is much less on cases of reverse shoulder replacement. Despite the incomparable advantages in reverse shoulder replacement, the use of this sort of prosthesis demands a clear learning curve, and has a range of related complications of its own. Upper limb surgeons must have sufficiently clear and accurate judgment in selecting joint replacement as the solution to the treatment of proximal humeral fractures, and be familiar with the surgical techniques and operation of the prosthesis.

9.4.2 Surgical Methods

9.4.2.1 Position and Approach

After administration of general anesthesia, the patient takes a beach chair position. Remove the bed board on the affected side after the position is set, so that the shoulder joint could be fully extended backward to facilitate installation of the prosthesis and determination of the retroversion angle of the prosthesis.

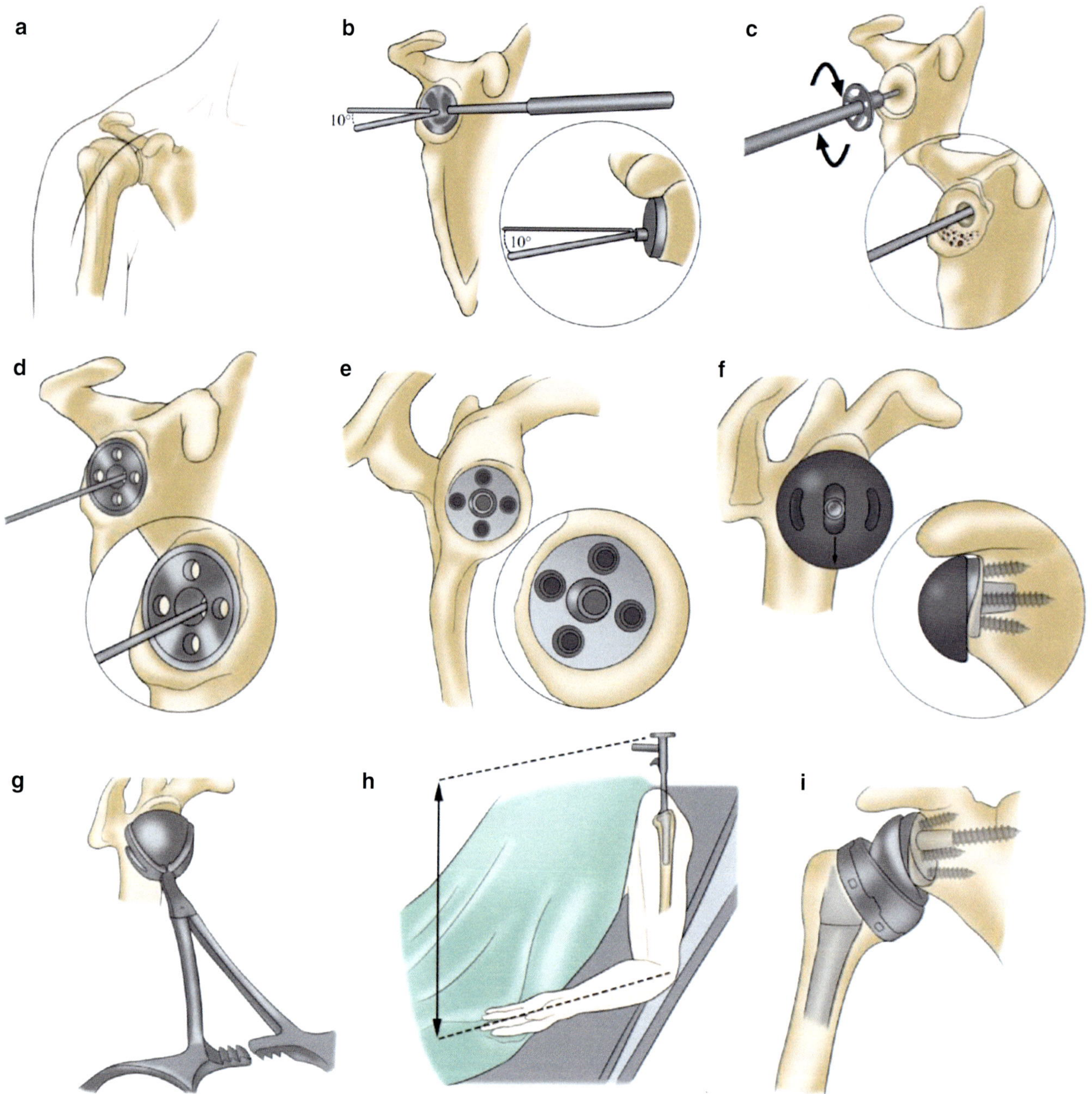

Fig. 9.37 Surgical operation of complex proximal humeral fracture in the elderly with reverse shoulder replacement with prosthesis. (**a**) "Beach chair" position, routine deltoid-pectoralis major approach; (**b**) Insert the Steinmann pin in the direction of the guide after exposure of the glenoid; (**c**) Polish the glenoid in the direction of the Steinmann pin until the subchondral bone is exposed below; (**d**) Install the base, with a secured downward inclination of at least 10°; (**e**) Fix the base with the central nail and the peripheral nails; (**f**) Measure the eccentricity of the glenoid ball; (**g**) Installation of the glenoid prosthesis; (**h**) Conventionally install the cemented stem on the humeral end with the retroversion angle set to 20°; (**i**) Reduction after installation of the humeral tray

The deltoid-pectoralis major approach (Fig. 9.37a) is adopted in all cases. Expose and protect the cephalic vein, paying attention to the ligation of cephalic vein branches; separate the deltoid from the pectoralis major, paying attention to protecting the insertion; look for the long head tendon of biceps brachii after opening the clavipectoral fascia, and then identify the intertubercular groove and find the greater and the lesser tubercles. Open the shoulder cuff space, detect the insertion of the supraspinatus tendon, the infraspinatus tendon, and the subscapular tendon at the greater and the lesser tubercles. Pass Non-Absorbable 5# ETHIBOND® Suture (Polyester, Ethicon Inc.) through the insertion of the shoulder cuff as traction line to pull the greater and the lesser tubercles apart to expose the humeral head. Osteotomy of the lesser tubercle may be executed if it is connected with the humeral head, but the integrity of the subscapular tendon should be preserved. Expose and take out the humeral head carefully to expose the glenoid fossa, cut off the long head tendon of the biceps at the insertion of the supraglenoid tubercle, and mark the distal end with a suture. Resect the supraspinatus tendon conventionally, leaving the muscle tissues retract randomly.

9.4.2.2 Installation of Glenoid Prosthesis

Fully expose the glenoid with the shoulder replacement retractor, and then clean the glenoid labrum. The electric knife is not recommended for cleaning the lower part, so as to avoid damage on the axillary nerve below the glenoid. When the cleaning is satisfactory, drive the Steinmann pin (Fig. 9.37b) in the direction of the introducer, and then polish the glenoid in the direction of the Steinmann pin until the subchondral bone is exposed as given below (Fig. 9.37c); install the base with a secured downward tilt of at least 10° (Fig. 9.37d), and then fix the base with the central nail and peripheral nails (Fig. 9.37e). Define eccentricity of the prosthesis with the trial, noting that the lower edge of the prosthesis should exceed that of the glenoid (Fig. 9.37f), and then install the shoulder glenoid prosthesis (Fig. 9.37g).

9.4.2.3 Installation of the Humeral End Prosthesis

Bone-cemented prosthesis is used for all humeral ends. The height of the prosthesis can be determined according to the height of the medial distance or 5 cm above the insertion of the pectoralis major, with posterior inclination angle set at 20° (Fig. 9.37h). Before installation of the humeral tray, the test membrane should be installed and the reduction should be tried, so as to determine the tightness of the prosthesis, the satisfaction of which is followed by installation of the humeral tray prosthesis and reduction of the shoulder joint (Fig. 9.37i). After this, use a number of Non-Absorbable 5# ETHIBOND® Suture (Polyester, Ethicon Inc.) to encircle and fix the greater and the lesser tubercles and strengthen the fixation, and use the cancellous bone graft of the humeral head between the greater and the lesser tubercles to promote the healing. After installation of the prosthesis, regulate the tension of the long head tendon of the biceps and fix it to the conjoint tendon. Negative pressure drainage tube is conventionally placed during the operation.

9.4.2.4 Tubercular Reconstruction During the Operation

This is also a step of critical importance as the reconstruction of the greater and the lesser tubercles during the operation will affect the rotational function later. It is similar to shoulder hemiarthroplasty in details, including the longitudinal and the transverse fixation of the tubercle to fix the tubercle around the humeral shaft and the prosthesis.

Of course, many ways are available for fixation of the tubercule, including this one. Firstly, lead in three Ethibond's non-absorbable 5# sutures (polyester, Ethicon) through the tendon-bone junction of the greater tubercle, with the one in the middle of the greater tubercle to pass through the suture hole on the medial side of the prosthesis neck (Fig. 9.38a). Then pass the upper and lower sutures in the greater tubercle through the upper and the lower foramina of the lateral wing of the prosthesis, respectively. Pass these sutures further through the tendon-bone junction corresponding to the lesser tubercle (Fig. 9.38b). Perform longitudinal suturing of the greater tubercle, lead in the suture into the hole reserved on the lateral side of the humeral shaft in advance, and place the longitudinal suture in the lateral hole of the humeral shaft before passing over the greater tubercle. Continue to pass the suture under that of the greater tubercle (Fig. 9.38c).

Fasten the sutures in the corresponding order. Firstly, fix the greater tubercle to the humeral shaft and then to the prosthesis (Fig. 9.38d). Then fix the lesser tubercle to the humeral shaft and then to the greater tubercle (Fig. 9.38e). Finally, perform the figure-of-8 suturing and, from the back to the front, pass the suture reserved, after passing through the humerus, before the insertion of the humeral stem through the shoulder cuff and close to the superior part of the tubercle, and then fix the tubercle to the humeral shaft (Fig. 9.38f). Implant the cancellous bone of the humeral head into under the tubercle to promote healing. Move the shoulder joint and observe stability of the tubercle.

9.4.2.5 Postoperative Management and Rehabilitation

Apply antibiotics conventionally for 1 day after the operation, and remove the drainage tube within 48 hours after the operation. Wear the shoulder brace (20° in shoulder abduction, 90° in elbow flexion, and neutral position of the forearm) conventionally after the operation for protection. Early pendulum movement of the shoulder joint as well as active motion of the elbow, the wrist and the fingers may begin under assistance of the rehabilitation doctor as early as Day 1 after the operation, with passive functional exercises to begin under the protection of the rehabilitation doctor in 6 weeks after the operation. Receive X-ray examination at Week 6 after the operation. Start active functional exercises upon confirmed desirable growth of the callus of the greater and the lesser tubercles. Strength training can be scaled up gradually 3 months after the operation. See Figs. 9.39 and 9.40 for typical cases and their functions.

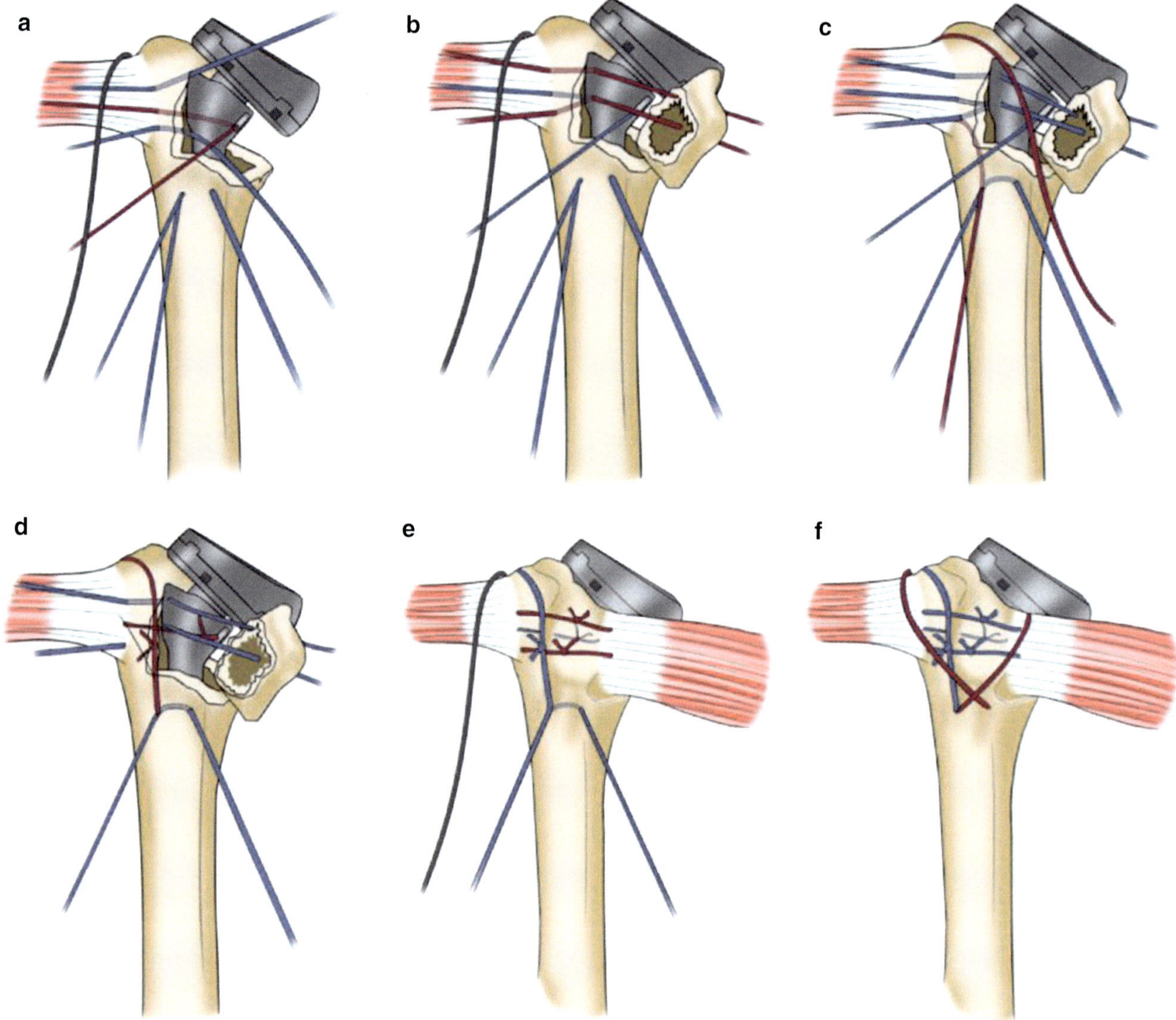

Fig. 9.38 Tubercular reconstruction in reverse shoulder joint replacement with prosthesis. (**a**) Lead in three Ethibond's non-absorbable 5# sutures (polyester, Ethicon) through the tendon-bone junction of the greater tubercle, with the one in the middle of the greater tubercle to pass through the suture hole; (**b**) Pass the upper and lower sutures in the greater tubercle through the upper and the lower foramina of the lateral wing of the prosthesis, respectively. Pass these sutures further through the tendon-bone junction corresponding to the lesser tubercle; (**c**) Perform longitudinal suturing of the greater tubercle; (**d**) Fix the greater tubercle to the humeral shaft and then to the prosthesis; (**e**) Fix the lesser tubercle to the humeral shaft and then to the greater tubercle; (**f**) perform the figure-of-8 suturing

9.4.3 Efficacy of Reverse Shoulder Joint Replacement with Prosthesis and Prevention of Complications

Initially, indications of reverse shoulder joint replacement with prosthesis were huge and irreparable shoulder cuff injuries. As clinical application proceeds, the indications have increased to complex proximal humeral comminuted fracture in the elderly, revision after shoulder hemiarthroplasty, prosthesis replacement after tumor resection, etc. Compared with shoulder hemiarthroplasty, reverse shoulder replacement is most superior in its definite curative effect and the lifting of the shoulder joint does not depend on whether the large tubercle is healed or not, of which the principle is to move the rotational center of shoulder joint inward and enable the lifting of the affected limb with the strength of the deltoid. However, it should be noted that the rotatory function of the shoulder joint still depends on the shoulder cuff structure. Therefore, the greater and the lesser also need to be reduced and fixed firmly even if it is a case of reverse shoulder joint replacement.

Kempton et al. point out that the postoperative complications of reverse shoulder joint replacement include hematoma formation, infection, prosthesis dislocation, acromion

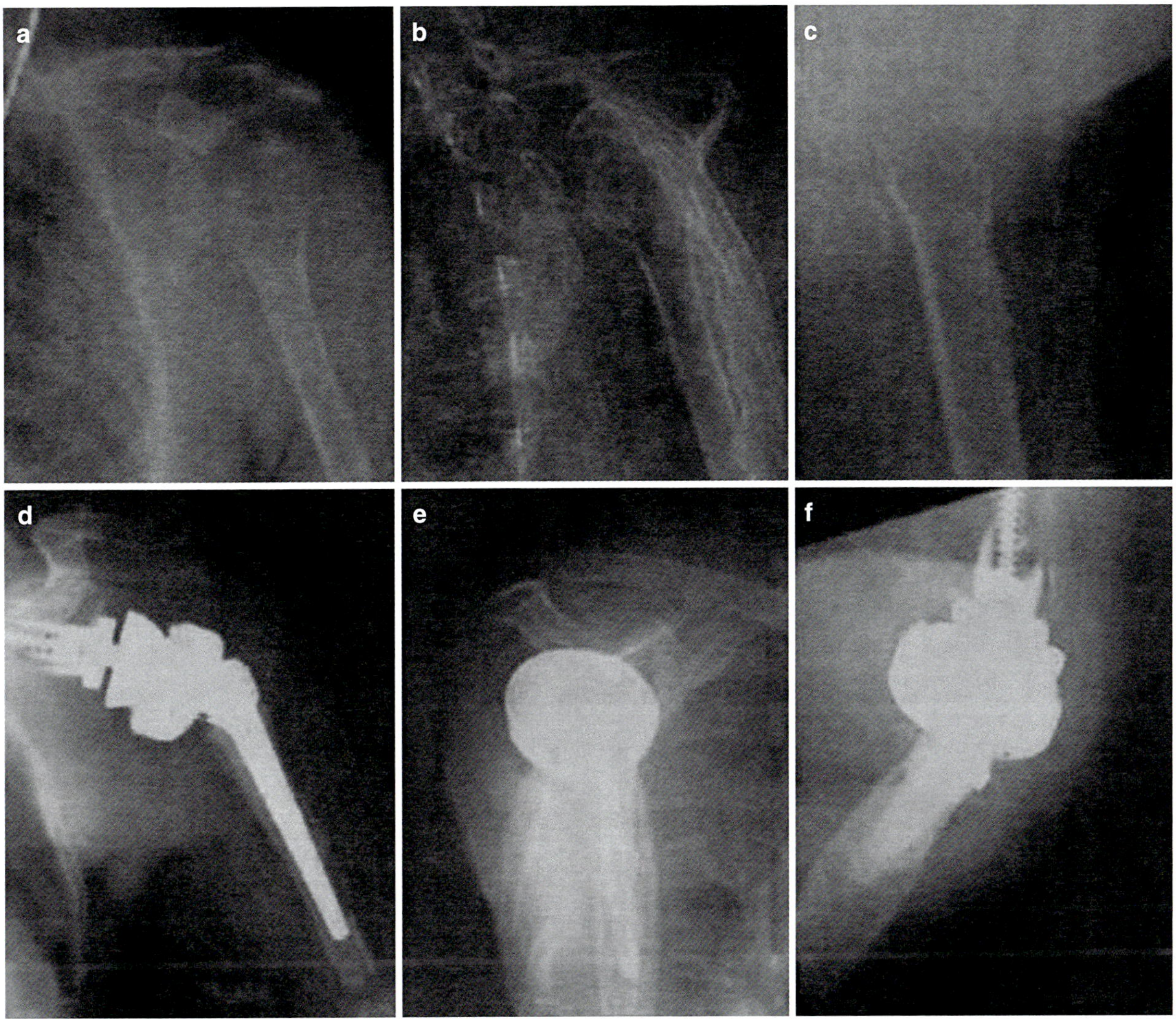

Fig. 9.39 A 72-year-old male with comminuted fracture and dislocation of the proximal humerus in a fall (4-part fracture under Neer Classification System). (**a**–**c**) X-ray films of the left shoulder joint in anterior-posterior, Y-position, and axillary position indicate comminuted fracture at the proximal end of the left humerus with dislocated glenohumeral joint. (**d**–**f**) X-ray films of the left shoulder joint in anterior-posterior, Y-position, and axillary position indicate satisfactory position of the prosthesis after comprehensive reverse shoulder joint replacement with prosthesis

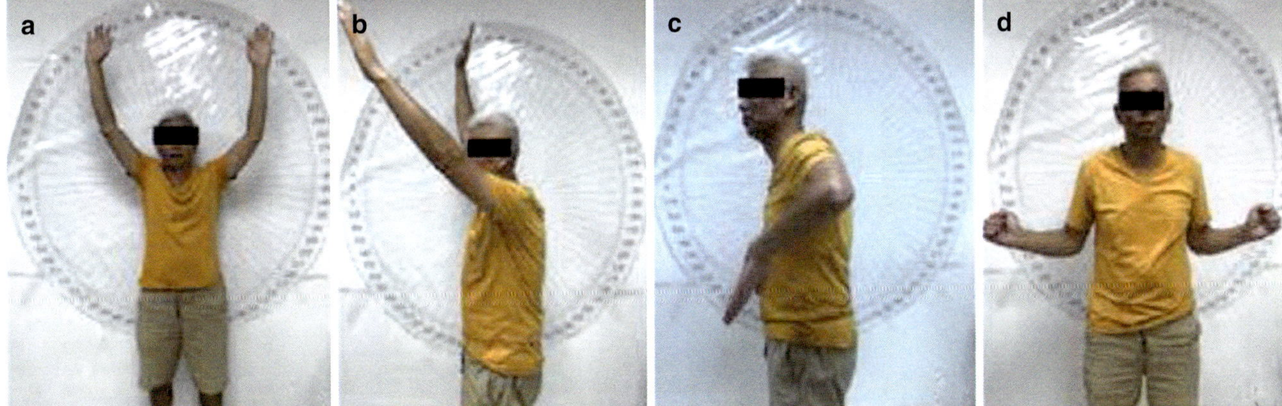

Fig. 9.40 Follow-up at Month 13 after the operation, left shoulder joint anteflexion and lifting up 130°, outward abduction and inward rotation 50°, outward lateral rotation 35°, Constant-Murley scores 91, VAS score 1, ASES score 85.8, satisfying functional recovery

stress fracture, scapula impingement, etc., which may occur at an incidence of 0%~68% [18]. However, the incidence decreases significantly after the surgeon has conducted 40 operations, indicating a long learning curve for reverse shoulder joint replacement. At the same time, the incidence of complications will also decrease with the progress in the design of prosthesis.

Postoperative complications of reverse shoulder joint replacement are mainly related to the surgeon's familiarity with the prosthesis and the specific operation details. Only when the surgeon has fully understood the steps to handle the prosthesis can the incidence of complications be reduced. Among these complications, prosthesis dislocation and acromion stress fracture are mainly due to the misjudgment on the tightness of the prosthesis during the operation. Much too loose prosthesis will lead to prosthesis dislocation, and much too tight prosthesis will result in acromial stress fracture. Scapular impingement is a special complication of reverse shoulder joint replacement, because when the shoulder joint is adducted, the humeral tray prosthesis collides with the lower edge of the scapular neck, which will cause loosening and even displacement of the glenoid prosthesis over time. Through biomechanical studies and imaging analysis, Nyffeler et al. and Roche et al. believed that the judgment on the glenoid eccentricity and downward tilt angle during the operation can reduce the incidence of scapular impingement [19–21].

Conclusively, reverse shoulder joint replacement can be applied to complex proximal humeral fractures among the elderly. Compared with shoulder joint hemiarthroplasty, it is less dependent on the repair of the shoulder cuff and healing of the tubercles and is used more and more frequently year by year. Many studies show that, among patients over 70 years old, particularly those with severe comminuted proximal humeral fractures, reverse shoulder joint replacement is evidently far more satisfactory in functional recovery than shoulder joint hemiarthroplasty or internal fixation. However, it requires a long learning process and only by fully understanding the principle and operative steps of the prosthesis can the best results be achieved.

Although the patients rely on the deltoid to complete lifting of the shoulder joint after reverse shoulder joint replacement, it should be noted that the rotatory function of the shoulder joint, especially the outward rotation function, still depends on the shoulder cuff structure. Therefore, in the reverse shoulder joint replacement, it is still essential to repair and fix the greater and the lesser tubercles by specific steps, during which the fixation is mainly fulfilled with multiple sutures from multiple directions for tight fixation. Therefore, the suturing technology is critical in the reverse shoulder joint replacement. Only by means of strong suture fixation techniques to repair the greater and the lesser tubercles to maintain their anatomical reduction can the rotatory function of the shoulder joint of patients be restored as much as possible.

9.5 Suturing Technique for Repair and Reconstruction of Peripheral Injury of the Shoulder Joint

Chen Jianhai and Fu Zhongguo

9.5.1 Repair of Rotator Cuff Injury

Abstract The rotator cuff injury is one of the common injuries of the shoulder joint, which often has a greater impact on the function of the shoulder joint, and the repair effect of rotator cuff injury is essential for the functional recovery of the shoulder joint. In this section, we will focus on the anatomy of the rotator cuff, the causes and diagnosis of the injury, and different surgical repair techniques to introduce the relevant contents of rotator cuff injury repair.

The rotator cuff is a cuff-like myoid structure formed by the tendons of supraspinatus, infraspinatus, subscapularis, and teres minor in the anterior, superior, and posterior parts of the humeral head (Fig. 9.41). The supraspinatus originates from the supraspinatus fossa of scapula and inserts at the superior part of greater tubercle of humerus through the

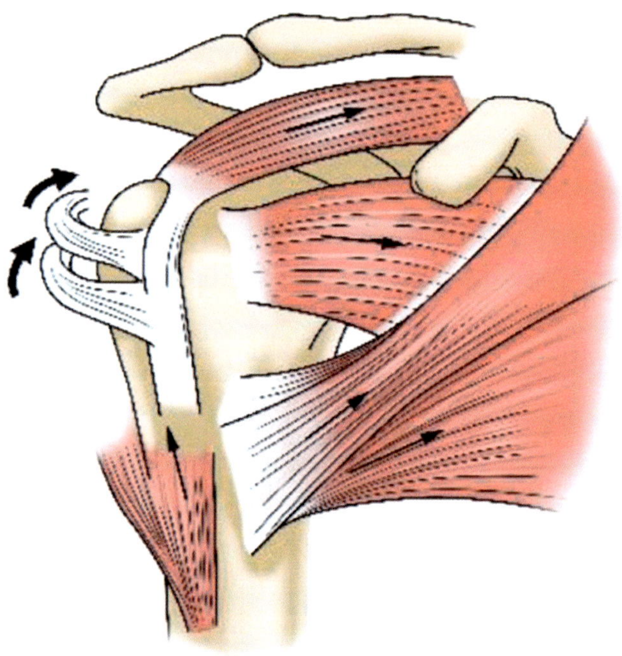

Fig. 9.41 Composition of rotator cuff

superior part of glenohumeral joint. It is innervated by the suprascapular nerve and mainly functions to abduct the upper arm and fix the humeral head on the glenoid to stabilize the glenohumeral joint; in addition, the supraspinatus can also prevent upward shifting of the humeral head during contraction of deltoid. The infraspinatus originates from the infraspinous fossa of scapula and inserts in the lateral middle of the greater tubercle of humerus through the posterosuperior part of the glenohumeral joint. It is also innervated by the suprascapular nerve and functions to externally rotate the upper arm in the drooping position of the upper arm. The subscapularis originates from the subscapular fossa and inserts anteromedially in the lesser tubercle of humerus through the anterior part of the glenohumeral joint. It is innervated by the subscapular nerve and has a function of medially rotating shoulder joint in the drooping position of the arm. The teres minor originates from the posterior part of the lateral margin of the scapula and inserts posteroinferiorly in the greater tubercle of humerus through the posterior part of the glenohumeral joint. It is innervated by the axillary nerve and functions to laterally rotate the upper arm.

The tendon ends, joint capsule, coracohumeral ligament, and glenohumeral ligament complex finally merge into a whole ending in the tubercle. The supraspinatus and infraspinatus tendons coalesce nearly 15 mm medial to their insertion and cannot be bluntly separated, the infraspinatus and teres minor tendons coalesce at the tendon-belly junction, the supraspinatus and subscapularis tendons form a sheath encompassing the long head tendon at the inlet of the long head tendon, wherein the infraspinatus tendons constitute the upper wall, and the subscapularis tendons constitute the lower wall. The coracohumeral ligament is a bundle of thick fibrous structures originating from the coracoid process, which runs on the surface of the joint capsule between the supraspinatus tendon and the subscapularis tendon, and inserts in the lesser and greater tubercles. This ligament is deep in the rotator cuff and constitutes the top of the long head tendon sheath with the joint capsule and the supraspinatus tendon. Another bundle of 1-cm-wide coracohumeral ligaments reaches the posterior margin of the infraspinatus tendon posteriorly between the joint capsule and the rotator cuff. There is also a bundle that covers the surface of the supraspinatus and infraspinatus tendons posteriorly and laterally.

Anatomy: The medial-to-lateral insertion widths of the rotator cuff (supraspinatus, infraspinatus, teres minor, subscapularis tendons) are 12.7 mm, 13.4 mm, 11.4 mm, and 17.9 mm, respectively. The minimum medial-to-lateral insertion width at the middle portion of the supraspinatus tendon is 14.7 mm. The distance from the articular surface margin to the lateral margin of the articular surface at the tendon insertion is also different and less than 1 mm from the articular surface margin with the range of 2.1 cm anterior to the supraspinatus and infraspinatus tendons. Then, this distance progressively increases posteriorly to reach 13.9 mm at the inferior margin of the teres minor. The anteroposterior distances of the rotator cuff insertions are 16.3 mm, 16.4 mm, 20.7 mm, and 24.3 mm, respectively.

Rotator cable: The anteroposterior diameter is 4.1 cm, and the medial-lateral diameter is 1.4 cm. The cable has a width of 1.2 cm and a thickness of 4.7 mm. Arthroscopically, it looks like a crescent-shaped structure from the anterior margin of the supraspinatus tendon to the inferior margin of the infraspinatus tendon, which has the effect of dispersing stress. This cable can be seen as the posterior coracohumeral ligament bundle. The majority of supraspinatus and supraspinatus tendon injuries occur distal to the cable.

The rotator cuff muscles jointly function to maintain the stability of the axis of rotation of the humeral head on the articular surface of the glenoid cavity in any moving or resting state, of which the balance of strength between the subscapularis and the infraspinatus and teres minor in medial and lateral rotation is particularly important to maintain the stability of the humeral head on the articular surface of the glenoid cavity.

9.5.1.1 Causes of Rotator Cuff Injury

The etiologies of rotator cuff injury are inconclusive. There are two best-known theories, one is exogenous mechanical impact, that is, subacromial impingement leading to rotator cuff injury; the other is endogenous degeneration leading to rotator cuff injury. In addition, there are also blood circulation effect and trauma-induced rotator cuff injury.

1. Degeneration theory. Yamanaka described the histopathological findings of tendon degeneration from autopsy specimens, cell deformation in the rotator cuff, necrosis, calcium deposition, fibrinoid thickening, hyaline degeneration, partial muscle fiber rupture, fibril formation, and disappearance of the wavy morphology of collagen, arteriolar proliferation, and appearance of chondroid cells in the tendon. Degeneration of the enthesis of the rotator cuff manifests as duplication and irregularity of the tidal line, irregularity or disappearance of a normal four-layered structure (intrinsic tendons, tidal lines, mineralized fibrocartilages, and bones), or granulation. These changes are rare in adults under 40 years of age, but tend to worsen with age.
2. The theory of blood supply. The critical zone, first described by Codaman, is located within 1 cm to the distal end of the supraspinatus tendon, and this avascular zone is the part where rotator cuff tear most often occurs. The perfusion study of cadaveric specimens has also confirmed the existence of the critical zone, blood supply for the bursal surface is better than that for the articular surface, and this finding matches the fact that articular sur-

face tear is more frequent than bursal surface tear. Brooks found an avascular zone within 1.5 cm to the distal end of the infraspinatus tendon as well. However, the incidence of supraspinatus tear is much higher than that of infraspinatus tendon tear, so there should be other factors in addition to the blood supply factor.

3. The theory of impingement. The concept of subacromial impingement syndrome was first proposed by Neer II in 1972, who concluded that rotator cuff injury is due to subacromial impingement. This impingement mostly occurs in the anterior 1/3 site of the acromion and the inferior acromioclavicular joint or the inferior part of the coracoacromial arch. Neer II classified supraspinatus tendon outlet impingement syndrome and non-outlet impingement syndrome according to the anatomical sites where impingements occurred. Neer II considered that 95% of rotator cuff ruptures are caused by impingement syndrome. The supraspinatus tendon passes between the acromion and the greater tubercle, and the long head tendon of biceps brachii is located deep to the supraspinatus and inserts in the top or the supraglenoid tuberosity of the shoulder over the humeral head. During movement of the shoulder joint, these two tendons move reciprocally underneath the coracoacromial arch. Degeneration or dysplasia of the acromion and the subacromial structures or glenohumeral joint instability due to dynamic causes may lead to impingement injuries of the supraspinatus tendon, the long head tendon of biceps brachii, and the subscapularis tendon. A bursal lesion emerges in the early stage, and degeneration and rupture of the tendons occur in the middle and late stages.
4. Trauma. Trauma has been widely accepted as an important etiology of rotator cuff injury. Labor injuries, sports injuries, and traffic accidents are all common causes of rotator cuff traumas. Traumas are classified into severe violent trauma and repeated minor trauma in terms of its magnitude of violence, and the latter is more important than the former in rotator cuff injury. Repeated minor injury during activities of daily living or sports causes micro-rupture of intratendinous muscle fibers, which is partial-thickness tendon or full-thickness tear. This pathological process is common in athletes engaged in throwing sports.

In summary, the intrinsic factor of rotator cuff injury is the tissue degeneration of the rotator cuff tendons that occurs with aging, as well as the inherent weakness of avascular areas existing on its anatomical structure. Additionally, trauma and impingement accelerate rotator cuff degeneration and contribute to the occurrence of ruptures. As Neviaser emphasized that 4 factors cause the rotator cuff degeneration process to varying degrees, none of them can alone cause rotator cuff injury, and the key factors should be analyzed on a case-by-case basis.

9.5.1.2 Pathology and Classification

1. *Partial-Thickness Rupture and Full-Thickness Rupture Classified According to the Degree of Injury*

   Partial-thickness rupture of the rotator cuff tendons may occur on the articular surface side (inferior) or bursal (superior) side of the supraspinatus tendon, as well as interlamellar tear of the tendons (Fig. 9.42). Partial-

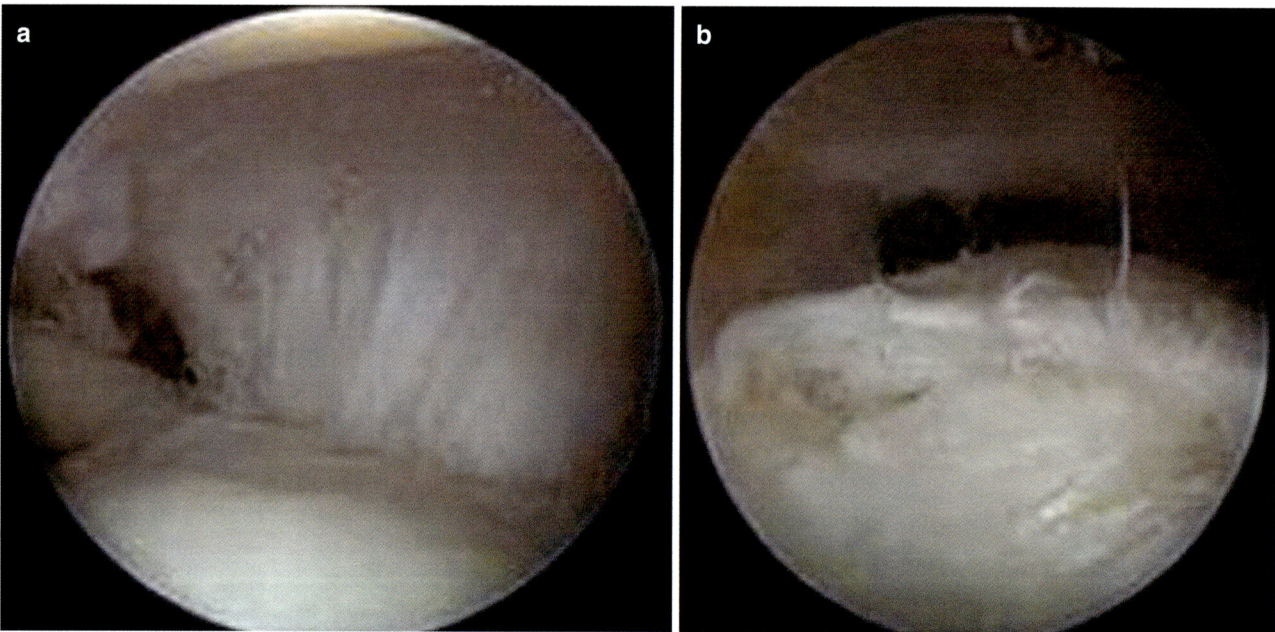

Fig. 9.42 Partial-thickness rupture of the rotator cuff. (**a**) Articular-sided tear; (**b**) Synovial-sided tear

thickness rupture may develop into full-thickness rupture if not treated properly or not repaired.

Full-thickness rupture is a full-thickness rupture of the tendon, which causes a penetrating injury between the glenohumeral joint and the subacromial bursa. This kind of injury is most common in the supraspinatus tendon, followed by the subscapularis tendon, and fewer in infraspinatus and teres minor tendons. It is not rare that the supraspinatus tendon and infraspinatus tendon are simultaneously involved, and the superior margin of the subscapularis tendon is torn in most cases.

The broken end of fresh tendon rupture is irregular accompanied with edematous muscle, fragile tissue, and exudate in the glenohumeral articular cavity. The broken end of the old rupture had formed a scar, which is smooth and dull, relatively hard, with a small amount of fibrinous exudate in the articular cavity, and the naked area of the articular surface proximal to the greater tubercle is covered with pannus or granulation tissue.

2. *Classification Based on Size of Tendon Rupture*

   Bateman classified the sizes of the rotator cuff tears measured intraoperatively: small tear <1 cm; medium tear = 1~3 cm; large tear = 3~5 cm; and giant tear >5 cm.

   Burkhart proposed classification according to tear morphology: classification is made according to the length of T2-phase coronal rotator cuff tears and the width of sagittal tears measured preoperatively through magnetic resonance imaging (MRI).

- Type 1: Length smaller than width and smaller than 2 cm.
- Type 2: Length greater than width, and width smaller than 2 cm.
- Type 3: Length greater than 2 cm, and width greater than 2 cm.
- Type 4: Significant glenohumeral arthritis, with disappearance of the scapulohumeral clearance.

9.5.1.3 Clinical Manifestation and Diagnosis

1. Clinical manifestation

   Pain: Most patients have severe shoulder joint pain, which lasts for a long time. Most of them present with anterior shoulder pain and dull and diffuse shoulder pain and cannot lie on the affected side. Nocturnal pain is a typical manifestation of rotator cuff injury. When the pain is severe, commonly used anti-inflammatory and analgesic drugs cannot significantly relieve the pain. Protraction of the shoulder joint will aggravate the pain. The majority of the pain is localized around the shoulder and deltoid region, and when associated with inflammation of long head tendon, the pain will radiate to the elbow.

   Common sites of tenderness are the anterior part of the shoulder, such as the intertubercular groove and the anterior greater tubercle.

   Limited range of joint motion: Due to long-term shoulder pain, the affected shoulder joint will cause frozen shoulder, manifested as reduced active and passive range of motion of shoulder joint adduction, lateral rotation and medial rotation; however, with the extension of time, the pain will be relieved, and the passive range of motion of the shoulder joint will be gradually improved. Most patients with complete rotator cuff tears have a basically normal passive range of motion of shoulder joint, but the active range of motion may be persistently limited.

   Decreased muscle strength: Those with full-thickness rotator cuff tears will experience a decrease in the strength of movement in the direction innervated by the injured muscle. For part of patients with tears, decreased muscle strength also occurs due to rotator cuff dysfunction caused by pain.

   Shoulder joint friction sensation: Rotator cuff injury is often accompanied by inflammatory hyperplasia and adhesion of subacromial and subdeltoid bursae. Passive movement of the shoulder joint may induce the friction sensation during joint movement.

2. *Special Examination*

   (1) Arm drop sign: Passively raise the affected arm by 90°~120°, then remove the support, and it is positive if spontaneous support of the affected arm fails to result in arm drop and pain.

   (2) Neer impingement sign: The examiner stabilizes the scapula with one hand and raises the affected arm with the other hand in the plane of scapula, and it is positive if the patient has anterior shoulder pain (Fig. 9.43).

   (3) Hawkins and Kennedy impingement sign: The examiner stabilizes the scapula with one hand and flexes the elbow at the angle of 90° with the other hand in the plane of scapula, and it is positive if the patient has anterior shoulder pain (Fig. 9.44).

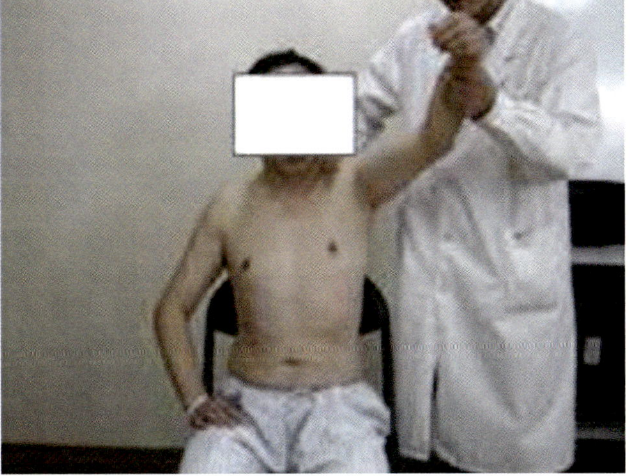

Fig. 9.43 Neer impingement sign

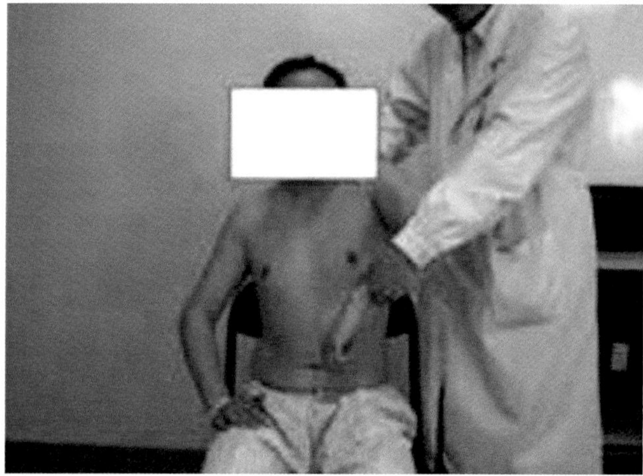

Fig. 9.44 Hawkins and Kennedy impingement sign

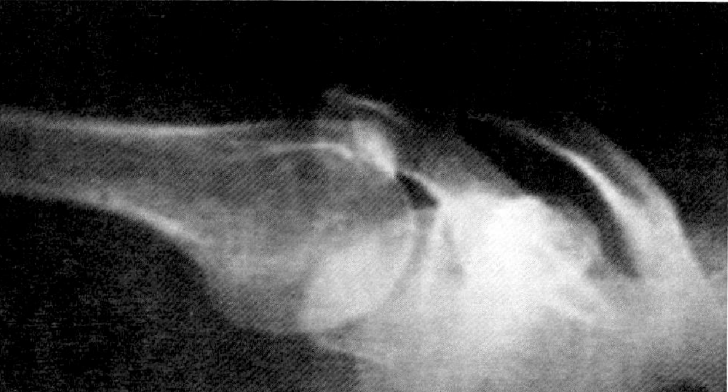

Fig. 9.45 Showing sclerosis of the subacromial articular surface

(4) Pain arc syndrome: Pain occurs in the anterior or subacromial region within the raising range of 60°~120° of the affected arm. It has some diagnostic significance for rotator cuff contusions and part of tears.

It is not easy to make a correct diagnosis of rotator cuff rupture. The possibility of rotator cuff tear should be considered in patients with a history of shoulder trauma, anterior shoulder pain accompanied with tenderness in the proximal greater tubercle or subacromial region, and patients with the presence of any of the above four special positive signs at the same time. If accompanied by muscle atrophy or joint contracture at the same time, it indicates that the lesion has already developed into a later stage, and further auxiliary examination should be done for suspected cases of rotator cuff rupture.

3. *Imaging Diagnosis*
   (1) X-ray radiography: X-ray plain film examination is not specific for the diagnosis of this disease. During projection made horizontally at a distance of 1.5 m, the separation distance between the acromion and the top of the humeral head shall not be less than 12 mm, and if it is less than 6 mm, it generally indicates the existence of a large rotator cuff tear. Under deltoid traction, upward shifting of the humeral head may be induced. The X-ray plain film shows a narrow subacromial clearance. In some cases, the cortical bone of the greater tubercle is sclerotic, the surface is irregular or exostosis is formed, and the cancellous bone presents atrophic and osteoporotic. In addition, X-ray findings such as too low acromion position, hook-like acromion, and sclerosis and irregularity of the subacromial articular surface provide a basis for proving the existence of impingement factors (Fig. 9.45).

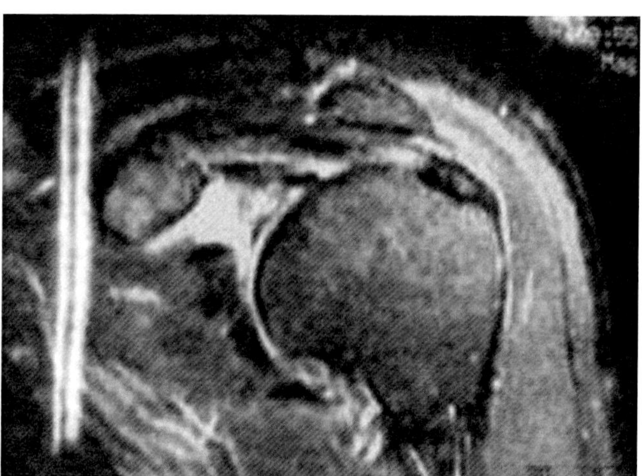

Fig. 9.46 Supraspinatus rupture showed by MRI

   (2) MRI: Magnetic resonance is an important method for the diagnosis of rotator cuff injuries. MRI can show pathological changes in tendon tissue based on different signals of damaged tendons in terms of edema, congestion, rupture, and calcium deposition (Fig. 9.46). MRI has the advantages that it is a noninvasive examination method, has repeatability, is sensitive to soft tissue injury, and has a very high sensitivity (95% or above).
   (3) Ultrasound diagnosis: The ultrasound diagnosis is also a non-invasive diagnostic method. It has the advantages of being simple, reliable, and capable of achieving repeated examination. Complete rotator cuff tears can be clearly distinguished. High-resolution probes can show contusive pathological changes such as rotator cuff edema and thickening, and show rotator cuff defects or atrophy and thinning for partial-thickness rotator cuff rupture. For complete rupture, the broken end, fissure and the extent of tendon defects can be showed. However, the accuracy of examination results depends on the technical level of the examiner.

9.5.1.4 Repair of Rotator Cuff Injury

Rotator cuff injuries, including partial-thickness or full-thickness, are mostly difficult to heal spontaneously once they occur and gradually increase with time. The aim of conservative treatment is to relieve symptoms and restore shoulder joint function by improving the function of the remaining rotator cuff with rehabilitation exercises. Already present rotator cuff tears cannot heal. Rotator cuff repair surgeries, including incisional repair and arthroscopic repair, are all required if the symptoms are not relieved after conservative treatment.

1. *Rotator Cuff Repair Methods with Small Incision*
   (1) Transosseous suturing technique: A small incision of about 3 cm is made inferiorly at the anterolateral corner of the acromion. The fibrous tissue between the anterior and medial bundles of deltoids is distinguished, the deltoid is longitudinally separated along the fiber bundles, and the subacromial bursa is incised. The humeral head is rotated medially and laterally to expose the rotator cuff tear site, which is generally located on the posterior side of the long head tendon and can be directly exposed in the surgical field. The footprint bone surface of the greater tubercle is cleaned, the sclerotic bone on the surface is removed by an osteotome, and bone tunnels are drilled by a 2 mm Kirschner wire from the lateral side of the greater tubercle to the margin of the articular surface, and the number of bone tunnels is determined according to the size of the rotator cuff tear, generally one bone tunnel needs to be drilled for every 1 cm of tear, and the rotator cuff is sutured after a suture passes through the bone tunnel. The suturing technique can be a figure-of-8 suturing or a NICE knot. Please note that the tension of each group of sutures should be even when knotting the sutures. The problem often occurs that the knot tied previously becomes loose after a latter suture is knotted. The solution is that suture knots are not tied at one time, continuous half-hitches in the same direction are locked first, and then knot tying is completed from the first knot after all sutures are locked.

   (2) Figure-of-8 suturing technique: A suture passes through a bone tunnel from the lateral side of the greater tubercle, the tendon is sutured from the articular side of the broken end of the rotator cuff to the synovial side, then the suture passes through the second bone tunnel from the lateral side of the greater tubercle, the broken end of the tendon is sutured again, and finally the suture is knotted on the lateral side of the greater tubercle to complete figure-of-8 suturing.

   (3) NICE knot suturing technique: A suture is sutured from the articular side of rotator cuff to the synovial side, and then from the synovial side to the articular side, both tail ends of the suture are pulled from the bone tunnel to the lateral side of greater tubercle. At this time, the suture is found on the tendon surface and a loop required to form a NICE knot is lifted up. The loop is pulled laterally for NICE knot fixation.

   (4) Anchor suturing technique:

      1) Single-row suturing: It is indicated for small and medium-sized tears, tears on the synovial side of the rotator cuff, and giant rotator cuff tears where severe retraction of the rotator cuff causes incomplete covering for the footprint bone surface. The surgical approach and management of the footprint bone surface are the same as those of the transosseous suturing method. The number of anchors is determined by the size of the rotator cuff tear, generally one anchor needed for 1 cm of tear. The anchor location is selected in the footprint bone surface of the greater tubercle, and the direction of anchor insertion is at a 45° angle to the direction of the rotator cuff. The rotator cuff anchors all have two different colored sutures.

         Simple suturing: One end of a suture passes through the tendon from the articular side of the rotator cuff, extracted from the synovial side, and then tied with the same-colored other end of the suture to complete the rotator cuff repair. This suturing technique is simple, but is insufficient in fixation strength.

         Modified Mason-Allen suturing technique: Two ends of a suture, respectively, pass through the rotator cuff tendon, and a suturing site is 1.5 cm from the margin of the broken end of the tendon, and the suture ends are apart about 1 cm anteroposteriorly when penetrating out of the tendon. One end of the other suture passes through the rotator cuff tendon in the midway of suturing of the first suture. The first suture is first knotted for fixation, so as to secure the second suture on the medial side of the first suture. The second suture is knotted after the first suture is knotted, so that the two sutures cross to maximize suturing strength.

      2) Double-row suturing: It is indicated for repairable full-thickness tears. The surgical approach and management of the footprint bone surface are the same as those of the transosseous suturing method. Double-row suturing requires double-suture anchors and lateral-row suture-free anchors. Medial-row anchors are implanted in the footprint bone surface at the margin of the articular surface,

and optimal holding strength may be obtained by screwing the anchors into the subchondral bone. The number of the medial-row anchors required is determined by the anteroposterior diameter of the rotator cuff tear, typically, one anchor is used for a tear of 1.5 cm or less, and 2 or more anchors are used for a tear of 2 cm or more, with an anchor distance of 1 cm. After complete release of the rotator cuff tendon, the anchor suture sequentially passes through the rotator cuff tendon body from posterior to anterior. The two ends of the same suture are knotted sequentially from posterior to anterior for fixation. The lateral soft tissue of the greater tubercle is then cleaned, and the sutures are pulled laterally to the greater tuberosity in two groups, respectively, and fixation is completed by the lateral-row anchors. The double-row suturing has the advantage that the broken end of the rotator cuff tendon can cover all the footprint bone surface, the fixation is stable, and there is no subacromial protruding suture knot, reducing the risk of subacromial impingement. Its disadvantages are increase of the number of anchors used compared with that of the single-row anchors and increase of the medical burden on patients.

2. *Arthroscopic Repair Method*

With the development and improvement of surgical instruments, arthroscopic treatment of rotator cuff injury has progressed from simple arthroscopic synovial shaving debridement to complete arthroscopic repair in the past 20 years. Compared with traditional incision surgery, the soft tissue injury of arthroscopic surgery is smaller, avoiding the stripping of deltoid; the postoperative pain is mild; the functional exercise may be done earlier; the glenohumeral joint cavity lesion may be evaluated in all directions at the same time, and the coexisting injury in the joint may be treated.

Technical key points of arthroscopic rotator cuff repair: Arthroscopic examination is first performed to understand the condition of injury in the shoulder joint and evaluate the size of rotator cuff tear and the degree of retraction. By using radio frequency and a shaver, the bone surface of the rotator cuff enthesis is cleaned to remove hyperplastic sclerotic bone, and part of the cortical bone of the enthesis is ground to expose the bleeding bone surface. For greatly retracted cuff tears, the tendon should be released so that it can be pulled back to the enthesis site without tension. Suture anchors are inserted close to the articular surface, and sutures pass through the rotator cuff tendon with a specially designed suturing instrument and then knotted for fixation. Arthroscopic knot tying is different from open surgical knot tying and requires a specially designed knot tying device, and there are several commonly used knot tying methods:

(1) Simple knot tying method: The two tails of a suture form a slip knot through two half-hitches in the same direction, a post is pulled to tighten the knot on the tendon surface, and then the fixation is completed through a reverse half-hitch.
(2) SMC method: One tail of a suture is selected as a post, and the other tail as an encircling suture. The two tails are tightened, and the encircling suture bypasses around the two tails a circle in a clockwise direction, then is turned around the post a circle, and finally passes through a middle hole. The knot may be pulled into the tendon surface by pulling the post, and by pulling the encircling suture, the suture knot may be locked to prevent loosening. Two half-hitches in the same direction and one reverse half-hitch are then used to achieve reliable knot tying (Fig. 9.47).
(3) Duncan method: An encircling suture encircles two tails for three turns in the clockwise direction, and then the tail end of the encircling suture passes through a loop formed proximally by the encircling suture. A knot can be tied on the tendon surface by pulling a post, and then the fixation is completed through two half-hitches and one reverse half-hitch (Fig. 9.48).

With the advancement of surgical techniques, arthroscopic rotator cuff repair is suitable for most rotator cuff injuries and achieves similar clinical results to open surgery.

3. *Tendon Transfer Surgery for Giant Rotator Cuff Injury*

The tendon transfer surgery for giant rotator cuff injury mainly includes pectoralis major transfer surgery for anterosuperior rotator cuff injury and latissimus dorsi or

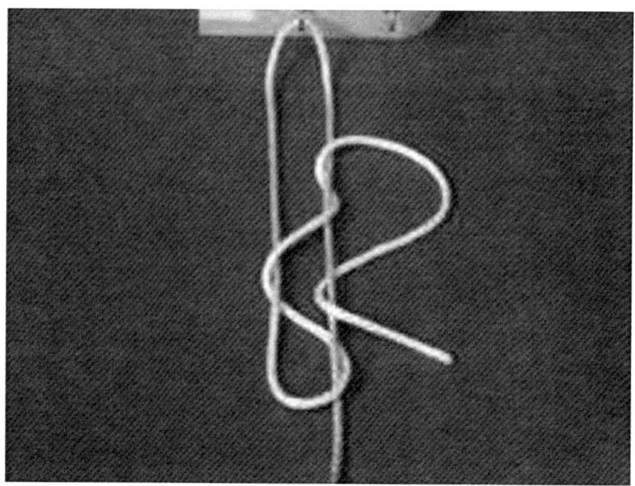

Fig. 9.47 Schematic diagram of SMC knot

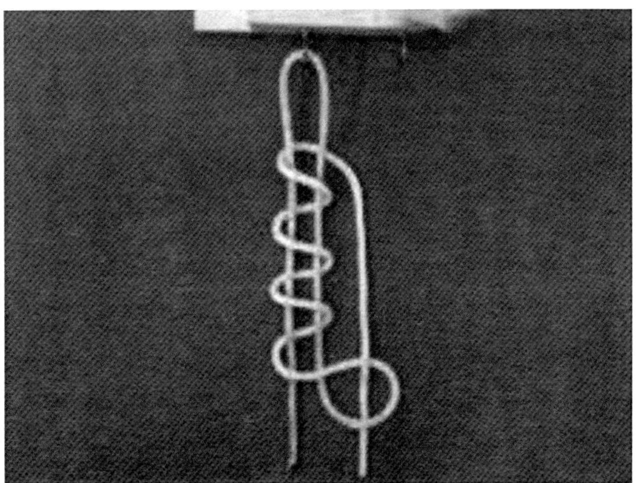

Fig. 9.48 Schematic diagram of Duncan method

teres major transfer surgery for posterosuperior rotator cuff injury.

Pectoralis major transfer surgery: It is indicated for irreparable subscapularis tendon injury accompanied with or without supraspinatus tendon injury.

Technical key points: An intermuscular groove approach between the deltoid and the pectoralis major is adopted to clean small nodules, remove scar tissue, and expose the bleeding bone surface. The pectoralis major is incised from the humeral shaft insertion, transferred to the lesser tubercle, and the pectoralis major tendon is fixed by an anchor suture fixed to the lesser tubercle.

Latissimus dorsi or teres major transfer surgery: It is indicated for irreparable injuries of the supraspinatus and infraspinatus tendons.

Technical key points: A posterior longitudinal approach to the shoulder joint is adopted to pull the deltoid open to expose the greater tubercle, and the tendon insertion is treated in the same way. The latissimus dorsi or teres major is localized and incised from the insertion, and the tendon is transferred to the greater tubercle and sutured and secured with an anchor suture (Fig. 9.49).

It should be pointed out that the rotator cuff function reconstruction surgery by the muscle transfer method has unstable postoperative results and great individual differences. Therefore, it is recommended to treat dysfunctional rotator cuff injury as early as possible and strive for anatomical or functional repair, so as to avoid progression of rotator cuff tear to the irreparable stage.

Correct diagnosis, early treatment, and postoperative systematic rehabilitation are the basic conditions for satisfactory treatment results. Conversely, if not repaired, it develops naturally and will eventually lead to rotator cuff arthropathy, joint instability, or secondary joint contracture, resulting in disability of joint functions.

9.5.2 Repair and Reconstruction of Shoulder Joint Capsule Injury

Zhuang Chengyu

Abstract The suturing technique of the shoulder joint mainly involves two types of diseases, one is the suture and repair problem of the joint capsule in shoulder instability, and the other is the giant rotator cuff rupture that needs a superior joint capsule suturing technique when cannot be repaired.

The treatment of early anterior shoulder joint dislocation is an open procedure that uses Putti-Platt's surgical method to achieve doubling suture of the joint capsule. Reconstruction of the avulsed joint capsule and glenoid labrum at the margin of the glenoid cavity was first proposed by Perthes in 1906 and is commonly referred to as Bankart repair, but its widespread use should be credited to Bankart. The recurrence rate reaches 19% after the Putti–Platt method is used alone, while it reduces to 2% after the Bankart procedure is introduced. So Bankart's technique is widely applied.

At present, for recurrent anterior shoulder joint dislocation, a conventional treatment means is arthroscopic capsulolabral repair. The current capsulolabral double-row anchor repair is such a means that the implantation of two rows of anchors at the anterior margin of the glenoid cavity and the scapular neck respectively, through which the joint capsule and glenoid labrum are pulled back into the glenoid cavity. Compared with single-row anchor repair, double-row anchor repair increases the contact surface between the joint capsule-glenoid labrum and the glenoid cavity, which is beneficial to promote healing of the joint capsule-glenoid labrum and the glenoid cavity. However, if the capsular ligament itself is problematic, the repair is less effective than that in a patient with a relatively intact capsule. The problems occurring in the arthroscopic capsular ligament are mainly classified into three types: the first is that there is also a tear on the side of the humeral head besides a tear of the capsular ligament involved with the glenoid labrum; the second is that the capsular ligament is severely flaccid; and the third is that the capsular ligament of the shoulder joint is absent in an arthroscopic finding. Therefore, for patients with shoulder joint dislocation in these three cases, in addition to repair of the glenoid labrum, repair of the joint capsule is further required.

9.5.2.1 Capsular Ligament Avulsion on the Attachment Surface of Humeral Head (HAGHL)

Usually, the capsular ligament along with the scapular glenoid labrum is avulsed from one side of the glenoid cavity during shoulder joint dislocation, but only a tiny minority of patients do have the capsular ligament avulsed off from the

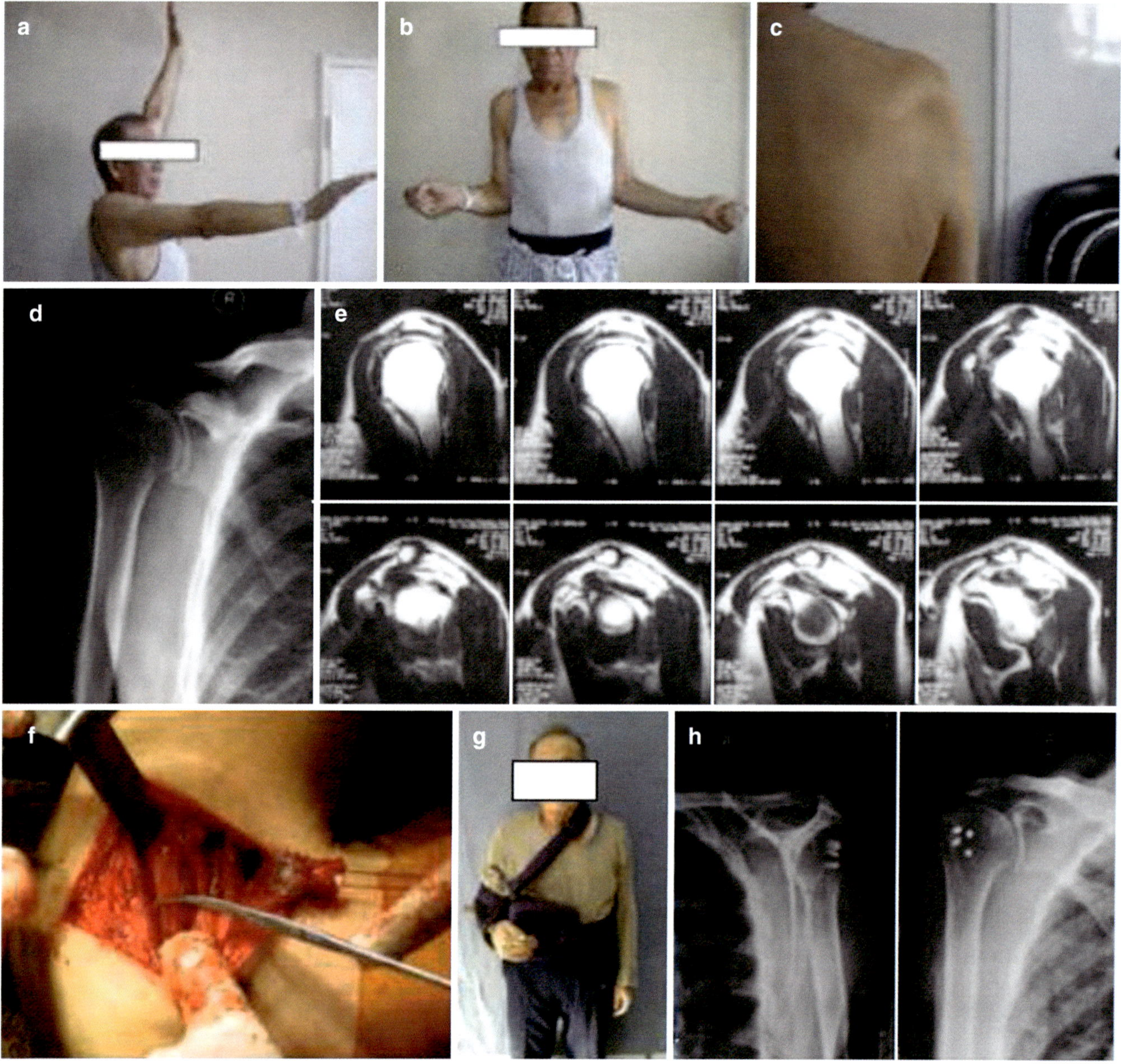

Fig. 9.49 Reconstructed posterior-superior rotator cuff injury by latissimus dorsi transfer. The elderly patient suffers from long-standing right shoulder pain and limited motion. (**a**, **b**) Preoperative limitation of motion; (**c**) Supraspinatus and infraspinatus atrophy; (**d**) Mild superior transfer of the humeral head; (**e**) Supraspinatus and infraspinatus tendon tears, retraction, severe muscle atrophy and steatosis showed through MRI; (**f**) Intraoperative latissimus dorsi transfer; (**g**) Postoperative immobilization position; (**h**) Postoperative film

attached side of the humeral head (humeral avulsion of the glenohumeral ligament, HAGHL), or a very small number of patients suffer from avulsion on both sides of the attachment. During arthroscopic exploration, reverse avulsion of the capsular ligament is relatively concealed and easily missed, especially in those patients with partial healing after avulsion. For the humeral avulsion of the capsular ligament, first, it needs to be fully recognized by a physician to improve the discovery rate. In surgical exploration, if it is found that the injury of the capsular ligament on one side of the glenoid cavity is not severe, the injury on the humeral side should be highly suspected. Second, once the injury is found, corresponding repair measures should be taken. The repair difficulty of the humeral avulsion of the capsular ligament lies in repair of the inferior glenohumeral ligament, because the injury site is located directly under the axilla and is difficult to operate; the broken end of the ligament is very close to the axillary nerve, leading to that the risk of axillary nerve injury is higher. Bilateral posterior arthroscopic approaches are generally required, with exposure of the axillary nerve followed by retraction of the glenohumeral ligament back to the humerus for repair using a transosseous fixation method.

9.5.2.2 Capsular Ligament Laxity of the Shoulder Joint

The capsular ligament laxity of the shoulder joint often does not occur alone, and is often a manifestation of generalized ligament laxity in the shoulder. There are five indicators for the diagnosis of generalized ligamentous laxity: elbow joint hyperextension; knee joint hyperextension; palpable forearm of the thumb; metacarpophalangeal joint dorsiflexion that allows the phalanges to be parallel to the forearm; and foot dorsiflexion of 45° or more. There are three indicators which can be used for diagnosing generalized ligament laxity. However, none of the indicators mentions a criterion for judging the capsular laxity of the shoulder joint. For the shoulder joint, the upper arm is attached to the chest wall, the elbow joint is flexed to 90°, the hand is rotated laterally from right front direction, and if the rotation angle exceeds 85°, it is diagnosed as the capsular ligament laxity of the shoulder joint. In such patients, the capsular ligament is often very thin and not easy to repair, even if the healing ability is poor after repair and the probability of re-tear is high, so it is indeed a treatment difficulty. For severe capsular ligament laxity, it is recommended to use a conjoint tendon transfer and subscapularis pressing technique while performing capsulolabral repair. This procedure requires partial osteotomy of the coracoid process of the conjoint tendon, approaching from the superior border of the subscapularis into the shoulder joint, with fixation to the glenoid cavity (generally fixed to the mid-superior glenoid cavity), known as the Trillat technique. As this tendon pushes the subscapularis anteriorly and inferiorly from the anterior side of the shoulder joint, it increases the obstruction of the subscapularis to the humeral head in the anteroinferior part of the shoulder joint. This procedure is much easier to perform arthroscopically than trans-subscapular conjoint tendon transfer fixation. For severe capsular ligament laxity, a glenohumeral ligament reconstruction surgery can also be used. The glenohumeral ligament is a thick fibrous band present in the shoulder joint capsule and an important structure to maintain shoulder joint stability, especially the inferior glenohumeral ligament. Therefore, reconstruction of the glenohumeral ligament is the most direct method when the capsular ligament is flaccid or defective.

9.5.2.3 Absence of Capsular Ligament

Absence of capsular ligament is the most serious type of capsular ligament problem of the shoulder joint, which is seen in patients who have originally had defects and have undergone surgery, and is also more common in patients with more recurrent dislocations, of which adolescents who love sports are in the majority. The degree of absence can range from a small part of defect to a large part of defect. For these patients, conventional glenoid labrum repair alone is less effective and other measures are required to prevent recurrence of dislocation. One such approach is to limit lateral rotation of the shoulder joint by the fixation of the subscapularis. One side of the subscapularis is attached to the humerus, and the other side is attached to the undersurface of the scapula. In the glenoid cavity plane, the subscapularis is always in a mediolateral sliding state. This procedure is to nail the subscapularis tendon on the glenoid cavity in the glenoid cavity plane and limit the lateral rotation of the shoulder joint by limiting the sliding of the subscapularis, thereby preventing shoulder joint dislocation. This procedure is similar to the incision surgery in the early years, and can prevent the recurrence of shoulder joint dislocation, but it affects the functions of the shoulder joint and can only be used as a backup means. For patients with severe absence of capsular ligament, some expert teams recommend glenohumeral ligament reconstruction surgery. This reconstruction procedure involves taking a tendon from another part of the body (usually the same calf), or using an allogenic tendon. The glenoid cavity and humerus are first tunneled, and then the glenoid cavity and humerus are connected with tendons to enhance or compensate for the original thin capsular ligament. In terms of surgical difficulty, reconstruction of the inferior glenohumeral ligament is similar to repair of humeral-sided avulsion of the inferior glenohumeral ligament, and the operating procedures are also similar. For these patients, we will perform both capsulolabral repair and conjoint trans-subscapular tendon transfer fixation, that is, "triple surgery for glenohumeral ligament reconstruction."

For patients with shoulder joint dislocation, while treating anteroinferior capsulolabral injury, some scholars believe that the treatment of a rotator cuff clearance is also conducive to consolidate the efficacy of Bankart repair and reduce the recurrence rate of dislocation. The method of suturing the rotator cuff clearance can be simple suturing or figure-of-8 suturing. Simple suturing technique: A suturing hook is used to pass the capsuloligamentous tissue on one side, and a Non-Absorbable 2# ETHIBOND® Suture (Polyester, Ethicon Inc.) is used for retention. On the other side, a suturing hook then passes through, with anAbsorbable 1# Antibacterial PDS®Plus Suture (polydioxanone, Ethicon Inc.). Non-Absorbable 2# ETHIBOND® Suture (Polyester, Ethicon Inc.) previously left in the joint and the Absorbable 1# Antibacterial PDS®Plus Suture (polydioxanone, Ethicon Inc.) are knotted together for threading. After that, another Non-Absorbable 2# ETHIBOND® Suture (Polyester, Ethicon Inc.) is used to repeat the previous operation. The two Non-Absorbable 2# ETHIBOND® Suture (Polyester, Ethicon Inc.) are knotted outside the joint, respectively, and the rotator cuff clearance is closed with the figure of-8 suturing technique.

Another suturing technique associated with joint capsule repair is used in the case of giant rotator cuff tears. When the rotator cuff ruptures to a certain extent, the retracted rotator cuff tissue gradually shrinks and fat infiltration is obvious. In the time when the remaining supraspinatus and infraspinatus tendons are not available for repair, surgeons encounter the embarrassing situation that one can't make bricks without straw. Although there are many surgical methods, including debridement, subacromial decompression, partial repair, muscle transposition, tendon transplantation and reverse shoulder replacement, none of the methods is considered most appropriate for irreparable rotator cuff.

9.5.2.4 About Superior Capsular Reconstruction (SCR) Technique

Dr. Mihata's team at Osaka Medical College in Japan has been exploring giant irreparable rotator cuff repair techniques since 2007, and has nearly 10 years of follow-up experience and good clinical results. Their improved superior capsular reconstruction technique has attracted international attention in recent years [22].

The clinical symptoms of giant irreparable rotator cuff tears are pain caused by subacromial impingement, muscle weakness of the shoulder joint, and limited arm lifting. The causes of the absence of stability of the superior glenohumeral joint are the upward shifting of the center of rotation of the shoulder joint and the loss of function of the rotator cuff muscle (supraspinatus). The superior joint capsule is also absent in patients with giant irreparable cuff tears, so arthroscopic superior capsular reconstruction (SCR) aims to restore the stability of the superior shoulder joint, push the humeral head back to its normal anatomical position, and rebalance the force couple of the shoulder joint. That is the concept of SCR surgery.

SCR Technical Key Points

1. Acromion shaping is required;
2. Subscapularis tear repair is required;
3. Measure the joint capsule with a probe, and please note that the measured length may be less than the actual length, because the joint capsule is arc-shaped while the probe is a straight;
4. A graft should be preferably large and thick;
5. Please note that the tension should not be too large when suturing the anterior side to prevent tearing, and if the medial, posterior, and lateral sides are well sutured, the anterior side does not need to be sutured;
6. In cases undergoing revision, where there are already many nails on the greater tubercle, a transosseous technique is recommended to fix a graft to the greater tubercle;
7. Open surgery for reconstruction of the superior joint capsule is also feasible if the surgeon is not skilled in arthroscopy;
8. Postoperative rehabilitation period of 6~12 months is needed;
9. Normal deltoid strength may improve postoperative shoulder joint function.

Since the creation of superior capsular reconstruction technique, there have been many other opinions. First, the superior capsular reconstruction technique does not restore the original dynamic structure of the tendon; second, the superior capsular reconstruction is equivalent to the spacer function under the acromion, and the increase of wear with time did not fundamentally solve the mechanical cause of upward shifting of the humeral head.

9.5.3 Repair of Acromioclavicular Joint Injury

Dong Jingming and Yao Qi

Abstract The acromioclavicular joint is composed of the medial surface of the acromion and the distal clavicle, it may be vertical or inclined more than 50°, and its stable structures include static stable structures and dynamic stable structures. Static stable structures include the acromioclavicular joint capsule and the acromioclavicular ligament (playing a role of strengthening the acromioclavicular joint capsule), and their main role is to control the movement of the clavicle in the horizontal direction. Dynamic stable structures include the anterior deltoid and the trapezius. Fibrocartilaginous discs are present in the acromioclavicular joint, but they gradually degenerate, disintegrate, or even disappear with age. When the shoulder joint is fully abducted and lifted, the clavicle should have a rotation of 40° to 45°, but due to the synergistic movement between the scapular and the clavicle, the clavicle actually has only a rotation of 5° to 8° relative to the acromion. Acromioclavicular joint injuries are very common in clinical practice and generally present with dislocation of the acromioclavicular joint. At present, although there are many kinds of surgical methods for acromioclavicular joint dislocation, the preferred methods are direct repair and reconstruction. The repair of the acromioclavicular joint helps to limit the movement of the clavicle in the horizontal direction and makes it be closer to the physiological state after the repair.

9.5.3.1 Anatomical Structure of the Acromioclavicular Joint

The acromioclavicular joint is located between the medial side of the acromion and the lateral side of the clavicle and belongs to the synovial joint. The joint structure includes the distal clavicle and acromion, with a large range of motion, which is connected by the articular disc to the middle site. The stability of the joint depends on the joint capsule, coracoclavicular ligament, and acromioclavicular ligament for maintenance. The stability of the anteroposterior plane is provided by the acromioclavicular joint ligament, which is the thickened part of the joint capsule, and the superior ligament is the strongest. The trapezoid and conoid ligaments maintain superior and inferior stability. The trapezoid ligament is located at the lateral end of the clavicle, with an average of 25.4 mm in men and 22.9 mm in women, and is more laterally attached to the subclavian surface, resisting the pressure of the acromioclavicular joint. The conoid ligament is inserted medial to the lateral border of the clavicle, with an average of 47.2 mm in men and 42.8 mm in women, and it limits anterosuperior shifting and rotation of the clavicle by approximately 60% (Fig. 9.50).

9.5.3.2 Mechanism of Joint Injury

Acromioclavicular joint injuries are very common in clinical practice and generally present with acromioclavicular joint dislocation, accounting for about 12% of all shoulder injuries. In fact, the true incidence of acromioclavicular joint injuries may be underestimated clinically, because many acromioclavicular joint injuries are not diagnosed or treated. Damage to the acromioclavicular joint is usually a direct injury to the shoulder due to contact movements during falls or arm adduction. When a straight hand or a bent elbow lands directly on the ground, a direct force may be transmitted superiorly through the humeral head to the acromioclavicular joint and enter the acromion. When the clavicle is maintained at an anatomical position, the force pushes the acromion downward, resulting in varying degrees of rupture of the acromioclavicular joint and clavicular ligament. The downward shifting of the clavicle is mainly resisted by the interlocking of the sternoclavicular joint and coracoclavicular ligament, while the anteroposterior shifting is mainly resisted by the acromioclavicular ligament. A more severe downward force may even tear the deltoid and trapezius attachments to the clavicle. Another uncommon mechanism of acromioclavicular joint injuries is that a traumatic force is formed through downward pulling of the upper limb or a lateral force during lateral rotation of the scapula.

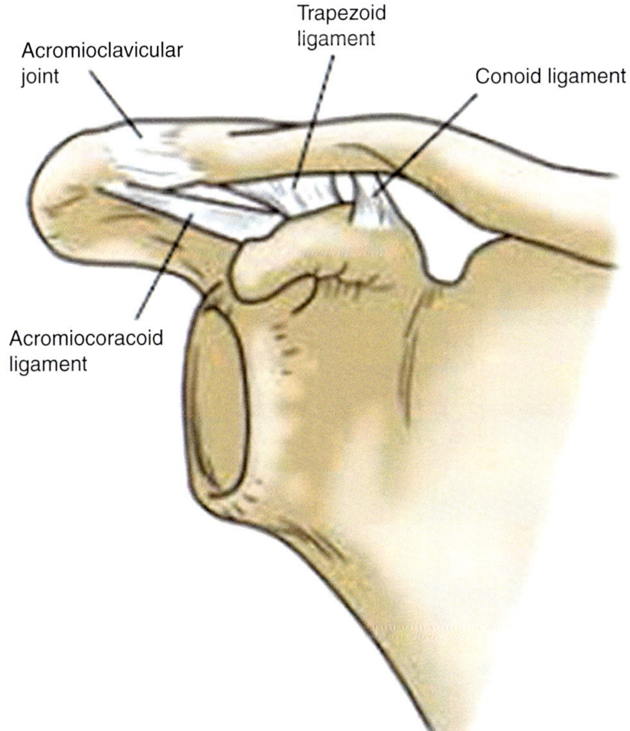

Fig. 9.50 Anatomical structure of the acromioclavicular joint

9.5.3.3 Assessment of Acromioclavicular Joint Injury

Clinical assessment: Acromioclavicular joint injuries should be considered for patients with shoulder trauma and pain near the acromion and clavicle. Most patients with acute acromioclavicular joint injuries experience that the pain may be relieved at an upper limb adducted supporting posture. Local pain, swelling, and point tenderness around the acromioclavicular joint are the most typical manifestations. Arm abduction and cross-inward retraction will increase the burden on the acromioclavicular joint and thus aggravate pain. X-ray assessment: When a plain film is taken, a tube ball is tilted by 10°~15° toward the head side, which can effectively avoid overlap of the acromion and scapula and take a bilateral comparison. For some patients, stress radiography may be performed under the condition of bilaterally lifting heavy weights of 10~15 kg. The bilateral comparison shows that the distance of distal clavicle shifting in a patient with dislocation is greater than or equal to the thickness of the clavicle (Fig. 9.51).

Classification of acromioclavicular joint dislocations: There are many clinical types of acromioclavicular joint dislocations, and Rockwood classification is basically selected at present. A classification system for acromioclavicular joint injuries is developed (Table 9.1, Fig. 9.52). Type I is acromioclavicular joint sprain without complete tear of the acromioclavicular joint ligament or coracoclavicular ligament. Type II is acromioclavicular ligament tear. Type III injuries include tears of the acromioclavicular joint and coracoclavicular ligament, which are displaced by 25%~100% compared with those on the other side. Type IV is an acromioclavicular joint injury in which the distal part of the clavicle penetrates posteriorly into the trapezoidal fascia. In type V injuries, both the acromioclavicular and coracoclavicular ligaments are completely torn, and the shift is greater than 100% compared with those on the other side. Type VI injuries are very rare; the distal clavicle is displaced inferiorly to the subaxillary position.

9.5.3.4 Therapeutic Regimens

1. *Conservative Treatment of Acromioclavicular Joint Injury*

   In recent years, with the deepening of the research on acromioclavicular joint injuries, most scholars at home and abroad believe that conservative treatment can be

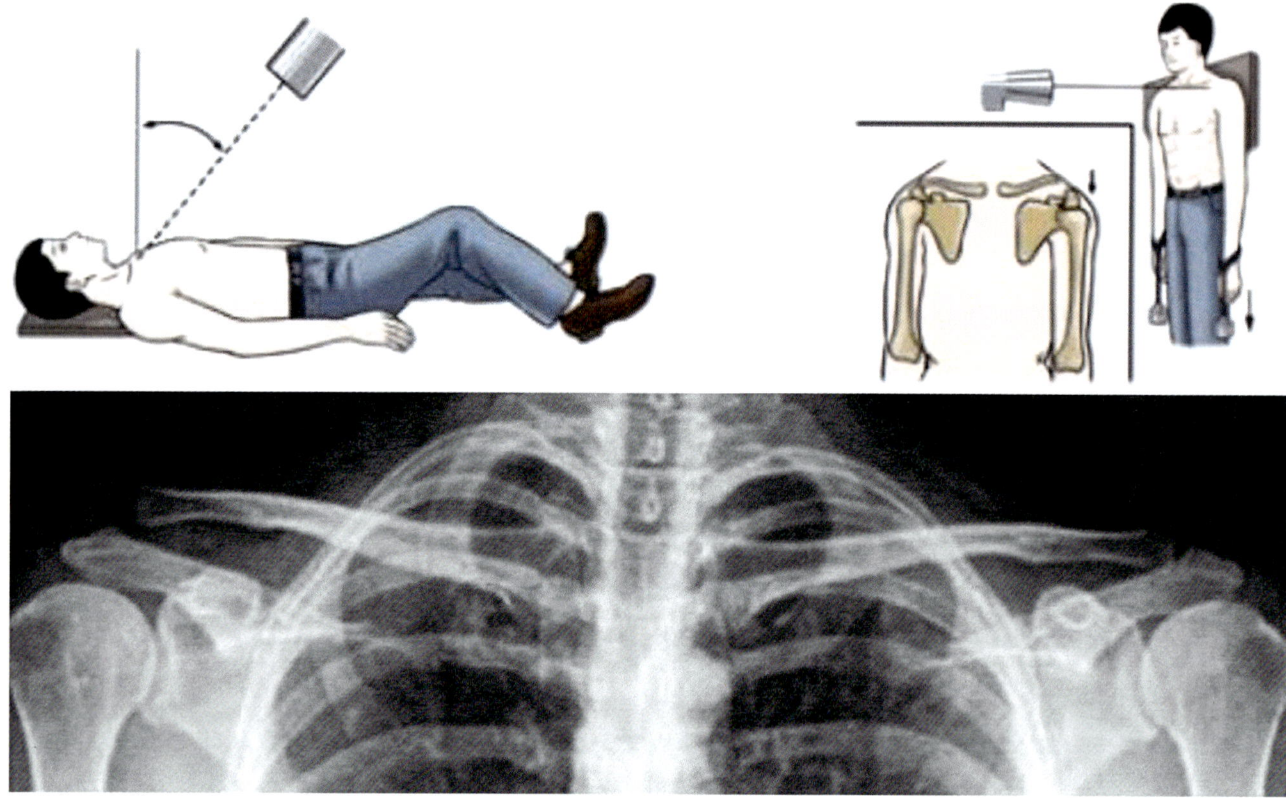

Fig. 9.51 X-ray radiographic angle, stress radiography, and typical X-ray manifestations of acromioclavicular joint injury

Table 9.1 Rockwood classification of acromioclavicular joint injuries

Type	Acromioclavicular ligament	Coracoclavicular ligament	Deltoid fascia	Coracoclavicular space distance[a]	Imaging manifestation of acromioclavicular joint
I	Sprained	Intact	Intact	Normal	Normal
II	Torn	Sprained	Intact	<25%	Enlarged
III	Torn	Torn	Torn	25%~100%	Enlarged
IV	Torn	Torn	Torn	Increased	Posterior shifting of clavicle (axillary)
V	Torn	Torn	Torn	100%~300%	
VI	Torn	Torn	Torn	Decreased	Clavicle shifting to inferior part of coracoid process

[a]Radiographically measured distance between the superior surface of the coracoid process and the inferior surface of the clavicle

tried for Rockwood type I and II acromioclavicular joint injuries, using a variety of methods for limiting shoulder joint activities, and common forearm slinging, fixation with adhesive tapes, shoulder and elbow fixation with straps and fixation with plaster supports are used to reduce the impact of the injured limb itself on the acromioclavicular joint, while giving appropriate pressure at the distal clavicle. While the therapeutic regimens for Rockwood type III are still controversial, Clavo et al. concluded that conservative treatment is not significantly different from surgical treatment, but Tuber et al. concluded that conservative treatment has the advantages of fewer complications and shorter fixation time compared with surgical treatment. Pereira et al. suggested that for patients with higher activity requirements, such as athletes, surgical treatment may be carried out to allow them to recover as soon as possible. In conclusion, type III patients should be treated individually in combination with their own conditions, such as type of injury, patient age, general condition, and amount of exercise.

2. *Surgical Treatment of Acromioclavicular Joint Injury*

Patients with types IV, V, and VI should be operated as early as possible to relieve symptoms and improve functions, and the surgical treatment of acromioclavicular joint injuries can be broadly classified into four categories: ① acromioclavicular fixation; ② coracoclavicular fixation; ③ non-anatomical reconstruction of the coracoclavicular ligament; and ④ anatomical reconstruction of the coracoclavicular ligament.

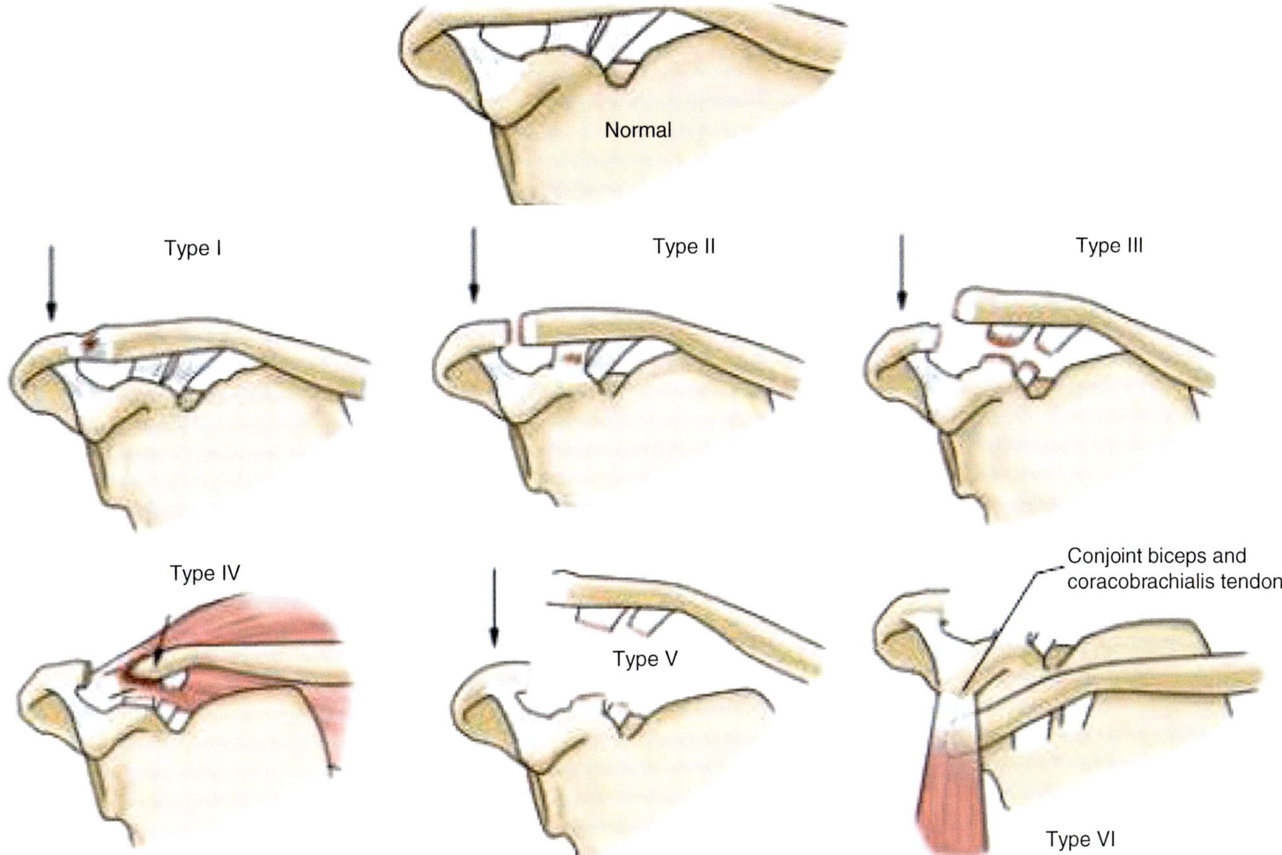

Fig. 9.52 Rockwood classification

A. Acromioclavicular fixation
 (1) Modified Phemister procedure (Kirschner wire fixation with tension band): The acromioclavicular joint is exposed through an anterior approach at the lateral end of the clavicle and coracoid process to observe whether the articular cartilage disc is damaged, and the disc is excised only when it is damaged. The coracoclavicular ligament is reinforced with anAbsorbable 0# VICRYL®Plus Suture (Polyglactin 910, Ethicon Inc.), which passes through a hole formed in the lateral clavicle to be slung in a figure-of-8 shape and tied under anatomical reduction of the acromioclavicular joint. The acromioclavicular ligament is then sutured. Finally, the injured acromioclavicular joint is traversed with a Kirschner wire, it should be noted that the tip of the Kirschner wire must drill through the posterior cortex of the clavicle, and its lateral end must be bent to prevent shifting. However, this method has been gradually abandoned due to the possible consequences of postoperative Kirschner wire shifting or even penetration.
 (2) Internal fixation of clavicular hook plate: This method has become the most important method for the treatment of acromioclavicular joint injuries. Surgery is performed under cervical plexus anesthesia or general anesthesia. The patient lies in the supine position, and a surgical incision is 5~7 cm from the medial and lateral 1/3 of the clavicle to a lateral-posterior curved incision of the acromion along the anterior margin of the clavicle. The plate is moderately pre-bent according to the shape of the clavicle, the posterior hook end of the clavicular hook plate is inserted into the space under the acromion close to the posterior part of the acromioclavicular joint, pressed down to attach to the superior part of the clavicle, and fixed with 3.5 mm cortical bone screw (Fig. 9.53). Repair of the acromioclavicular ligament and acromioclavicular joint capsule. After operation, the affected limb is suspended using a neck and wrist strap or triangular bandage. The functional exercise of the shoulder joint begins after 3 days, and the shoulder joint can move freely after 6~8 weeks.

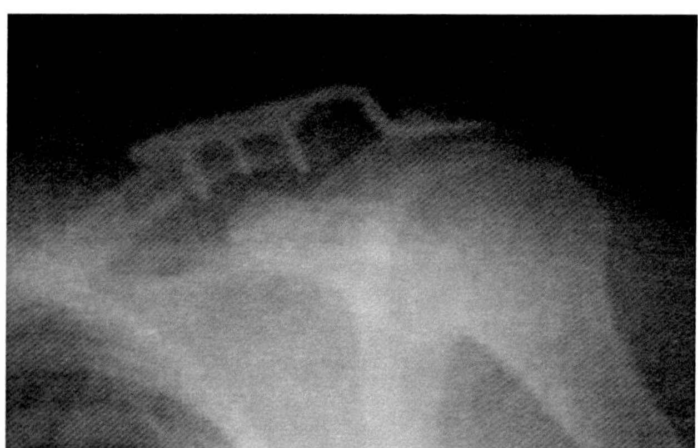

Fig. 9.53 X-ray film taken after internal fixation of clavicular hook plate

B. Coracoclavicular fixation: The primary coracoclavicular fixation technique now is the placement of a synthetic loop between the clavicle and the coracoid process or the cooperative use of Fiberwire sutures with Endobutton for fixation.

Surgical techniques: The procedure should be performed in a beach chair position without arm traction. Routine disinfection and draping are needed for arthroscopic surgery. The acromioclavicular joint is reduced by manual traction, and temporary fixation is performed using a Kirschner wire with 1.8 mm diameter. Shoulder joint reduction should be performed before arthroscopy to correctly identify bone landmarks. A 30° arthroscope is then inserted into the glenohumeral joint through a standard posterior approach. A 7 mm soft plastic stamp passes through the anterior mid-joint approach with an outside-in technique. This approach must allow the instrument to reach the anteroinferior part of the base of the coracoid process, traverse between the superior and middle glenohumeral ligaments, and pass from the superior border of the subscapularis tendon to the lateral side. A standard anterosuperior approach should be created, switching the extent and targeting the medial side to visualize the base of the coracoid process. The anteroinferior surface of the base of the coracoid process is completely exposed with a radiofrequency ablation instrument. The tip of a femoral guide for posterior cruciate ligament reconstruction passes through the anterior approach and inserted into the center of the base of the coracoid process. A 6 mm skin incision should be made in the superior part of the clavicle, at the site 3 cm medial to the acromioclavicular joint, and a needle guard of the femoral guide for posterior cruciate ligament reconstruction is located between the anterior 1/3 and the middle 1/3 of the clavicle, so as to avoid anterior shifting of the bone. The Kirschner wire is drilled through the clavicle and coracoid process. Correct location of the tip of the Kirschner wire at the base of the coracoid process is determined by arthroscopy, in which the tip of the guide should be already carefully kept in an appropriate place to prevent shifting. The femoral guide is removed and a 4.5 mm Endobutton cannulated drill (Smith and Nephew INC, Largo, FL) is used to create the bone tunnel. The guide wire is then removed, the cannulated drill bit is left in place, and an Absorbable 1# Antibacterial PDS®Plus Suture (polydioxanone, Ethicon Inc.) is threaded into it and accessed through the anterior glenoid anterior approach. A 5# Fiberwire suture and a 2# Fiberwire suture (Arthrex, Inc. Naples, Florida, USA) encircle the inner eyelets of both Endobuttons. The implantation into the coracoid process is achieved by sliding the first Endobutton through the bone tunnels in the clavicle and coracoid bone with two additional Ethibond No. 2 (Ethicon Endo-Surgery, Inc., Cincinnati, OH) sutures. These sutures are inserted into the side holes of the inferior button plate and removed through the Absorbable 1# Antibacterial PDS®Plus Suture (polydioxanone, Ethicon Inc.) from the anterior glenoid approach. Once the first Endobutton is flipped and secured at the base of the coracoid process, the Fiberwire suture would be locked in the second Endobutton on the superior part of the clavicle. The channel is monitored arthroscopically. Finally, the suture is removed (Fig. 9.54).

C. Non-anatomical reconstruction of coracoclavicular ligament: For complete tear of coracoclavicular ligament and acromioclavicular ligament caused by Rockwood type III or above acromioclavicular joint

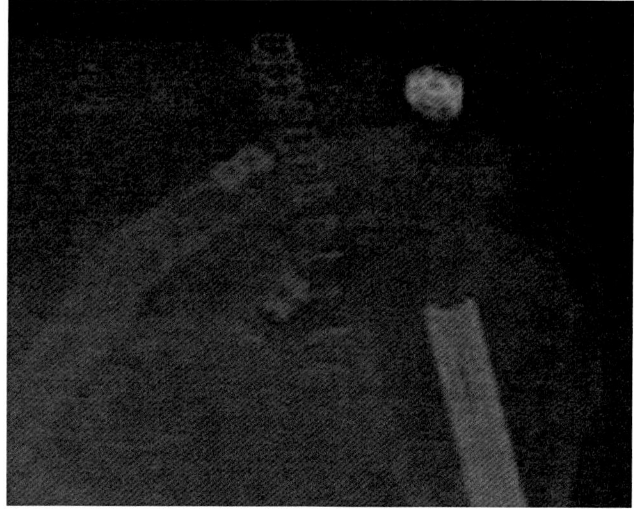

Fig. 9.54 X-ray film taken after coracoclavicular fixation with Endobutton and FiberTape suture

dislocation, Weaver and Dunn firstly proposed a method of distal clavicle resection and cutting, suture and fixation of the distal coracoacromial ligament to the distal clavicle for the treatment of acromioclavicular joint dislocation. After modification, a Weaver–Dunn surgical method using sutures, autologous or allogeneic free tendons, screws, and steel cables is formed. On this basis, Weinstein further proposed the modified Weaver–Dunn surgical method to strengthen the fixed coracoclavicular ligament with non-absorbable suture, which has become the main surgical method for non-anatomical reconstruction of the coracoclavicular ligament.

Surgical techniques: The patient is placed in a beach chair position and under general anesthesia. The skin incision is directed from the posterior part of the acromioclavicular joint to the coracoid process (Fig. 9.55). The lateral clavicle and the acromioclavicular joint are exposed. The 1 cm lateral end of the clavicle is removed. The resection direction of distal clavicle is from posterosuperior and lateral to anteroinferior and medial. The coracoacromial ligament and its border are identified (Fig. 9.56a). The bone fragment at the attachment point is preserved, and the coracoacromial ligament is separated from the acromion attachment to enhance bone-to-bone healing (Figs. 9.56b and 9.57). The medullary cavity is opened from the lateral end of the clavicle using a small curette. The two drill holes are 5~6 mm apart and 5~7 mm from the lateral border of the clavicle. It should be noted that the holes are neither too close to the resected end of the clavicle nor too close to each other. Two Absorbable 1# Antibacterial PDS®Plus Suture (polydioxanone, Ethicon Inc.) pass through the inferior coracoid process for future use as coracoclavicular ligament reinforcements. The free coracoacromial ligament is pulled into the medullary cavity of the clavicle together with Non-Absorbable 2# ETHIBOND® Suture (Polyester, Ethicon Inc.) through two holes that had been drilled in the lateral clavicle (Figs. 9.56b and 9.57) and fixed to the clavicle. Two PDS®Plus Suture (polydioxanone, Ethicon Inc.) pass through the inferior coracoid process and are strapped to the clavicle for reinforcement (Figs. 9.56d and 9.58). The arm is suspended for 6 weeks, and the stitches are removed after 10~14 days, at which stage, active movements of the elbow, wrist, and fingers are allowed. From 6th to12th week, the shoulder joint is mobilized following a rehabilitation exercise program in order to restore the range of motion of the shoulder joint.

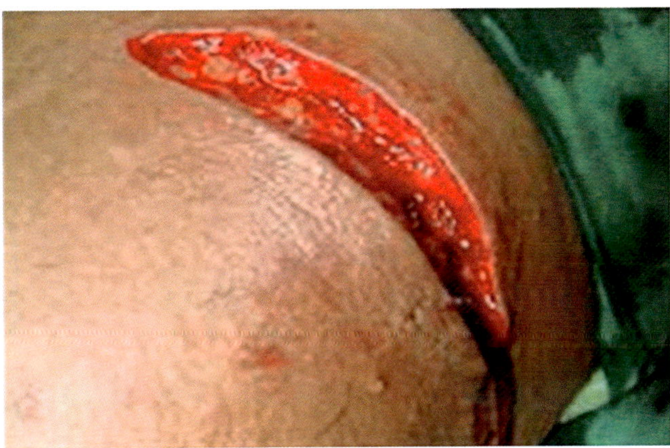

Fig. 9.55 Surgical incision from the acromioclavicular joint to the coracoid process

D. Anatomic reconstruction of coracoclavicular ligament: Plate fixation and coracoclavicular ligament repair are the main means of clinical treatment of acromioclavicular joint dislocation, but after fixation, the patient has strong pain and experienced limiting of shoulder joint activities. Non-anatomical repair and reconstruction of coracoclavicular ligament likely cause traumatic arthritis. Therefore, arthroscopic treatment of the complications of acromioclavicular joint dislocation has not widely used. Arthroscopic treatment of acromioclavicular joint dislocation is mostly used for types IV~VI dislocation (Fig. 9.59).

Surgical techniques: Check the position of the acromioclavicular joint, and assess the vertical instability of the acromioclavicular joint by pulling down on the upper limb. The patient lies in a beach chair position and under general anesthesia. After determining the anatomical reduction, a 2.4 mm Kirschner wire passes through the acromioclavicular joint from the posterior border of the acromion to the clavicle instead of penetrating the acromioclavicular joint. Arthroscopy is performed through an anterolateral or posterior approach to the inferior surface of the coracoid process. Soft tissue is removed during exposure of the coracoid process through an anterior approach using radio frequency and a shaver. An approximately 2 cm skin incision is made in the superior conoid tuberosity of the clavicle 3–4 cm from the acromioclavicular joint, and the tip of the drill guide is placed on the inferior surface of the base of the coracoid process through the anterior approach. The cannulated drill guide is placed in the superior clavicle, and the position of the guide tip is confirmed by intraoperative fluoroscopy. Later, the coracoid and clavicular bone tunnels are drilled with a cannulated drill through the guide. A 2-0 Nylon suture is attached to a Leeds–Keio synthetic ligament (3.0 mm wide × 50.0 cm long) with an

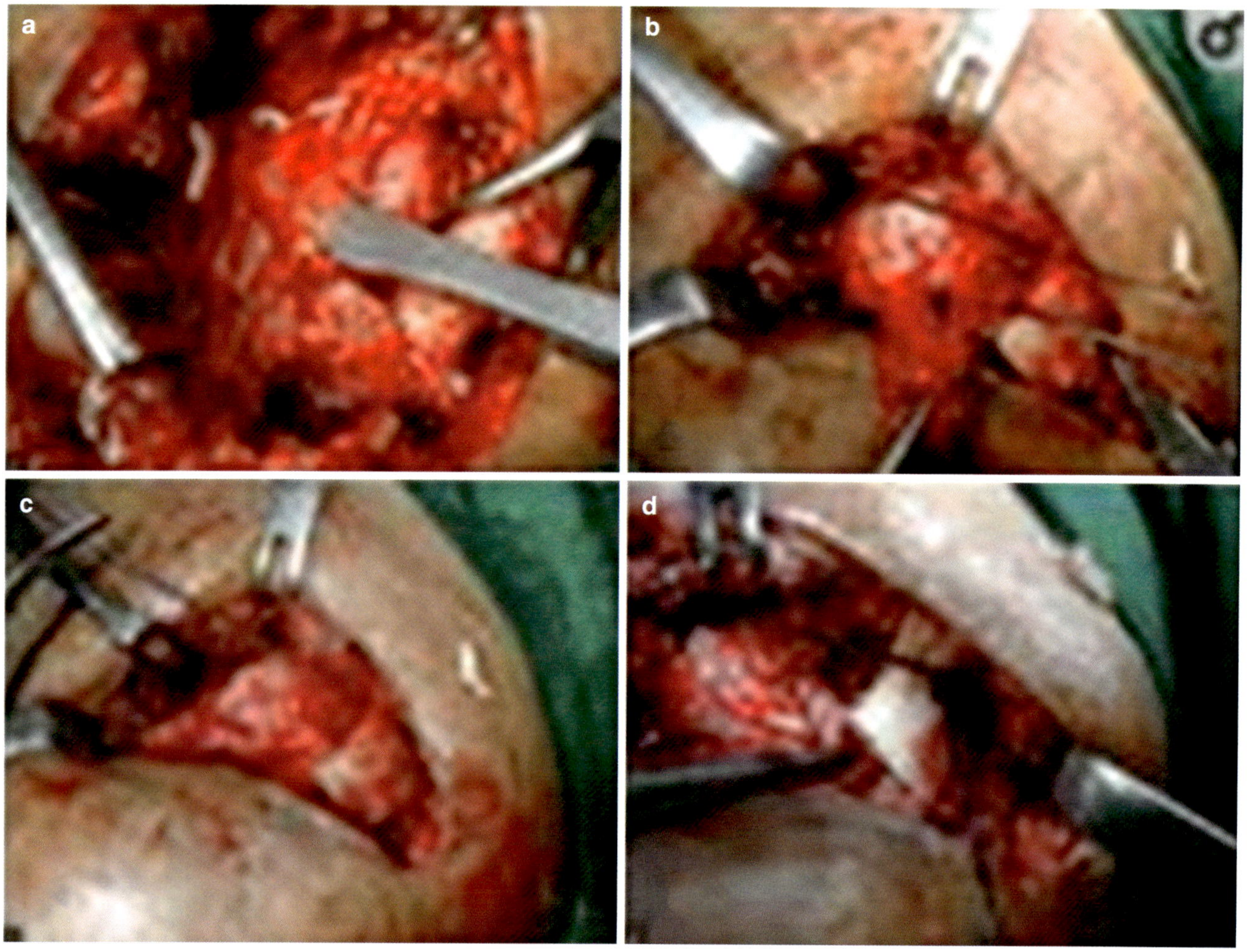

Fig. 9.56 (**a**) Identification of the coracoacromial ligament; (**b**) Coracoacromial ligament and PDS® Plus loop separated around the coracoid process; (**c**) Reconstruct the coracoacromial ligament with lateral clavicle. (**d**) Reinforce construction with PDS® Plus loop

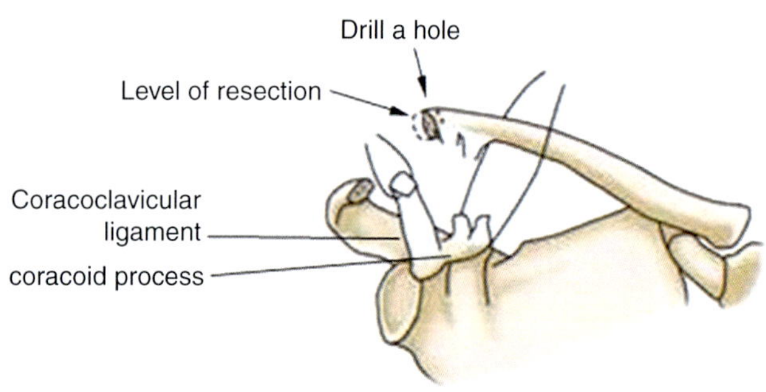

Fig. 9.57 Resect the lateral clavicle, obtain the coracoacromial ligament with bone fragment, and leave PDS® Plus Suture in the inferior coracoid process for reinforcement

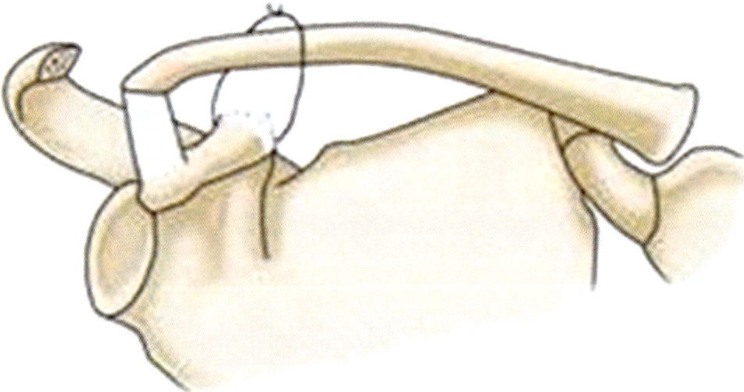

Fig. 9.58 Acromioclavicular joint with modified Weaver–Dunn reconstruction

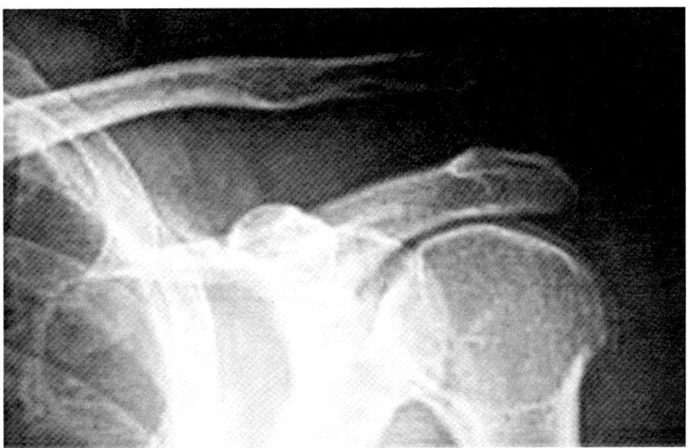

Fig. 9.59 X-ray film showing Rockwood Type V acromioclavicular joint dislocation

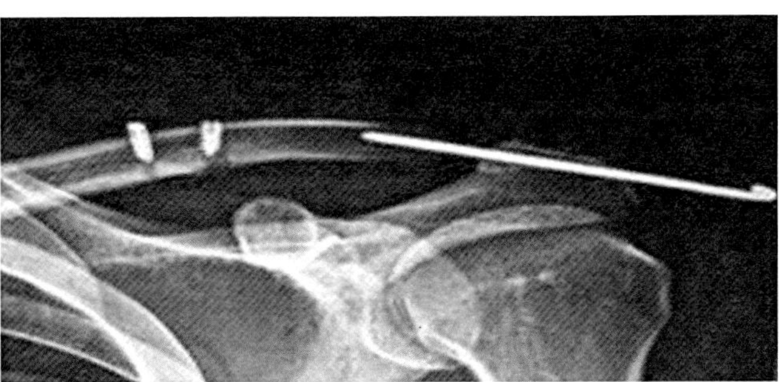

Fig. 9.60 Postoperative anteroposterior X-ray film showing arthroscopic coracoclavicular ligament reconstruction with synthetic ligament fixed by Endobutton, door-shaped screw and interference screw

Endobutton (4.0 mm × 12.0 mm) and pulled from the clavicle to the inferior surface. The process of obtaining the clavicular and coracoid tunnels by the cannulated drill is repeated for the trapezoid tuber osity. After pulling out the cannulated drill bit, the nylon suture with the synthetic ligament and the Endobutton is pulled to the clavicle via the anterior approach. The Endobutton is secured to the inferior surface of the coracoid process when the synthetic ligament is tightened. The synthetic ligament pulled out through the clavicular tunnel is fixed to the supraclavicular surface using a door-shaped screw (5.0 mm wide × 10.0 mm long) and an interference screw (TJ screws 4.0 mm × 9.0 mm) (Fig. 9.60). The stability of the acromioclavicular joint and the range of shoulder motion should be carefully examined. A Kirschner wire is implanted subcutaneously to close the wound.

9.5.4 Repair and Reconstruction of Coracoclavicular Ligament Injury

Zhuang Chengyu

Abstract There are two main categories of surgical methods in the treatment of acromioclavicular joint dislocation: one is to seek strong fixation between the coracoid process and the clavicle; the other is to seek methods for reinforcing or reconstructing the coracoclavicular ligament. At present, the coracoclavicular ligament is anatomically reinforced and reconstructed using soft tissue grafts, and a variety of fixation methods are used. Many modifications have been made for each technique, and reports have shown their good clinical efficacy.

In addition to the injuries and rupture of the acromioclavicular ligament, the rupture of the coracoclavicular ligament is the main cause of acromioclavicular joint dislocation. There are two main ways to manage coracoclavicular ligament injuries: one is rigid fixation; the other is ligament reconstruction technique.

Rigid fixation is mainly performed by using rigid materials such as screws to fix the coracoid process and clavicle. After acromioclavicular joint dislocation, the ruptured coracoclavicular ligament is usually torn to be of a horsetail shape without transection-like rupture, such that it brings difficulties to repair and suturing, and suturing with sutures is usually not possible. Bosworth first used lag screws to fix the clavicle to the base of the coracoid process for fixation. This screw may be implanted through an incising or percutaneous way, but it is important to have bicortical fixation. The percutaneous screw technique has a failure rate of about 32%, and for type VI acromioclavicular joint dislocation, incision can also allow the repair of deltoid and trapezius fascia to be completed. The screws are usually removed 6–8 weeks after surgery. Rigid fixation of the coracoid process with the clavicle also has many complications: early degeneration of the acromioclavicular joint; dissolution of the distal clavicle; and ossification between the coracoid process and the clavicle.

9.5.4.1 Reconstruction Technique of Ligament Between Coracoid Process and Clavicle

Reconstruction of the acromioclavicular and coracoclavicular ligaments can restore vertical stability between the coracoid process and the distal clavicle, there are also many surgical techniques, and a variety of grafts are used to restore the coracoacromial ligament after injury. These surgical approaches can be graded into: non-anatomical reconstruction, that is, coracoacromial ligament transfer with or without coracoclavicular suspension augmentation; and anatomical reconstruction of the coracoclavicular ligament. A number of techniques involving reconstruction of the acromioclavicular joint capsule ligament with grafts or suture materials have also been reported recently. In addition, there is also the possibility of simultaneous use of multiple surgical methods.

9.5.4.2 Non-Anatomical Reconstruction of Coracoclavicular Ligament

In 1968, Neviaser first proposed the method of repairing the acromioclavicular joint using the coracoacromial ligament, which separates and transfers the ligament from the coracoid process to the distal clavicle, in which acromioclavicular joint fixation can be enhanced. Subsequently, Weaver and Dunn proposed a modified technique for old acromioclavicular joint dislocation: the coracoacromial ligament is separated and transferred from the acromion, the distal clavicle is resected, and the coracoacromial ligament is transferred to the distal clavicle. Such method later named the Weaver–Dunn technique. However, earlier biomechanical tests showed that the strength of the coracoacromial ligament provided by the Weaver–Dunn technique was only 25% of the strength of the original ligament.

Since then, further technical improvements have been made, including the addition of high-tensile sutures, synthetic ligaments, allogeneic tendons, and autologous tendons. Lee and his colleagues compared the load torque and migration of the Weaver–Dunn technique with the modified Weaver–Dunn technique (with sutures, braided straps, semitendinosus allograft reinforced) using a cyclic test method and found that the allograft tendon technique is superior to several other methods.

In reconstruction, the graft or suture material encircles or passes through the base of the coracoid process, which predisposes to axillary nerve injury, and a curved suturing device is placed from medial to lateral of the coracoid process, so that the risk of neurovascular injury can be reduced. Once the graft or a suture tunnel is perforated, various methods can be used for the distal clavicle, including cerclage fixation, bone tunnel passing, or internal fixation (with button plates or interference screws). The complications of this technique are mainly due to the relative concentration of internal fixation stresses, including suture cut-out, internal fixation failure, clavicular osteolysis as well as coracoid process fracture.

The suture anchor fixation technique achieves coracoclavicular space fixation and avoids resection of the inferior structure of the coracoid process, and follow-up studies have shown that this technique has a higher incidence of dislocation. However, the use of suture anchors in the modified Weaver–Dunn technique can maintain stability in the anterosuperior direction of the acromioclavicular joint with better postoperative outcomes.

Non-rigid fixation of the coracoclavicular ligament reconstruction by the button plate technique is widely used, and high-tensile strength solid suture materials provide stability by means of closed loops. In addition, a rotational motion of the clavicle is theoretically allowed. Button plates increase the areal distribution of tension transmission, and it is reported that they are used mostly in anterior cruciate ligament reconstruction. Biomechanically, the strength of in vitro reconstruction is basically the same as that of the original ligament, and for acute acromioclavicular joint injuries, the reconstructed ligament can maintain stability and promote healing of the original ligament. For old injuries, reconstruction with allogeneic tendon can provide biological basic parts to reconstruct the coracoclavicular ligament, and many studies have shown that this reconstruction method can obtain better outcomes. However, the incidence of complications is also high, including clavicular-end plate shifting, suture breakage, and button plate prolapse. It is important to drill a bone tunnel in the middle of the base of the coracoid process, and it is reported that eccentric tunnels lead to the occurrence of coracoid fractures.

The reconstruction can be completed by both incision and arthroscopy, and there is no evidence that either is more advantageous. Open reduction allows direct visualization of the reduction and determination of drilling sites. For highly violent injuries, the deltoid and trapezius fascia may be repaired, but there is a greater risk theoretically.

Advocates of arthroscopic technique believe that it is minimally invasive and avoids dissection of the deltoid and trapezius fascia. Complete intra-articular examination can be used for assessing whether there is an accompanied pathological condition. However, this reconstruction method requires a higher arthroscopic technique, which can well expose the coracoid process and precisely drill a coracoid tunnel, and even for experienced physicians, the eccentricity of the bone tunnel may also lead to the aforementioned technique failure. Lateral decubitus or beach chair position may be adopted according to surgeon's preference. The posterior or anterolateral approach can be used for observation, and full visualization can be achieved with a 30° lens, while the inferior surface of the coracoid process can be fully visualized with a 70° lens.

In order to accurately locate a tunnel passing through the coracoid process, a predrilling guide wire is required, and it also depends on the surgeon's technique. The guide wire is inserted from the anterior approach, located at the base of the coracoid process using an aiming device for approximate reduction, and the guide wire drills through the coracoid process and clavicle for temporary reduction. After the aiming device is removed, the guide wire is fixed using a shaver head to prevent shifting during expansion. A reconstruction device is introduced with its attached steel wire or lifting wire. During the introduction process, it is necessary to use such assistance as a guide wire, ring forceps or holding forceps, so as to ensure that the tension direction is consistent with the direction of bone tunnel. A force is exerted to the device for reduction, knot tying for fixation is made on the supraclavicular surface, and if a graft is used, an interference screw is used for fixation after an appropriate tension is maintained.

9.5.4.3 Anatomical Reconstruction of Coracoclavicular Ligament

Simultaneous reconstruction of the conoid ligament as well as "anatomical" reconstruction of the trapezoid ligament can improve the situation that there is still loss of reduction after various reduction techniques aforementioned. This technique has led to a tendency to "anatomical" reconstruction, namely, reconstruction of the supraclavicular insertion of the coracoclavicular ligament with biological materials. A precise description on the location of the supraclavicular insertion is based on a previous analysis of the bony structure. The insertions of the conoid ligament and the trapezius muscle on the supraclavicular surface are 46.3 mm and 24.9 mm from the lateral end of the clavicle, respectively. It is considered that the medial bone tunnel during conoid ligament reconstruction should be established on the posterior side of the supraclavicular surface, about 30% of the total length from the distal clavicle; and the bone tunnel of the trapezoid ligament should exceed the middle clavicle, with its length 17% of the total length from the distal clavicle.

It is widely used that non-biomaterials such as sliding plates and suture anchors are used for anatomical reconstruction. The two-anchor technique and the one-anchor technique have similar rate of loss of reduction of the acromioclavicular joint. Wellmann and his colleagues reported radiographic and clinical results in a small series of 15 patients that showed excellent short-term results. They recommended anatomic sliding plates in acute injuries, and allotransplants in injuries undergoing revision and chronic injuries. Long-term follow-up visit is currently not available, but increasing biomechanical strength does not ultimately reduce the incidence of loss of reduction. With the advent of multiple tunnels on the coracoid process, theoretically, the incidence of coracoid process fractures also increases, and the possibility of fractures also increases when a fixation device produces greater stress on the bone structure than physiological one.

Biological reconstruction allows restoration of the anatomy of the coracoid process. Carofino and Mazzocca described the early use of free tendons encompassing the coracoid process and supraclavicular figure-of-8 fixation. The high-tensile and non-absorbable suture stitched tendons reinforce fixation. Once the clavicle is fixed, the caudal end of the transplanted tendon can laterally reinforce the acromioclavicular joint capsule. This is the currently recommended technique. It is suitable for patients with acute type IV and type V injuries as well as old type III injuries, as well as patients undergoing revision, because its biological reconstruction is similar to natural anatomy.

During surgery, the patient is required to be supine for adequate exposure of the surgical field on the medial side of the clavicle. A surgical drape or pad is placed on the medial border of the scapula to extend the scapula. Intraoperatively, a semitendinosus graft and high-strength sutures are prepared by braiding them on a rear preparation table, and pretensioning is performed on a tendon transplanting table to decrease folding. If necessary, the graft needs to be trimmed to make sure it is easy to pass through a 5 mm catheter. The clavicle is measured, and the location of the clavicle tunnel is temporarily marked. For adult patients, the conoid ligament insertion is located 45 mm distal to the clavicle on the surface of the posterior 1/3 of the clavicle; the trapezoid ligament insertion is 15 mm distal to the conoid ligament insertion and is centered on the superior surface. Along the Langer line, a longitudinal incision is made from the coracoid process to the posterior border of the clavicle, reaching the deep fascia, and the skin flap is turned over. The deltoid and trapezius fascia are longitudinally incised, extending from the supraclavicular surface to the distal clavicle as previously described. A full-thickness deltoid trapezius muscle flap is isolated under the periosteum for repair. A wide blunt retractor is placed below the muscle flap to expose the coracoid process. The braided band passes from medial to lateral in the inferior part of the coracoid process using a suture passer to preserve the acroclavicular ligament insertion on the lateral surface of the coracoid process, and the braided band can slide gently in the posterior part of the base of the coracoid process.

The location of the tunnel is again measured, and a hole is drilled anterior to the posterior cortex of the conoid ligament. Two cortical layers are taken using a 5.5 mm cannulated drill, and a blunt retractor is placed in the inferior part of the clavicle to protect its deep structure. The braided band and three auxiliary solid sutures pass through the inferior coracoid process through the allograft tendon, the graft and one suture pass through the clavicular tunnel, while the other two pass the posterior clavicle with hemostatic forceps or a suture passer. Under direct vision, a downward force is applied to the clavicle to reduce the acromioclavicular joint and hold the elbow to stabilize the upper limb. The loop sutures are knotted to ensure stability. The lateral limb is first stabilized with a 0.5 mm × 8 mm polyetherketone tenodesis screw, and the stabilization can extend into the acromioclavicular joint capsule. Tendon tension can prevent excessive reduction. The medial limb is secured with another tenodesis screw. The third suture is tied, and the tissue of the remaining medial tendon is sutured together with the lateral limb or repaired with the acromioclavicular joint capsule.

9.5.5 Reconstruction of Rotator Cuff Functions in Artificial Shoulder Arthroplasty

Zhou Junlin

Abstract The main surgical purposes of artificial shoulder arthroplasty are to relieve shoulder joint pain, improve shoulder joint functions, and remove the lesions for patients with shoulder joint tumors. Rotator cuff functions play an important role in artificial shoulder arthroplasty. How to reconstruct rotator cuff functions is a key factor affecting the efficacy of artificial shoulder arthroplasty. This section will explain the rotator cuff functions and how to reconstruct the rotator cuff in total shoulder arthroplasty.

In 1893, the French physician Jules Emile Pean first applied a hinged artificial shoulder joint in clinical practice and pioneered the history of shoulder arthroplasty [23]. In 1951, Boron et al. successfully performed acrylic prosthesis replacement of glenohumeral joint, which enriched the material choices of artificial joint prostheses [24]. At present, artificial arthroplasty is graded into hemiarthroplasty, total shoulder arthroplasty, and reverse shoulder arthroplasty. According to different types of prostheses, prostheses are further classified into restrictive joint prostheses, semi-restrictive joint prostheses, and non-restrictive joint prostheses. The main surgical purposes of artificial shoulder arthroplasty are to improve shoulder joint functions, relieve shoulder joint pain, and remove the lesions for patients with shoulder joint tumors. No matter which kind of shoulder arthroplasty and joint prosthesis is adopted, the surgical efficacy is related to the prosthesis design, surgical methods, surgical indications, postoperative functional exercise, and the conditions of peripheral soft tissues. Among them, the conditions of peripheral soft tissues, especially the rotator cuff conditions, not only affect the selection of surgical methods but also affect the postoperative shoulder joint functions of patients. If the assessment of rotator cuff functions is not accurate, the intraoperative treatment of rotator cuff is not appropriate, which will seriously affect the functional recovery of patients. So, for artificial shoulder arthroplasty, the reconstruction of rotator cuff functions is essential.

9.5.5.1 Role of Rotator Cuff in Shoulder Joint Movement

The shoulder joint is the joint with the highest requirement and the strongest dependence of motor function and stability on the peri-articular soft tissues, and the rotator cuff is important for the motor function of the shoulder joint. The rotator cuff is a group of muscle and tendon complexes that encompass the shoulder joint to form a covering around the humeral head. The anterior part of the humeral head is the subscapularis tendon, the superior part of the humeral head is the supraspinatus tendon, and the posterior part of the humeral head is infraspinatus tendon and the teres minor tendon. The movements of these tendons lead to the medial and lateral rotation and elevating activities of the shoulder joint. However, more importantly, these tendons stabilize the humeral head on the glenoid cavity and play an extremely important role in stabilization and activities of the shoulder joint. Because the constrained joint prosthesis provides the mechanical fulcrum to compensate for the rotator cuff functions, subluxation or dislocation is prevented through the mechanical combination, so that the affected limb can achieve stable functions such as lateral rotation, abduction, and forward flexion. However, because the interface between the prosthesis and a bone may cause a high abnormal stress, it is prone to result in prosthesis loosening, shedding or breakage, increasing the failure rate. Therefore, constrained joint prostheses have been rarely adopted at present. Also, the non-constrained or semi-constrained joint prostheses relatively rely on the functions of the peripheral soft tissues.

Kralinger et al. conducted a multi-center study in 12 Austrian hospitals. A total of 167 patients with 3- and 4-part proximal humerus fractures and fracture dislocations were included. All patients had undergone hemiarthroplasty. The follow-up visit lasted for at least 1 year. Patients' Constant scores and subjective satisfaction were recorded. It was found that whether the greater and lesser tubercles of the humerus anatomically healed severely affected the prognosis of the patients. It is believed that the reconstruction of the rotator cuff insertion in artificial shoulder hemiarthroplasty is very important, and anatomic reduction and secure fixation of the greater and lesser tubercles should be done as much as possible. Hashiguchi et al. conducted a follow-up study on the clinical and radiological results of artificial shoulder hemiarthroplasty. Thirty-five patients with a mean age of 75.1 years were included. The patients' intraoperative rotator cuff conditions, postoperative shoulder Constant scores, and X-ray examination findings 12 months after surgery were recorded. It was found that the rotator cuff functions and the healing status of the greater and lesser tubercles were very important for patients' prognosis. It is recommended to reconstruct the rotator cuff functions during surgery, repair the injured rotator cuff, and anatomically reduce the greater and lesser tubercles as much as possible [25].

9.5.5.2 Reduction of the Greater and Lesser Tubercles of the Humerus and Rotator Cuff Functions

The greater tubercle of the humerus serves as the insertion for the supraspinatus, infraspinatus, and teres minor, while the lesser tubercle serves as the insertion for the subscapularis. Therefore, the reconstruction of the rotator cuff is closely related to the reduction of the greater and lesser tubercles of the humerus. The reconstruction of the rotator cuff enthesis is closely related to the location of repairing and reducing the greater and lesser tubercles. Malunion or nonunion of the greater and lesser tubercles of the humerus seriously affects the functions of the shoulder joint after artificial shoulder arthroplasty.

Abu-Rajab et al. compared the security of three humeral tubercle suturing fixation techniques. The first suturing technique is suturing between the tubercles, including suturing between the tubercles and the humeral shaft, in which the greater and lesser tubercles are connected by two sutures. One bypasses the humeral stem, and the other passes through a suture hole in the humeral stem. The second method differs from the first method in that the sutures connecting the greater and lesser tubercles all pass through the suture holes in the humeral stem. The third suturing technique does not adopt direct connection of sutures between the greater and lesser tubercles. Additional abduction stress is applied to the proximal humerus by biomechanical testing to measure the angulation and transfer conditions of the tubercles. It is found that the first two suturing fixation methods are more secure than the third fixation method. It indicates that the directly connected suturing fixation sutures are needed between the greater and lesser tubercles [26].

This article introduces a suturing fixation method: Pre-placing sutures before a humeral-sided prosthesis is implanted. Two holes are drilled horizontally in the humeral shaft, and two fixation sutures pass through. Four sutures pass through the aponeurosis on the surface of the greater tubercle. The humeral stem is then implanted. A modified reconstruction technique is adopted. That is, medial and lateral horizontal sutures bypass the neck part of the prosthesis for cerclage fixation, then reserved sutures located vertically at the proximal humerus are ligated for fixation, and finally the medial and lateral rotator cuffs are overlapped and sutured. During the operation, the tightness of the rotator cuff is generally detected preferably by slightly tightening the lateral side and slightly loosening the medial side (Fig. 9.61).

Several suture knot tying methods are introduced as follows: The first is Weston knot. It was proposed by Weston in 1991 as a basic knot for continuous suturing, which is safe and reliable, small in size, and easy to operate. In knot tying, a sliding suture is held with the left hand, a looping suture is held with the right hand, the suture held with the left thumb and index finger and the suture held with the right hand bypass

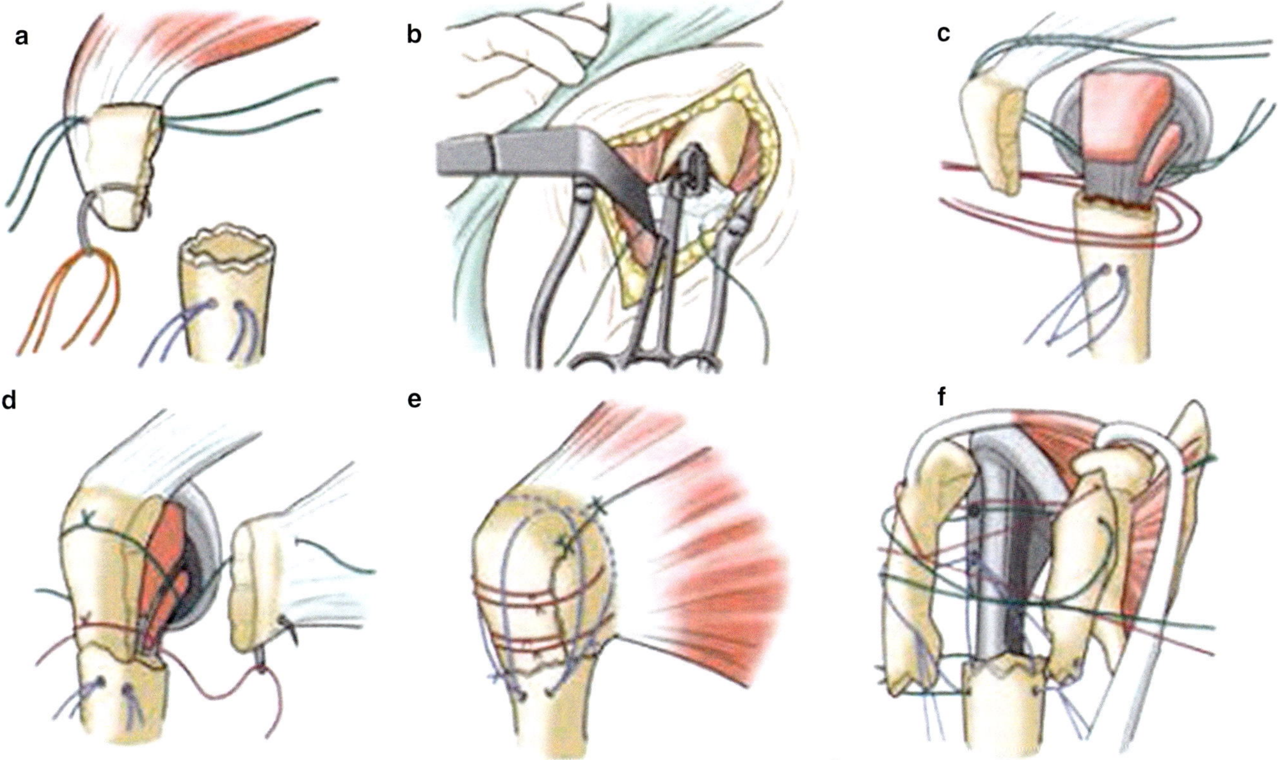

Fig. 9.61 Novel suturing fixation method. (**a**) Place reserved sutures; (**b**) Implant the humeral stem; (**c**) Sutures bypass the humeral stem for cerclage fixation; (**d**) Connected sutures between the greater and lesser tubercles; (**e**) Vertical fixation; (**f**) Spatial schematic diagram of all the fixation sutures

from the lower part of the straight suture to the front, and then pass out through the lower part of the suture held with the right hand, that is, an ascending single knot is made. After the tail of a side looping suture is wound around the looping suture half a turn counterclockwise first, it passes between the two sutures from front to back and then is wound around the double sutures half a turn clockwise, the suture tail passes through the loop closest to the suture-holding hand from back to front. The suture knot is tightened by gradually tightening the straight suture held by the left hand, and with the help of an auxiliary knotter, the suture held in the right hand is tightened after tightening to obtain a knot with satisfactory tension, and the suture knot is locked. Thereafter, 3 or 4 single knots are tied to complete final locking. For double-row fixation of the rotator cuff, the lateral structures are reduced and fixed first, and then the medial structures are repaired. The Weston knot is a low-resistance sliding knot that is strong when the suture is monofilament or multifilament (Fig. 9.62).

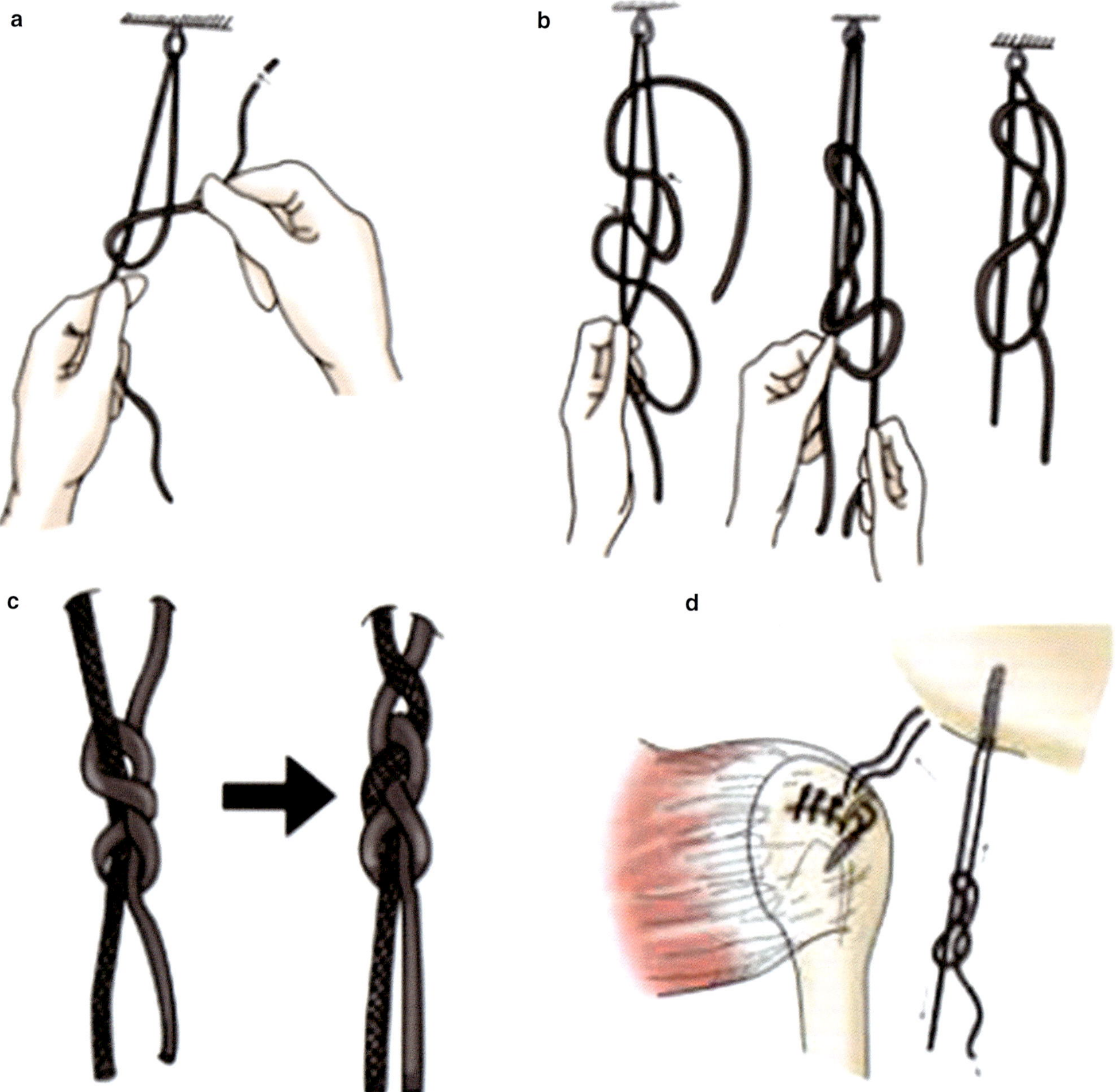

Fig. 9.62 Schematic diagram showing Weston knot making process. (**a**) During knot tying, hold a sliding suture with the left hand, hold a looping suture with the right hand to make an ascending single knot; (**b**) Perform winding and threading according to the steps to complete the basic knot; (**c**) Tighten the sliding suture and the looping suture successively to lock the basic knot, and then tie 3–4 knots for fixation; (**d**) Use the Weston knot for rotator cuff repair

The second is Giant knot. The novel Giant knot, reported by Basim et al. in 1999, is a self-locking sliding knot with simple structure, easy operation, small size, and with no need for additional single-knot fixation. It is commonly used for the repair of rotator cuff injury and surgical treatment of Bankart injury and shoulder capsule. A sliding suture is held with the left hand, and a looping suture is held with the right hand. First, an upper knot is completed by enabling the looping suture clockwise to be wound around the sliding suture 2 turns. The tail of the looping suture is drawn between the two sutures from back to front. The looping suture is then wound clockwise around the sliding suture below the completed knot 2 turns to complete a lower knot. The two sutures are gradually tightened to complete the base knot (Fig. 9.63).

The third is Nice knot. This knot is characterized by being particularly practical for open reduction and reconstruction of the fracture site, and this technique is emphasized here. This suture knot was invented by Dr. Pascal Boileau, Nice, France. The knot is of a double-suture structure, with the suture tail part held by the left hand and the looping suture part held by the right hand; first, the looping suture part is wound around the suture tail part to form an ascending single knot. The two suture tails then pass though the loop. The two sutures are gradually tightened to complete the base knot, and 3 to 4 additional single knots may be added as needed to achieve secure fixation (Fig. 9.64).

9.5.5.3 Free Soft Tissue Protection as well as Prosthesis Position and Rotator Cuff Functions

It is very important for the protection of peripheral soft tissues in shoulder arthroplasty. The neurovascular distribution is more concentrated in the local anatomy of the shoulder joint, and if not managed properly, it will cause injury and seriously affect the prognosis. The axillary nerve is a branch of the posterior bundle of the brachial plexus and contains fibers from the anterior branches of C5 and C6 nerve roots. After derived from the posterior bundle of the brachial plexus, it passes posteriorly and laterally through the quadrangular foramen with the posterior humeral circumflex artery, and runs around the surgical neck of the humerus in the deep surface of the deltoid. It innervates the skin of the

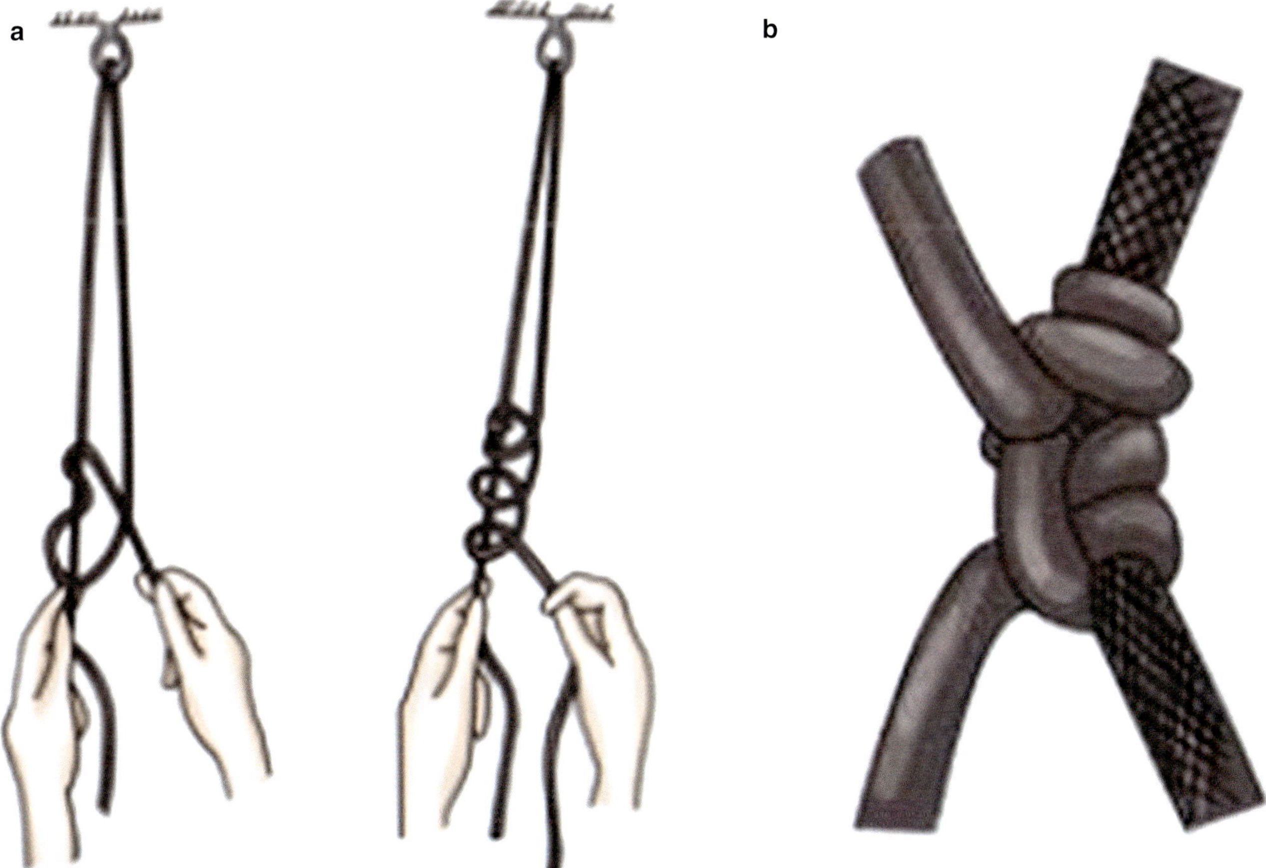

Fig. 9.63 Schematic diagram showing Giant knot making process. (**a**) Use the right suture as a looping suture to be wound around the sliding suture clockwise 2 turns to complete the upper knot, and then draw out the looping suture between the two sutures to be wound around the sliding suture 2 turns to complete the lower knot; (**b**) Tighten to complete the making of this knot

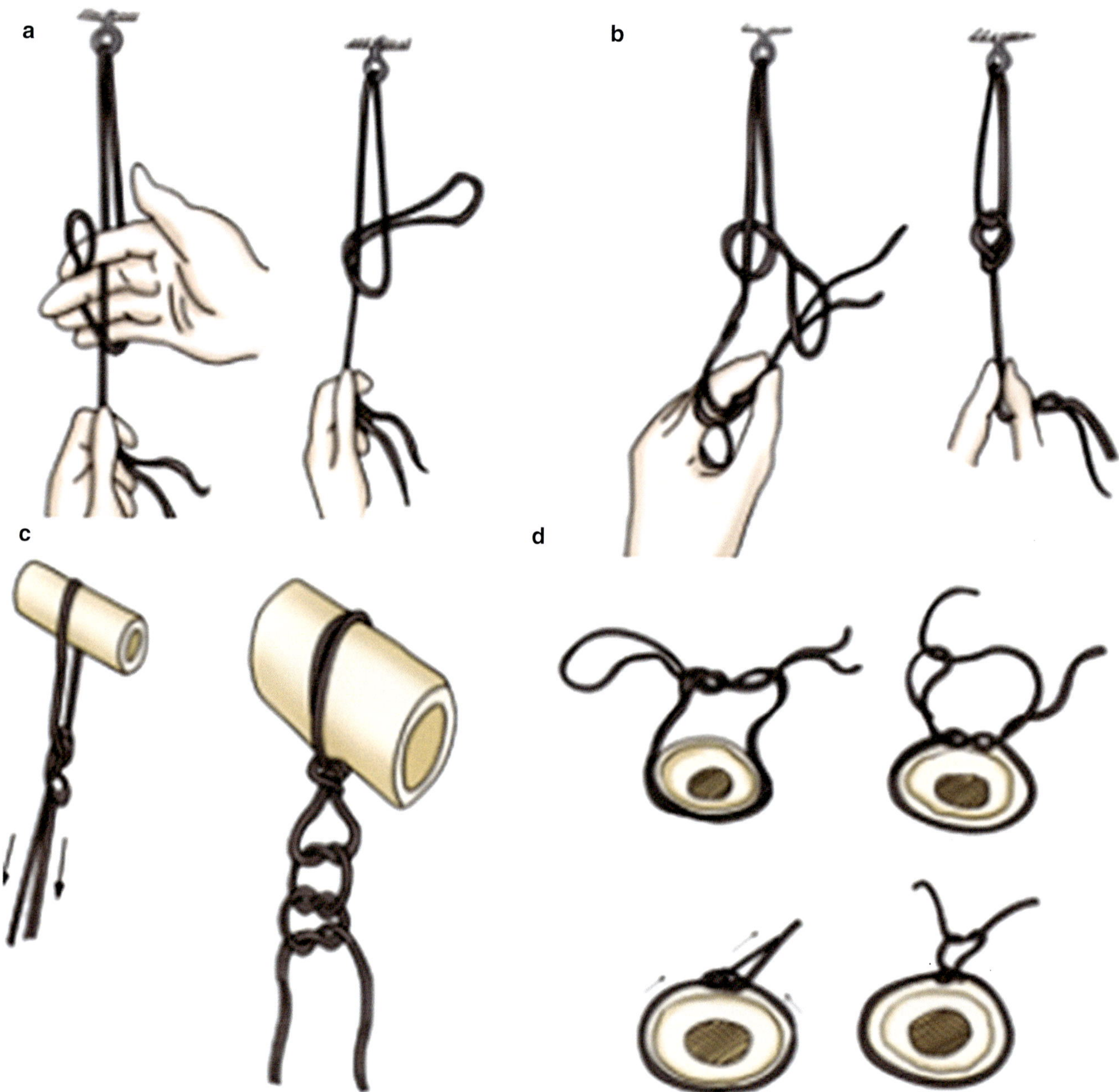

Fig. 9.64 Schematic diagram showing Nice knot making process. (**a**) Make a double-suture knot by selecting a long suture to form the structural feature with a loop on one side after folding in half, use double sutures to tie a single knot first; (**b**) Enable the double tail sutures to pass through the suture loop, so as to complete the main structure of knot. Gradually and forcefully pull the double tail sutures to make the knot slide to the bundled tissue, then separate the double tail sutures, hold one suture with each hand, respectively, and forcefully pull them until the knot tension is satisfactory; (**c**) End the operation with 3–4 single knots; (**d**) Tie a square knot in the same way, so that the knot can be tightened with a single suture instead of the double sutures, and the high tension can also be maintained

teres minor and the anterior and posterior deltoid, the posteroinferior deltoid, and the long head of the triceps brachii. Deltoid atrophy will occur when the axillary nerve is injured. The shoulder joint should be laterally rotated in operation to increase the distance between the surgical field and the axillary nerve, which is conducive to the protection of the axillary nerve. For dissection of the muscle from the joint capsule, please take care not to damage the deltoid during surgery if the patient has a rotator cuff injury. The rotator cuff should be gently pulled because the rotator cuff on the surface of the greater and lesser tubercles forms aponeurosis. Please remember not to detach and split the aponeurosis; otherwise, an iatrogenic rotator cuff injury will be caused. In patients with proximal humeral fractures, the fractured bone fragments of the greater and lesser tubercles are connected to the aponeurosis, so that the greater and lesser tubercles can be reduced and fixed by tractive assistance from sutures pre-implanted in the aponeurosis. The joint capsule and subscapularis insertion can serve as a whole for dissection to maintain the strength of the soft tissue flap, facilitate the suturing of the joint capsule and strength maintenance, and perform functional exercise in the early postoperative period. Blunt dissection and release of the joint capsule from the peripheral soft tissue should be performed as much as possible, and if a rotator cuff tear requires repair, suturing and repair should be conducted without tension, and the arm may be placed in a rotationally neutral position. Moderate rotator cuff tears may be repaired in situ; extensive tears may be repaired by freeing the proximal subscapularis when a prosthesis has not been implanted after humeral head resection. When it is necessary to extend the subscapularis for repair, the subscapularis can be incised from the joint capsule, sharply dissected to make its transverse section in a "Z" shape, or its proximal part may be moved upwards to repair the ruptured supraspinatus tendon. If the rotator cuff is severely torn, the muscle should be freed from the base of the coracoid process and joint capsule, and the defect should be repaired by end-to-end alignment. When the supraspinatus or infraspinatus is defective, it may be replaced by the pectoralis major or minor muscle, drilling and suturing may be performed on the humerus to fix the rotator cuff.

For proximal humeral fractures, especially severe 3- and 4-part fractures, mostly accompanied by rotator cuff injuries, it is appropriate to reduce the fractures and repair the rotator cuff during treatment. Old injuries should be repaired or reconstructed as appropriate. Reverse shoulder arthroplasty may be used if necessary. For proximal humeral tumors, most of the rotator cuff and its attached bones are damaged due to tumor erosion to varying degrees, and some patients require partial or even total resection of the deltoid and rotator cuff in order to completely remove the tumor tissue as much as possible during the operation, so that the rotator cuff is further damaged. During the operation, the residual rotator cuff and muscle tissue should be sutured to the corresponding positions on the prosthesis as much as possible, and attention should be paid to the muscle tension after suturing.

For the position and selection of prosthesis for artificial shoulder arthroplasty, the humeral prosthesis should be slightly higher than the level of the greater tubercle, so that there will be a certain clearance between the rotator cuff and the acromion, avoiding the collision between the acromion and the greater tubercle of the humerus in the initial stage of upper arm abduction. The humeral head should be appropriately sized to avoid postoperative deltoid laxity, difficulty in lifting of the patient's arm, and subluxation of the joint prosthesis. The use of a thick-padded glenoid prosthesis as well as a large-diameter humeral head will increase the traction force of the subscapularis and predisposes to postoperative soft tissue damage in anterior part of the joint as well as anterior dislocation of the joint prosthesis.

9.5.5.4 Reverse Shoulder Arthroplasty and Functional Substitution of Rotator Cuff

Reverse shoulder arthroplasty is defined as an artificial total shoulder arthroplasty in which the spherical articular surface of a shoulder prosthesis is placed on the glenoidal side of the scapula, while the glenoid cup is placed in the proximal humerus. At present, the reverse shoulder prosthesis widely used in clinical practice is designed by Paul Grammont, a French physician, and is a semi-constrained artificial joint prosthesis. Reverse shoulder arthroplasty is characterized by using the deltoid to functionally substitute the rotator cuff. The anterior bundle of the deltoid can anteriorly flex and slightly medially rotate the shoulder joint during contraction, abduct the shoulder joint synergistically with the supraspinatus during contraction of the middle bundle, and posteriorly extend and slightly laterally rotate the shoulder joint during contraction of the posterior bundle. The glenoidal-sided spherical prosthesis of the Grammont prosthesis is a collarless 1/3 sphere. The collarless design allows the spherical prosthesis to be in direct contact with the base and medialize the center of rotation, thereby decreasing the shear force at a prosthesis–bone interface and loosening of the glenoidal side of the prosthesis. Differing from the normal humeral collodiaphyseal angle, the collodiaphyseal angle of the reverse shoulder prosthesis is about 155°. By increasing the collodiaphyseal angle to shift the humeral shaft slightly downward, the tension of the deltoid is increased, such that the deltoid can functionally substitute the rotator cuff for shoulder elevation and abduction (Fig. 9.65).

9.5.5.5 Recovery of Rotator Cuff Functions After Artificial Shoulder Arthroplasty

The functional exercise program after shoulder arthroplasty is an important factor determining the efficacy of patients. Correct functional exercise can promote the recovery of rotator cuff functions and increase the range of motion of artificial joints. Basti proposed that postoperative rehabilitation and patient compliance are extremely important for the prognosis of artificial shoulder arthroplasty. Repair of the shoulder joint may be more challenging and more difficult than any other joint in the body. The activity of the glenohumeral joint depends on the peripheral soft tissues, including joint capsule, ligaments, rotator cuff, and deltoid. Postoperative functional rehabilitation protocols vary from person to person. The specific rehabilitation plan should be based on the stability of the prosthesis and the conditions of the rotator cuff and deltoid. Cahill established a target system for rehabilitation after artificial shoulder arthroplasty in 2014. It is divided into four stages. The first stage is postoperative 4 weeks, which is called conservative period. It mainly includes controlling soft tissue swelling and assisting the limb in passive lateral rotation, forward flexion, and other movements. Pendulum-like movements may be performed

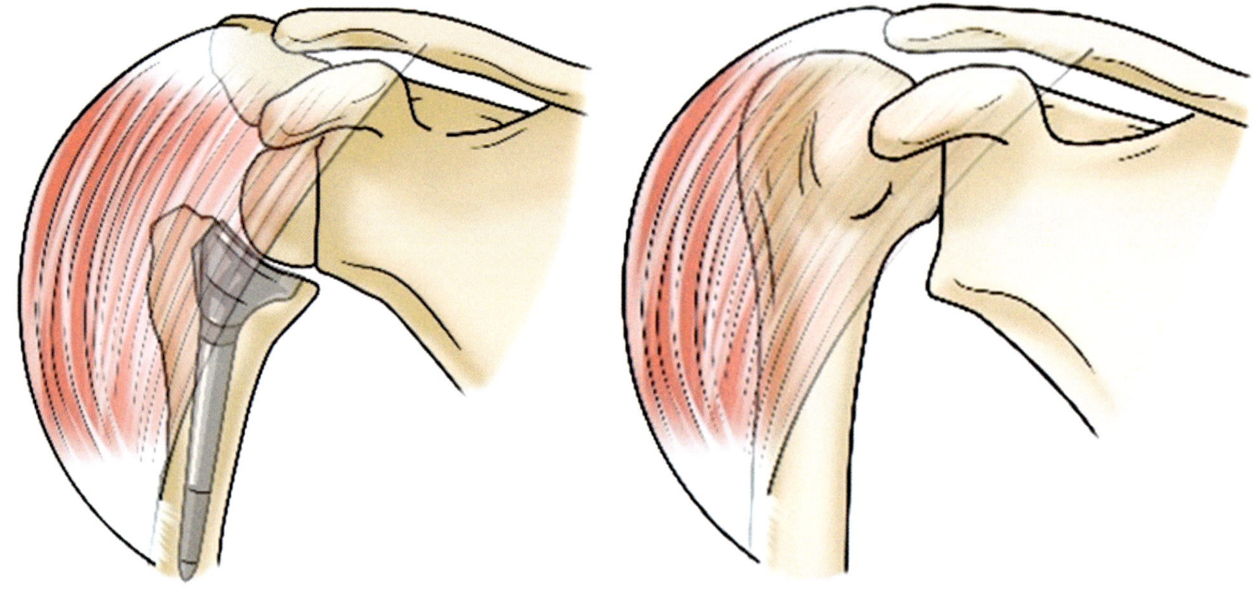

Fig. 9.65 Reverse shoulder arthroplasty and deltoid

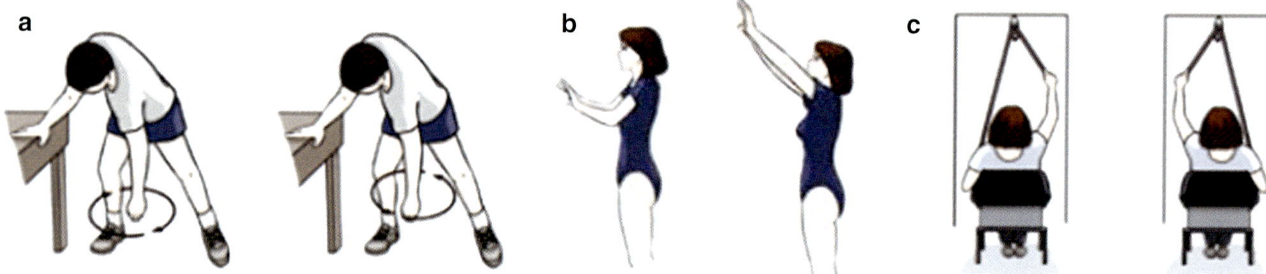

Fig. 9.66 Rotator cuff exercise. (**a**) Pendulum-like movements; (**b**) Standing reach movements; (**c**) Assisted joint movements

depending on the patient's condition. The range of joint motion can be gradually increased in the second and third stages. In the fourth stage, the strength and flexibility of the joint are increased (Fig. 9.66) [27].

9.6 Suture Techniques for Repair and Reconstruction of Injuries Around the Elbow Joint

9.6.1 Repair and Reconstruction of Ulnar Collateral Ligament Injuries of the Elbow Joint

Xing Danmou, Peng Zhengren, and Ren Dong

The ulnar collateral ligament plays an important role in the valgus stability of the elbow joint. When the elbow joint flexes between 20° and 120°, the main static restraint structure for valgus stress is the anterior bundle of the ligament. Callaway et al. confirmed in cadaveric models that when the anterior bundle of the ulnar collateral ligament is damaged, valgus instability will occur at either 30°, 60°, 90° or 120° of flexion. The instability will reach the highest at 90°of flexion. The radial head joint is a secondary static restraint structure. The flexor-pronator muscle group provides dynamic stability for the elbow valgus stress. Waris first described ulnar collateral ligament injury of the elbow joint in 1946. Few papers are published over the next 40 years. Until 1986, Jobe and his colleagues described the reconstruction of the ulnar collateral ligament for the first time.

Injuries of the ulnar collateral ligament can be caused by acute trauma (i.e., dislocation, terrible triad) or chronic injuries (i.e., overhead throwing of athletes). Acute injuries can be treated conservatively or by direct repair. For chronic injuries, reconstructions are more effective than repair due to pathological anatomical characteristics.

9.6.1.1 Direct Repair of Ulnar Collateral Ligament Ruptures of the Elbow Joint

The traumatic valgus instability caused by acute injury is related to two factors: (1) the avulsion of the ligament at the origin of the medial epicondyle of humerus, (2) the rupture of the superimposed part of the flexor-pronator muscle. The pathological anatomy is unique. It can be treated by direct repair of the ulnar collateral ligament and the flexor-pronator origin. Its main indication is acute traumatic valgus instability of the elbow joint. For valgus instability caused by acute trauma, valgus stress radiography (X-ray and MRI) can be conducted, which helps to confirm the avulsion of the ulnar collateral ligament from the medial epicondyle, and the pathological anatomy status (rupture and retraction) of the flexor-pronator muscle which is attached to the medial epicondyle (Figs. 9.67a, b and 9.68). Pathological findings can be confirmed by medical histories, imaging examinations, and intraoperative findings. The direct repair of the ulnar collateral ligament is suitable for patients who are physically young, active, without chronic injury, and hope to regain the valgus stability and mobility of the elbow joint. Contraindications for direct repair include original defects of the medial collateral ligament, in that condition the medial soft tissue is not suitable for direct repair. Relative contraindications are the concurrent presence of both posterolateral and varus instabilities, such as combined fractures of capitulum radii or ulna coracoid process. To rule out these injuries, imaging results should be carefully studied. In this case, it is recommended to focus on fractures and lateral ligaments. The repair of medial collateral ligament should be considered only if necessary.

1. *Surgical Technique*

The patient lies in supine position, lays the limb flat on the operating table. The pneumatic tourniquet is tied on the upper arm. After routine disinfection, a 12 cm long skin incision is made above the cubital tunnel and centered on the medial epicondyle (Fig. 9.69). Only sharp dissection is performed. The branches of the medial forearm cutaneous nerve are identified and preserved by blunt dissection. These nerve branches locate on the superficial surface of the fascia, perpendicular to the incision. Although there are often anatomical variations, two branches are the most commonly seen: one is from the proximal end to the medial epicondyle, and the other is from the distal end to the medial epicondyle. Two automatic retractors are placed to expose structures of the inside of the elbow joint. Muscles should be carefully examined. Rupture areas of superficial muscles and distal retraction condition of the flexor-pronator teres are exposed (Fig. 9.70). Injuries usually involve the first 2/3 parts of the muscles. It is not rare to find hematoma in the cubital tunnel.

The bottom of the cubital tunnel is the posterior bundle of the ulnar collateral ligament. Therefore, the ulnar collateral ligament, which locates beneath the ulnar never, can be better exposed by moving the nerve. Anterior transposition of the ulnar nerve should be routinely performed. The ulnar nerve can be easily distinguished in the proximal end of the cubital tunnel and behind the medial intermuscular septum. If it cannot be seen directly, you can touch its cord-like structure in the proximal end of the medial epicondyle in a forward and backward direction

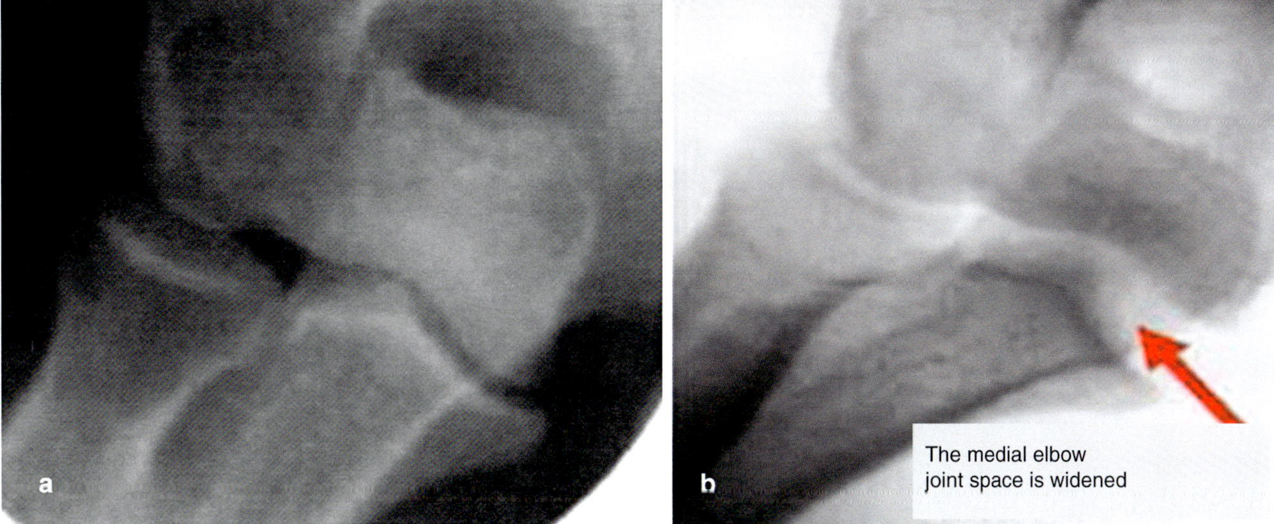

Fig. 9.67 Valgus stress radiograph of the elbow joint. (**a**) The preoperative elbow joint on the anterior-posterior film, valgus stress test not conducted. (**b**) The medial joint space is widened under the valgus stress test, confirmed by the anterior-posterior film

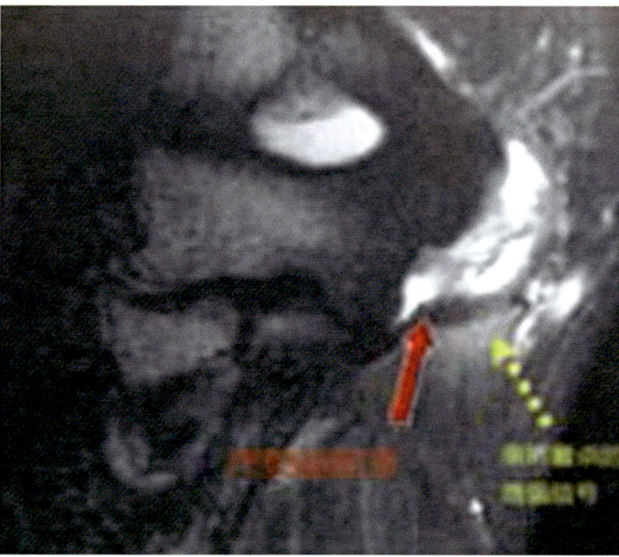

Fig. 9.68 T2-weighted fat suppression image of the elbow joint MRI. The ulnar collateral ligament is avulsed from the medial epicondyle origin. The flexor-pronator muscle is also avulsed and retracted distally. There are increased signals at the original attachment points

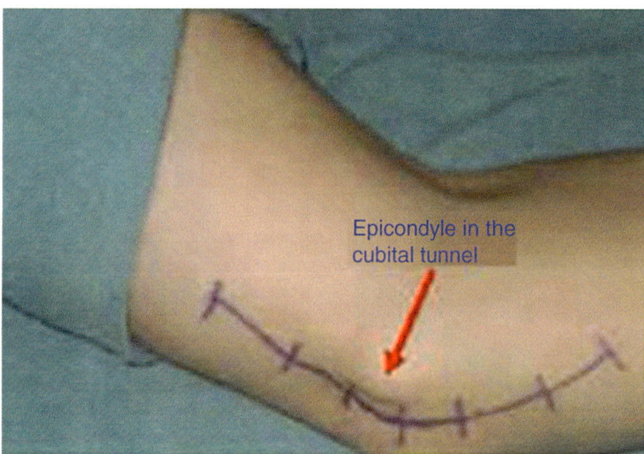

Fig. 9.69 The incision is in the center of the medial cubital tunnel. The distal end of the incision is slightly forward in an arc. Determine the anatomic landmarks of the medial epicondyle of the humerus and the olecranon of the ulna

with your fingers. When exposing the proximal end of the ulnar nerve, in order to reduce the damage caused by the retraction of the nerve, surgical clamps should not be used. A rubber ring can be used to pull and preserve the nerve. Loosen the Osborne ligament, and remove the distal end of the ulnar nerve from the cubital canal. The dissection begins from the distal end of the fascia layer above the flexor muscles, until the nerve is seen to enter deep into the both heads of the muscle. Gently pull the ulnar nerve, and check the ulnar collateral ligament. It is often avulsed from the exposed medial epicondyle in the form of a sleeve (Fig. 9.71a, b, c).Usually, due to the injuries of the flexor-pronator muscle, the ulnar collateral ligament can be better exposed without further dissection. Sometimes, the ulnar collateral ligament is found embedded in the ulnohumeral joint. In order to check internal injuries of the joint, the ulnar collateral ligament can be pulled aside. At this time, the ulnar collateral ligament is ready to be attached to the medial epicondyle of the humerus.

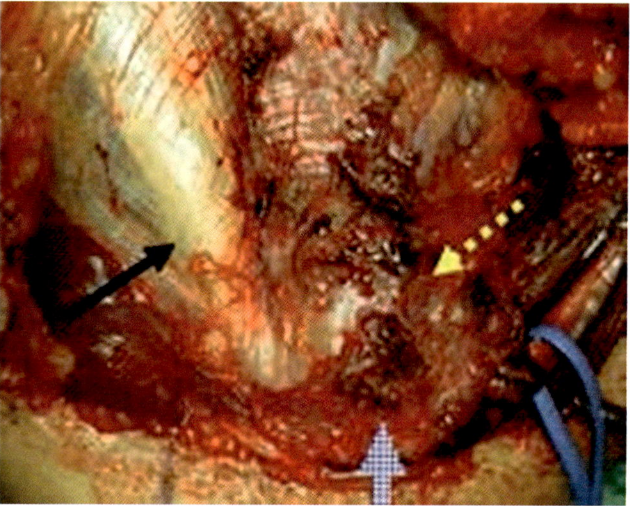

Fig. 9.70 The whole skin flap is lifted. The flexor-pronator muscle of the medial epicondyle is damaged. The black arrow shows the undamaged part of the flexor-pronator muscle, and the yellow arrow shows the ruptured part of the flexor-pronator muscle

(1) Continuous locking suture: Repair the ligament with two Non-Absorbable 2# ETHIBOND® Suture (Polyester, Ethicon Inc.) (Fig. 9.72). A transverse suture should be placed as far as possible into the anterior bundle of the ulnar collateral ligament and inserted close to the sublime tubercle of the ulna. After confirming that the two strands are equally long, the suture passes through the ulnar collateral ligament from distal to proximal along the edge of the ligament, with a parallel and continuous locking manner. The key of the suture is to make sure the sutures are not slacked. Only in that condition, the repaired area will not loosen, and be firmly fixed on the bone bridge. At last, each suture must pass through the proximal end of the ligament, so that one suture is in front of the ligament and the other one is behind it. Prepare the bone tunnel with a 2.0 mm drill bit. First, under the inner epicondyle, create a repair entrance at the attachment point of original ligament. The drill hole should be placed as deep as possible into the medial epicondyle and as close as possible to its junction with the inner wall of the trochlea. A drill cover should be used each time, so as to reduce the risk of ulnar nerve injury. In order to form a bone bridge on

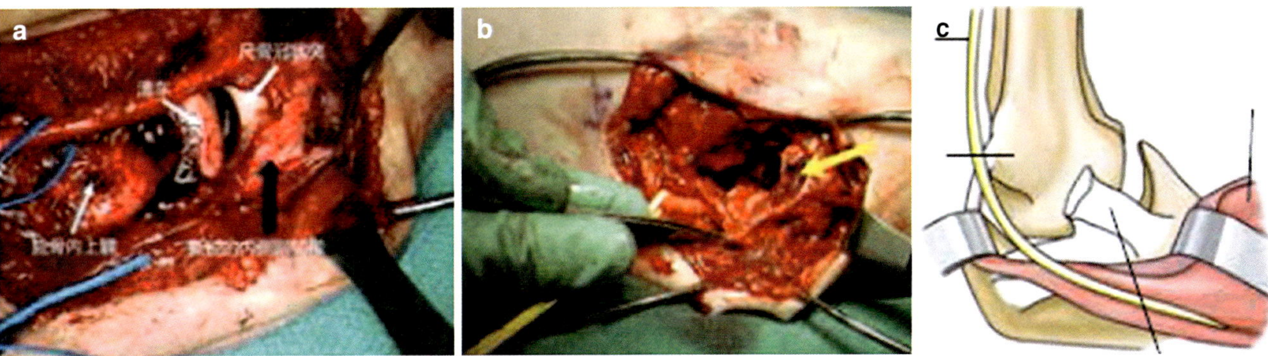

Fig. 9.71 Surgical method. (**a**) During the operation, it is found that the medial epicondyle of the left elbow joint is exposed, and the ulnar collateral ligament and flexor-pronator muscle are avulsed. Deep injuries of the ulnohumeral joint could be seen. The ulnar nerve (in the rubber ring) moved forward; (**b**) It is easy to identify the avulsed ulnar collateral ligament held by forceps. Note that it may be embedded in the ulnohumeral joint. The avulsed and contracted flexor-pronator muscles can result in the valgus instability of the elbow. (**c**) The avulsed ulnar collateral ligament injury results in its avulsion from the proximal origin. The flexor-pronator muscle group is also avulsed from its humerus origin and retracted distally

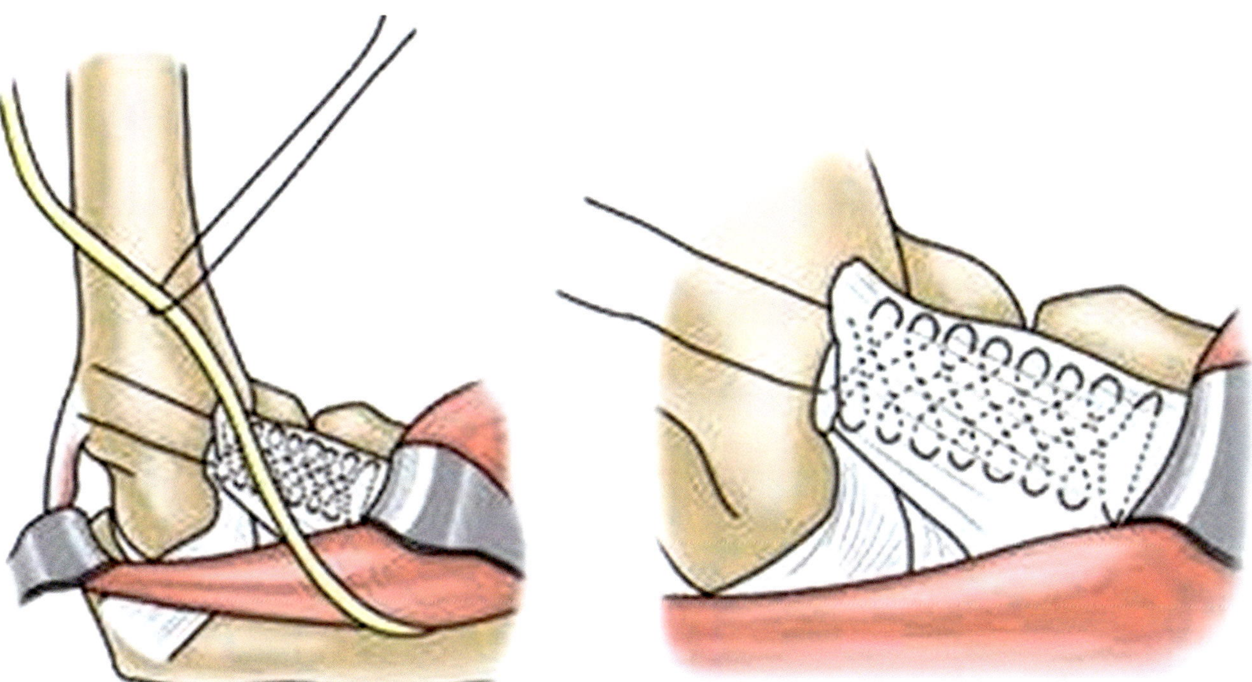

Fig. 9.72 Repair the ulnar collateral ligament with Non-Absorbable 2# ETHIBOND® Suture (Polyester, Ethicon Inc.). The horizontal suture is at the distal side of the ligament, near the insertion. The two strands are of equal length. The suture goes forward to the proximal end in a continuous locking manner, until the origin of the ligament

which sutures can be knotted, both the two tunnels should be drilled proximally through the same entrance. One tunnel leads to the supracondylar ridge to form an anterior exit, and the other one is to form a posterior exit. To avoid fractures during the fixation, the width of the bone bridge should be 2 cm. The anterior and posterior strands pass through their own bone tunnels, respectively. The position of the elbow and forearm is very important to reconstruct the tension of the ulnar collateral ligament. As it is an anatomical repair of original tissues, problems associated with repair techniques will be minimal (Fig. 9.73a–e). When constructing a bone tunnel, a relatively small drill bit is selected to avoid bringing the ulnar collateral ligament into the tunnel. We placed the elbow joint in about 70° flexion and supinator position of the forearm, with a bit varus stress at the elbow joint during the suture. Once the ulnar collateral ligament

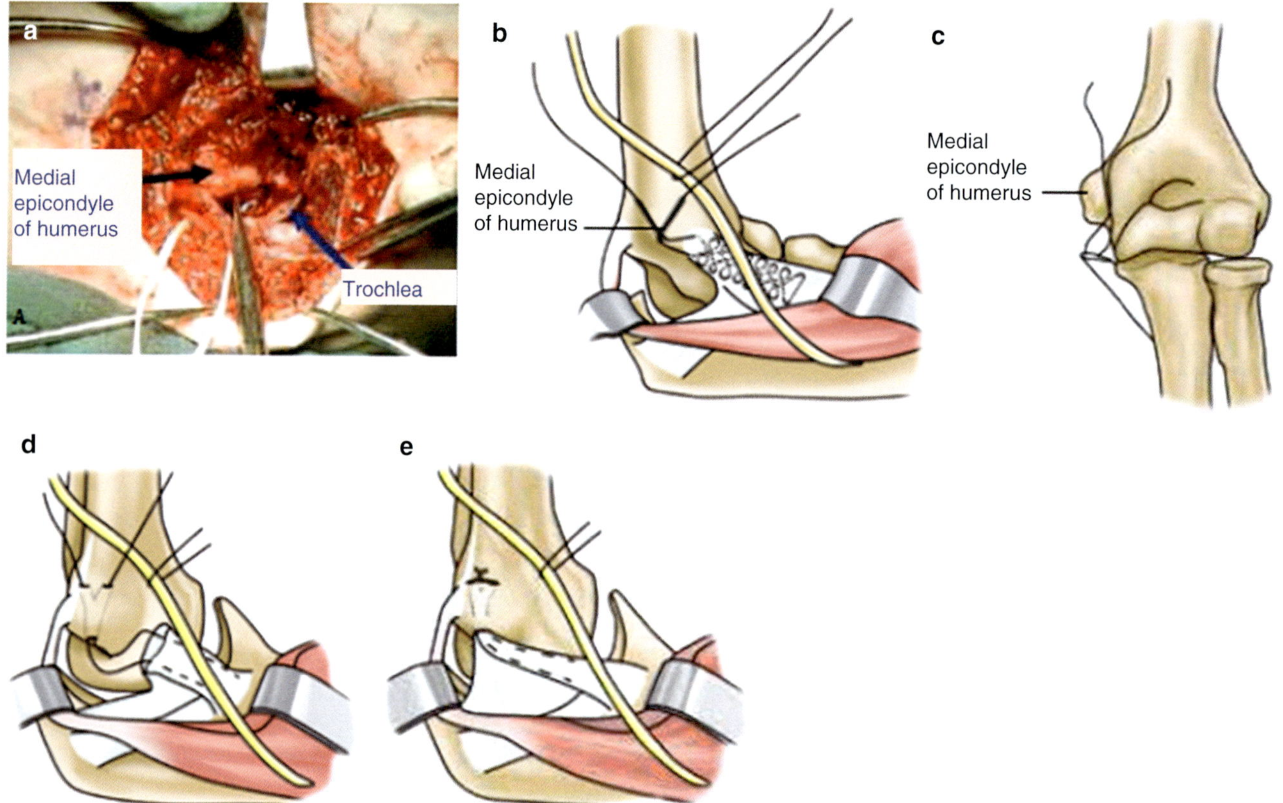

Fig. 9.73 Continuous locking suture technique. (**a**) The scissors are pointing to the entry point of the repair. It is the anatomical starting point of the ulnar collateral ligament. The lower part of the medial epicondyle is connected with the internal wall of the trochlea; (**b**) Schematic diagram; (**c**) The entry point of the medial epicondyle of humerus depicted in the coronal plane; (**d**) Surgical repair uses 2# double-strand non-absorbable suture. It passes through the ulnar collateral ligament in a continuous locking manner. Then the two strands pass through their corresponding bone tunnels, which drilled in the anterior and posterior side of the medial epicondyle, respectively; (**e**) After passing through the bone tunnels, the two strands are knotted on the bone bridge formed between the tunnels. Keep the elbow joint in the state of mild varus and flexion when knotting

is sutured safely, the flexor-pronator muscle can be repaired with figure-of-8 suturing technique (Fig. 9.74).

Finally, evaluate whether anterior transposition of the ulnar nerve should be performed. If there are any problems in the cubital tunnel that can cause instability, or if there are such stimulating factors as suture knots in the repair site, anterior transposition of the ulnar nerve should be performed. Usually a subfascial technique is used; attention should be paid to loosening the arched structure and removing part of the medial intermuscular septum, so as to avoid compression of the ulnar nerve. Lift the anterior and posterior fascia flaps from the flexor-pronator muscle. The anterior fascial flap is based on the distal end, and the posterior fascial flap is based on the proximal

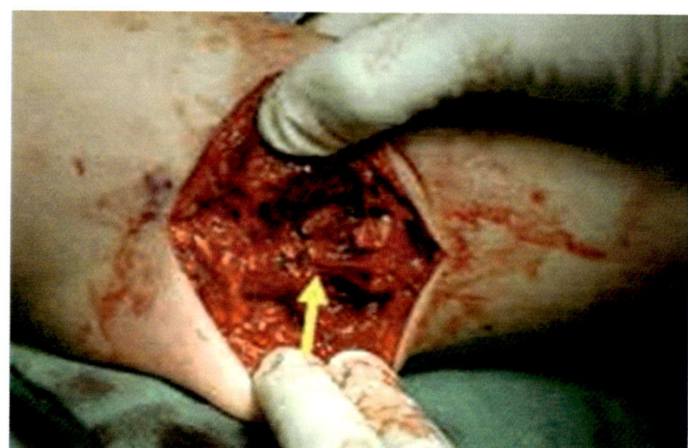

Fig. 9.74 Knot the suture on the bone bridge while keeping the elbow joint slightly varus and in 70° flexion. The yellow arrow points to the repaired ulnar collateral ligament

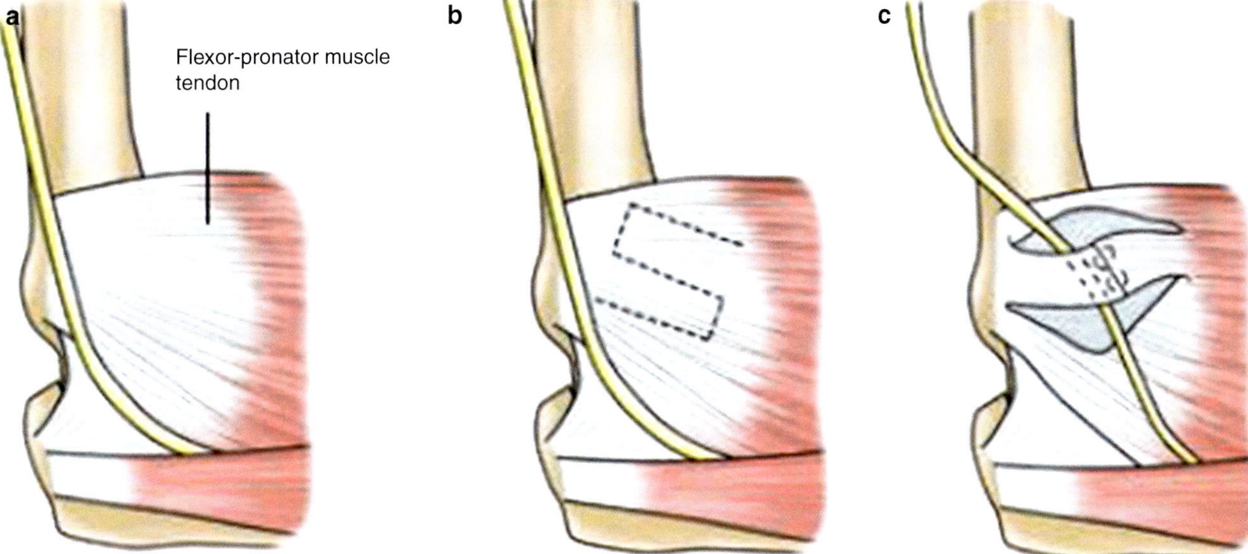

Fig. 9.75 Operation schematic diagram. (**a**) The fascia covering the common origin of flexor-pronator muscles is determined by lifting the anterior full-thickness skin flap; (**b**) The anterior and posterior fascia flaps that are lifted are in the same direction as the muscle fibers. The anterior flap is based on the distal end, and the posterior flap is based on the proximal end; (**c**) The fascia flap is placed above the ulnar nerve and fixed with 2-0 absorbable sutures. Then fully flex and extend the elbow joint to ensure that the ulnar nerve can slide properly

end. The formed fascial flap should have enough length, so as to avoid compression of the ulnar nerve when suturing with 2-0 absorbable sutures (Fig. 9.75a, b, and c). After anterior transposition of the ulnar nerve is performed (Fig. 9.76), the elbow joint can be flexed and extended to confirm that the nerve can slide without compression. Loosen the tourniquet to obtain abundant blood flow at the surgical site. Hemostasis is carefully performed by using a bipolar electrocoagulator. The subcutaneous layer of the incision is discontinuously sutured with absorbable sutures, and then the skin is sutured with nylon sutures.

(2) Anchor locking suture: For avulsion injuries of the ulnar collateral ligament, the anchor locking suture can be used. The avulsed tissues can be directly sutured with the sutures attached to the anchor. The most important step of the successful repair is to place the anchor on the coaxial point of the elbow joint rotation center, that is, the central point of the medial epicondyle. Then overlap the avulsed ulnar collateral ligament and flexor-pronator muscle on the trauma plane by 5 mm, and use 4 sutures of the anchor to pass through the deep surface of ruptured tissues. The two strands are knotted on the surface of the tissue to make the ruptured ulnar collateral ligament and flexor-pronator muscle tightly attached to the original origin (Fig. 9.77a–f).

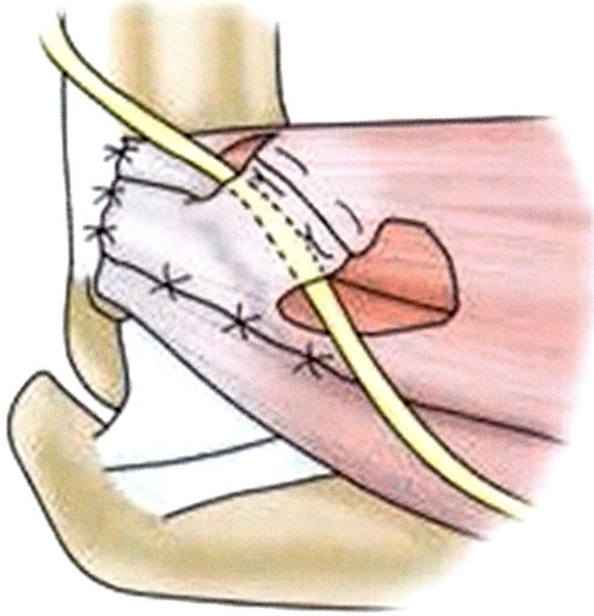

Fig. 9.76 The flexor-pronator muscle group is repaired by using irregular figure-of-8 stitching, and anterior transposition of the ulnar nerve is performed by using fascia strip

2. *Postoperative Treatment*

Fix the elbow joint with a well-padded splint when the elbow joint is in 90° flexion and the forearm is in the neutral position. At the first follow-up, the sutures are

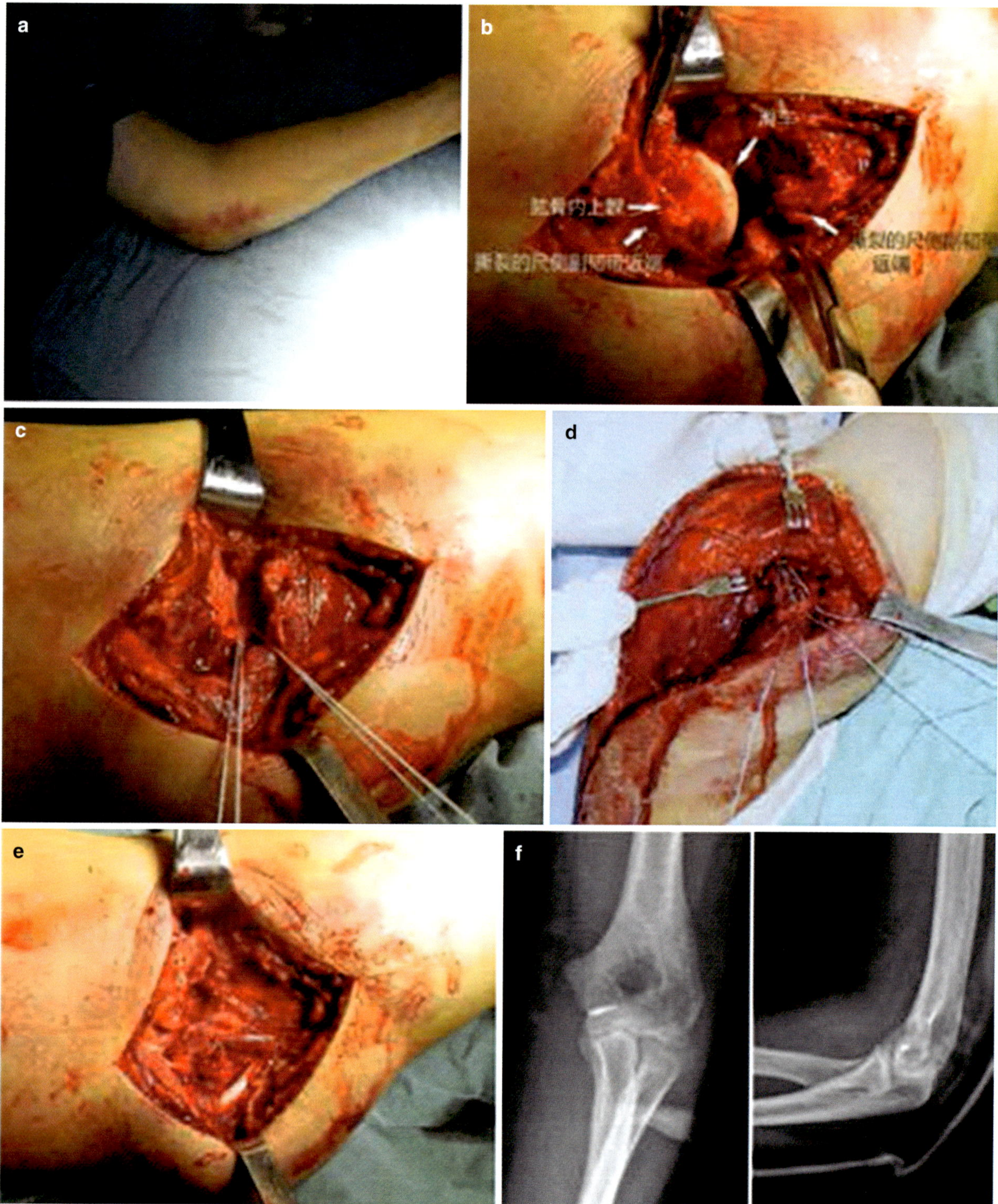

Fig. 9.77 Anchor locking suture. (**a**) The left elbow joint is dislocated with subcutaneous bruise and valgus instability; (**b**) The ulnar collateral ligament and flexor-pronator muscle are avulsed from the medial epicondyle of humerus. (The thin white arrow points to the medial epicondyle of humerus. The thick white arrow points to the proximal end of the ruptured ulnar collateral ligament. In the gray arrows, the thin one points to the trochlea of humerus, and the thick one points to the stump of proximal flexor-pronator muscle); (**c**) Insert anchoring sutures in the central point of the medial epicondyle, in the direction of the elbow joint rotation axis; (**d**) The four sutures on the anchor pass through the deep surface of ruptured tissues. The two respective strands are knotted on the surface of the tissue to make the ruptured ulnar collateral ligament and flexor-pronator muscle tightly attached to the origin; (**e**) After repair of the ulnar collateral ligament and the origin of the flexor-pronator muscle of the elbow joint; (**f**) Postoperative elbow joint X-ray (anteroposterior and lateral positions) shows that the normal anatomy is restored

removed, and a hinged elbow orthosis is used. Keep the elbow in 90° flexion and the forearm in a neutral position until the third week after surgery. At the third week after surgery, the orthosis is unlocked, and protected elbow exercise is encouraged. At the sixth week after surgery, the orthosis is removed, and the patients begin to strengthen the forearm rotation function gradually. Strengthening exercise of the flexor-pronator muscle should be postponed until the forearm rotation can be performed perfectly. During the 12-week exercise, not only the elbow joint is exercised, the flexibility and strength of the shoulders should be paid attention to avoid shoulder stiffness. After the full range of motion of the elbow joint is restored, the flexor-pronator muscle is strengthened, and no pain occurs under valgus stress are confirmed through clinical examination, the overhead exercises can be allowed. The average time allowing overhead exercises is the 19th week (18~22 weeks).

9.6.1.2 Reconstruction of Ulnar Collateral Ligament Old Injuries of the Elbow Joint

Old injuries of the ulnar collateral ligament of the elbow joint are serious injuries that can affect the joint stability and cause pain. They are most common in athletes who exercise overhead throwing and can also occur after treatment of dislocation and terrible triad of the elbow. Pain and instability of the elbow may result in the loss of normal function and decreased athletic performance. Such injuries were initially treated with non-surgical methods with suboptimal results. It would threaten the athletes' careers and affect the lives and work of patients. A large number of studies have shown that for patients with old injuries in the ulnar collateral ligament, the prognosis will improve after reconstruction.

The diagnosis of old injuries of the ulnar collateral ligament is based on clinical signs and imaging. It is often associated with occupation or major trauma history. The main signs are postural pain and fear. Its onset is gradual. It is usually manifested as pain on the medial elbow when overhead throwing or planking. The physical examination mainly includes mobility and valgus stress test.

During the examination, when the elbow is valgus unstable, the patient can sit, fix the hands and wrists under the examiner's axilla, flex the elbow over 25°, and palpate the ulnar collateral ligament under valgus stress (Fig. 9.78).The following signs in the test indicate the presence of valgus instability of the elbow joint (old injuries of the ulnar collateral ligament): local pain and/or tenderness; fricative on medial ulnohumeral joint, humeroradial joint, the inner posterior part of olecranon-humerus; arthrochalasis of the elbow joint.

Anteroposterior and axial radiographs of the elbow joints should be performed to evaluate the joint space stenosis, osteophytes, loose bodies, and calcification of the ulnar collateral ligament. Valgus stress film can be used to measure the opening of medial joint space. The opening length >3 mm indicates valgus instability, compared with the application of stress. For chronic injuries, traditional MRI can identify the thickening of ligaments and some obvious full-thickness tears. MRI arthrography is recommended to diagnose partial tears inferior to the ulnar collateral ligament (Fig. 9.79).

If the goals are joint stabilization and pain relief, non-surgical treatment usually meets the requirements. However,

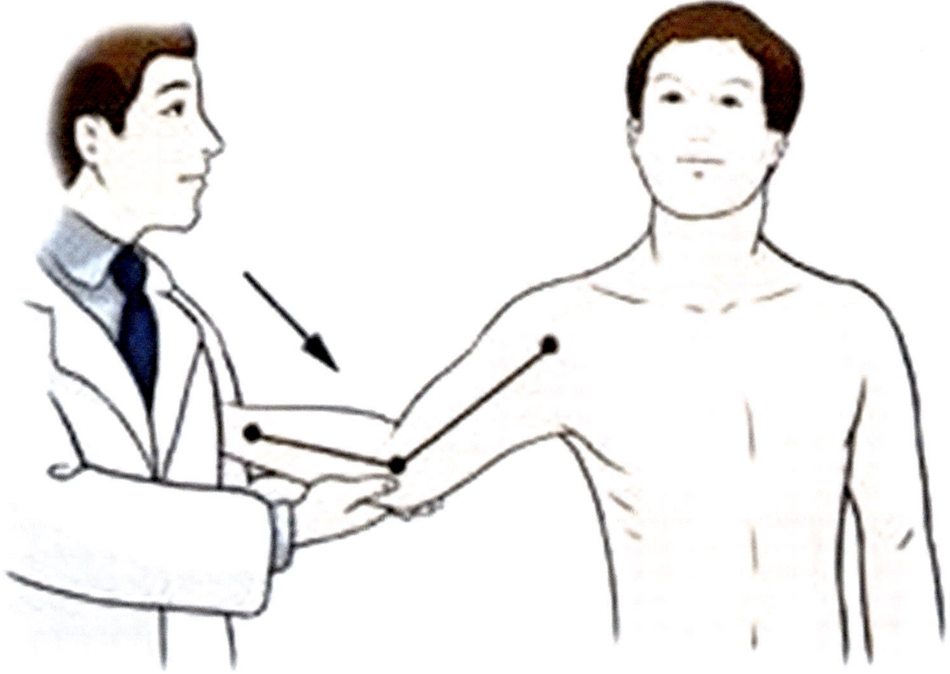

Fig. 9.78 Valgus stress test. Continuous pain and tenderness in the ulnar ligament of the elbow

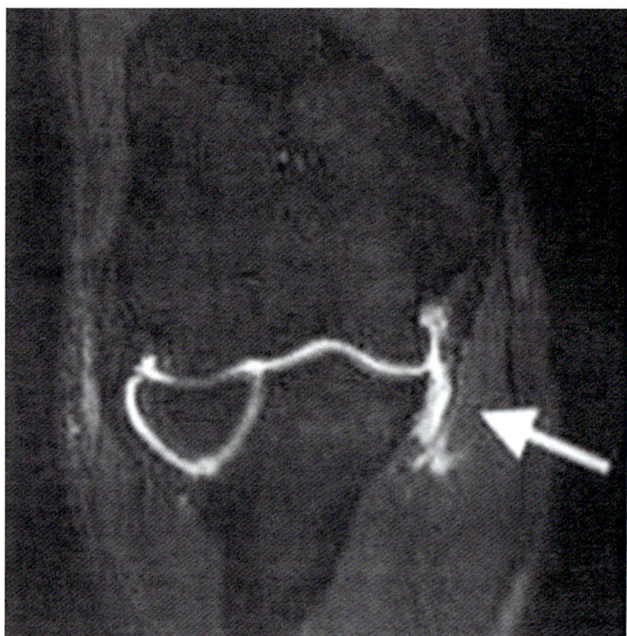

Fig. 9.79 MRI shows continuity interruption and fluid extravasation of ulnar collateral ligament

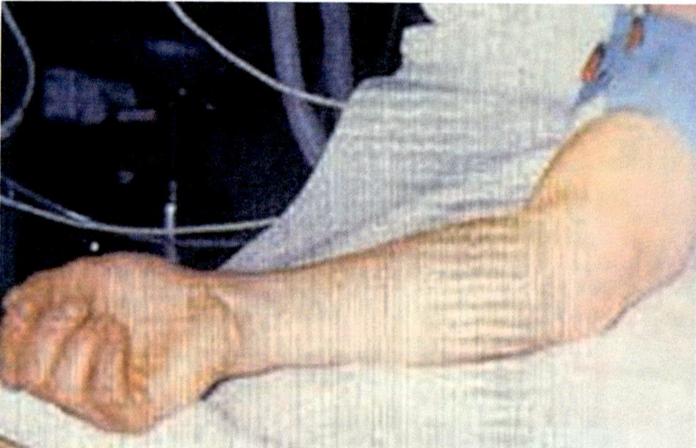

Fig. 9.80 The forearm is placed on the plate, and the shoulder joint is externally rotated to reveal the inner side of the elbow

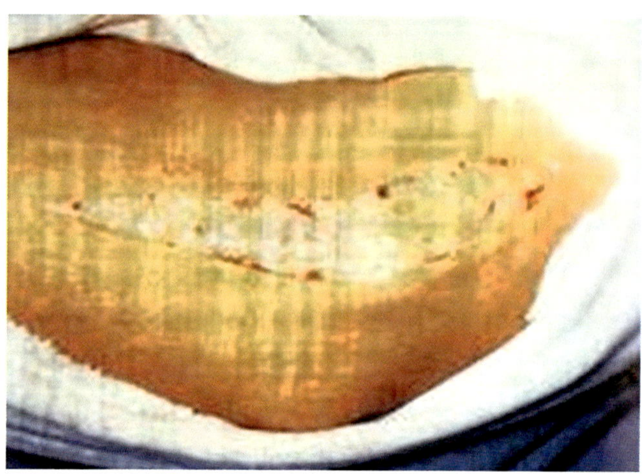

Fig. 9.81 The incision is at the front edge of the distal end of the medial epicondyle, 8~10 cm in length, centered on the medial epicondyle

if the patient needs to restore overhead or throwing exercise and the non-surgical treatment fails, then surgery should be performed.

1. Surgical techniques

   Since Jobe first described the reconstruction of the ulnar collateral ligament of the elbow in 1986, there have been a number of modified reconstruction surgeries for better functional outcomes.

   The operation is performed under general anesthesia or brachial plexus anesthesia. The pneumatic tourniquet is tied on the upper arm. The forearm lies on the forearm operating table in abduction position (Fig. 9.80). The operation uses the medial elbow approach (Fig. 9.81). Protect the ulnar nerve and the branches of cutaneous sensory nerve carefully (Fig. 9.82a, b). The fascia is incised along the fibers. The submuscular approach is adopted. The interspace of flexor carpi ulnaris, which is considered to be the ulnar fascia interspace of the flexor-pronator muscle group, is firstly incised. Separate the muscle group bluntly along the longitudinal direction of muscle fibers. Retractors are placed on the distal, ulnar, and radial sides, respectively, so as to expose the anterior bundle of the ulnar collateral ligament at the base of the medial epicondyle of humerus (Fig. 9.83a, b). Identify the ulnar nerve at the posterior edge of the ulnar collateral ligament and protect it. Sterile dressings are bound on the lateral condyle, so as to facilitate the application of valgus stress. When the ulnohumeral joint is open, confirm the affected ligament tissues, including avulse on the ulnar and humeral side, and medial parenchymal injuries. If there are calcifications or/and osteophytes in local soft tissues and ligaments, they should be removed (Fig. 9.84a, b).

   (1) Jobe surgical technique: Carefully separate the ulnar nerve from the sulcus for ulnar nerve. Place it above the medial epicondyle. Use a 6.4 mm Penrose drainage tube to retract and protect it. A portion of the proximal muscle septum is removed to avoid impaction and compression of the ulnar nerve when it is subject to anterior transposition. Special care must be taken to protect the motor branches of the ulnar nerve.

   Use a low-speed drill to form bone tunnels. Drill a 3.4 mm diameter bone tunnel at the medial epicondyle of humerus and the sublime tubercle of the ulna coracoid process, that is, the corresponding attachments of the residual ligament, under the protection of the drill cover (Fig. 9.85a). These drilled sites

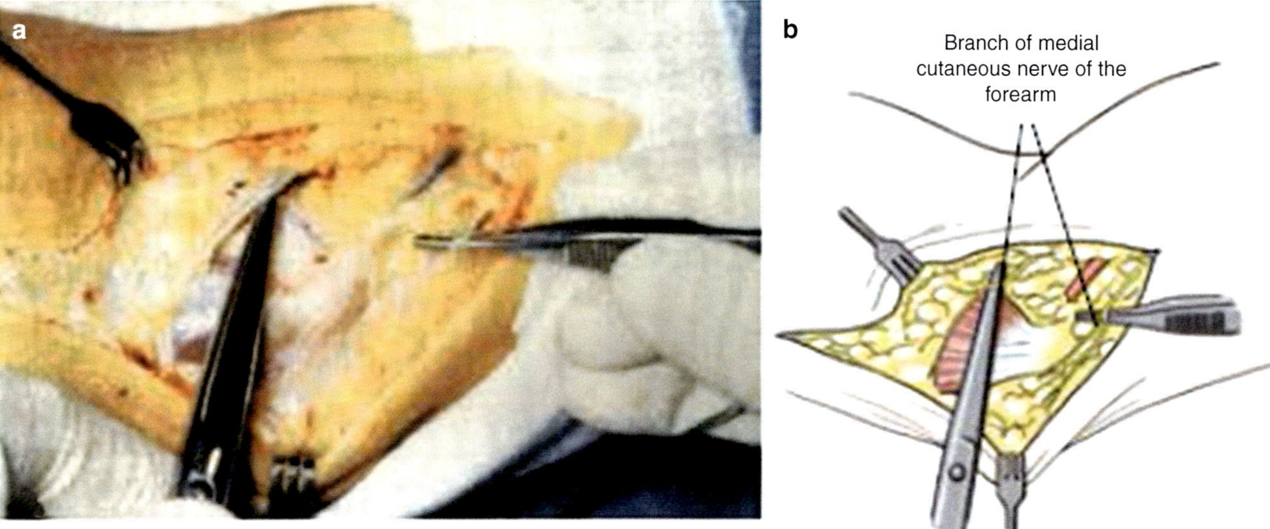

Fig. 9.82 Operation schematic diagram. (**a**, **b**) Identify the medial cutaneous nerve of the forearm. Protect it when it passes through the surgical field. Below the nerve is the common tendon of the flexor-pronator group. Note: The variation of this nerve branch, but it is usually located at the anterior and distal end of the medial condyle

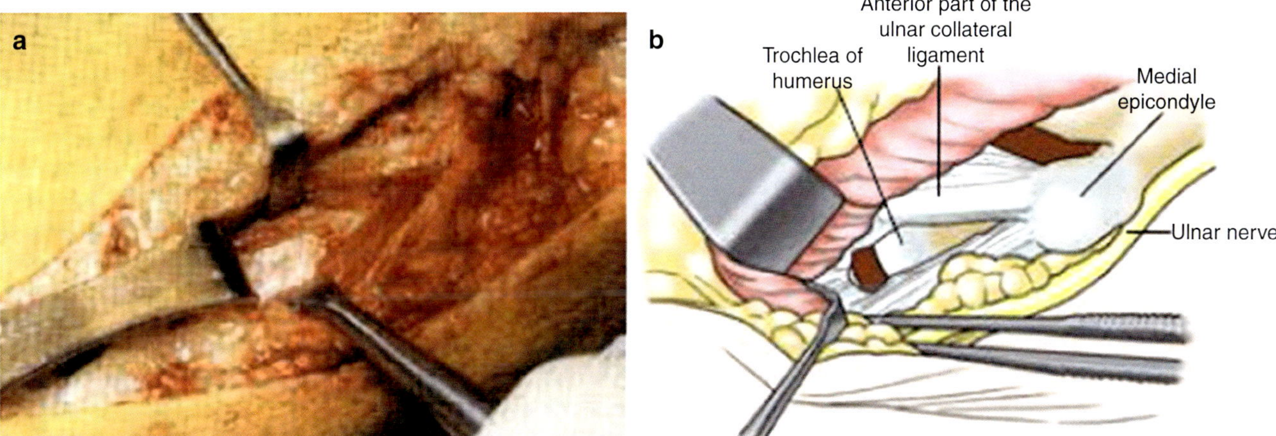

Fig. 9.83 Expose the ulnar collateral ligament. (**a**, **b**) Separate bluntly and retract the muscle group along the longitudinal direction of muscle fibers. Expose the damaged anterior bundle of the ulnar collateral ligament at the base of the medial epicondyle of humerus

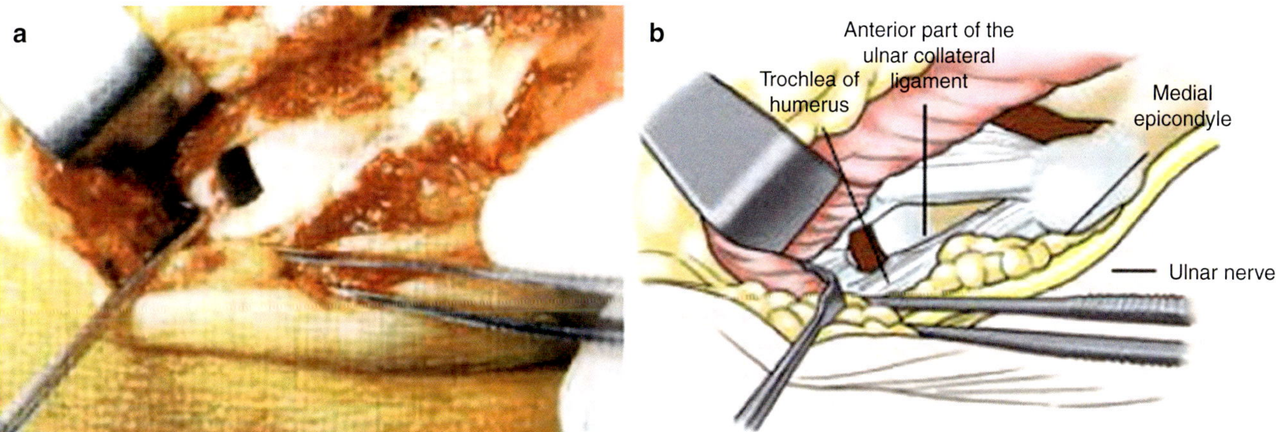

Fig. 9.84 (**a**, **b**) Dissect the ulnar collateral ligament. Open the medial side of the ulnohumeral joint under valgus stress

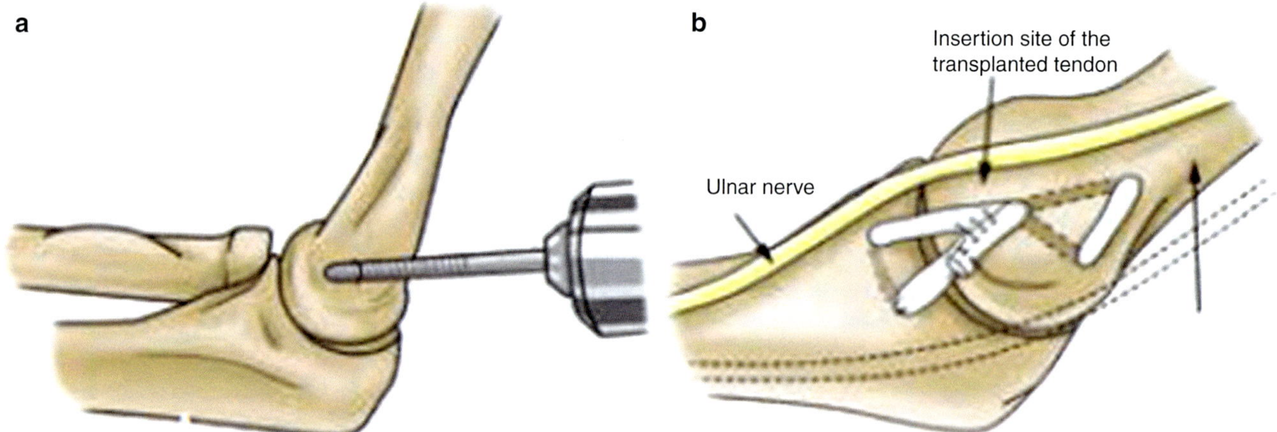

Fig. 9.85 Reconstruction of the ulnar collateral ligament of the elbow joint (Jobe operation). (**a**) Drill a bone tunnel at the sublime tubercle of the ulna coracoid process and the medial epicondyle of humerus, respectively, for the introduction of the transplanted tendon; (**b**) Pass the transplanted tendon through the bone tunnel in a figure-of-8 shape. Anterior transposition of the ulnar nerve

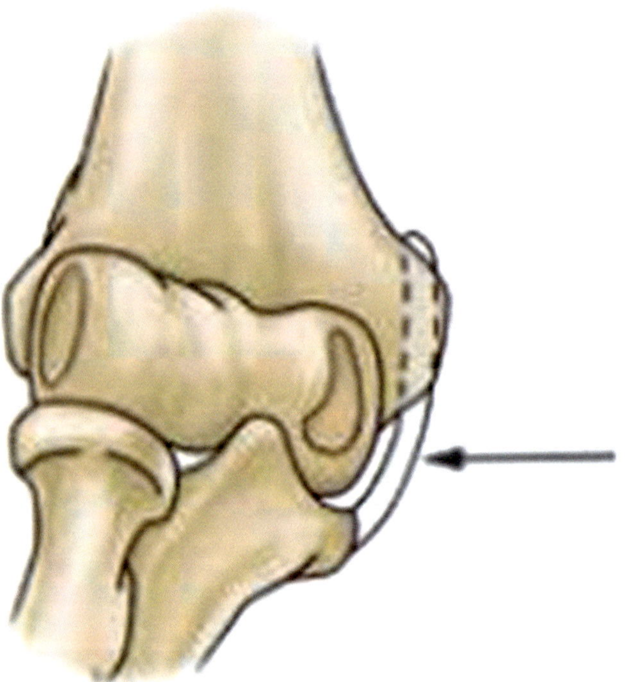

Fig. 9.86 Front view of the transplant site. The arrow points to the insertion site of the transplanted tendon. This prevents the tendon from rubbing against the humerus and ulna ridges

allow the transplanted tendon to be inserted without friction with either the medial epicondyle of humerus or the sublime tubercle of the ulna coracoid process (Fig. 9.86). To reconstruct the lacking part of the ulnar collateral ligament, a transplanted tendon should be used. The donor sites for the transplanted tendon are mostly from the palmaris longus muscle, followed by the plantaris muscle. If both of them are absent, the Achilles tendon (3 mm in width, 15 cm in length) can also be used.

Pass the obtained tendon through the bone tunnel in a figure-of-8 shape (Fig. 9.85b). Let it function as the anterior bundle of the ulnar collateral ligament. The transplanted tendon should be tightened and sutured with itself. Any residual ligament tissue should be sewn over the transplanted tendon, so as to increase the tensile strength of the reconstructed ligament. Displace the ulnar nerve to the front of the medial epicondyle of humerus (Fig. 9.85b), then cover it with the flexor-pronator muscle (this helps to keep the nerve in this anterior position). Re-suture the flexor-pronator muscle with the residual tendinous tissues on medial epicondyle of humerus. After surgery, the elbow joint is fixed at 90° flexion with a postpositional splint, and the wrist joint can move freely. The upper arm does not require additional support because of the inherent stability of the elbow joint.

(2) Modified Jobe operation: Since only two transplanted tendons are used to cross the ulnohumeral joint in the Jobe operation, the strength of the reconstructed ulnar collateral ligament is insufficient. In order to increase the strength of the reconstructed ligament, many modified operations have been developed. The focuses of these modified operations are on the formation of the bone tunnel in the medial epicondyle of humerus, and strand number of the transplanted tendons that cross the medial side of the ulnohumeral joint.

The strand number of the transplanted tendons that cross the medial side of the ulnohumeral joint is three. The construction of the bone tunnel is shown in Fig. 9.87. The ulnar nerve should be carefully protected throughout the ulnar tunnel drilling. Choose a 3.2 mm or 3.5 mm drill bit according to the size of the transplanted tendon. Under the protection of the drill cover, drill a bone tunnel at the sublime tubercle of the ulna coracoid process along the anterior and posterior directions. The distance between the tunnel entrance is 5 mm. The bone bridge formed between the two tunnels is 2~4 mm from the articular surface. The risk of ulnar nerve damage is extremely high when the tunnel is drilled posteriorly. Therefore, a protective hook should be placed between the drill bit and the ulnar nerve. Use an angled curette to scrape through the medullary cavity, and remove sharp corners. If a larger size graft such as the gracilis is used, select a 3.5 mm drill bit and implant the looped suture into the tunnel for future use.

Drill on the medial epicondyle of humerus using a 4.5 mm drill bit with cannula. The locating point is at the anatomical insertion of the anterior bundle of the ulnar collateral ligament. Be careful not to penetrate the posterior cortex. If the transplanted tendon of a larger size is used, a 5.0 mm drill bit

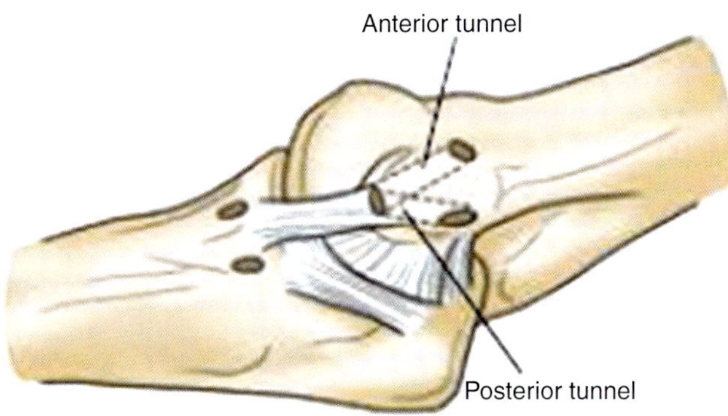

Fig. 9.87 Drill a hole at the base of the medial epicondyle as the entrance for the transplanted tendon. Pass the tendon through the anterior and posterior parts of the medial epicondyle to form a "Y"-shaped tunnel. The ulna drill hole is located at the plane of the coronal tubercle. The two holes are 1 cm apart

is used. Incise the fascia above the medial condyle to expose the front of the medial epicondyle. Use a 3.2 mm drill to drill a hole in front of the attachment of the medial septum to connect it to the previous 4.5 mm tunnel. Note that a bone bridge of sufficient width should be reserved to accommodate the posterior tunnel (Fig. 9.87). Protect the ulnar nerve, and expose the posterior attachment of the muscle septum. Drill the second 3.2 mm tunnel 1 cm away from the first one, and connect the two tunnels. Use an angle curette to link the three tunnels, and smooth the tunnel walls. To facilitate the passage of the graft, implant the looped suture into the proximal tunnel (Fig. 9.88).

The tendon of the ipsilateral palmar longus is then incised (Fig. 9.89). At the distal end of the wrist crease, a 5~10 mm long transverse incision is made at the most obvious site of the palmar longus tendon. Identify the palmar longus tendon, separate it from underlying tissues, and clamp it with small forceps. Make two same additional transverse incisions at 7.5 cm and 15 cm of the distal wrist to separate and expose the full tendon. Then dissect the palmar longus tendon from distal to proximal. After the incision, perform continuous locking suture with 1# non-absorbable sutures at both ends of the tendon. The ipsilateral lower limb should be routinely prepared before surgery in cases of the absence of the palmar longus tendon, which may affect the reconstruction surgery.

Pull the transplanted tendon into the proximal ulna bone tunnel from proximal to distal, and then cross through the bone tunnel in the medial epicondyle of humerus in a figure-of-8 shape (Fig. 9.90a, b). Tighten the transplanted tendon in the state of 40°~60° flexion, varus of the elbow joint and supination of the forearm. Suture the ulnar side of the tendon with the stump of the ulnar collateral ligament. The proximal end of the graft is sutured with the medial muscle septum. Flex and extend the elbow joint to adjust the isometricity of the reconstructed ligament, and then suture the cross part of

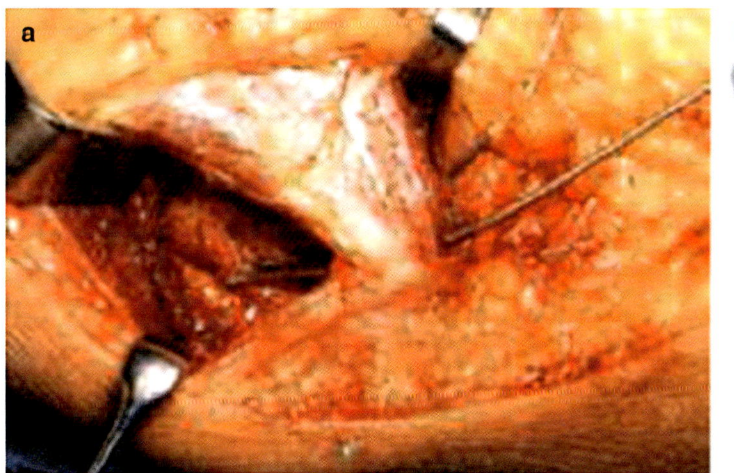

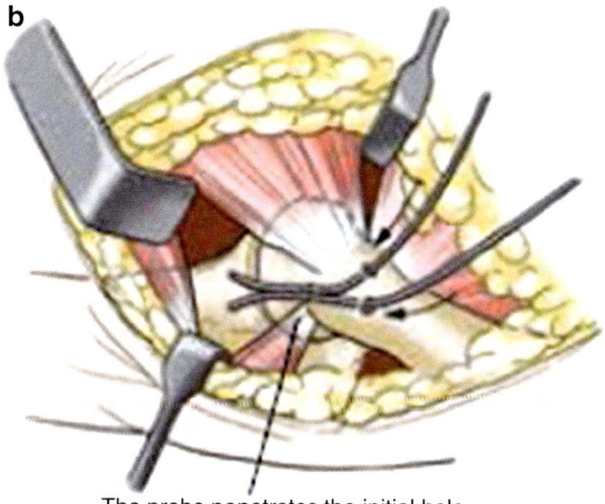

Fig. 9.88 (**a**, **b**) Drill the medial epicondyle of humerus from the anterior to the posterior muscular septum, then penetrate the hole with the probe

the transplanted tendon with 0# non-absorbable sutures. Repair the adjacent ligament, and suture it with the transplanted tendon. Use 2-0 absorbable sutures to close the fascia. Routinely close the skin.

2. *Postoperative Treatment*

   The elbow joint is flexed at 60° and fixed by orthosis for 7~10 days to facilitate wound healing. Then change the orthosis to a hinged one, which can restrict full elbow extension. Active exercise of the shoulder, elbow, and wrist joints can start. Strengthening exercise starts after the 4th~6th week, but valgus orientations should be avoided within 4 months after surgery. After 4 months, recovery exercise can start and then gradually increase the amount. At the 7th month, gradually increase the range of motion, increase strength exercise and systemic exercises; gradually increase the throwing speed and training time. Athletes can return to the sports field after 8~9 months, and gradually increase the exercise amount in the next 2~3 months until a simulation match can be completed. Competitive throwing can be resumed at about 1 year if there is no pain in the shoulder, elbow, and forearm during the throwing and the strength and range of motion are restored. The entire rehabilitation takes about 18 months to return to preoperative competitive level. During the rehabilitation, patients should be carefully supervised, so as to prevent adverse outcomes. The rehabilitation time varies with profession and person.

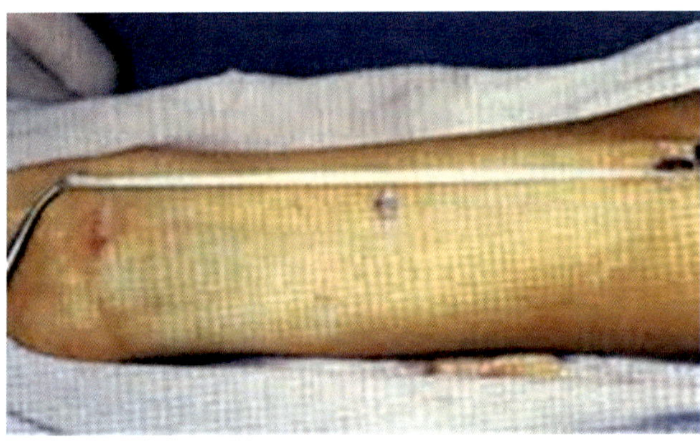

Fig. 9.89 A 15~20 cm long metacarpus longus tendon is obtained as a transplanted tendon to reconstruct the ulnar collateral ligament through a small incision

3. *Key Points*

   The ulnar nerve should be carefully protected throughout the operation. Anterior transposition of the ulnar nerve should be considered if the ulnar nerve is subluxated or may be stimulated after the ulnar collateral ligament repair. Since the ulnar collateral ligament is sutured in a continuous locking manner, when the sutures are knotted on the bone bridge, the force applied to each knot should be estimated in advance, so as to avoid any loose suture in repair sites. It should be ensured that the bone tunnel is drilled on the medial epicondyle, and that the bone bridge has sufficient width to achieve anatomical repair and minimize the risk of fracture caused by suturing and knotting.

9.6.2 Repair and Reconstruction of Lateral Collateral Ligament Complex Injuries of the Elbow Joint

Xing Danmo and Ren Dong

Abstract The lateral collateral ligament complex is the main stable structure limiting the posterolateral dislocation and varus of the elbow joint. Lateral collateral ligament injuries are mostly caused by elbow trauma, such as the combined effect of axial compression, external rotation, and valgus stress on the elbow; the second is iatrogenic injury,

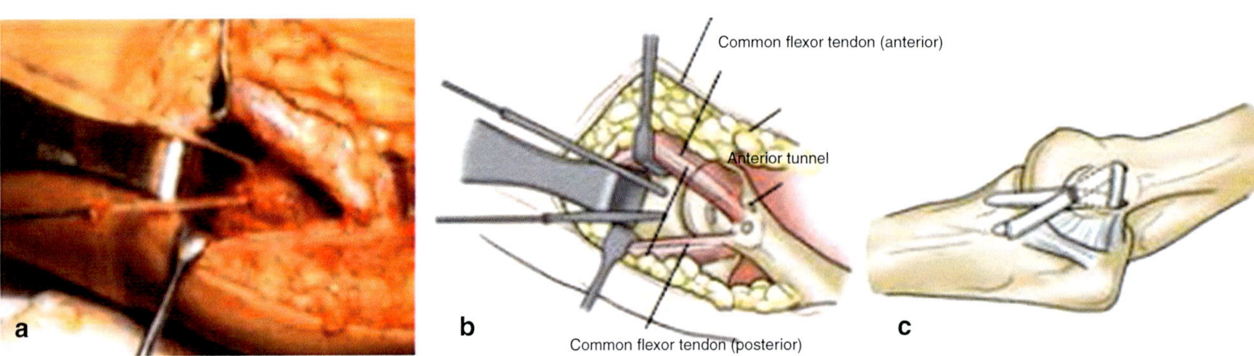

Fig. 9.90 Transplanted tendon. (**a~c**) After the transplanted tendon passes through the ulnar tunnel (1 → 2), the longer end passes through the basal bone hole of the medial epicondyle (2 → 3). Then pull it out from the proximal tunnel (3 → 4). It passes through the basal bone hole again (5 → 3) after bypassing the ridge of the medial epicondyle. Tighten the tendon and suture it with itself under varus stress and 45° flexion of the elbow. Three strands should be crossing the medial part of the ulnohumeral joint after suturing

such as extensive debridement of the lateral soft tissues of the tennis elbow, or injuries of the lateral ulnar collateral ligament during resection or fixation of the capitulum radii.

Although the old lateral collateral ligament complex injury is rare to cause instability of the elbow joint, it often has serious impacts on daily life. Surgical reconstruction can significantly improve the prognosis.

This section introduces the diagnosis, surgical approach, direct repair, and reconstruction methods (classic reconstruction of LUCL, reconstruction of figure-of-8 Yoke technique, transplant and reconstruction with anconeus fascia dissection and reconstruction of annular ligament) and postoperative rehabilitation training of lateral collateral ligament injuries.

The lateral collateral ligament complex (LCLC) of the elbow joint is a complex structure of capsular ligaments (Fig. 9.91), including the radial collateral ligament (RCL), the lateral ulnar collateral ligament (LUCL), and the annular ligament (AL). The lateral collateral ligament complex is the main stable structure limiting the posterolateral dislocation and varus of the elbow joint. Although the old lateral collateral ligament complex injury is rare to cause chronic instability of the elbow joint, it often has serious impacts on daily life. The stability assessment should include medical history, physical examination, and imaging examination. For chronic instability of the posterolateral rotation, the main surgical method is to reconstruct the lateral ulnar collateral ligament by tendon transplantation.

Lateral collateral ligament injuries are mostly caused by elbow trauma, such as the combined effect of axial compression, external rotation, and valgus stress on the elbow; the second is iatrogenic injury, such as extensive debridement of the lateral soft tissues of the tennis elbow, or injuries of the lateral ulnar collateral ligament during resection or fixation of the capitulum radii.

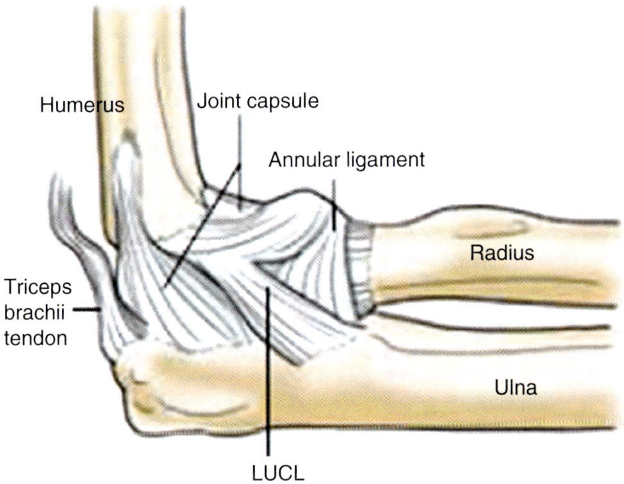

Fig. 9.91 The lateral collateral ligament complex of the elbow joint

In 1881, Eduard Albert first described a case of recurrent dislocation of the elbow joint. The radius and ulna of the patient shifted inwards. Bloch reported a case of recurrent posterior dislocation in 1900. Osborne and Cotterill described in detail the injury mechanism of acute and recurrent dislocation of the elbow joint in 1966. They found that acute dislocation happens when the elbow joint is slightly flexed when falling. Patients then get injured when the hands touch the ground. The violence causes avulsion of the lateral ligaments and posterolateral joint capsule. For recurrent dislocation, it is caused by the failure of the injured posterolateral ligament and joint capsule which are not repaired after the initial dislocation. In 1991, O'Driscoll et al. promoted the famous concept of "posterior lateral rotation instability" (PLRI) [28]. In this theory, when the patient falls, the hand touches the ground and the elbow joint is slightly flexed. Then the elbow joint suffers stress of axial, valgus, and external rotation at the same time. The stress damages stable structures (including the joint capsule and ligaments around the elbow joint) from the outside to the inside, eventually leading to posterior dislocation of the elbow joint (Fig. 9.92). The lateral ulnar collateral ligament was considered to be the most important stable structure of the lateral elbow joint. Schreiber et al. objected to this opinion, arguing that there are other mechanisms of elbow joint instability. After analyzing 62 cases of elbow joint dislocation, they pointed out that the most common mechanism of elbow joint dislocation should be the valgus stress when the elbow joint is straight. In this condition, the medial collateral ligament is mainly injured.

9.6.2.1 Diagnosis of Lateral Collateral Ligament Injuries of the Elbow Joint

Most patients have a history of trauma and dislocation. Some patients have a history of external humeral epicondylitis or surgery. Patients often report snapping and slippage sense when the elbow joint is supinated and straight.

Physical examination: Tissue edema often exists in acute injuries and not obvious in old injuries.

Posterolateral rotatory pivot shift test: When the elbow joint is slightly flexed, the capitulum radii can be pressed to dislocation or subluxation. When the elbow joint flexes more than 40°, the capitulum radii can be repositioned, and often accompanied by snapping.

Push-up test: Positive if it causes fear or the patient cannot complete it [29].

Table pushing relocation test: Positive when it causes pain or fear when the elbow joint is flexed at 40°.

Drawer test for the elbow joint: Positive if the ulnohumeral joint is subluxated.

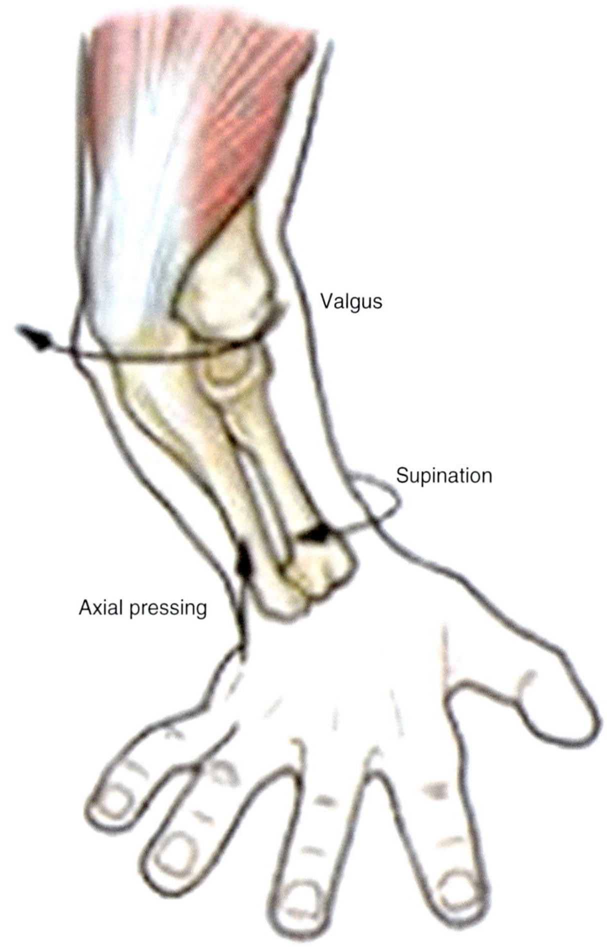

Fig. 9.92 Typical mechanism of elbow joint dislocation. It shows the stress on the elbow joint

Anteroposterior and lateral radiographs of the elbow joints under stress can show the widening of brachioradial space and posterior subluxation of the capitulum radii. MRI can show the damage of LCL complex, but MRI signals can also be abnormal during repair after the injury, so MRI cannot be completely relied on (Fig. 9.93).

9.6.2.2 Surgical Technique

The Kocher approach on the lateral side of the elbow (Fig. 9.94a) is routinely selected. Open the space between the anconeus and the extensor carpi ulnaris (Fig. 9.94b). The LUCL locates just below the two tendons. This intermuscular space can be identified by the fat zone of deep fascia.

1. *Direct Repair of LUCL*
   (1) Identify the origin of LUCL: In acute injury, avulsion usually begins at the distal origin of the humerus. This point locates at the center of the rotation of the capitellum, also known as the "isometric point." The position can be confirmed by holding the sutures while flexing and extending the elbow joint (Fig. 9.95a).
   (2) Drill holes at the isometric point with a 2.0 mm drill bit. Make two bone tunnel exits on the anterior and posterior sides of the lateral column. The two exits are connected to the bone tunnel at the isometric point in a "Y" shape (Fig. 9.95b).
   (3) Pass a 2# non-absorbable suture through the bone tunnel, and pull it out at the isometric point. Perform Krackow locking suture along the anterior and posterior sides of the ligament. Pass by the insertion of the supinator trochanter ligament. Pull back the suture to the origin of the ligament, and pass through the bone tunnel. Knot when the elbow joint flexes 30° and the forearm is under pronation and valgus stress (Fig. 9.95c).
2. *Reconstruction of LUCL*
   (1) Bone tunnel preparation

   Peel the origin of the ulnar supinator on the posterior edge of the capitulum radii, and expose the supinator crest. Make two bone tunnels at the level of the capitulum radii at a distance of 1.25 cm with a 3~4 mm drill. The tunnel depth should reach 1 cm. A small curette can be used to connect the tunnels [20]. The connection of the two entrances should be perpendicular to the direction of the reconstructed ligament (Fig. 9.96a). ① Pass a suture through the two holes, knot one end to the suture, hold the other end to the lateral epicondyle of the humerus. Determine the isometric point of the ligament by repeatedly flexing and extending the elbow joint. The suture will not move with the joint if it is at correct isometric point (Fig. 9.96c). ② Make a Y-shaped bone tunnel in the lateral epicondyle (Fig. 9.96b). The method is similar to the humeral bone tunnel described in the previous repair of LUCL. The exit of the ligament is the isometric point. ③ Widen the tunnel at the isometric point with a 4.5 mm drill bit to accommodate three transplanted tendons at the same time [31].

   (2) Passing and tension control of transplanted tendons

   ① Transplanted tendons usually come from the palmar longus or gracilis tendon, and allogeneic tendons can also be used. ② One end of the graft is braided with Non-Absorbable 2# ETHIBOND® Suture (Polyester, Ethicon Inc.) by the Krackow suture. ③ Pass one end of the transplanted tendon through the two holes in the ulna, and suture it with itself (Fig. 9.96d). The other end passes through the isometric point and is pulled out from the anterior bone hole of the distal humerus. It then enters the tun-

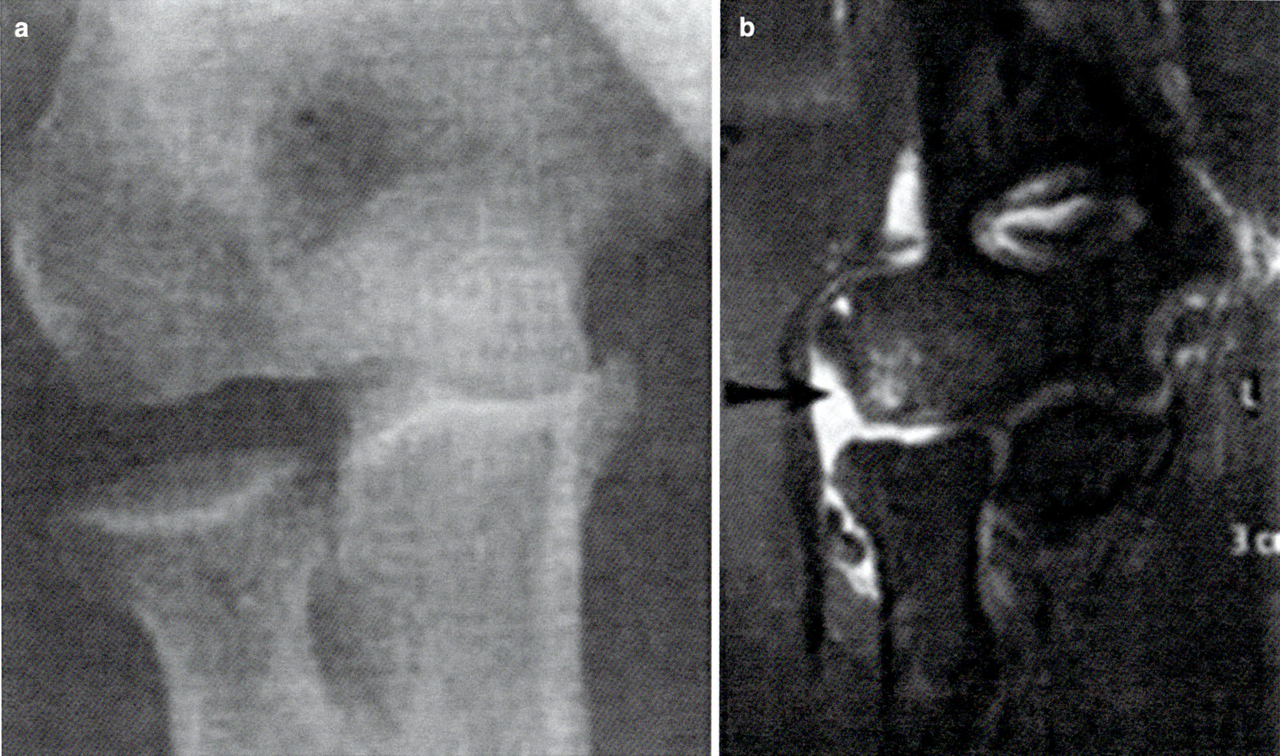

Fig. 9.93 Diagnosis diagram. (**a**) Varus stress anteroposterior radiograph of the elbow joint shows that the brachioradial space is widened; (**b**) CL fracture can be observed on coronal MRI (arrow)

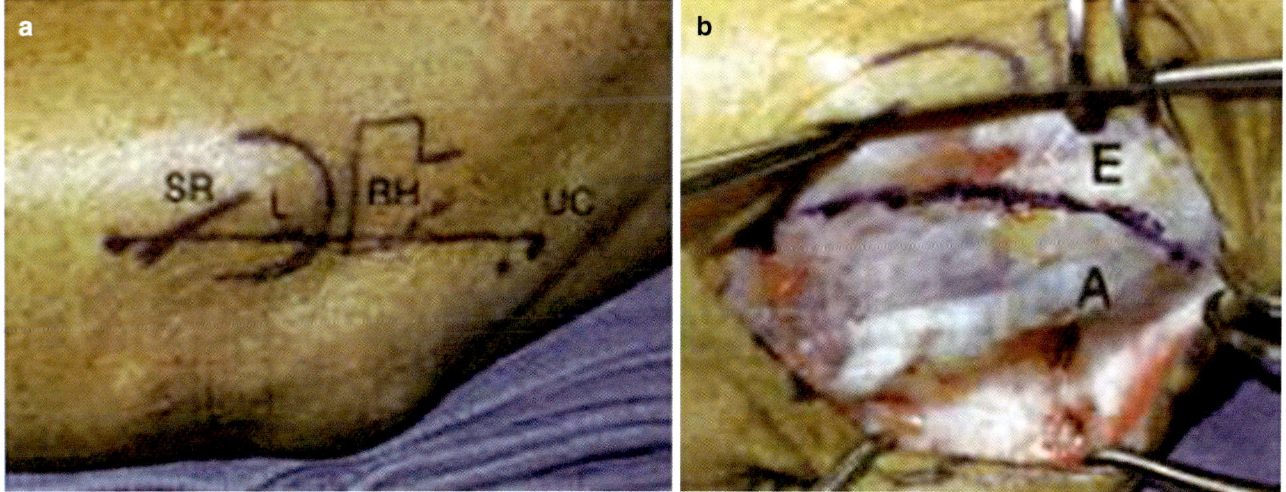

Fig. 9.94 The intermuscular space between the anconeus and the extensor carpi ulnaris in the Kocher approach

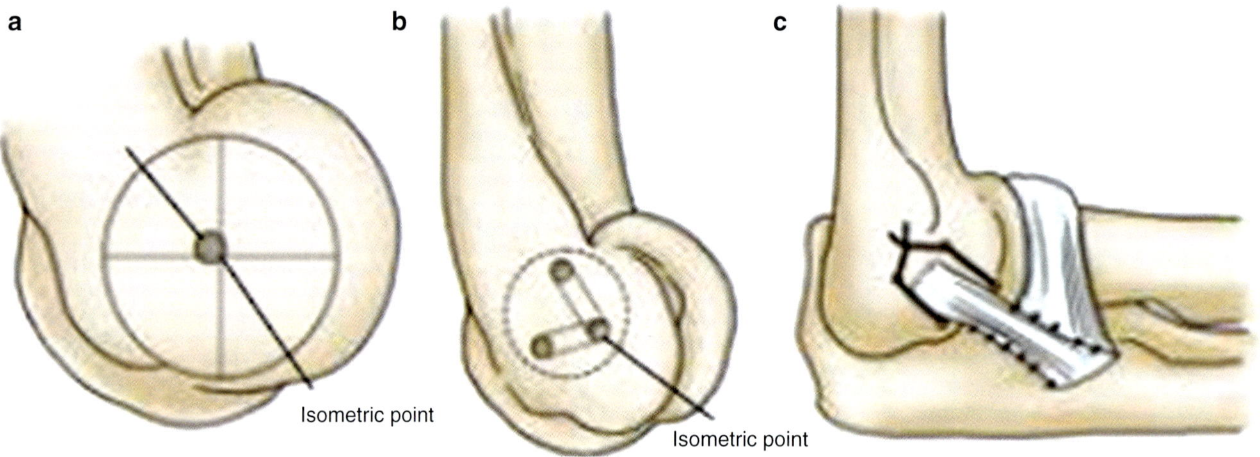

Fig. 9.95 Direct repair of LUCL. (**a**, **b**) The isometric point of LUCL is the center of rotation of the capitellum. Ensure that the ligament is repaired at the isometric point; (**c**) The suture is pulled out from the isometric point. Suture along the ligament with the Krackow locking suture, pull back the suture and knot at the origin

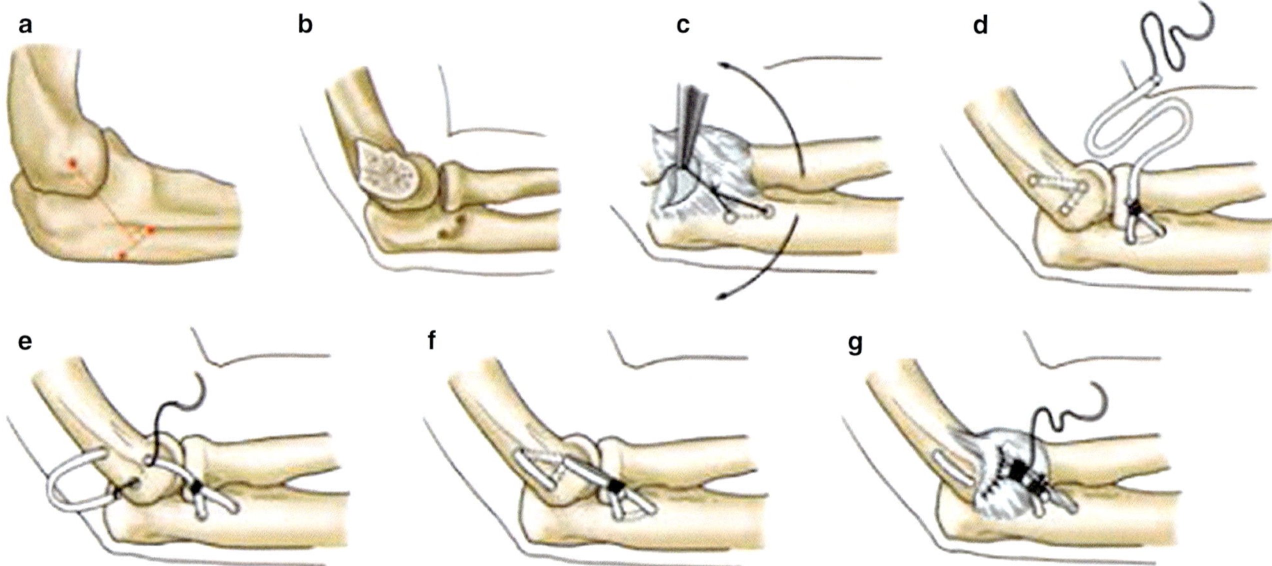

Fig. 9.96 Reconstruction and repair of bone tunnels in LUCL. (**a**) The connection between the two ulnar tunnels is perpendicular to the direction of the reconstructed ligament; (**b**) The two bone tunnels at distal humerus are located on the anterior and posterior sides of the lateral column. They are connected to the isometric point in a "Y" shape; (**c**) The suture passes through the ulnar tunnel, place the other end of the clamp at the isometric point, and the suture does not move when flexing and extending the elbow joint to determine the position of the isometric point; (**d**) One end of the transplanted tendon passes through the two ulnar holes and is sutured with itself; (**e**) The other end passes through the isometric point and is pulled out from the anterior bone hole of the distal humerus. It then enters the tunnel again through the posterior bone hole of the humerus. Pull it out from the isometric point; (**f**) When the elbow joint flexes 40° and the forearm is under pronation and valgus stress, tighten the tendon and suture with itself with 2# non-absorbable sutures; (**g**) Pull the transplanted tendon forward, and suture it to the superficial surface of the joint capsule

nel again through the posterior bone hole of the humerus. Pull it out from the isometric point (Fig. 9.96e). ④ When the elbow joint flexes 40° and the forearm is under pronation and valgus stress, tighten the tendon and suture with itself with Non-Absorbable 2# ETHIBOND® Suture (Polyester, Ethicon Inc.) (Fig. 9.96f) [32]. ⑤ Overlap and suture the joint capsule, and stitch the graft to the joint capsule (Fig. 9.96g). Note that the joint capsule must be closed on the deep side of the graft, so as to prevent friction between the capitellum and the radial head.

3. *Reconstruction of LUCL with Figure-of-8 Yoke Technique*

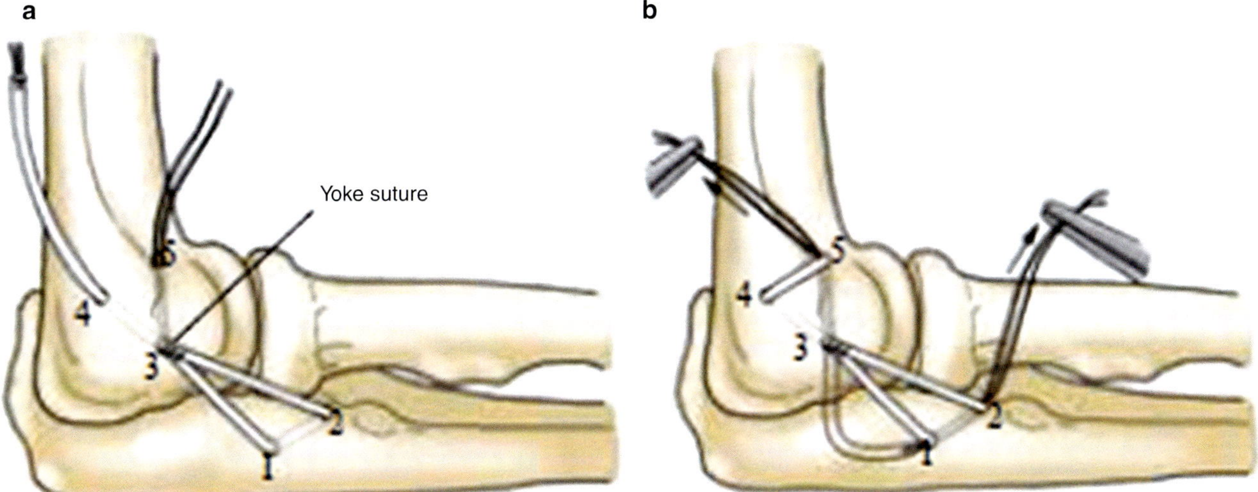

Fig. 9.97 (**a**, **b**) Reconstruction of LUCL with figure-of-8 Yoke technique

(1) Bone tunnel preparation: Similar to the bone tunnel described in the previous repair of LUCL.
(2) Passing and tension control of transplanted tendons
① Pass the transplanted tendon through the ulnar tunnel, place the short end at the isometric point, pull the long end through the isometric point and exit through the proximal humeral tunnel. The short end is braided to the long end (Yoke suture) (Fig. 9.97a) [33].
② The longer end bypasses the lateral epicondyle crest. It passes through the bone tunnel in distal humerus and is pulled out from the isometric point again, and then pull it into the ulnar tunnel (Fig. 9.97b).
③ When the elbow joint flexes 40° and the forearm is under pronation and valgus stress, braid the tendon from distal to proximal in a figure-of-8 shape with 2# non-absorbable sutures. In this way, the transplanted tendons are sutured to each other, so as to strengthen the reconstructed ligament.

4. *Transplant and Reconstruction of LUCL with Anconeus Fascia Dissection*
(1) Graft preparation: ① Select the Kocher approach. Enter the gap between the flexor carpi ulnaris and the anconeus, expose and separate the annular ligament. Separate the anconeus and the distal fascia of the triceps brachii as a whole (Fig. 9.98a). Cut a 1 cm wide and 8 cm long deep fascia strip pedicled at the distal end, and separate its distal end to the ulnar attachment point (Fig. 9.98b). ② Divide the fascia strip into two bundles with equal width along the longitudinal axis (Fig. 9.98c, A is the anterior bundle and P is the posterior bundle). The anterior bundle (shown by the thin arrow) passes through the deep surface of the annular ligament (AL), and the posterior bundle (shown by the thick arrow) passes through the deep surface of the anconeus (A) (Fig. 9.98d). Braid two bundles with 0# non-absorbable suture by the Krackow suture. Bone tunnel preparation: ③ Make a Y-shaped bone tunnel in the lateral epicondyle. The method is similar to the humeral bone tunnel described in the previous repair of LUCL. The exit of the ligament is the isometric point. ④ Widen the tunnel at the isometric point with a 4.5 mm drill bit [34].
(2) Insertion and tension control of transplanted tendons:
① Pass the two sutures of the anterior and posterior fascia strips through the tunnel at the isometric point. Pull them out from the anterior and posterior bone holes of the distal humerus, respectively. ② Place the proximal ends of the two fascia strips into the humeral bone tunnels. When the elbow joint flexes 40° and the forearm is under pronation and valgus stress, tighten the fascial bundle, and knot the sutures on the distal humerus crest (Fig. 9.98e) [35].

Notes:
(1) Keep the forearm in pronation position during the operation, so as to avoid injuries of the posterior interosseous nerve.
(2) Identify the isometric point of the lateral epicondyle of the humerus carefully; the ulnar tunnel should be perpendicular to the direction of the reconstructed ligament.
(3) The bone bridge between the tunnels should be wide enough to avoid apical fracture. Smooth the tunnel walls to avoid friction with the graft.

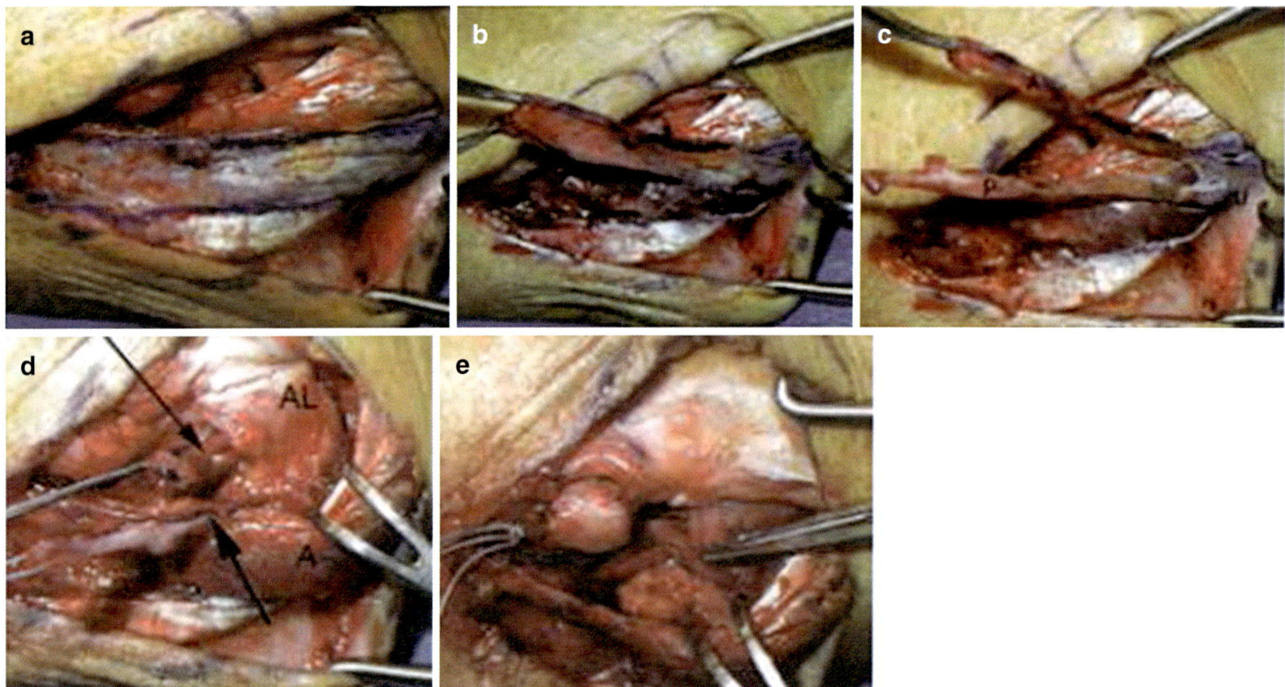

Fig. 9.98 (**a**, **b**, **c**, **d**, **e**) Transplant and reconstruction of LUCL with anconeus fascia dissection

5. *Reconstruction of the Annular Ligament*

   In children with old Monteggia fracture, the radial head is overgrown after dislocation due to the lack of the restriction and pressure of the normal humeroradial joint. The capitellum is dysplastic, and the radius is significantly longer than the ulna, resulting in instability of the lateral elbow joint and deformity, and traumatic arthritis is prone to occur in late stage. Surgery should be actively performed in an early stage. As for the materials for the reconstruction of the annular ligament, autologous palmar longus tendon, fascia lata, and allogeneic tendon have been reported. The author recommends deep forearm fascia, which is available locally without additional incision and bone tunnel [36].

   The surgery still uses the approach which inters the gap between the flexor carpi ulnaris and the anconeus. A fascia strip with 8 cm length and 1 cm width is cut from the anconeus surface to the distal direction at the capitulum radii plane (Fig. 9.99). After osteotomy at the ulnar malunion to correct the angle and fixed with a nail plate, reposition the radial head, and pass the fascia strip through the anconeus to the supinator trochanter in the deep side. Pass the fascia strip around the radial head and neck from inside to outside, and tighten it. Passively rotate the forearm to confirm that the radial head and the capitellum are in good alignment. Keep the elbow joint in 90° flexion and neutral rotation. Suture the fascia strip with itself with 2# non-absorbable suture [37].

9.6.2.3 Postoperative Management

Stage I (0~3 weeks)

- Fix the elbow joint at 40° flexion with plaster slab or brace;
- Equal-length movement of the wrist and hand within a tolerable range;
- Active and passive movement of the shoulder joint [38].

Stage II (3~6 weeks)

- Fix the elbow joint with a hinged elbow orthosis. The doctor sets ranges of restricted and active activities: 20°~120° flexion of the elbow joint and the forearm always in the pronation position;
- Begin equal-length movement of the forearm flexor and pronator teres;
- Begin strength exercises of the wrist and hand;
- The shoulder joint movement is the same as before.

Stage III (6~12 weeks)

- Passive and auxiliary active movement within the full range of joint motion, including supination;
- Begin unrestricted strength exercises of the flexors and extensors [39];
- Intermittent immobilization;

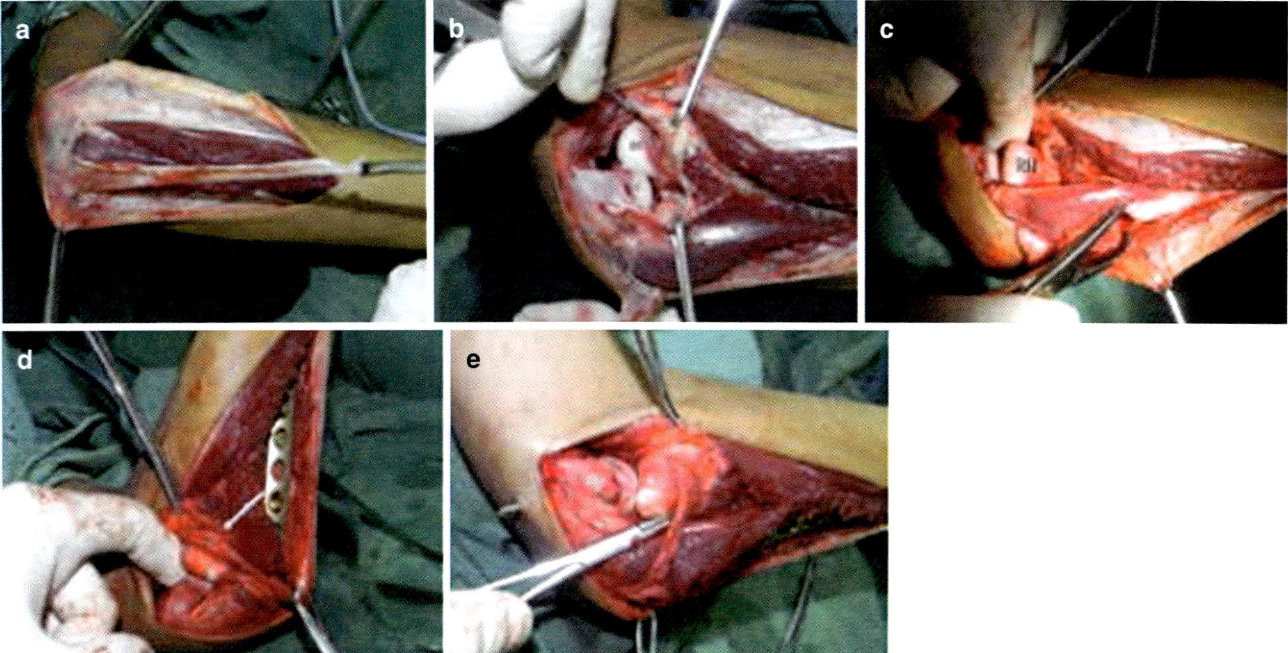

Fig. 9.99 Reconstruction of the annular ligament. (**a**) Cut a fascia strip with 8 cm in length and 1 cm in width from the anconeus surface. The pedicle is at the radial head level; (**b**) The radial head (RH) is dislocated forward, and loses its alignment with the capitellum (C); (**c**) Pass the fascia strip through the anconeus to the deep side after radial head reduction; (**d**) Pass the fascia strip around the radial head and neck (shown by the arrow) from inside to outside; (**e**) Tighten the fascia strip and suture with itself

Stage IV (3~6 months)

- Avoid varus stress or heavy activities when the elbow joint is in extreme flexion and extension positions;
- Begin resistance exercises of the should joint;
- Begin systemic exercises;
- Stretch after elbow joint exercise;
- Resistance exercises of the elbow joint within a tolerable range [40].

9.6.2.4 Complications

- Reappearance of elbow instability;
- Stiff elbow joint;
- Infection;
- Donor site injury of the transplanted tendon;
- Stress fracture of the bone tunnel [41].

9.6.3 Repair and Reconstruction of the Triceps Brachii Tendon Insertion Rupture

Xing Danmou and Chen Yan

Abstract The triceps brachii is not only the main reliance of the extension of the elbow joint. It also contributes to active external stabilization of the elbow joint. The causes of distal injuries of the triceps tendon can be summarized as traumatic, pathological, and iatrogenic. The injury mostly occurs at tendon insertion, with or without bone avulsion. Anatomical characteristics of this injury determine that it is difficult to perform direct repair and fixation.

Patients with acute and complete rupture of the distal triceps brachii tendon often present with limited active elbow extension, fatigue, and pain. In this condition, the triceps tendon needs to be repaired to restore its normal extension function. Classic repair techniques include the Bunnell suture and Krackow suture techniques. With the development of biomechanics and materials, various methods for the repair and fixation of the triceps tendon have emerged. The article introduces classic repair techniques, modified surgeries, and the application of suture bridge technique and anchor.

In the old complete injury of the distal triceps brachii tendon, the tendon usually retracts in muscle belly and causes secondary scars. It makes the surgery difficult. The degree of tendon retraction should be evaluated during the operation. If the retraction is not serious, the V-Y tendon lengthening, tendon subvolution, and anconeus transposition can be used to repair the injury. For more serious tendon rupture with defects, it cannot be repaired with local tendon flaps or muscle flaps. In this condition, it is necessary to use transplanted tendons such as autologous tendons, allogeneic tendons, and allogeneic Achilles tendon with calcaneus. Indications for surgical reconstruction of chronic injuries include obvious dysfunction in daily activities or failed conservative treatment and rehabilitation training for 3 months. The purpose and possible results of surgical treatment must be explained to the patient, as well as the long-term training plan after surgery.

Rupture of the distal triceps brachii is extremely rare. It is reported that the incidence of distal triceps rupture accounts for less than 1% of all tendon injuries. Distal biceps tendon rupture is more common in males, while the distal triceps tendon rupture occurs in a male-to-female ratio of 3:2. The average onset age is 33 years (7~80 years). There are multiple mechanisms and risk factors for triceps tendon rupture. The main causes are overload, strong eccentric contraction, or direct trauma of the triceps tendon. These include falling with upper arm straight, weight training, swinging baseball bat, push-ups, bodybuilding, rugby, etc. It can also because of the weakness of the tendon-bone junction, such as metabolic diseases (diabetes, chronic renal failure, osteogenesis imperfecta, rheumatoid arthritis, and hyperparathyroidism), systemic use or local injection of steroids. As many as 25% of professional athletes have triceps rupture after receiving local steroid injections for olecranon bursitis. Triceps tendon rupture associated with previous elbow joint surgery is being increasingly recognized, especially in the case of total elbow replacement, which may be as high as 29%. A thorough review of medical history and risk factors is essential to determine the potential cause of tendon rupture [42].

The main symptoms include swelling and tenderness at the triceps insertion, the palpable defects (Fig. 9.100), and significantly weakened elbow extension. The most reliable examination method is to raise the upper arm and flex the elbow at 90°. Meanwhile, let the patient extend the elbow against gravity. The strength of the elbow extension is very important, because in a triceps injury, complete anatomical rupture does not necessarily lead to complete loss of elbow extension function. Old triceps ruptures can be diagnosed with a loss of elbow extension over 30° [43].

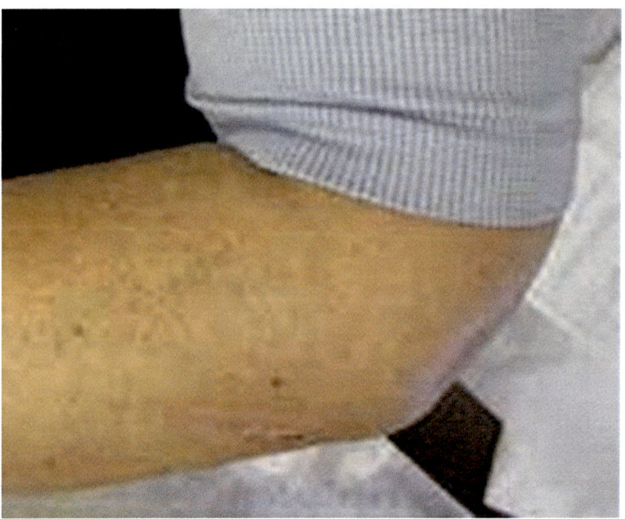

Fig. 9.100 The depressed area of tissue defect can be palpable behind the elbow

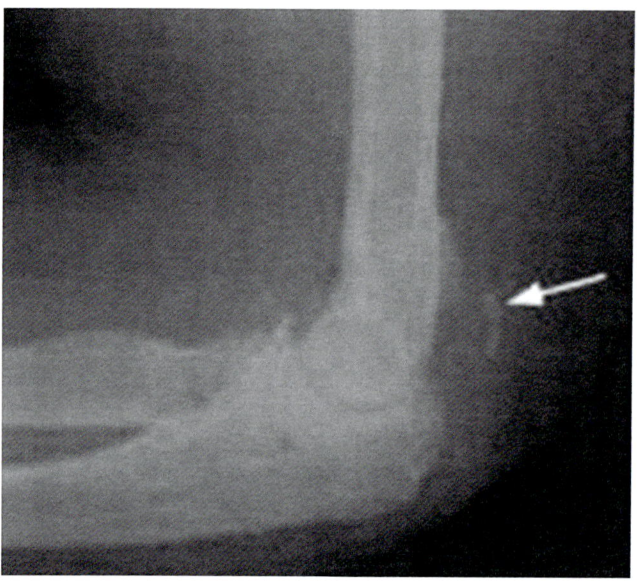

Fig. 9.101 Lateral X-ray of the elbow joint. The arrow shows a fractured piece avulsed from the olecranon tip

X-rays are used to rule out olecranon fractures. The lateral X-ray (Fig. 9.101) can show the avulsion fracture of the olecranon tip. Ultrasonography can find triceps rupture, but MRI is preferred. MRI can distinguish between complete avulsion and partial avulsion, evaluate tendon retraction, and help making surgical plan (Fig. 9.102) [44].

Partial rupture of the triceps tendon is self-healing, so conservative treatment can be applied. Conservative treatment includes fixing the affected arm with brace, plaster, or splint. Avoid lifting heavy objects and elbow extension of the affected arm, until the injury is completely healed. The fixing period is 3–8 weeks according to the patient's injury condition. For patients with high functional requirements (such as athletes), early individualized rehabilitation exercises can be considered.

After 3 months of the treatment, the pain should be obviously relieved, and the patient is able to carry out daily activities and voluntary activities. Before the avulsion is completely healed, intensive movement of the elbow joint may cause partial or complete rupture. In this condition, the patient may present with elbow extension weakness that cannot be improved. If the symptom persists, it indicates that the conservative treatment has failed. Surgical treatment can be considered based on the patient's own needs [45].

9.6.3.1 Direct Repair of Triceps Tendon Injuries

Complete rupture and severe partial rupture of the triceps brachii require surgical intervention. The therapeutic effect of direct repair is the best if the injury is within 3 weeks. The posterior midline incision is generally used. Identify and

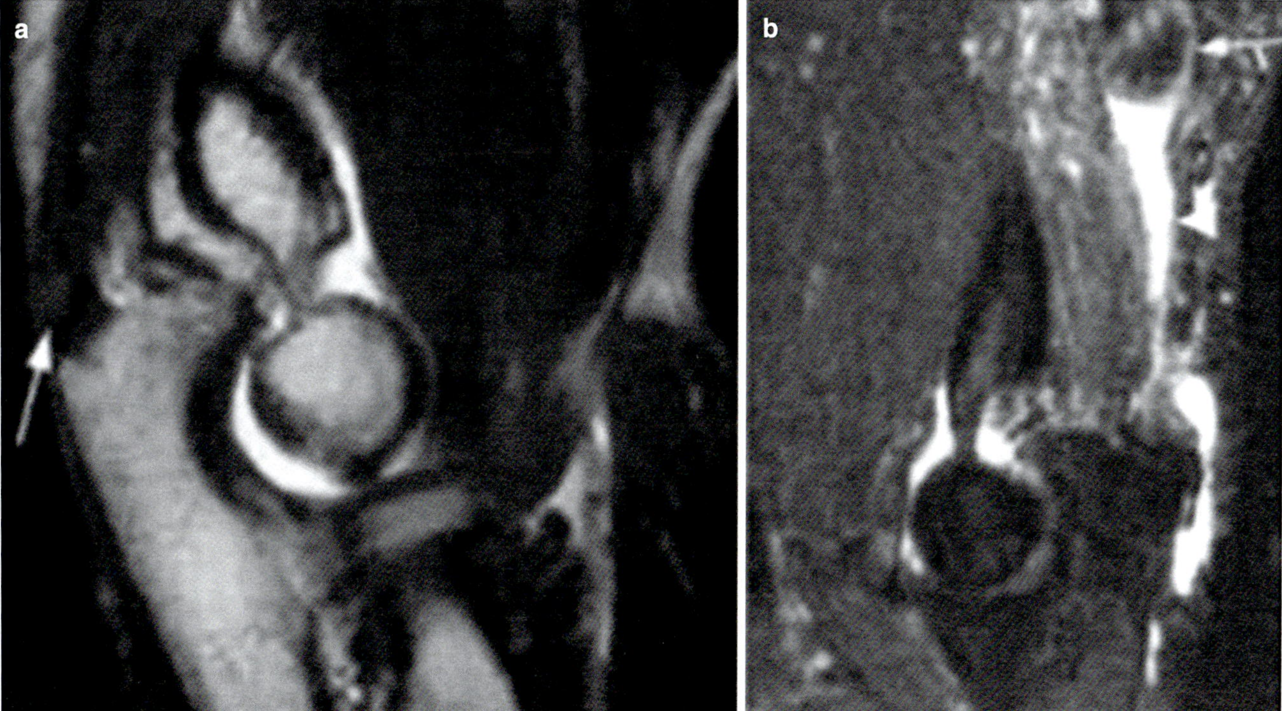

Fig. 9.102 MRI examination. (**a**) The T1 image of MRI. The arrow shows a partial rupture of the distal triceps. (**b**) The T2 image of MRI. The distal triceps brachii is completely ruptured and retracted (small arrow). Fluid remains around the stump (large arrow)

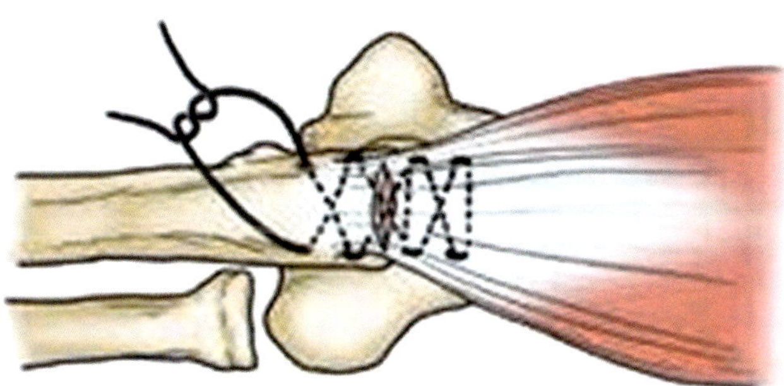

Fig. 9.103 The Bunnell suture technique for acute triceps rupture repair. Pass a non-absorbable suture through the tendons. The sutures are knotted through the pre-drilled holes in the olecranon to reattach the triceps to the insertion

loosen the ulnar nerve in the cubital area, debride the tendon stump and freshen the olecranon bed to promote the healing of the bone and tendon. If the fragment is large enough to be fixed by a plate, it can be treated as olecranon fractures. Small fragments can be sutured or excised. Reconstruct the tendon insertion in one-stage operation [46].

Classical repair techniques include the Bunnell (Fig. 9.103) or Krackow locking suture. With the development of biomechanics, various methods for repair and fixation of the triceps brachii have emerged. With the development of materials, intraosseous suture anchors have also been widely applied in the triceps tendon repair.

Recently, some modified repair techniques, such as double-row suture technique (Fig. 9.104), have achieved better repair effects with greater contact area and better repair status in physiological anatomy [47].

After biomechanical testing, some scholars recommended that the triceps be repaired with continuous Krackow suture plus a double-row suture bridge which is fixed by passing through bone tunnels (Figs. 9.105 and 9.106) [48].

This technique uses a routine posterior approach of the elbow joint. Remove the granulation tissue around the tendon stump (Fig. 9.105a). Remove the granulation tissue around anatomical insertion of the triceps on the olecranon. Use an oscillating saw to remove local bone on the surface with a thickness of 2~4 mm. Insert two single-suture anchors with 2# non-absorbable sutures into the olecranon tip and then put the sutures aside (Figs. 9.105b and 9.106a). Pass the 2# non-absorbable sutures through the middle structure of the Krackow suture (Fig. 9.105c). Place a straight needle in the central of the triceps insertion after two crossed Kirschner wires passing through the rotation hole in the olecranon (Figs. 9.105d and 9.106b). Pass the Krackow suture through the tail hole of the needle, and pass through the rotation hole in the olecranon introduced by the needle (Fig. 9.105c). Before tightening the suture through the olecranon, pass the sutures of the previous anchors through the distal triceps tendon at a distance of 2~3 cm from the edge. The Krackow suture is tightened and fixed on the hole to cover the insertion

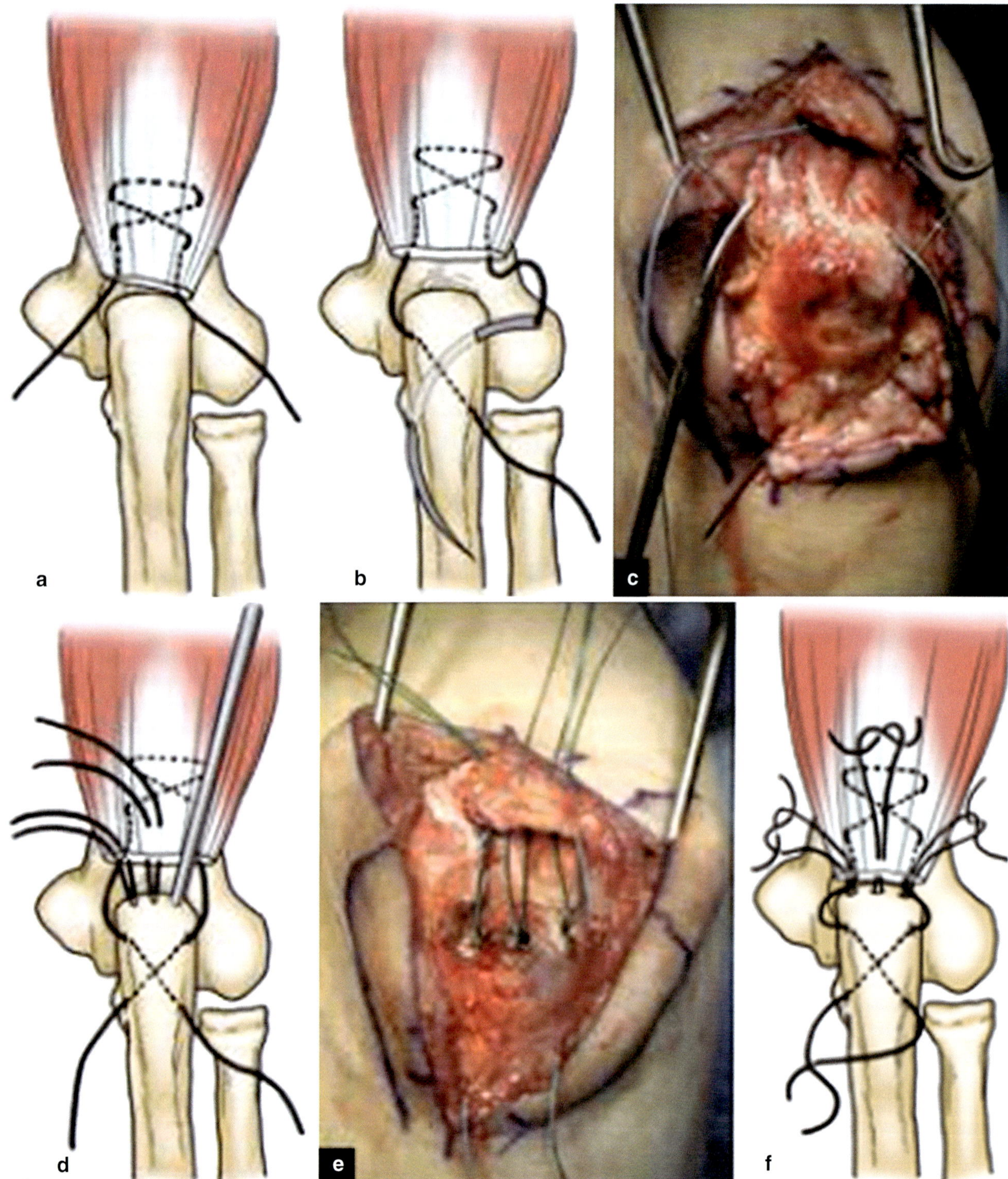

Fig. 9.104 Modified repair technique for triceps tendon injuries. (**a**) Pass the ETHIBOND® Suture (Polyester, Ethicon Inc.) through the distal triceps tendon with the Bunnell suture technique; (**b**, **c**) Pass the ETHIBOND® Suture (Polyester, Ethicon Inc.) through bone tunnels crossing the olecranon; (**d**) Insert 3 anchors with sutures into the olecranon; (**e**) Pass the anchor sutures through the triceps tendon; (**f**) Knot the ETHIBOND® Suture (Polyester, Ethicon Inc.) and then the anchor sutures; (**g**) Fix the triceps tendon at the olecranon; (**h**) Suture finished

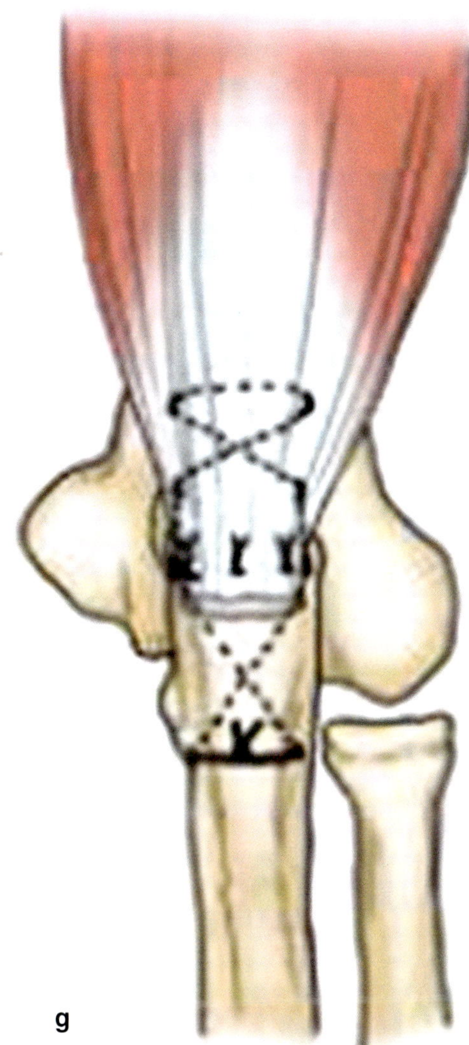

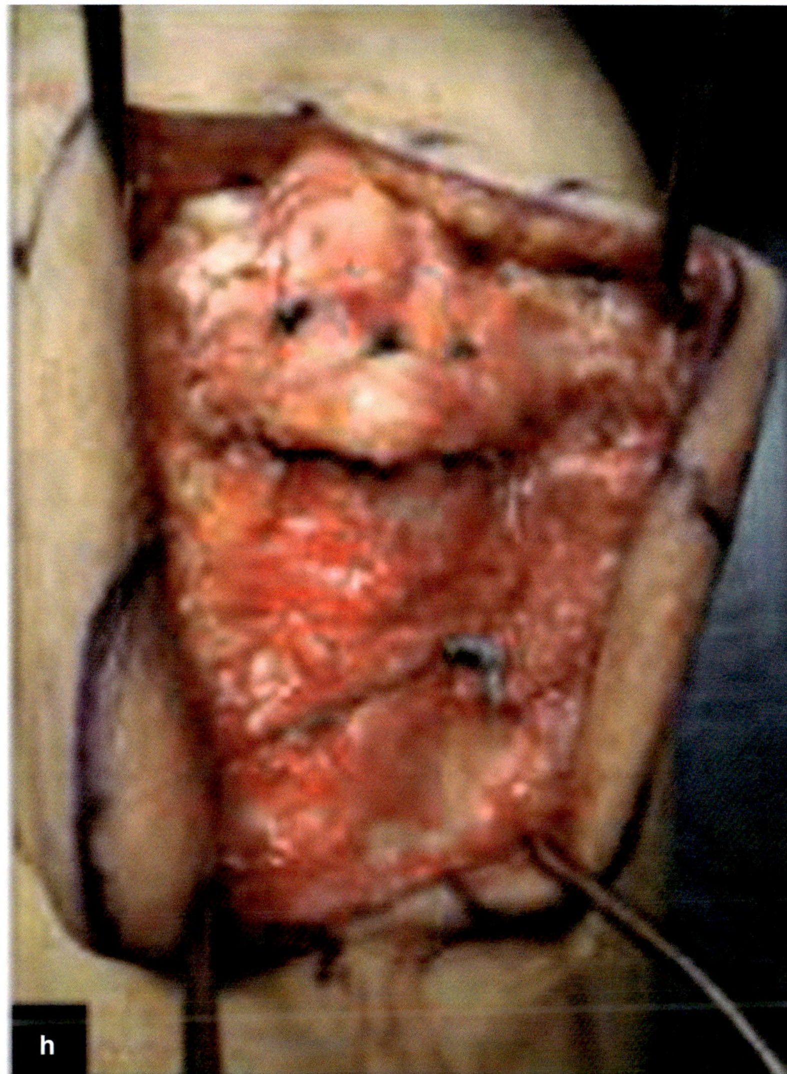

Fig. 9.104 (continued)

area on the dorsal olecranon. Knot the sutures of the anchors to the triceps tendon, leaving the remaining sutures long (Fig. 9.105f). At the distal bone tunnel, transverse the hole to form the third bone tunnel (Fig. 9.105g). Cross the remaining sutures of the anchors through the bone tunnels and knot. After that, these cross sutures compress the distal triceps tendon at the triceps insertion (Figs. 9.105h and 9.106c) [49].

Since the triceps tendon insertion on the olecranon is located directly behind the elbow joint and soft tissue coverage is weak here, the above-mentioned repair method with non-absorbable sutures cannot avoid pain around the knot. Many surgeons begin to use wireless repair techniques which are fixed by anchors. These include knotless suture bridge technique with two anchors (Figs. 9.107 and 9.108) and the knotless repair technique with single anchor of distal insertion of the triceps tendon (Figs. 9.109, 9.110, 9.111 and 9.112) [50].

9.6.3.2 Repair Techniques for Chronic Injuries with Partial Loss and Retraction of the Tendon

Acute triceps brachii injury generally does not have severe tendon retraction or loss. However, old tendon rupture of more than 3 weeks is often accompanied by tendon loss and retraction, which is almost impossible to repair directly. In such cases, the ulnar nerve must be loosened sufficiently to allow greater movement of the distal triceps tendon. When direct repair is infeasible, several options are usually available. These include the V-Y plasty of the triceps tendon, triceps subvolution, and anconeus transposition [51].

The V-Y plasty of the triceps tendon is a technique to lengthen the triceps tendon in situ to compensate for the contracture or loss of the tendon. Yazdi reported and described this procedure: Use the routine posterior approach, identify and protect the ulnar nerve. The apex of the

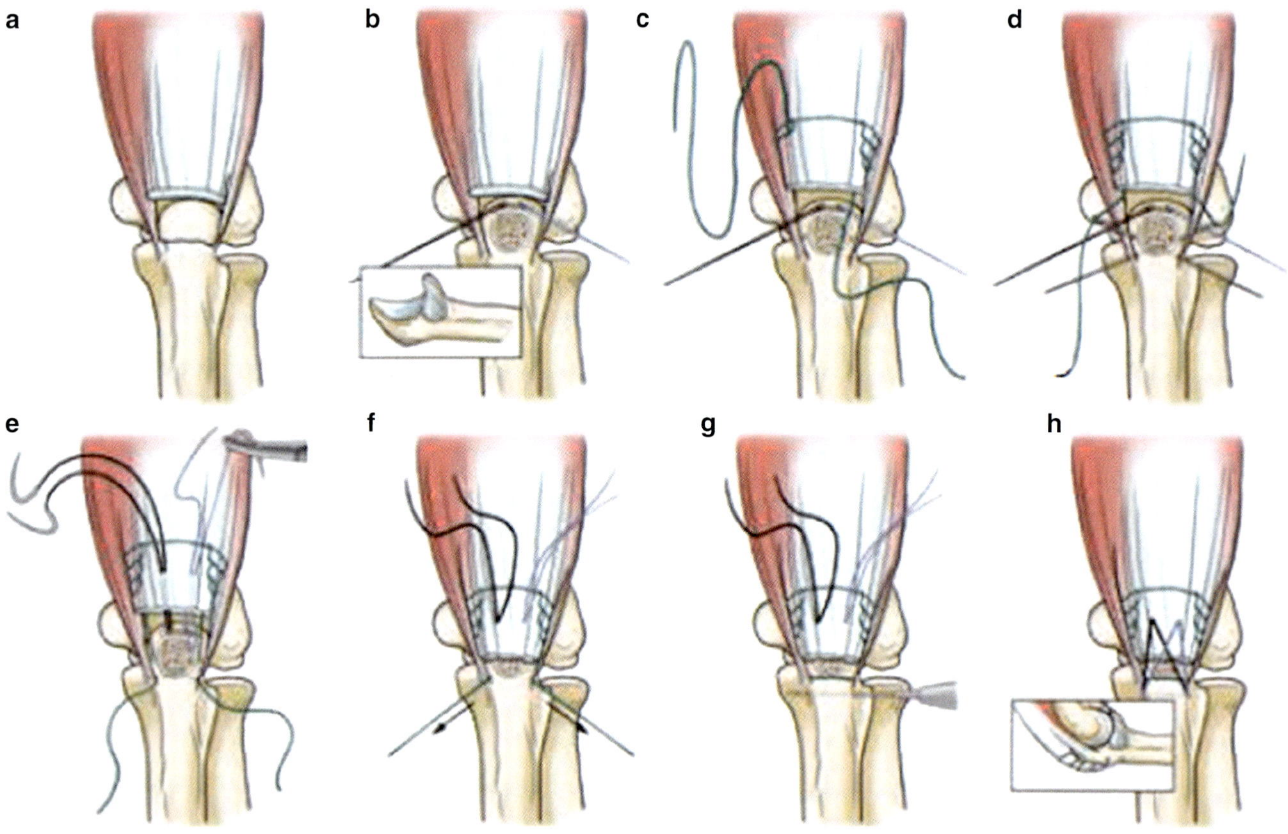

Fig. 9.105 (**a–h**) Modified repair technique for triceps tendon injuries

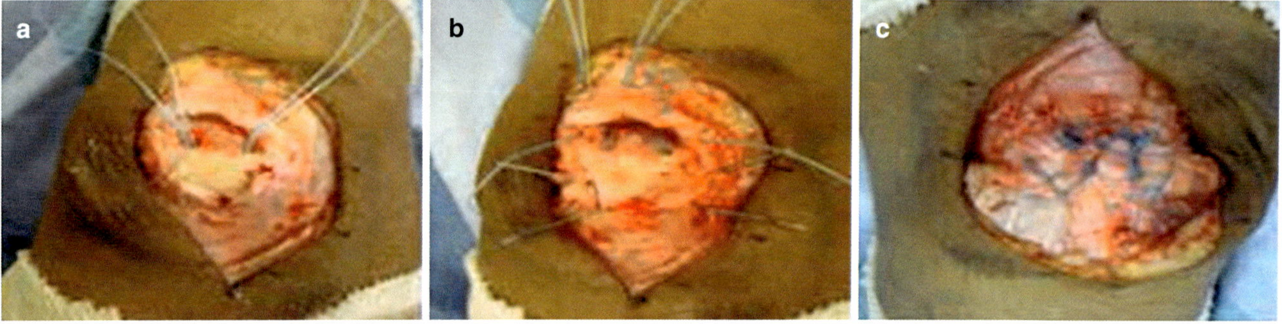

Fig. 9.106 (**a–c**) Modified repair technique for triceps tendon injuries

V-shaped incision of the triceps tendon should be at the distal side of the musculotendinous junctions. A V-shape is formed by making two longitudinal incisions on both sides of the distal tendon stump, the medial and lateral retinacula of the triceps. Preserve the deep fascia under the tendon when the two incisions converge. The two longitudinal incisions finally converge to form the apex of the V shape (Fig. 9.113a). To ensure sufficient aponeurosis and blood supply around the V-shaped flap for closure after the operation, the length of the two sides of the V-shaped incision is usually 8~10 cm. The V-shaped flap should be wide enough to ensure that the distal tendon stump can completely cover the original insertion of the triceps on the olecranon, while ensuring there are enough tissues for repair on the two sides. Pull the tendon forward to its original insertion when the elbow joint flexes at about 70° (Fig. 9.113b). If the stump is retracted or the defect is large, the triceps brachii and the V-shaped flap may need additional loosening. Note that enough muscles attaching to the distal tendon and aponeurosis should be retained to maintain the blood supply. Then fix the Y-shaped flap with the Krackow suture and a double-row suture bridge which is fixed by passing through bone

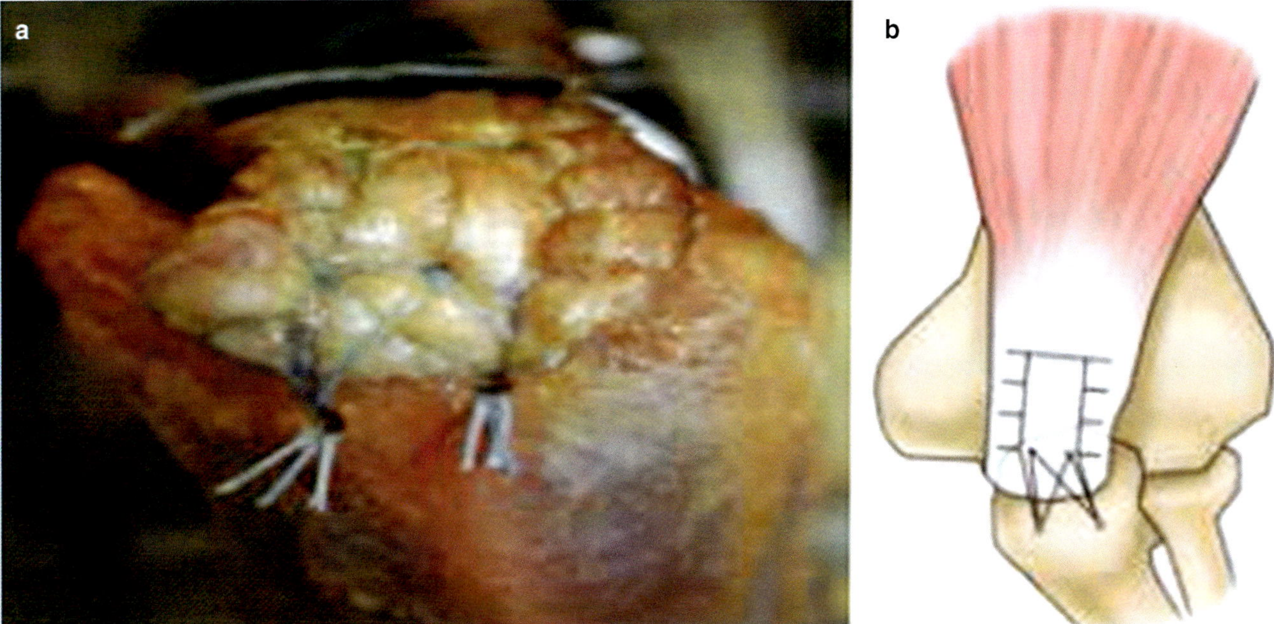

Fig. 9.107 (**a–b**) Use the Krackow suture technique on the distal triceps brachii. One about 13 mm from the distal olecranon, insert one 3.0 mm anchor with suture into the medial and lateral edge of the tendon insertion, respectively. Take one suture from each anchor, pass them through the triceps tendon and knot. Drill two holes on the ulnar shaft, take the Krackow suture of one side and the suture of anchor of the same side, pass them through the hole of the 3.5 mm knotless anchor, and insert the anchor into the hole to fix the knot

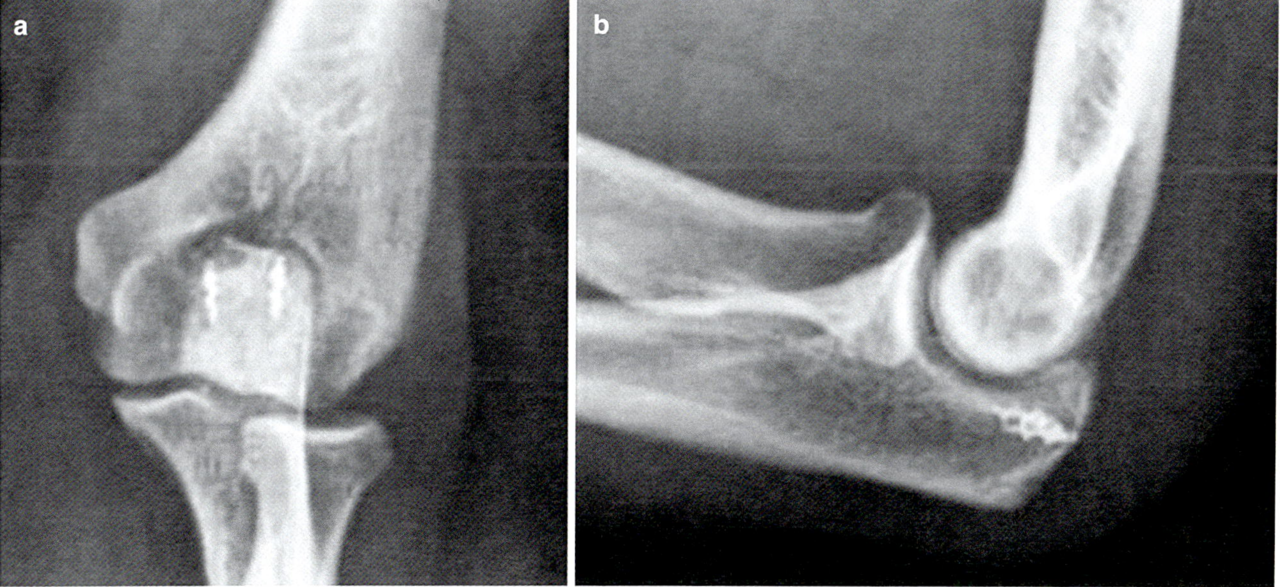

Fig. 9.108 Anteroposterior X-rays after surgery. (**a**, **b**) The anchors are inserted into the insertion of the triceps brachii on the olecranon

tunnels (Fig. 9.113c). Handle the knots carefully, as they may cause local irritation [52]

The subvolution of the triceps tendon is another option to repair the defect. First, cut the tendon flap with the same thickness as the distal triceps. Most tendon flaps are square. Turn over the distal tendon flap at around 2~3 cm from the stump. The width of the tendon flap is determined by the area of the triceps insertion behind the olecranon (Fig. 9.114a). Ensure that the tendon flap is continuous with the residual tendons at the distal end, and the junction is stable enough to withstand a certain amount of tension without avulsion. Insert two anchors with 2# sutures into the triceps tendon

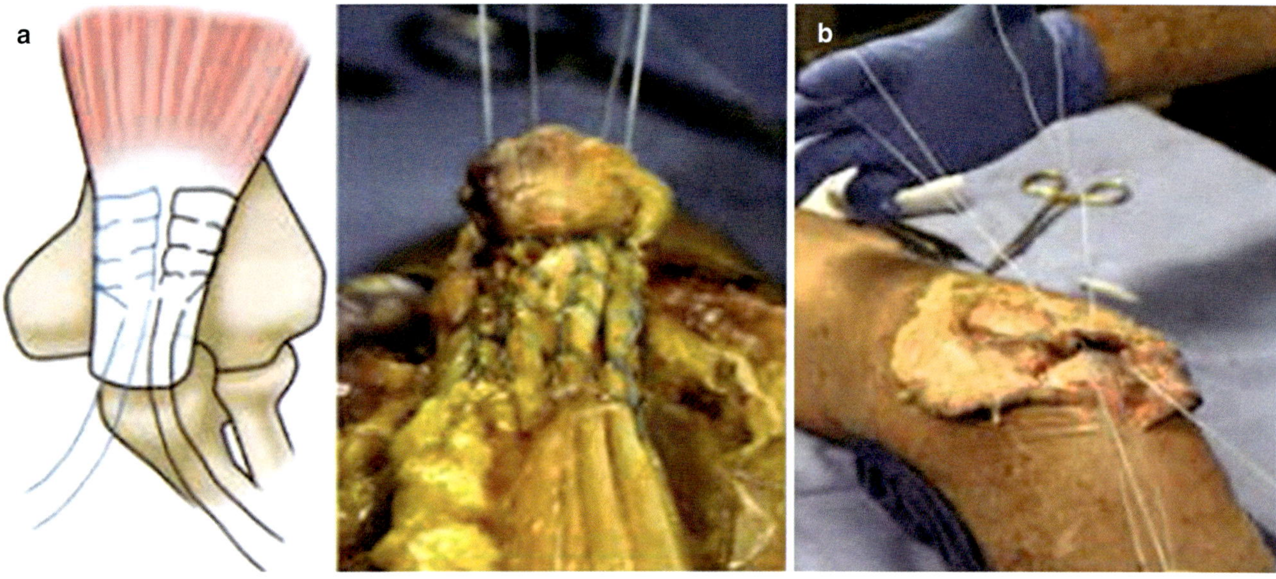

Fig. 9.109 The Krackow suture technique. (**a**) Use the Krackow suture technique on both the medial and lateral edges of the triceps brachii; (**b**) Pass a FiberLink suture through both the medial and lateral sides of the triceps insertion, with the loop end located behind the tendon

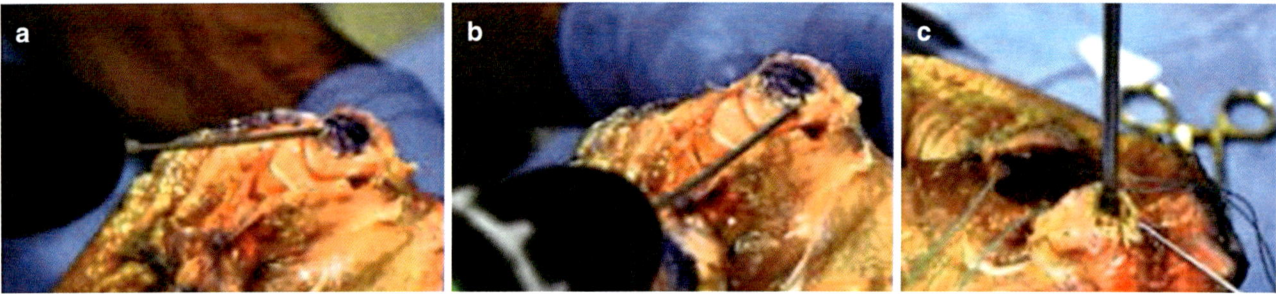

Fig. 9.110 Bone preparation. (**a**, **b**) Reserve 2 mm bone tunnels on both medial and lateral sides of the olecranon; (**c**) Drill a hole between the two tunnels, and then insert a 4.75 mm anchor

insertion. Suture the turned tendon directly with the residual tendon on the olecranon. Finally, use the 2# suture on the anchor to pass through the turned tendon, tighten the knot to compress it to the triceps insertion (Fig. 9.114b) [53].

Anconeus transposition: First, loosen and expose the anconeus and the extensor carpi ulnaris. Separate and loosen the anconeus along the edge of the intermuscular space of the extensor carpi ulnaris. Separate the anconeus attached to its radius insertion. Pull and rotate the anconeus belly and the triceps tendon stump to the insertion on the olecranon (Fig. 9.115a). The proximal ends of the anconeus and triceps and the stump of the olecranon insertion of the broken triceps are directly sutured for repair (Fig. 9.115b, c). If the anconeus cannot completely cover the middle defect after transposition, its proximal and distal ends need to be further fully loosened until completely covering the defect wound of the triceps tendon [54].

9.6.3.3 Repair Technique of Old Triceps Brachii Rupture

In the old complete rupture of the triceps brachii tendon, the tendon usually retracts in muscle belly and causes serious scars. It makes the surgery difficult. The same posterior incision is applied. Tendon transplantation will be considered if (1) the stump is retracted or the defect area is large, (2) it cannot be sutured even after full release, and (3) anconeus transposition is not available. Both autologous and allogeneic transplantation can be used. The grafts include tendons of palmaris longus, plantaris or hamstring, as well as allogeneic tendon of the Achilles/calcaneus [55].

Tendon braiding repair technique: Choose a transplanted tendon with sufficient length. Braid the tendon through the two sides of triceps stump, leaving enough length on both sides to pass through the gap and the bone tunnel across the olecranon. At the same time, the transplanted tendon should

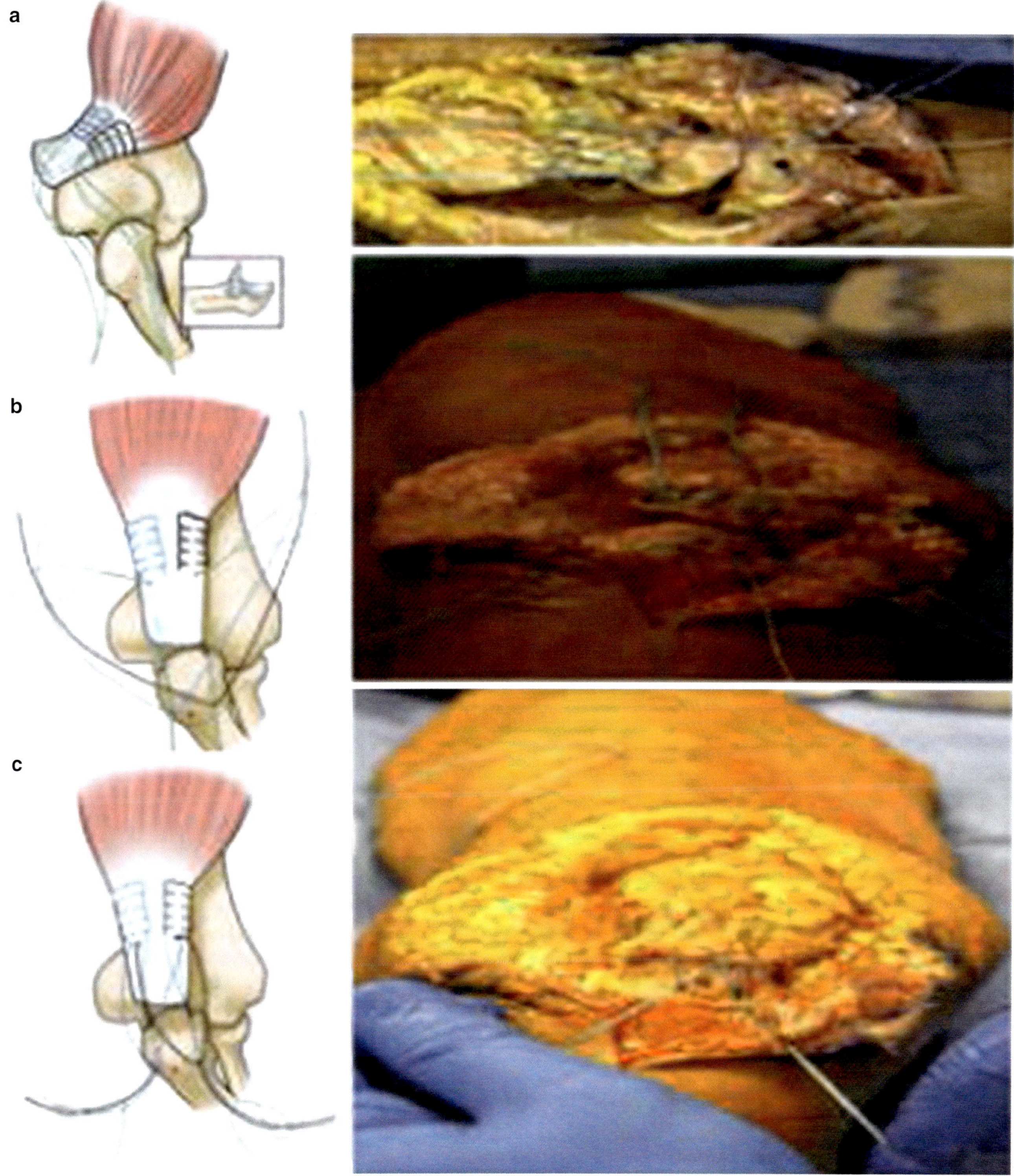

Fig. 9.111 Trend of suture. (**a**) On the lateral side, the two Krackow sutures and the FiberLink tail pass through the lateral bone tunnel. The same operation on the medial side; (**b**) Take one Krackow suture from both medial and lateral sides. Insert them into the lateral FiberLink ring and pass through the lateral bone tunnel. The same operation on the medial side; (**c**) Form a box and X configuration locally

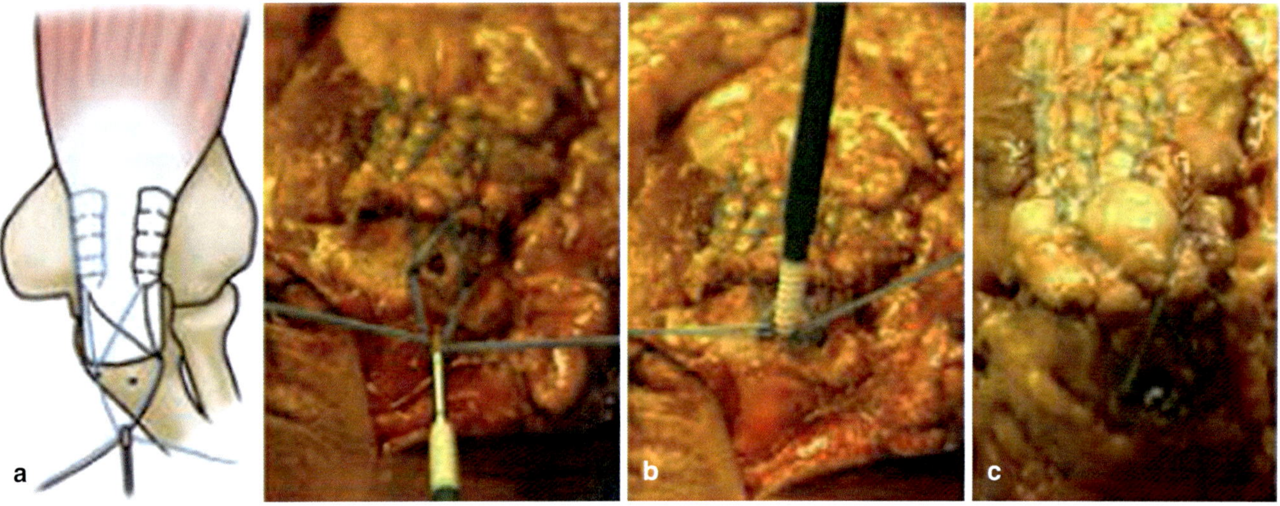

Fig. 9.112 Final fixation. (**a**) Pass 4 sutures through the anchor; (**b**) Insert the anchor into the reserved hole; (**c**) Final form

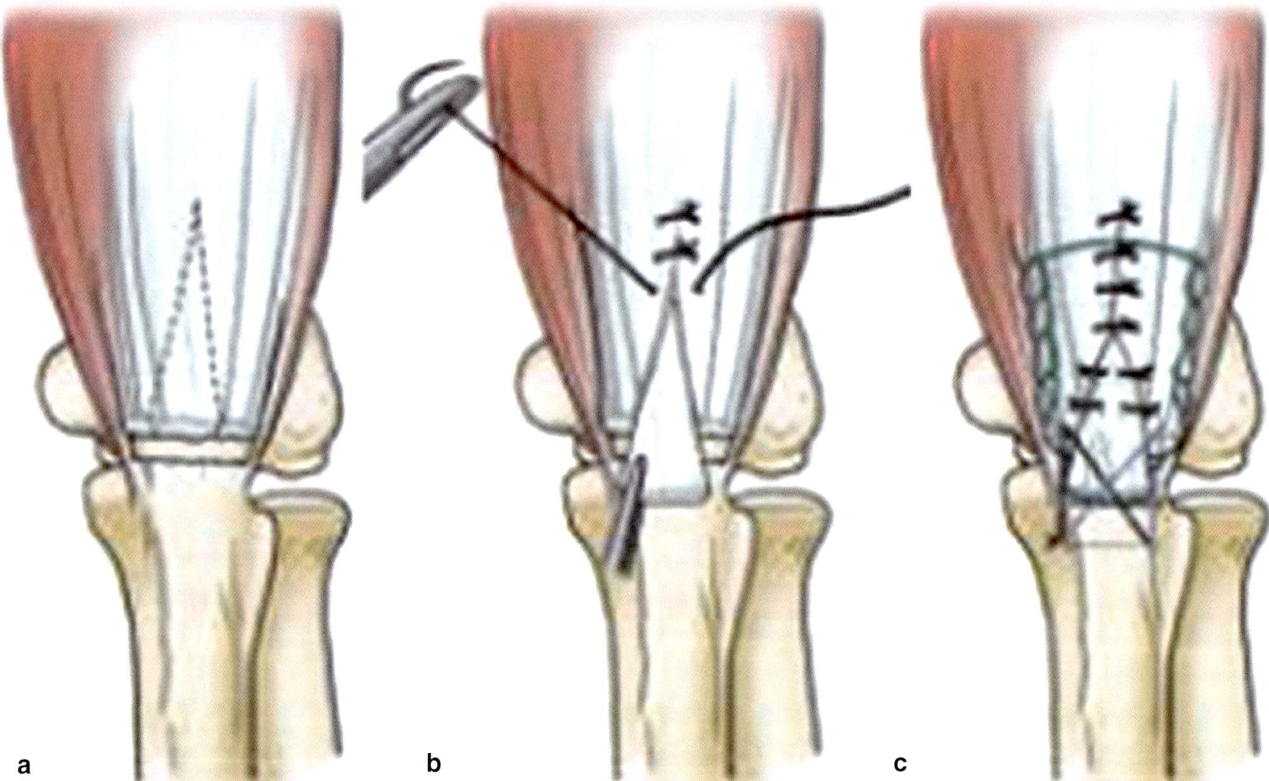

Fig. 9.113 (**a–c**) V-Y plasty of the triceps tendon

have sufficient width and strength to enhance and replace the defective triceps. The transplanted tendon passes through the two sides of triceps stump in an X shape and is braided inside the tendon (Fig. 9.116a). Drill bone tunnels at equal distances on the dorsal side and the proximal cortex of the olecranon. The width of the tunnels matches the width of the transplanted tendon, while avoiding damage to joint surface. The two ends of the tendon pass through the tunnel in opposite directions (Fig. 9.116b). Tighten the triceps and transplanted tendon, and fix the transplanted tendon with non-absorbable sutures (Fig. 9.116c, d). The extra tendon is used to strengthen the suture to fill the defect area of the triceps brachii. If the transplanted tendon is too short to pass through the olecranon tunnel, fix it to the olecranon insertion of the triceps brachii with the squeezing screw technique [56].

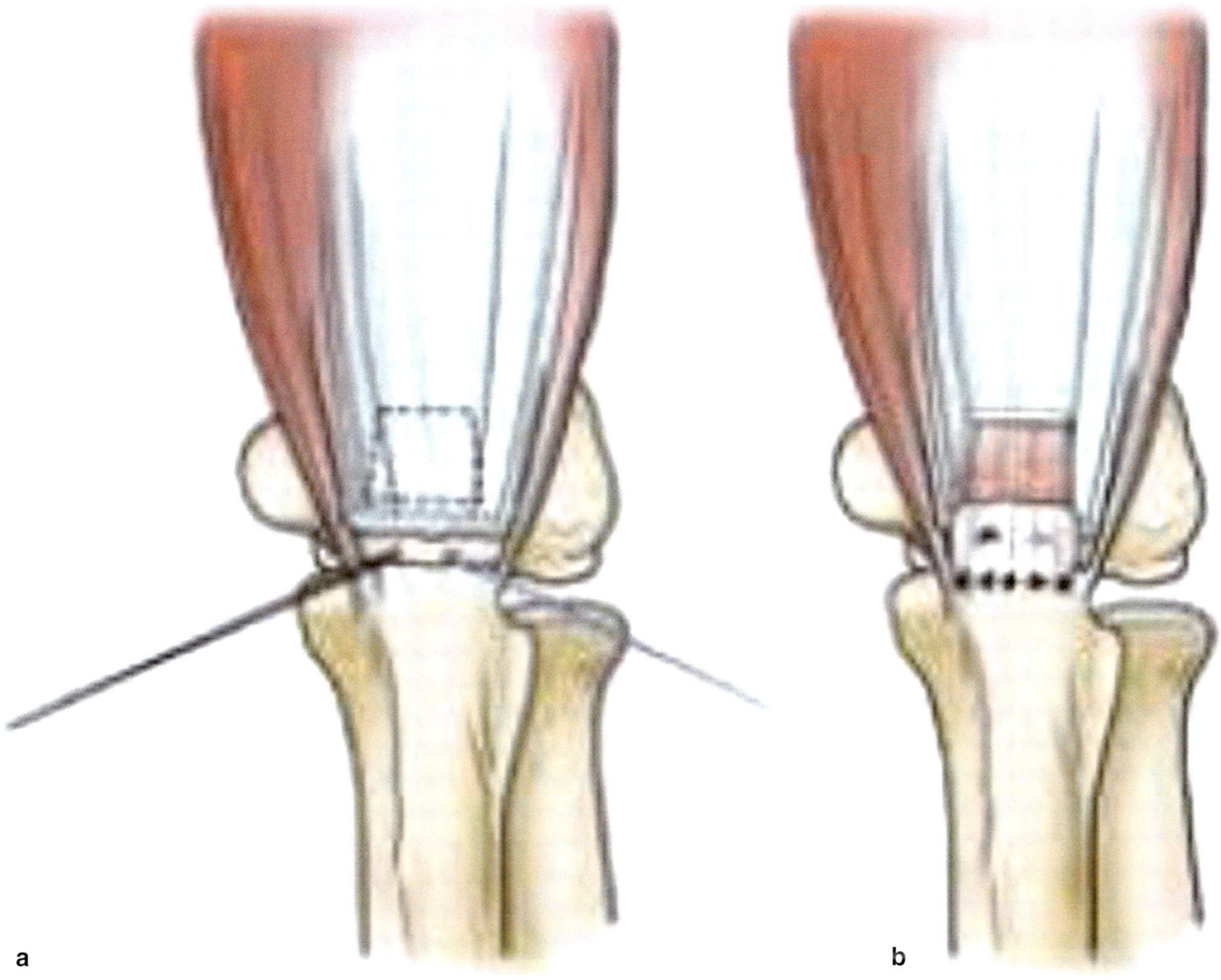

Fig. 9.114 (**a, b**) Subvolution of the triceps tendon

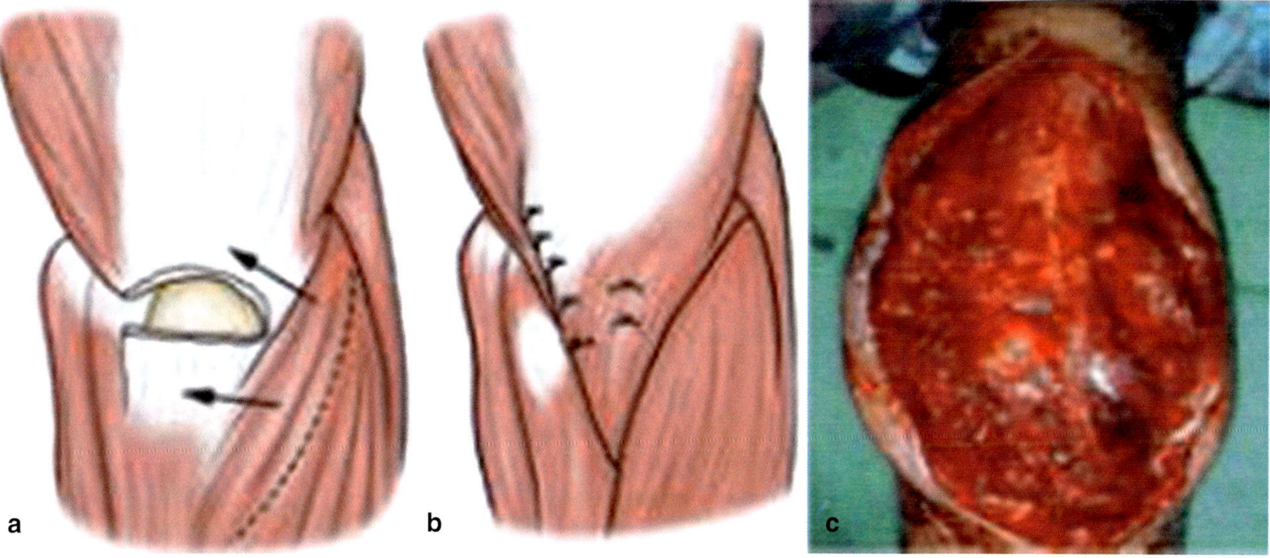

Fig. 9.115 (**a–c**) Anconeus transposition

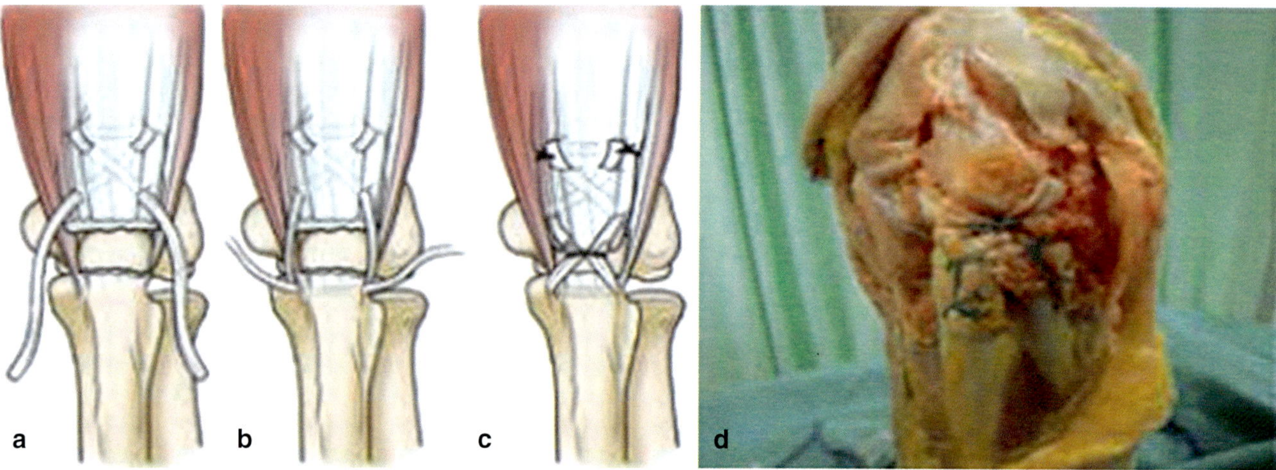

Fig. 9.116 Braiding repair of the tendon

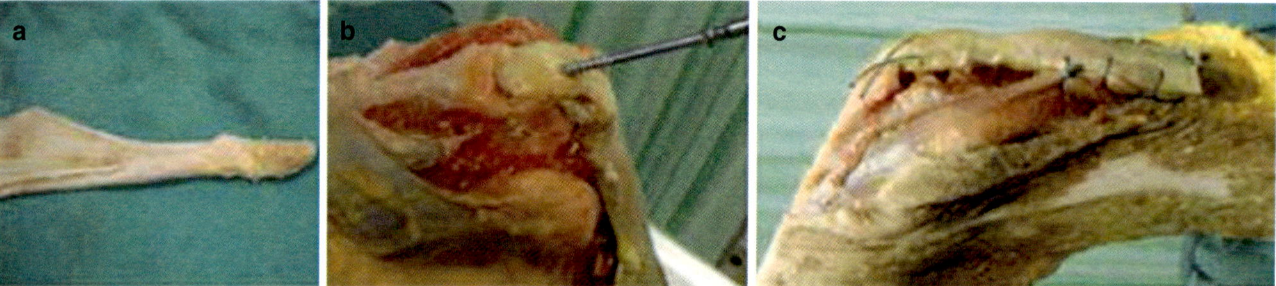

Fig. 9.117 (**a–c**) Achilles tendon transplantation with bone fragment

Achilles tendon transplantation with bone fragment: This surgery transplants the Achilles tendon with calcaneus. Remove the cortical bone with a drill at the olecranon top, so as to provide a contact area with the bone fragment of the transplanted tendon. The transplanted bone fragments are mostly wedge-shaped. Retain the bone fragment with a thickness of about 1.5 cm. Use an arc oscillating saw to trim the bones in order that the arc fits the olecranon surface (Fig. 9.117a). Trim the tendons and muscle tissues. Use 4.5 mm half-threaded cancellous screws to fix the bone graft (Fig. 9.117b). A washer can be used when necessary. After the graft is fixed at the distal end, cover the triceps gap and the proximal triceps fascia with part of the tendon. Adjust the tension, and suture the transplanted tendon in place with 2# non-absorbable braiding suture. Then flex the elbow joint 20°~30°, pull the triceps distally as far as possible, suture the triceps brachii with the Achilles tendon stump, and suture the remaining Achilles tendon to the medial and lateral edges of the triceps belly (Fig. 9.117c) [57].

9.6.3.4 Postoperative Rehabilitation and Prognosis

One-stage repair

1. Remove the splint 10~14 days after surgery, and change to a hinge bracket with a flexion range of 30°~45°.
2. Active elbow flexion and passive elbow extension are allowed.
3. If it is difficult to reach full elbow extension by passive activities, the elbow extension splint can be used for fixation at night.
4. Gradually increase the flexion range within the 3rd~6th weeks. Allow full-range active extension and flexion of the elbow joint after the 6th week and passive elbow flexion after the 8th weeks.
5. Triceps isometric contraction training can be performed during the 10th~12th week until complete recovery.
6. No restrictions on activities 5 months after surgery.

Delayed repair

The postoperative rehabilitation of the anconeus transposition, V-Y plasty of the triceps tendon, triceps subvolution and autologous or allogeneic tendon transplantation are just the same with the one-stage repair. If tendon transplantation is chosen, in order to achieve adequate revascularization of the transplanted tendon, all the steps must be postponed by 2 weeks compared to the one-stage repair [58].

Prognosis

The effect of surgery depends on the type of injury. Acute injury has a good surgery effect. For most patients who undergo one-stage repair within 3~4 weeks after injury, the loss of elbow extension function is expected to be 5°~10°, and muscle strength can be restored to 90% of the normal level. In cases of professional American football players, 10 out of 11 patients restored their original exercise level without significant strength loss or limited mobility. A paper with the largest case number on triceps injury reported that all the patients achieved satisfactory results. During our long-term follow-up, we found that delayed surgery did not affect the final outcome. For injuries more than 3 weeks, reconstruction surgery and longer recovery time were required.

The prognosis of patients with pathological injuries varies greatly, depending on the quality of the damaged tissues and other local and systemic factors. The result of iatrogenic injury is not as good as traumatic injury, but it can still achieve relatively ideal outcomes. For these patients, the success rate of direct repair is lower than that of reconstruction (e.g., anconeus transposition or allogeneic Achilles tendon reconstruction) [59].

9.6.3.5 Complications and Key Points

The main complication is the re-fracture of the repair site. It has been reported that 3 of 23 patients had re-rupture after repair, and 1 had temporary ulnar nerve palsy after tension band fixation of the olecranon fracture.

For triceps tendon rupture, direct repair has the best effect. It should be noted that, before the final fixation of any repair and fixation technique, the triceps brachii must be pulled, so that the damage at the original anatomical insertion is completely repaired. To test whether the intraoperative tension of the triceps brachii is appropriate, the arm should be supported, and the forearm should be kept relaxed. It is recommended to repair and fix the triceps tendon when the elbow joint is flexed at 20°, and then check whether the tension of the forearm is appropriate within the motion range of 0°~90°. Too tight or too loose tension of the triceps brachii can also affect elbow recovery after surgery [60].

9.6.4 Repair and Reconstruction of Distal Rupture of the Biceps Tendon

Xing Danmou and Feng Wei

Abstract Distal biceps tendon rupture is relatively rare in clinical practice, accounting for 3% to 5% of biceps tendon ruptures. Improper diagnosis and treatment will usually result in weakened forearm flexion and supination, which affects the daily work and life. Therefore, early diagnosis and treatment are very important. Acute rupture of the distal biceps tendon should be fixed to the radius tubercle if possible. Usually, patients engaged in heavy physical work or activities are prone to suffering from the distal biceps tendon rupture. The biceps tendon is mostly ruptured from its attachment to the radius tubercle, so its function is almost completely lost. This article introduces several surgical approaches and repair techniques in detail. Surgical approaches include the modified Henry approach or the Boyd-Anderson double-incision approach. The advantage of the modified Henry approach is the small possibility of heterotopic ossification, but the disadvantage is that there is a risk of radial nerve injury. The advantage of the double-incision approach is to reduce the possibility of radial nerve injury. The initial Boyd-Anderson approach exposes the ulna, which may result in heterotopic ossification. In recent years, the modified MAYO–Boyd–Anderson approach has been widely applied. This technique does not expose the ulna, which will rarely cause heterotopic ossification [61].

Distal biceps tendon rupture is relatively rare in clinical practice, accounting for 3% to 5% of biceps tendon ruptures. It mostly happens when the elbow joint is in flexion position and suffers eccentric force. Improper diagnosis and treatment will usually result in weakened forearm flexion and supination, which affects the daily work and life. Therefore, early diagnosis and prompt treatment are very important (Fig. 9.118). Recent research has focused on the early diagnosis, reduction principles, and surgical incision selection of distal biceps tendon rupture. [62]

9.6.4.1 Direct Repair Method of Distal Biceps Tendon Rupture

Acute rupture of the distal biceps tendon should be fixed to the radius tubercle if possible. Usually, patients engaged in heavy physical work or activities are prone to suffering from the distal biceps tendon rupture. The biceps tendon is mostly ruptured from its attachment to the radius tubercle, so its function is almost lost. Surgical approaches

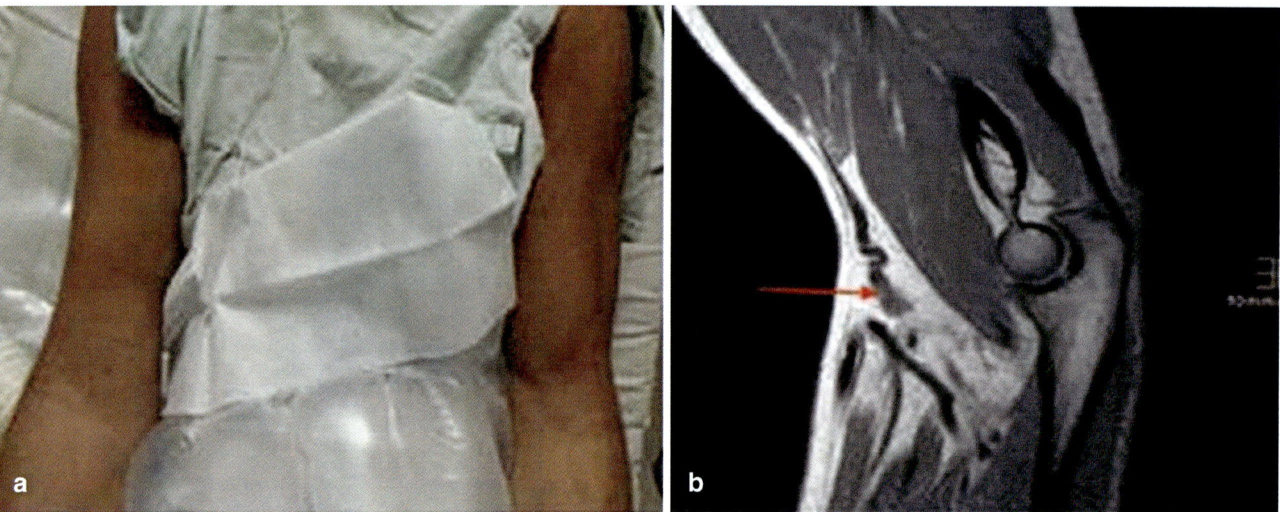

Fig. 9.118 Distal biceps tendon rupture. (**a**) Comparing the right upper arm with the uninjured left upper arm, the anti-Popeye sign appears; (**b**) MRI. The red arrow indicates that the distal biceps tendon is completely ruptured and the stump is retracted

include the modified Henry approach and the Boyd–Anderson double-incision approach. The advantage of the modified Henry approach is the slim possibility of heterotopic ossification, but the disadvantage is that there is a risk of radial nerve injury. The advantage of the double-incision approach is to reduce the possibility of radial nerve injury. The initial Boyd–Anderson approach exposes the ulna, which may result in heterotopic ossification. In recent years, the modified MAYO–Boyd–Anderson approach has been widely used. This technique does not expose the ulna, which will rarely cause heterotopic ossification [63].

The tendon contracture makes the delayed fixation difficult. If this happens, it is better to fix the tendon to the radius tubercle than to the brachialis.

For patients without obvious dysfunction, delayed fixation is contraindicated. This situation often occurs in patients with less activities, however, such patients rarely suffer this injury. For those who have been delayed for 3 weeks before fixation, comprehensive consideration should be taken. At this time, the biceps tendon has retracted into the muscle belly, and there is no sufficient length to reach the radius tubercle. Furthermore, the path to the radius tubercle has been scarred and adhered, which makes the surgery rather difficult [64].

If the injury exceeds 4 weeks, a more detailed separation is required in the anterior elbow area. If the tendon has retracted into the muscle belly, it is the best choice to restore its length with an allogeneic Achilles tendon. These possible situations must be evaluated and prepared ahead of the surgery [65].

Delayed reconstruction is complicated and requires experienced orthopedic surgeons. Allogeneic Achilles tendon transplantation would be an option.

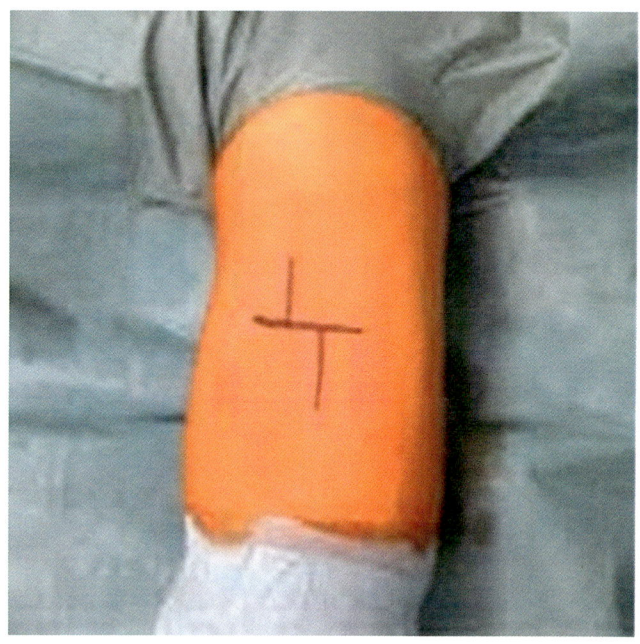

Fig. 9.119 The S-shaped incision with a length of 4 cm on the antecubital fossa

1. *Surgical Techniques and Methods*

   Under brachial plexus anesthesia, the patient is in a supine position with upper limb routinely disinfected. A 4 cm long S-shaped incision is made on the antecubital fossa (Fig. 9.119) [66].

   Preparation of the tendon stump: Identify the tendon stump by palpating and separating the surrounding fascia tissues. Separate the tendon stump from the incision (Fig. 9.120). The tendon end curls into a ball and needs to be trimmed into the shape suitable for fixation at the tubercle. After the tendon is trimmed (Fig. 9.120), pass two 5#

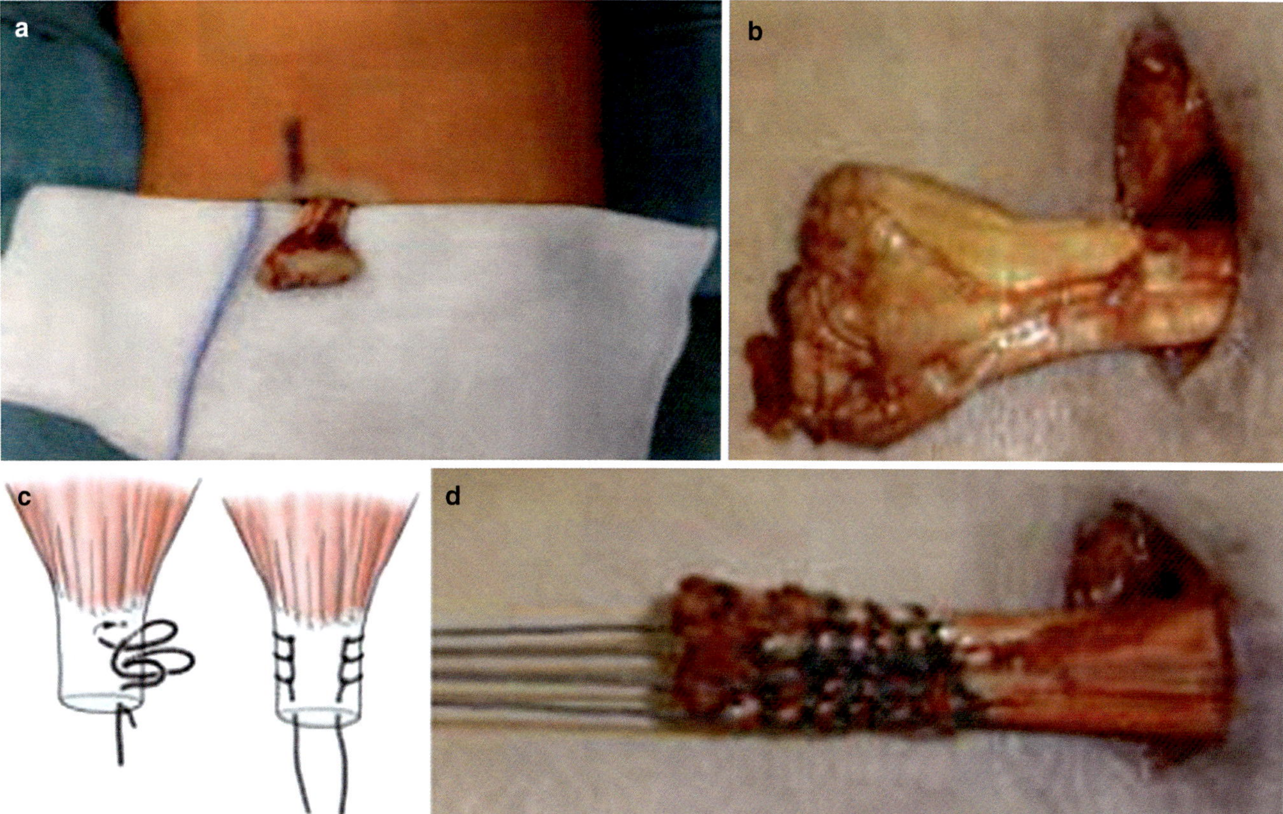

Fig. 9.120 Preparation of the tendon stump. (**a**) Identify the tendon by palpation. Separate it from the incision, showing the spherical degeneration of the raptured end of the tendon; (**b**~**d**) Pass two 5# non-absorbable sutures through the tendon stump, and suture with the Bunnell cross suture or the Krackow locking suture

silk sutures through the tendon stump and enter the tendinous tissue. Use cross suture (Bunnell method) or locking suture (Krackow method, Fig. 9.120). Insert a hemostatic forceps into the original path of the biceps tendon. Cross over the radius tubercle through the interspace between the ulnar and radius, and contact the tendon stump. Rotate the forearm, so as to ensure the proper position of the radial fixation on the ulnar side. The hemostatic forceps moves forward until it penetrates the muscle layer and subcutaneous tissue to the radial dorsal side of the proximal forearm (Fig. 9.121). Cut and separate the extensor and supinator muscles on the protrusion (Fig. 9.122). The forearm is completely pronated to determine the radial tubercle and clear the surrounding soft tissues [67].

Fixation: Use a high-speed drill to remove the cancellous bone at the midpoint of the tubercle. Drill a hole with a size of (10~12) cm × (7~8) cm as the implantation site for the tendon. Then drill 3 small holes on the radial side of the tubercle (Fig. 9.123). The forearm is slightly supinated to facilitate the drill and keep the holes of radial tubercle in good alignment. The small holes drilled should retain sufficient bone to prevent bone splitting or suture avulsion (Fig. 9.124).

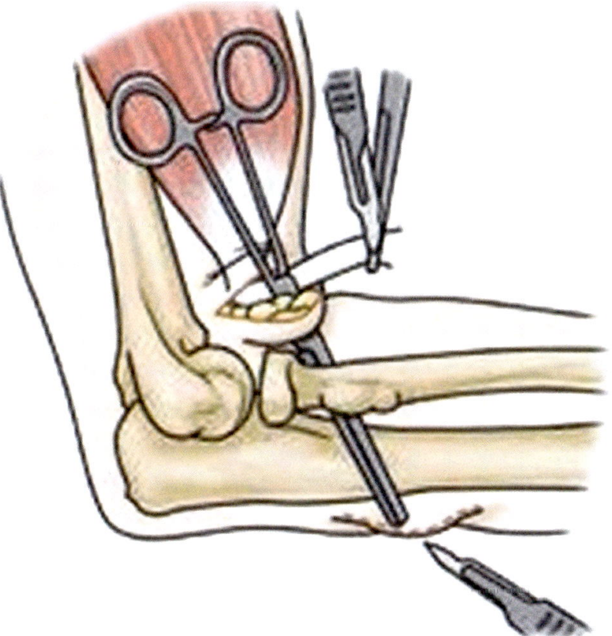

Fig. 9.121 The hemostatic forceps moves between the ulna and the radial tubercle, passing through the muscle belly of extensor digitorum to the lateral skin of the proximal forearm

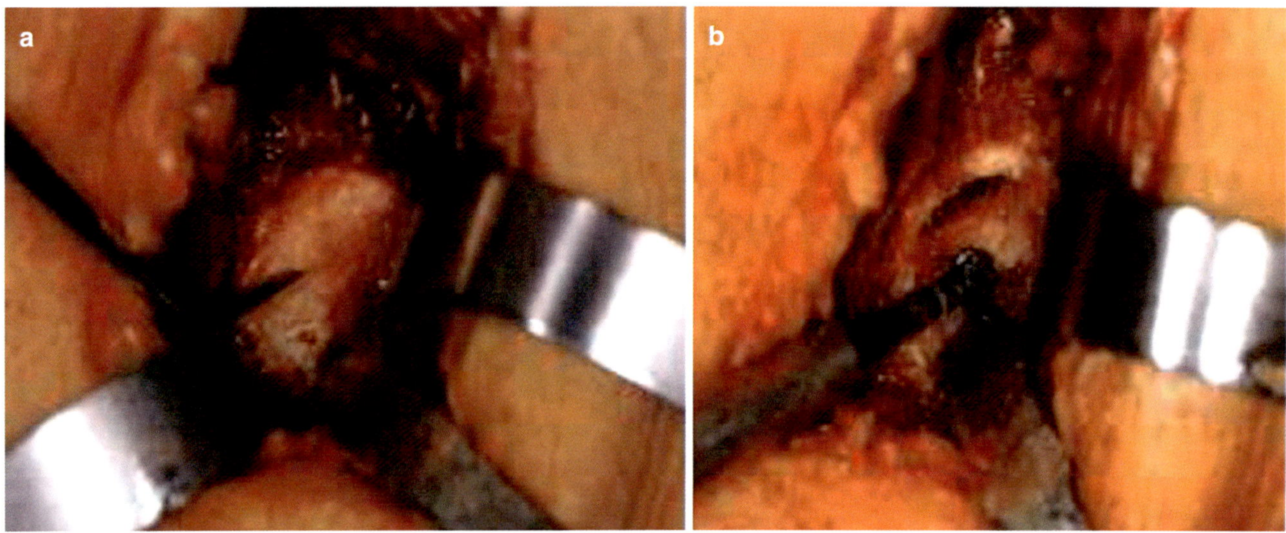

Fig. 9.122 Preparation of tendon stump. (**a**) Cut and separate the muscles on the protrusion. The forearm is fully pronated to reveal the tubercle; (**b**) Drill a hole on the radial tubercle with a high-speed drill to provide the implantation site for biceps tendon

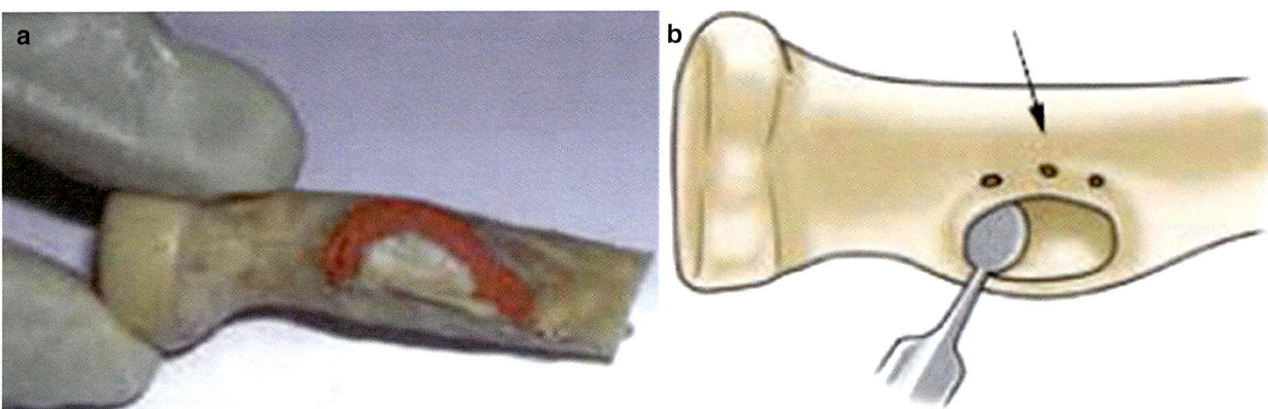

Fig. 9.123 (**a–b**) Drilling on the radial side of the radial tubercle

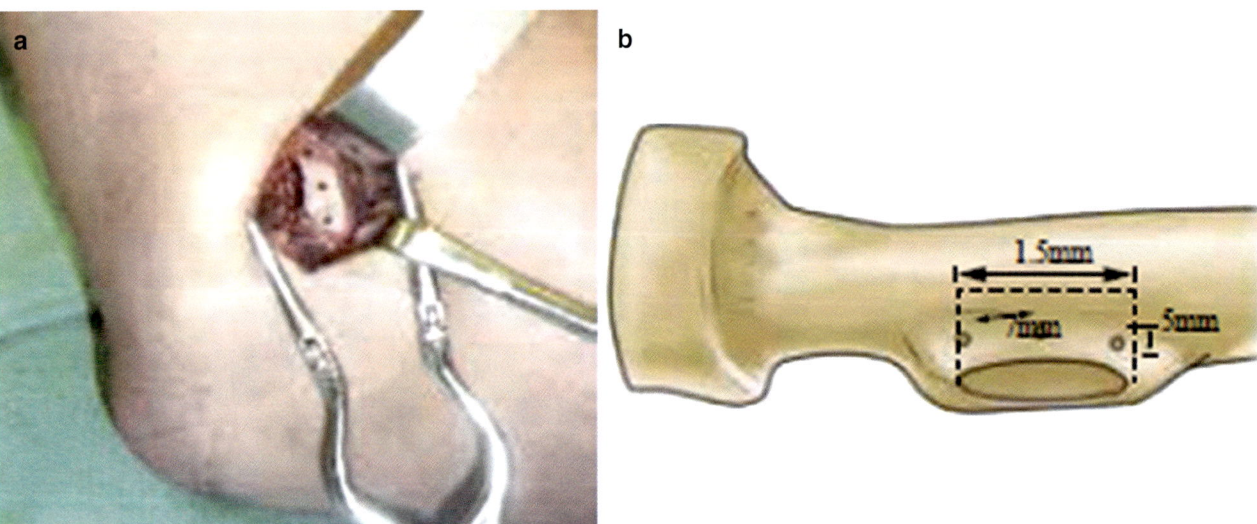

Fig. 9.124 (**a–b**) Pay attention to keep sufficient hole spacing for suture fixation

Tendon fixation: Hold the suture with hemostatic forceps and place back the biceps tendon through the anterior incision of the elbow. Pull the fixed end from the second incision along the tunnel (Fig. 9.125). The tendon is then pulled along the tunnel from the anterior elbow area and through the ulnar side of the radial tubercle (Fig. 9.126). The anterior area passes the suture on the ulnar side of the tubercle and passes through the small holes on the tubercle edge. One suture passes through the proximal end and the middle hole, and the other suture passes through the middle and distal holes (Fig. 9.127). The biceps tendon is inserted into the tubercle, while the forearm is slightly supinated. With the forearm kept slightly supinated, the sutures are knotted (Fig. 9.128).

Incision suture: Confirm that slight pronation or supination does not affect ulnar rotation. Straighten the forearm to ensure there is no excessive contraction of the biceps. Separate the fascia on the muscles of proximal forearm, and suture it with Absorbable 2-0 VICRYL®Plus Suture (Polyglactin 910, Ethicon Inc.). After the in-situ suture of the anterior elbow, place a drainage tube. Routinely suture the subcutaneous tissues and the skin. Suture the posterior lateral incision layer by layer [68].

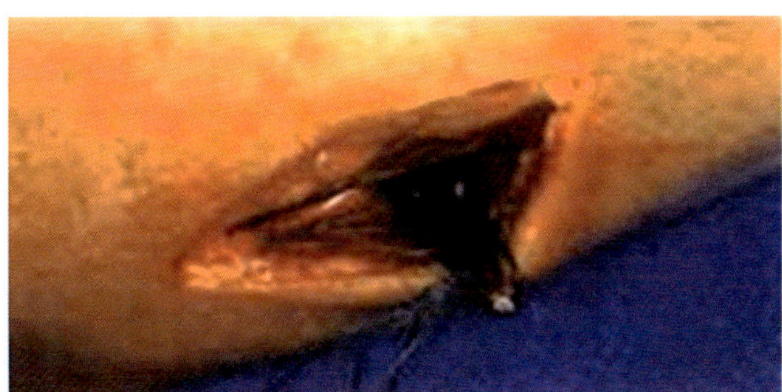

Fig. 9.125 Pull the suture with hemostatic forceps through the biceps tendon tunnel

Surgical Technique: Suture Using Anchors with Sutures Use the Henry or modified Henry incision when fixing with anchors with sutures (Fig. 9.129). It reveals that the radial nerve reaches distal supinator on lateral biceps brachii (Fig. 9.130). Separate the fascia and ligate the radial reverse artery to expose the radial tubercle (Fig. 9.131). When using the anchors with sutures, part of the bone is removed from the tubercle, and two anchors with sutures are inserted into the tubercle base where part of the bone is removed (Fig. 9.132). Pass the suture through the tendon stump and suture at the proximal end of the tendon. Trim the stump and implant it into the prepared fixation hole (Fig. 9.133). Knot while the forearm rotated in a neutral position [69].

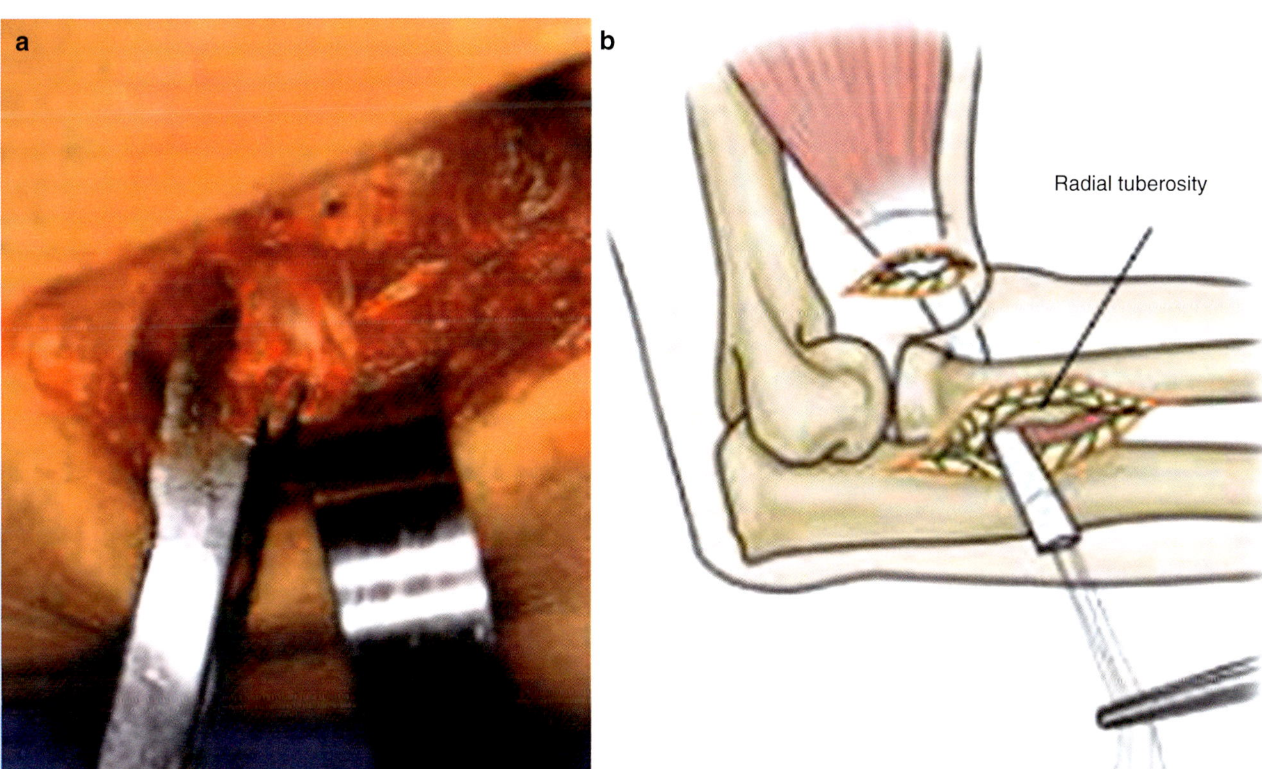

Fig. 9.126 (**a–b**) The tendon passes through the forearm incision

9.6.4.2 Delayed Reconstruction

When the tendon is retracted and cannot be directly fixed to the radial tubercle, an allogeneic Achilles tendon can be applied to increase the tendon length.

When using the allogeneic Achilles tendon transplantation, the exposure should be extensive, and the biceps brachii must be exposed (Fig. 9.134). Confirm that the biceps tendon is not sufficient for re-fixation (Fig. 9.135). Separate bluntly and expose the radial tubercle. Confirm the forearm incision location with hemostatic forceps (Fig. 9.136). Expose the radial tubercle, and remove part of the bone (Fig. 9.137). The calcaneus part of the allogeneic Achilles tendon complex must be carefully trimmed to be small enough and implanted into the radial tubercle and maintain the tendon-osseous integration at the same time (Fig. 9.138). Pass 5# non-absorbable suture through the small holes of the Achilles tendon complex and suture with the Krackow technique (Fig. 9.139), then fix it on the radial tubercle through the holes on the tubercle edge (Fig. 9.140). Flex the elbow at 45° and fix the Achilles tendon fascia around the biceps edge. In this way, the biceps brachii is pulled distally and enough to maintain proper tension (Fig. 9.141).

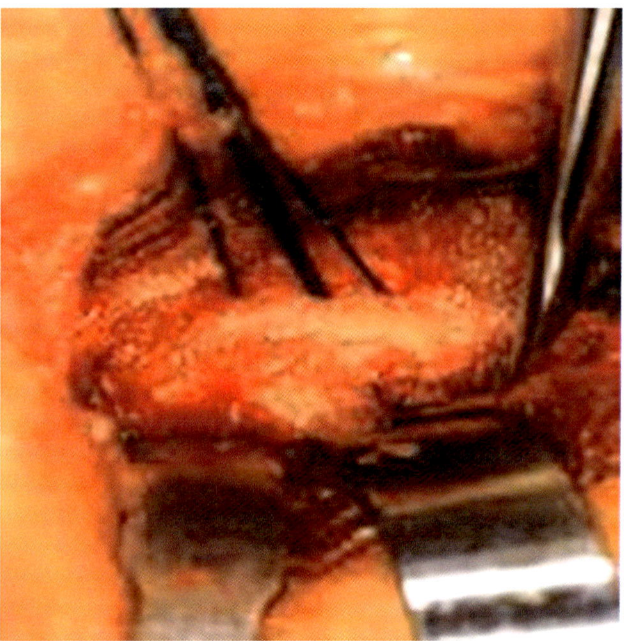

Fig. 9.127 Insert the distal biceps tendon into the hole in the radial tubercle where the cancellous bone is excavated. The suture passes through three small holes, with one end of each suture passes through the middle bone hole

9.6.4.3 Postoperative Management

1. *Acute Repair*

   The hinged external fixation orthosis is used to fix the elbow at 90°. The forearm rotates to a neutral position. Keep this position for 3~7 days. Remove the orthosis after about 1 week, and allow mild passive flexion. Active extension of the elbow to 30° after 1 week is encouraged. Four weeks after surgery, the patient is allowed to resist the tolerable gravity and practice extension and flexion. Mild strength exercise of flexion can be performed at 6 week. Tolerable activities are allowed at 3 months. Activities without limit are allowed at 6 months after surgery.
2. *Allograft Reconstruction*

   For patients with allogeneic tendon transplantation, they will be trained on the CPM within 3 weeks after surgery. Passive activities begin from the 3rd week till the 6th week. Complete straighten of the elbow joint is not allowed until the 6th week. Active daily activities are allowed during 6~12 weeks. Tolerable activities are allowed during 3~6 months [70].

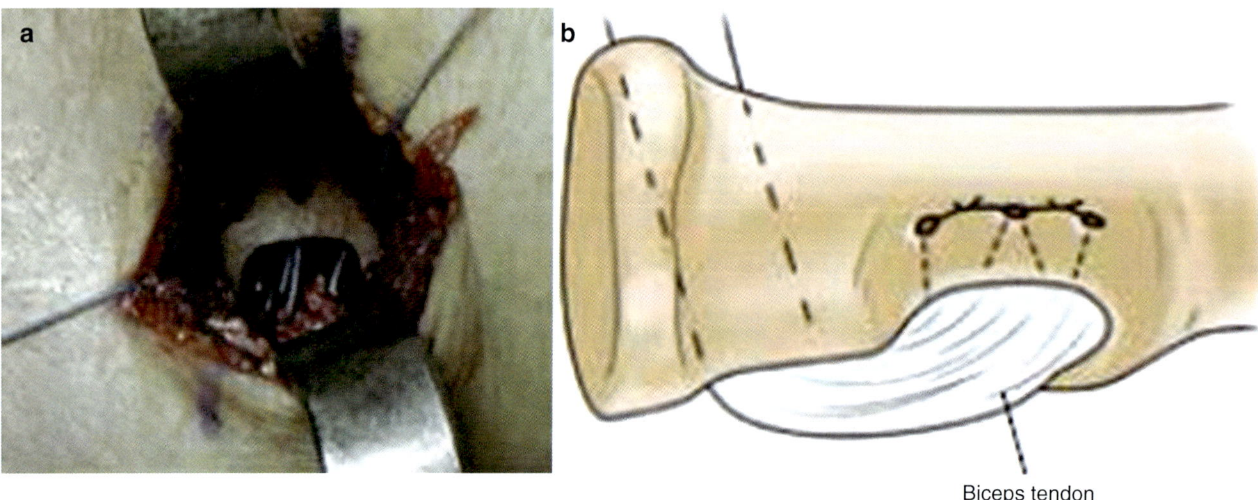

Fig. 9.128 (**a–b**) The forearm is slightly supinated to facilitate knotting

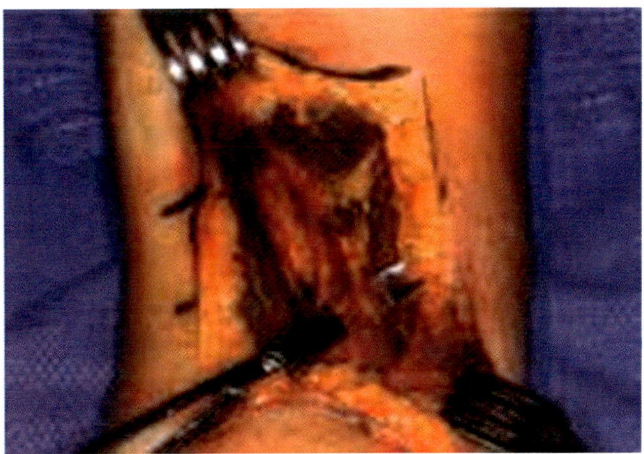

Fig. 9.129 Expose the tendon and aponeurotic fibrous tissue with the Henry technique

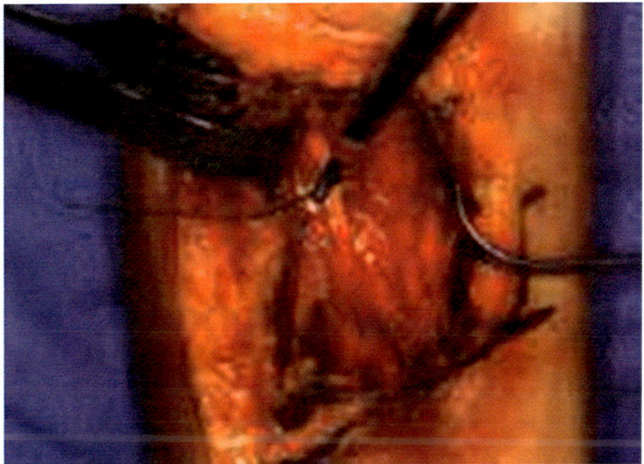

Fig. 9.130 The radial nerve runs between the brachioradialis and the lateral biceps brachii. Identify and ligate the radial reverse artery

9.6.5 Suture Techniques for Repair of Articular Cartilage Fractures Around the Elbow Joint

Xing Danmou and Wang Huan

9.6.5.1 Overview

Cartilage fractures around the elbow joint are a group of special types of intra-articular fractures. They include fractures of the capitellum and/or humeral trochlear or other fractures containing articular cartilage, such as the epicondyle of humerus, the lateral condyle, and the capitulum radii. The damaged structure is relatively superficial. It mainly involves the cartilage surface and is usually connected to only a small amount of the subchondral bone. This type of fracture is essentially a shell-shape exfoliation of the articular cartilage, with or without a small amount of the subchondral bone.

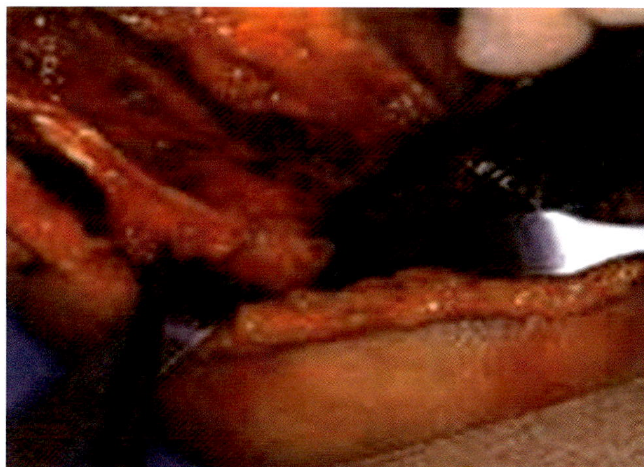

Fig. 9.131 Expose the radial tubercle

Treatment of this type of fracture is challenging. Fragments which are small and completely separated from articular surface, subchondral bones, small bone fragments, and multiple bone fragments should all be repaired. Due to the characteristics of the anatomical structure and limited space, the fixation difficulty increases greatly. However, each orthopedist has limited experience in dealing with such injuries due to its relatively low incidence [71].

For the treatment of articular cartilage fractures of the elbow joint, early scholars advocated the removal of the fragments, while other scholars advocated joint prosthesis replacement. With the further understanding of the anatomical structure and biomechanics of the elbow joint, the open reduction and internal fixation with the preservation of articular cartilage surgery is booming. Various internal fixation materials are currently used, mainly including micro plates, micro screws, absorbable rods, and self-reinforced absorbable cartilage screws. However, it is difficult to find suitable internal fixation materials to fix small cartilage fragments separated from articular surface, partially tilted articular surface cartilage and collapsing fractures of articular surface cartilage. With the development of suture-assisted fixation technique, these problems are being solved gradually.

9.6.5.2 Suture Techniques for Various Cartilage Fractures Around the Elbow Joint

1. *Suture-Assisted Plate Repair of Complex Radial Head and Neck Fractures*

   In the treatment of complex radial head and neck fractures with open reduction and internal fixation, proper auxiliary fixation with sutures can achieve satisfactory therapeutic effects. First, fix the large fragment from the

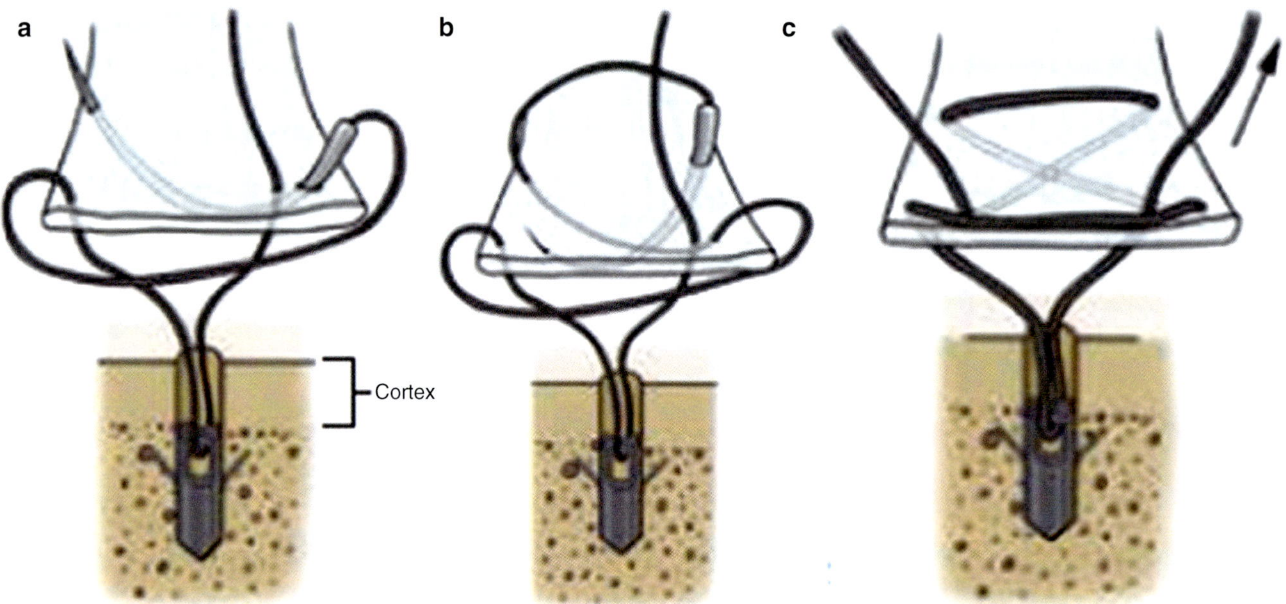

Fig. 9.132 (**a**~**c**) Excavate part of the bone in the radial tubercle. Two anchors with sutures are fixed into the radial tubercle

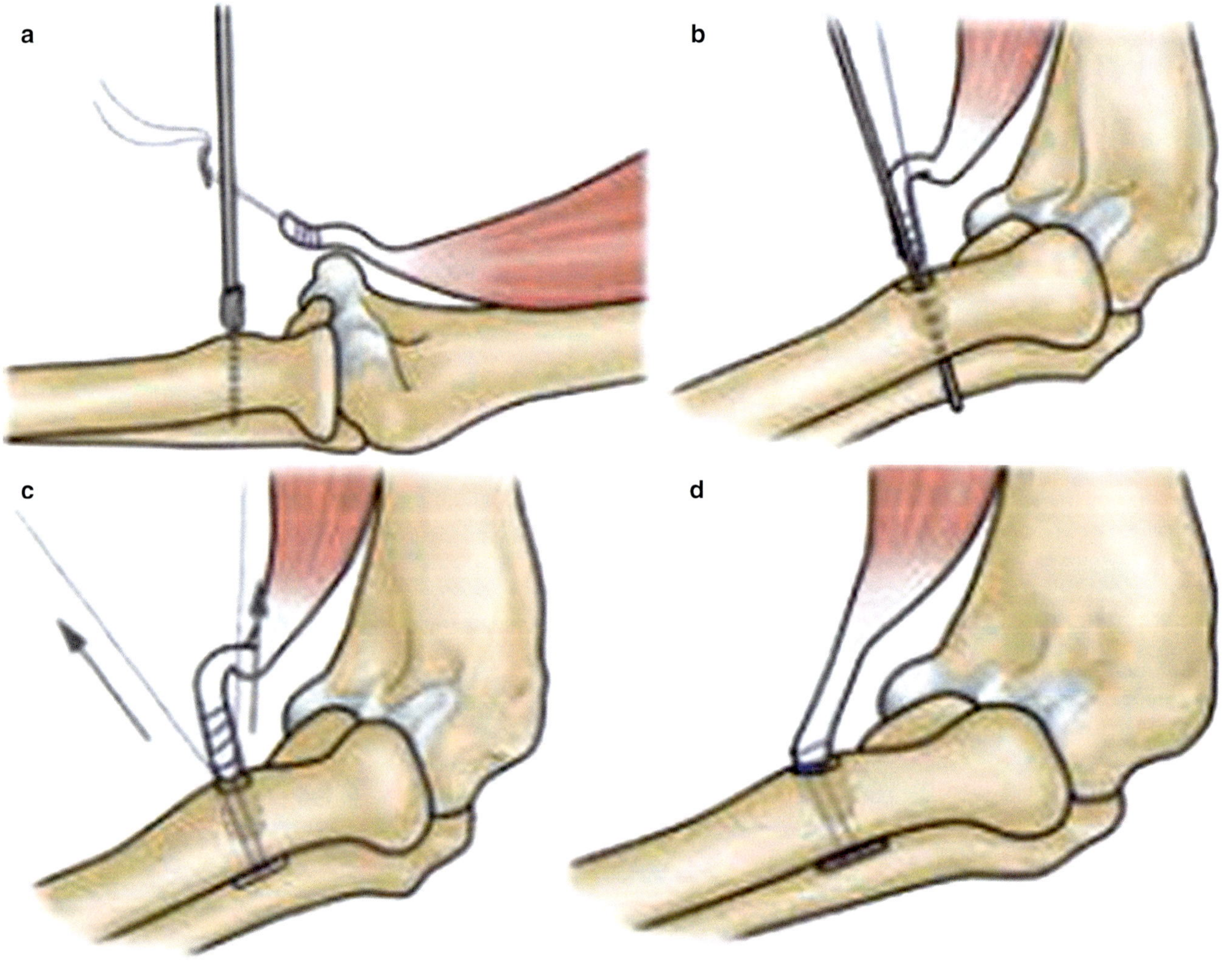

Fig. 9.133 Suture the tendon with cross suture or the Krackow technique, and then fix it to the radial tubercle (**a**~**d**)

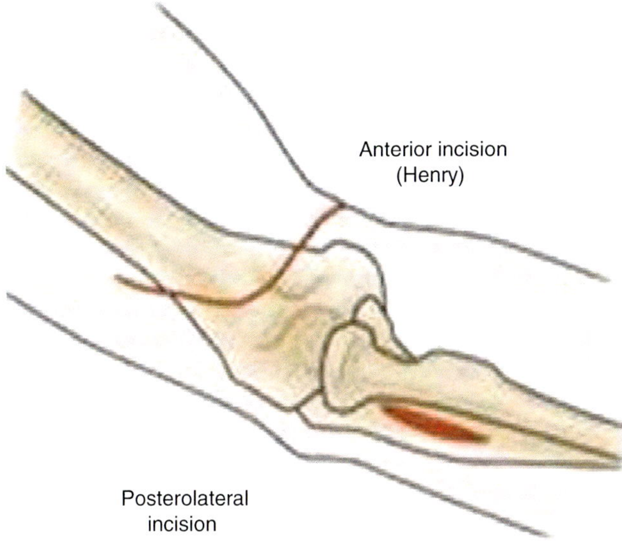

Fig. 9.134 Application of double-incision technique, the anterior elbow incision of the Henry technique, the posterolateral 4 cm incision on the proximal forearm: the incision on the anterior elbow area needs to be extended to expose the biceps brachii

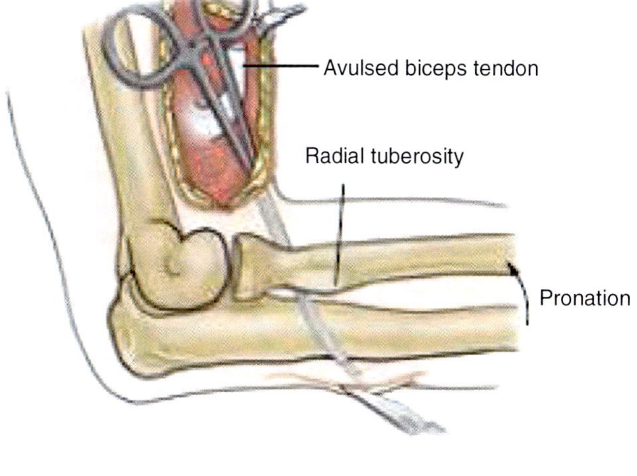

Fig. 9.136 The hemostatic forceps moves between the ulna and the radial tubercle, passing through the muscle belly of extensor digitorum to the lateral skin of the proximal forearm

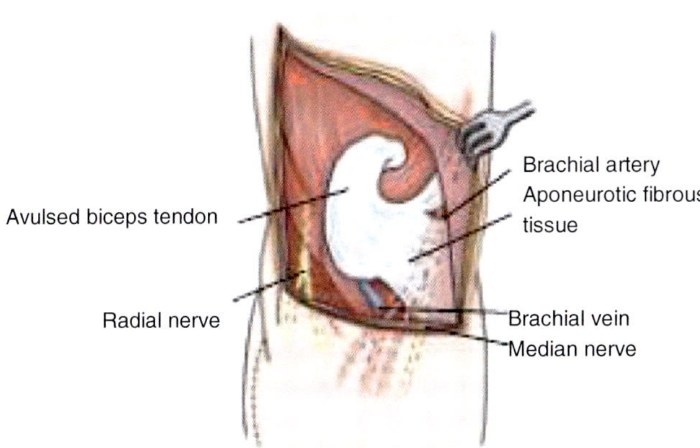

Fig. 9.135 The biceps tendon is usually retracted and varies in length, but its stump is sufficient to anastomose with various kinds of allograft tendons

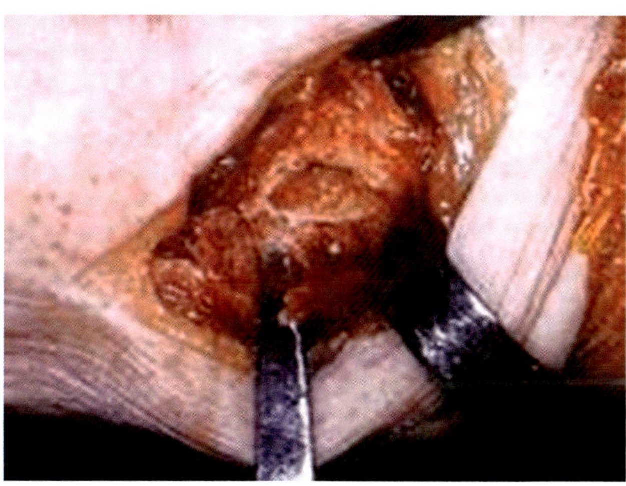

Fig. 9.137 Radial tubercle exposure and preparation

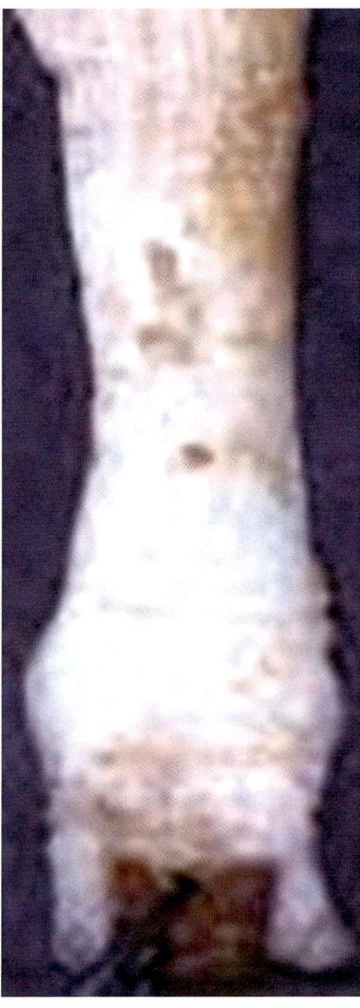

Fig. 9.138 The calcaneus part of the allogeneic Achilles tendon complex is complete and trimmed small enough to be completely implanted into the prepared hole in the radial tubercle

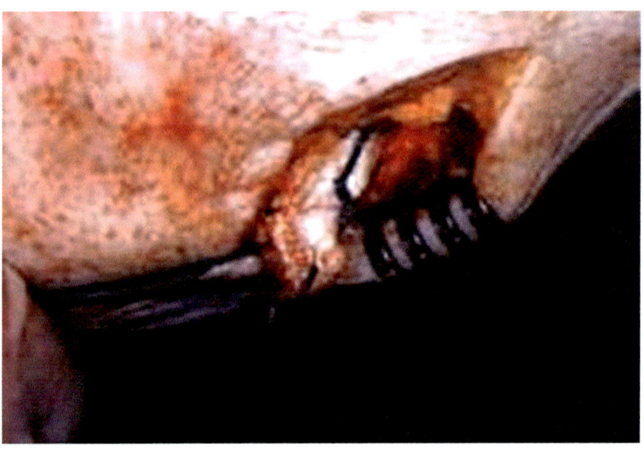

Fig. 9.139 The suture passes through the calcaneal hole. Fix the tendon with the Krackow technique

radial head with cartilage screws, and then fix the radial head and neck with the locking compression plate (LCP). For the cartilaginous or annular articular surface of the radial head which is still lifted after plate internal fixation, absorbable sutures can be used to pass through the plate holes or nail holes for auxiliary fixation (Fig. 9.142).

2. *"Suture Anchoring" Fixation Technique for Bone Fragments Separated from Articular Surface and Partially Lifted Articular Cartilage Surface* [72]

   In fractures of the capitellum, humeral trochlear, and capitulum radii, it is difficult to find suitable internal fixation materials to fix small cartilage fragments separated from articular surface, subchondral bones, small bone fragments, multiple bone fragments, and partially tilted articular surface cartilage. In this condition, the "suture anchoring" technique for suture fixation can be used.

   For example, when the cartilage surface or the annular articular surface of the radial head is lifted, the Absorbable 4-0 VICRYL®Plus Suture (Polyglactin 910, Ethicon Inc.) "suture anchoring" is used for fixation. That is, drill holes at the two ends of the lifted cartilage surface with 0.8 mm Kirschner wires. Introduce the absorbable suture by inserting a 7# syringe needle into the hole. Tighten and knot the suture to fix the cartilage surface on the bone surface (Fig. 9.143) [73].

   For example, for capitellum fracture which has small complete lifting on the articular cartilage surface, the "suture anchoring" technique can be used. Drill several holes with Kirschner wires on the lateral condyle to the defected edge of the cartilage. Insert a 7# syringe needle, and introduce an Absorbable 4-0 VICRYL®Plus Suture (Polyglactin 910, Ethicon Inc.) from the articular surface. Cross the surface of the free cartilage fragments and re-introduce the sutures to the lateral condyle through another hole. Tighten the suture and knot to fix the cartilage fragments to their original locations and main the integrality of the articular surface cartilage (Fig. 9.144).

3. *Suture Fixation Technique of Collapsing Fractures of Articular Surface Cartilage*

   In lateral dislocation of the elbow joint, the articular cartilage of the internal and external condyles of the humerus is directly hit by the ulna and radius, and collapsing fractures may occur. This type of fracture is special. The bone fragment is crescent-shaped, and the subchondral cancellous bone compresses and collapses. The crescent-shaped cartilage fragment is difficult to fix after the articular cartilage is reduced. The "suture anchoring" technique can also fix this type of fracture effectively [74].

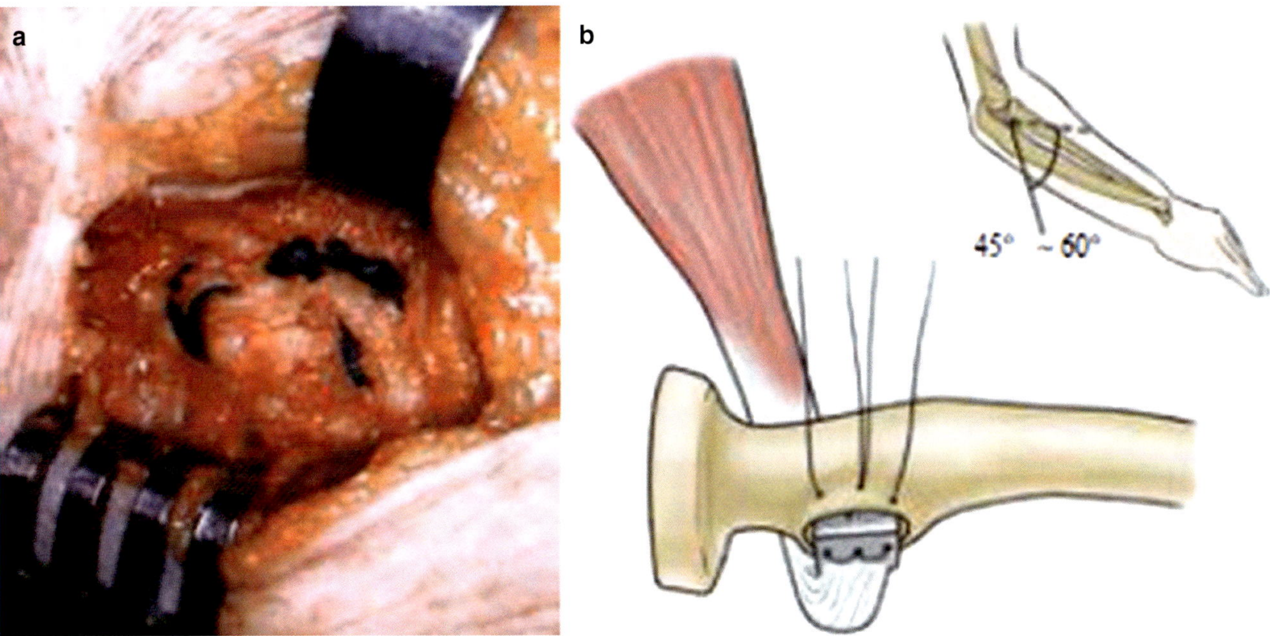

Fig. 9.140 (**a**, **b**) The calcaneal fragment is inserted into the hole in the radial tubercle. It passes through the tubercle edge and gets fixed

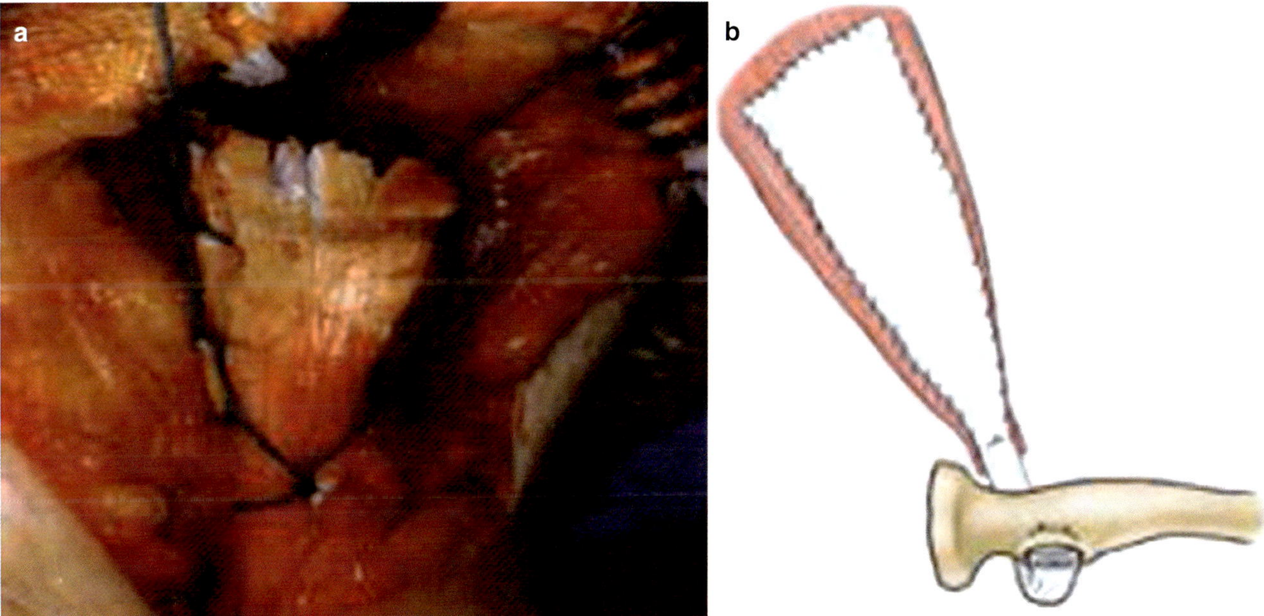

Fig. 9.141 (**a–b**) The Achilles tendon fascia is fixed around the belly of the biceps brachii with the elbow flexed at 60°

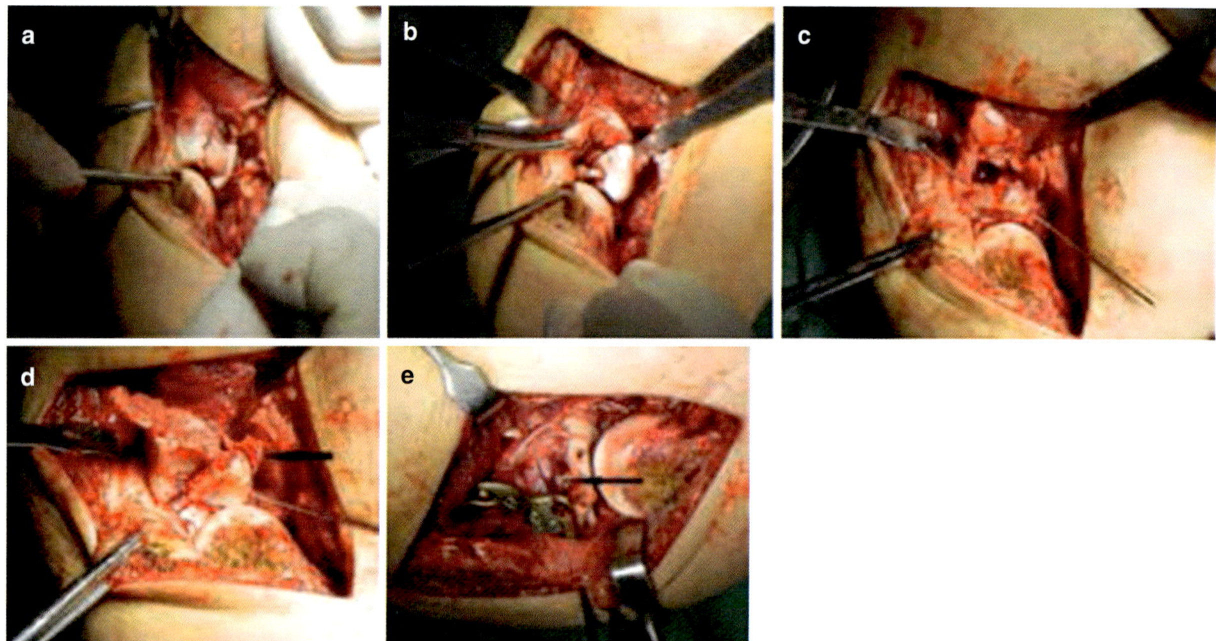

Fig. 9.142 Complex radial head and neck fracture **a**, **b**. (**a**, **b**) Comminuted fracture of the capitulum radii, forming several bone fragments; (**c**) Firstly reduce the larger bone fragment, and temporarily fix it with Kirschner wire; (**d**–**e**) Fix the reduced capitulum radii fragments with absorbable cartilage screws. Fix the radial head and neck fracture with LCP. For the cartilaginous or annular articular surface of the radial head which is still lifted after the fixation, absorbable sutures can be used to pass through the plate holes or nail holes for auxiliary fixation

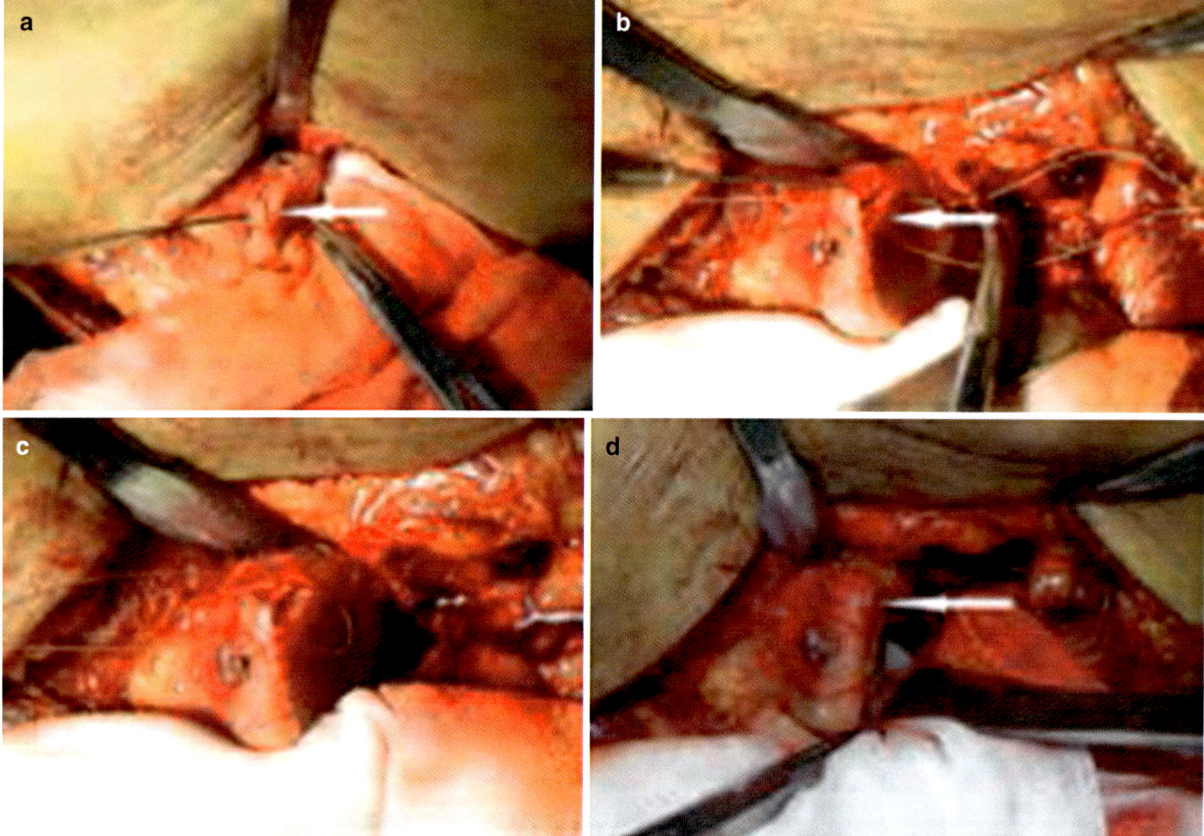

Fig. 9.143 The "suture anchoring" fixation technology. (**a**) Fix capitulum radii fracture with absorbable screws. There is still cartilage lifted on the annular articular surface; (**b**, **c**) Drill holes with 0.8 mm Kirschner wires at the two ends of the lifted cartilage surface and introduce sutures; (**d**) Tighten and knot the sutures to fix the lifted cartilage surface

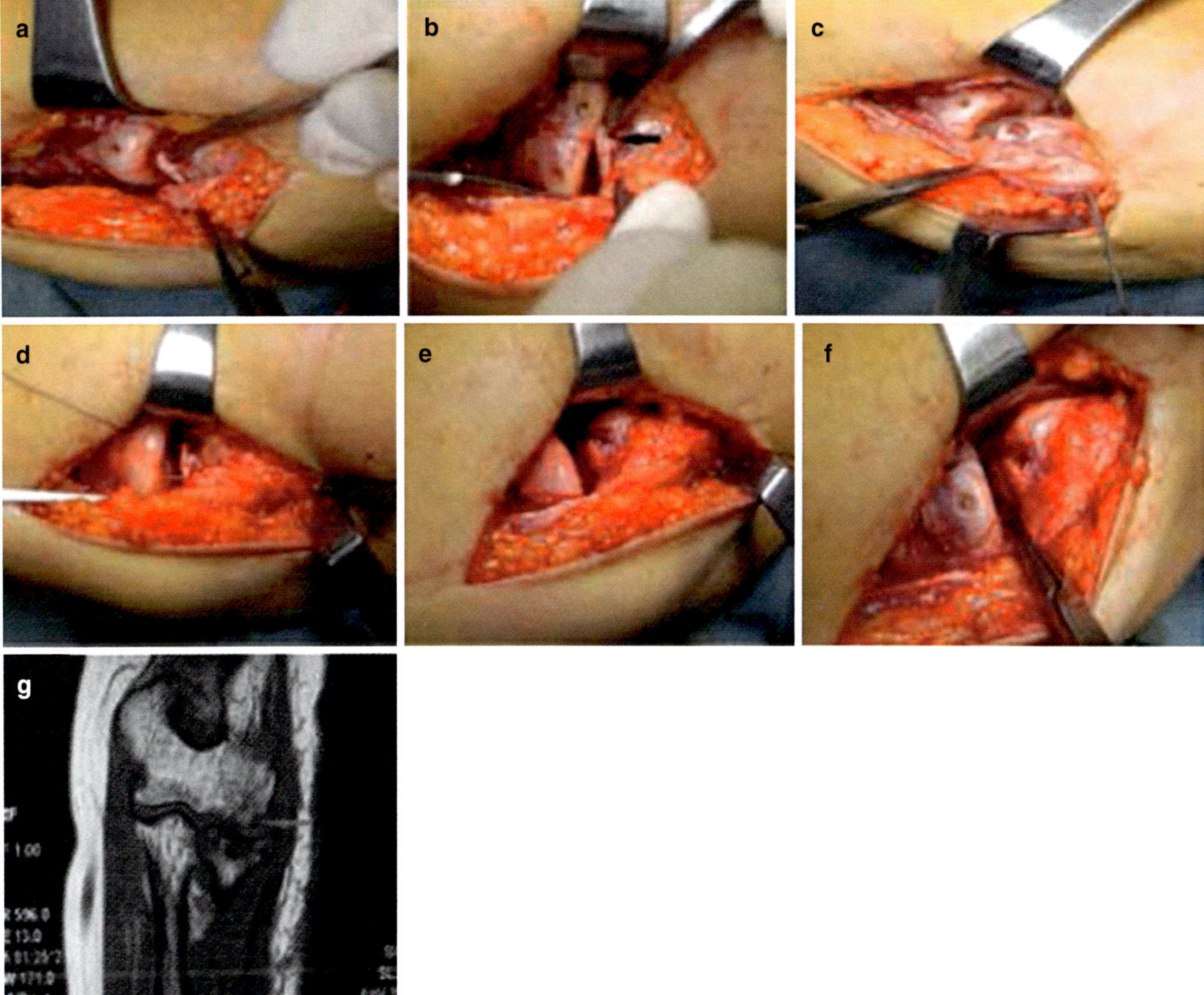

Fig. 9.144 Capitellum fracture. (**a**, **b**) Capitulum radii fracture combining capitellum fracture. The articular cartilage surface of the capitellum is lifted without subchondral bones. (**c**, **d**) Drill several holes with Kirschner wires on the lateral condyle to the defected edge of the cartilage. Insert a 7# syringe needle, and introduce 4-0 absorbable braiding sutures from the joint surface to the lateral condyle. Cross the surface of the free cartilage fragments. (**e**, **f**) Introduce the suture to the lateral condyle side of humerus. Tighten the suture and knot to fix the cartilage fragments to their original locations. (**g**) MRI shows that the articular cartilage surface is smooth without exfoliation at the 8th week after surgery

Take the crescent-shaped collapsing fracture of the trochlear edge of the internal condyle, for example. Reduce the collapsed cartilage fragment. Drill several holes I parallel from the lateral side of the medial condyle to the cartilage edge on the medial side of the fracture. Insert a 7# syringe needle, and introduce the Absorbable 4-0 VICRYL®Plus Suture (Polyglactin 910, Ethicon Inc.) to the articular surface. It crosses the surface of the cartilage fragment and binds the cartilage fragment with locking and continuous suture techniques. Tighten the suture on the lateral side of the medial condyle, and knot it to fix the bone fragment (Fig. 9.145) [75].

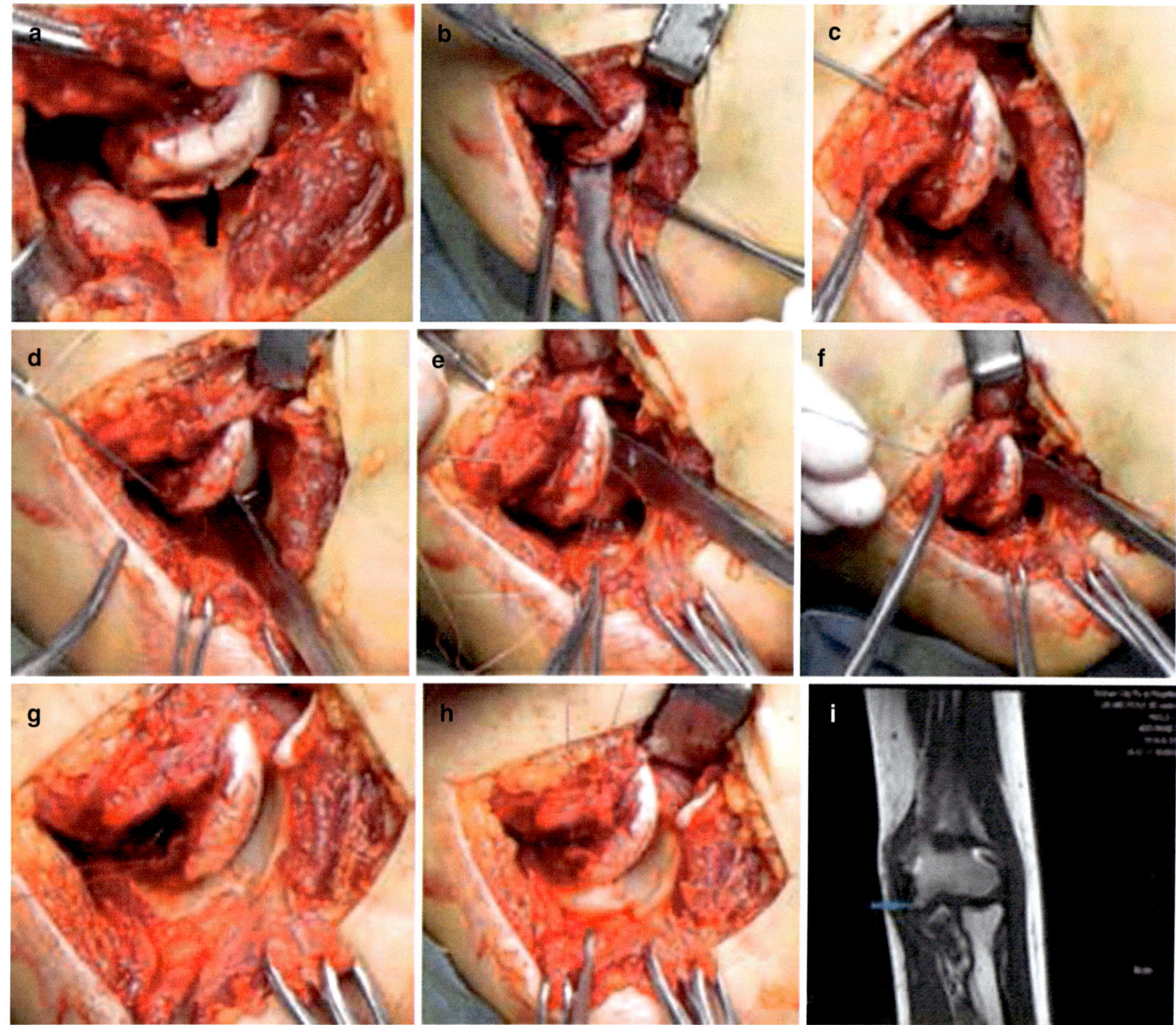

Fig. 9.145 Collapsing fractures of articular surface cartilage. (**a**, **b**) The crescent-shaped collapsing fracture of the trochlear edge of the internal condyle. The bone fragment collapses and shifts to the lateral side. The cancellous bone under the articular cartilage is compressed and collapsed. Lift and reduce the collapsed cartilage fragment. (**c**, **d**) Drill several holes in parallel from the lateral side of the medial condyle to the articular surface. Insert a 7# syringe needle, and introduce the 4-0 absorbable braiding suture to the articular surface. (**e**, **f**) Bind the cartilage fragment with locking and continuous suture techniques with the introduced suture. (**g**, **h**) Tighten the suture on the lateral side of the medial condyle and knot it to fix the bone fragment. 5 J. MRI shows the cartilage fragment heals well and the articular surface is smooth six months after surgery

References

1. Wilk KE, Obma P, Simpson CD, Cain EL, Dugas J, Andrews JR. Shoulder injuries in the overhead athlete. J Orthop Sports Phys Ther. 2009;39:38.
2. Buckley RE, Moran CG, AO. Principles of fracture management. 3rd ed. New York: Thieme; 2017.
3. Wiesel BB, Shaffer B, Williams GR. The shoulder. Orthop Surg Princ Diagnosis Treat. 2011.
4. Momma D, Nimura A, Muro S, Fujishiro H, Miyamoto T, Funakoshi T, Mochizuki T, Iwasaki N, Akita K. Anatomic analysis of the whole articular capsule of the shoulder joint, with reference to the capsular attachment and thickness. J Exp Orthop. 2018;5.
5. Lea MA, Makaram N, Srinivasan MS. Complex shoulder girdle injuries following mountain bike accidents and a review of the literature. BMJ Open Sport Exerc Med. 2016;2.
6. Jain NB, Wilcox RB, Katz JN, Higgins LD. Clinical examination of the Rotator Cuff. PM R. 2013.
7. Iyer KM. The shoulder. In: Iyer K, editor. Trauma management in orthopedics. London: Springer; 2013.
8. Beach H, Gordon P. Clinical examination of the shoulder. N Engl J Med. 2016;375:e24.
9. Azar FM, Beaty JH, Canale ST. Campbell's operative orthopaedics. 13th ed. London: Elsevier; 2017.
10. Tornetta P, Williams GR, Ramsey ML, Hunt TR, Wiesel SW. Operative techniques in orthopaedic trauma surgery; 2012.

11. Bakhsh W, Nicandri G. Anatomy and physical examination of the shoulder. Sports Med Arthrosc. 2018;26:e10.
12. Kates SL, Mears SC. A guide to improving the care of patients with fragility fractures. Geriatr Orthop Surg Rehabil. 2011;2(1):5–37.
13. Sandstrom CK, Kennedy SA, Gross JA. Acute shoulder trauma: what the surgeon wants to know. Radiographics. 2015;35:475–92.
14. Jarraya M, Roemer FW, Gale HI, Landreau P, D'Hooghe P, Guermazi A. MR-arthrography and CT-arthrography in sports-related glenolabral injuries: a matched descriptive illustration. Insights Imaging. 2016;7:167–77.
15. Buckley AT, Richard E, Moran Christopher G, AO. Principles of fracture management. 3rd ed. New York: Distribution by Georg Thieme Verlag; 2017.
16. Pouliquen L, Berhouet J, Istvan M, Thomazeau H, Ropars M, Collin P, Popeye sign: frequency and functional impact. Orthop Traumatol Surg Res. 2018.
17. Boileau P, Krishnan SG, Tinsi L, et al. Tuberosity malposition and migration: reasons for poor outcomes after hemiarthroplasty for displaced fractures of the proximal humerus. J Shoulder Elb Surg. 2002;11:401–12.
18. Kempton LB, Ankerson E, Wiater JM. A complication-based learning curve from 200 reverse shoulder arthroplasties. Clin Orthop Relat Res. 2011;469:2496–504.
19. Nyffeler RW, Werner CM, Gerber C. Biomechanical relevance of glenoid component positioning in the reverse Delta III total shoulder prosthesis. J Shoulder Elb Surg. 2005;14:524–8.
20. Roche C, Flurin PH, Wright T, et al. An evaluation of the relationships between reverse shoulder design parameters and range of motion, impingement, and stability. J Shoulder Elb Surg. 2009;18:734–41.
21. Roche CP, Marczuk Y, Wright TW, et al. Scapular notching in reverse shoulder arthroplasty: validation of a computer impingement model. Bull Hosp Jt Dis. 2013;71:278–83.
22. Mihata T, McGarry MH, Pirolo JM, Kinoshita M, Lee TQ. Superior capsule reconstruction to restore superior stability in irreparable rotator cuff tears: a biomechanical cadaveric study. Am J Sports Med. 2012;40(10):2248–55.
23. Qingwei Y, Yi J. Historical review and prospect of artificial shoulder arthroplasty. Chin J Bone Joint Injury. 2007;22(7):612–4.
24. Kanglai T, Qihong L, Yang L. Research progress of artificial shoulder joint. Chin J Orthop Surg. 2005;13(14):1099–101.
25. Kralinger F, Schwaiger R, Wambacher M, et al. Outcome after primary hemiarthroplasty for fracture of the humeral head. A retrospective multicentre study of 167 patients. J Bone Joint Surg-Br. 2004;86(2):217–9.
26. Abu-Rajab R, Stansfield BT, Nicol A, et al. Re-attachment of the tuberosities of the humerus following hemiarthroplasty for four part fracture. J Bone Joint Surg. 2006;88(11):1539–44.
27. Cahill JB, Cavanaugh B, et al. Total shoulder arthroplasty rehabilitation. Tech Should Elbow Surg. 2014;15(1):13–7.
28. O'Driscoll SW, Bell DF, Morrey BF. Posterolateral rotatory instability of the elbow. J Bone Jt Surg Am. 1991;73:440–6.
29. Shukla DR, McAnany S, Pean C, Overley S, Lovy A, Parsons BO. The results of tension band rotator cuff suture fixation of locked plating of displaced proximal humerus fractures. Injury. 2017;48(2):474–80.
30. Hinds RM, Garner MR, Tran WH, Lazaro LE, Dines JS, Lorich DG. Geriatric proximal humeral fracture patients show similar clinical outcomes to non-geriatric patients after osteosynthesis with endosteal fibular strut allograft augmentation. J Shoulder Elbow Surg. 2015, 24:889–96.
31. Gavaskar AS, Bhupesh Karthik B, Tummala NC, Srinivasan P, Gopalan H. Second generation locked plating for complex proximal humerus fractures in very elderly patients. JINJ. 6867:5.
32. Neer CS II. Displaced proximal humeral fractures. II. Treatment of three- part and four-part displacement. J Bone Joint Surg Am. 1970;52:1090–103.
33. Gallinet D, Clappaz P, Garbuio P, et al. Three or four parts complex proximal humerus fractures: hemiarthroplasty versus reverse prosthesis: a comparative study of 40 cases. Orthop Traumatol Surg Res. 2009;95:48–55.
34. Longo UG, Petrillo S, Berton A, et al. Reverse total shoulder arthroplasty for the management of fractures of the proximal humerus: a systematic review. Musculoskelet Surg. 2016;100:83–91.
35. Ross M, Hope B, Stokes A, et al. Reverse shoulder arthroplasty for the treatment of three-part and four-part proximal humeral fractures in the elderly. J Shoulder Elbow Surg. 2015;24:215–22.
36. Passaretti D, Candela V, Sessa P, et al. Epidemiology of proximal humeral fractures: a detailed survey of 711 patients in a metropolitan area. J Shoulder Elb Surg. 2017;26:2117–24.
37. Yuksel HY, Yilmaz S, Aksahin E, et al. The results of non operative treatment for three- and four-part fractures of the proximal humerus in low-demand patients. J Orthop Trauma. 2011;25:588–95.
38. Smith CD, Guyver P, Bunker TD. Indications for reverse shoulder replacement: a systematic review. J Bone Joint Surg Br. 2012;94(5):577–83.
39. Huegel J, Williams AA, Soslowsky LJ. Rotator cuff biology and biomechanics: a review of normal and pathological conditions. Curr Rheumatol Rep. 2015;17(1):476.
40. Micallef J, Pandya J, Low AK. Management of rotator cuff tears in the elderly population. Maturitas. 2019;123:9–14.
41. Thigpen CA, Shaffer MA, Gaunt BW, Leggin BG, Williams GR, Wilcox RB 3rd. The American Society of Shoulder and Elbow Therapists' consensus statement on rehabilitation following arthroscopic rotator cuff repair. J Shoulder Elb Surg. 2016;25(4):521–35.
42. Adams CR, DeMartino AM, Rego G, Denard PJ, Burkhart SS. The rotator cuff and the superior capsule: why we need both. Arthroscopy. 2016;32(12):2628–37.
43. Lewis JS. Rotator cuff tendinopathy. Br J Sports Med. 2009;43(4):236–41.
44. Gombera MM, Sekiya JK. Rotator cuff tear and glenohumeral instability: a systematic review. Clin Orthop Relat Res. 2014;472(8):2448–56.
45. Mazuquin BF, Wright AC, Russell S, Monga P, Selfe J, Richards J. Effectiveness of early compared with conservative rehabilitation for patients having rotator cuff repair surgery: an overview of systematic reviews. Br J Sports Med. 2018 Jan;52(2):111–21.
46. Pagnani MJ, Deng XH, Warren RF, Torzilli PA, Altchek DW. Effect of lesions of the superior portion of the glenoid labrum on glenohumeral translation. J Bone Joint Surg Am. 1995;77(7):1003–10.
47. Glasgow SG, Bruce RA, Yacobucci GN, Torg JS. Arthroscopic resection of glenoid labral tears in the athlete: a report of 29 cases. Arthroscopy. 1992;8(1):48–54.
48. Rowe CR. Recurrent transient subluxation of the shoulder. J Bone Joint Surg Am. 1981;63A:863–72.
49. Gill T. Open repairs for the treatment of anterior shoulder instability. Am J Sports Med. 2003;31:142–53.
50. McFarland E. The effect of variation in definition on the diagnosis of multidirectional instability of the shoulder. J Bone Joint Surg Am. 2003;85A:2138–44.
51. Henry JH, Genung JA. Natural history of glenohumeral dislocation revisited. Am J Sports Med. 1982;10:135–7.
52. Arciero RA, Wheeler JH, Ryan JB, McBride JT. Arthroscopic Bankart repair versus nonoperative treatment for acute, initial anterior shoulder dislocations. Am J Sports Med. 1994;22:589–94.

53. Kim SH, Ha KI, Cho YB, Ryu BD, Oh I. Arthroscopic anterior stabilization of the shoulder. Two to six-year follow-up. J Bone Joint Surg Am. 2003;85A(8):1511–8.
54. Miniaci A, McBirnie J. Thermal capsular shrinkage for treatment of multidirectional instability of the shoulder. J Bone Joint Surg Am. 2003;85A(12):2283–7.
55. Hartzler RU, Burkhart SS. Superior capsular reconstruction. Orthopedics. 2017;40:271–80.
56. Pallis M, et al. Epidemiology of acromioclavicular joint injury in young athletes. Am J Sports Med. 2012;40(9):2072–7.
57. Cisneros LN, Reiriz JS. Management of chronic unstable acromioclavicular joint injuries. J Orthop Traumatol. 2017;18(4):305–18.
58. Mazzocca AD, Spang JT, Rodriguez RR, Rios CG, Shea KP, Romeo AA, Arciero RA. Biomechanical and radiographic analysis of partial coracoclavicular ligament injuries. Am J Sports Med. 2008;36:1397–402.
59. Rios CG, Arciero RA, Mazzocca AD. Anatomy of the clavicle and coracoid process for reconstruction of the coracoclavicular ligaments. Am J Sports Med. 2007;35:811–7.
60. Cadenat FM. The treatment of dislocations and fractures of the outer end of the clavicle. Int Clin. 1917;1:145–69.
61. Rockwood CA. Disorders of the acromioclavicular joint. In: Rockwood CA, Matsen FA, editors. The shoulder. 4th ed. Philadelphia: WB Saunders; 2009. p. 453–526.
62. Spencer HT, Hsu L, Sodl J, Arianjam A, Yian EH. Radiographic failure and rates of re-operation after acromioclavicular joint reconstruction: a comparison of surgical techniques. Bone Joint J. 2016;98(B):512–8.
63. van Bergen CJA, van Bemmel AF, Alta TDW, van Noort A. New insights in the treatment of acromioclavicular separation. World J Orthop. 2017;8(12):861–73.
64. Cook JB, MD, Kevin P. Krul, MD. Challenges in treating acromioclavicular separations: current concepts. J Am Acad Orthop Surg. 2018;26:669–77.
65. Weaver JK, Dunn HK. Treatment of acromioclavicular injuries, especially complete acromioclavicular separation. J Bone Joint Surg Am. 1972;54:1187–94.
66. Millett PJ, Horan MP, Warth RJ. Two-year outcomes after primary anatomic coracoclavicular ligament reconstruction. Arthroscopy. 2015;31:1962–73.
67. Woodmass JM, Esposito JG, Ono Y, et al. Complications following arthroscopic fixation of acromioclavicular separations: a systematic review of the literature. Open Access J Sports Med. 2015;6:97–107.
68. Beitzel K, Cote MP, Apostolakos J, et al. Current concepts in the treatment of acromioclavicular joint dislocations. Arthroscopy. 2013;29:387–97.
69. Scheibel M, Dröschel S, Gerhardt C, Kraus N. Arthroscopically assisted stabilization of acute high- grade acromioclavicular joint separations. Am J Sports Med. 2011;39:1507–16.
70. Scheibel M, Ifesanya A, Pauly S, Haas NP. Arthroscopically assisted coracoclavicular ligament reconstruction for chronic acromioclavicular joint instability. Arthrosc Tech. 2016;5(6):e1239–46.
71. Beitzel K, Obopilwe E, Apostolakos J, et al. Rotational and translational stability of different methods for direct acromioclavicular ligament repair in anatomic acromioclavicular joint reconstruction. Am J Sports Med. 2014;42:2141–8.
72. Fukuda K, Craig E, An K, Cofield R, Chao E. Biomechanical study of the ligamentous system of the acromioclavicular joint. J Bone Joint Surg Am. 1986;68:434–40.
73. Oki S, Matsumura N, Iwamoto W, et al. The function of the acromioclavicular and coracoclavicular ligaments in shoulder motion: a whole-cadaver study. Am J Sports Med. 2012;40:2617–26.
74. Weinstein D, McCann P, McIlveen S, Flatow EL, Bigliani LU. Surgical treatment of complete acromioclavicular dislocations. Am J Sports Med. 1995;23:324–31.
75. Lafosse L, Baier GP, Leuzinger J. Arthroscopic treatment of acute and chronic acromioclavicular joint dislocation. Arthroscopy. 2005;21:1017.e1–8.

Incision Suture Technique After Total Hip and Knee Arthroplasty

10

Wei Chai, Ming Ni, Weijun Wang, Jun Fu, Minghui Sun, Yonggang Zhou, Jinyu Zhu, and Rui He

Abstract

Total hip arthroplasty and total knee arthroplasty (THA and TKA) are surgeries to replace severely damaged hip and knee joints in the human body by artificial joints. THA and TKA can significantly alleviate the pain of the patient's joints, improve function and the quality of life. As China is gradually becoming an aging society, according to the figures published by the National Bureau of Statistics of China, as of 2019, the data on the elderly population in our country is: the population over 60 years old account for 17.9% of the total population, and is growing rapidly at a rate of nine million per year; the population over 65 years old account for 12.6% of the total population. In 2022, it will become a deep aging society with the percentage of more than 14%, a super-aging society with the percentage of more than 20% in 2033, and then continue to rapidly increase to about 35% in 2060. Due to the large basic population, China has a huge number of the elderly population, and the number of elderly patients suffering from bone and joint diseases is increasing year by year, and the demand for THA and TKA is also gradually increasing. Kurtz et al. (J Bone Joint Surg Am 89(4):780–785, 2007) predicted in 2007 that the demand for hip and knee arthroplasty in the United States in 2020 would reach 380,000 and 1,520,000, and by 2030, it would reach 570,000 and 3,480,000. According to statistics from Professor Weng Xisheng of Peking Union Medical College Hospital, the number of hip and knee arthroplasty in China in 2019 was 577,000 and 375,000 respectively, an increase of 31% and 50% compared with 2018.

With the increase THA and TKA, surgical complications also receive increasing attention, one of which is incision complications. Common incision complications after THA and TKA include drainage, swelling, ecchymosis, blisters, dehiscence, superficial and deep infections, etc. The incidence reported in the literature ranges from 0.2%–21% (Saleh et al., J Orthop Res 20(3):506–515, 2002; Patel et al., J Bone Joint Surg Am 89(1):33–38, 2007; Adelani et al., Bone Joint J 96-B(5):619–621, 2014; Wagenaar et al., J Arthroplast 34(1):175–182, 2019). Once there is surgical incision complication, more dressing changes, debridement, and even repeated surgeries may be indicated, which will prolong the patient's hospital stay and treatment time, delay early functional exercise, increase the incidence of periprosthetic joint infection (PJI) (Atkins et al., J Arthroplast 34(2S):S85–S92, 2019), lead to lower patient satisfaction, medical resource consumption, lower hospital operation efficiency, increased workload of doctors and increased risk of medical disputes. On the contrary, good incision healing can also shorten the patient's hospital stay and reduce medical expenses. At the same time, a beautiful incision can also significantly increase the patient's satisfaction with the surgical effect. Therefore, in artificial joint arthroplasty surgeries, we need to pay attention to the incision and suturing technique of the surgical incision and select the appropriate materials to close the incision to obtain the best incision healing and reduce complications.

This chapter will focus on the incision and closure in hip and knee arthroplasty surgeries, taking the commonly used posterolateral approach, lateral approach, anterior approach of the hip arthroplasty, and medial parapatellar approach of the knee arthroplasty as examples, and intro-

W. Chai (✉) · M. Ni · J. Fu · Y. Zhou
Department of Orthopedics, The First Medical Center of PLA General Hospital, Beijing, China
e-mail: zhouyg@263.net

W. Wang · M. Sun
Nanjing Drum Tower Hospital, Nanjing, China

J. Zhu
Shenzhen University General Hospital, Shenzhen, China

R. He
The Southwest Hospital of AMU, Luzhou, China

P. Tang et al. (eds.), *Tutorials in Suturing Techniques for Orthopedics*, https://doi.org/10.1007/978-981-33-6330-4_10

duce the techniques of the surgical incision, soft tissue closure, and related precautions, as well as the prevention and treatment of complications.

Keywords

THA · TKA · Suture · Incision complication

10.1 Hip and Knee Joint Replacement Surgical Approach

10.1.1 Hip Joint Replacement Surgical Approach

10.1.1.1 Posterolateral Approach

The posterolateral hip approach was born on the European battlefield in the nineteenth century to treat hip infections and war trauma. It was originally advocated by Kocher and Langenbeck and was widely used for acetabular posterior wall fractures, artificial femoral head replacement after femoral neck fracture, total hip arthroplasty, etc. Later it was modified and popularized by Gibson and Moore in 1950 [1, 2]. This approach can expose the extended incision with trochanter osteotomy, extended greater trochanter osteotomy, etc. The abductor muscles are preserved during the surgery, and the incidence of postoperative claudication is low; repairing the posterior joint capsule and external rotation brevis muscles after the surgery could reduce the risk of postoperative joint dislocation. And it is currently one of the commonly used approaches for primary hip arthroplasty and revision in clinical practice.

The patient with posterolateral approach adopts a standard lateral decubitus position. A slightly curved incision is made centered by the apex of the greater trochanter (Fig. 10.1). The proximal incision is made along the gluteus maximus muscle fibers, and the distal incision is extended along the longitudinal axis of the femoral shaft with a total length of about 10–15 cm. The incision can be extended or shortened appropriately according to the patient's body shape or the needs of prosthesis implanting. Incise the skin and subcutaneous tissue layer by layer to the fascia lata and the fascia of the gluteus maximus (Fig. 10.2). At the surface of the center of the greater trochanter incise the fascia along the skin incision. Bluntly split along the direction of the gluteus maximus muscle fibers at the proximal end, and fully extend to the attachment point of the gluteus maximus tendon on the posterior edge of the femur at the distal end.

Use deep and shallow muscle retractors or Charnley retractors to retract the tensor fascia lata and gluteus maximus respectively, resect the bursa around the greater trochanter, flex the knee, internally rotate and straight hip joint to

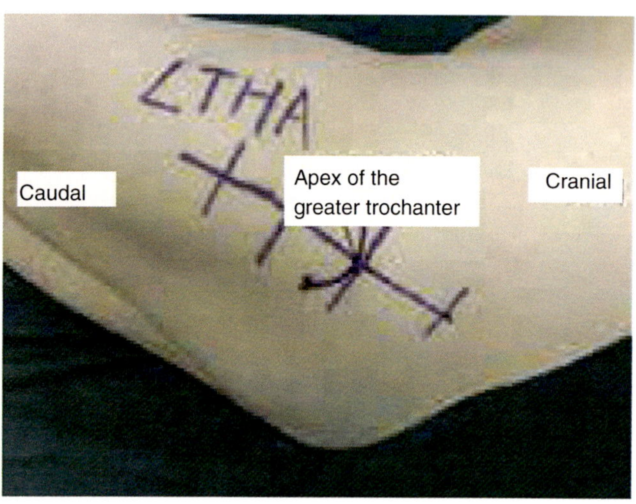

Fig. 10.1 Posterolateral approach skin incision

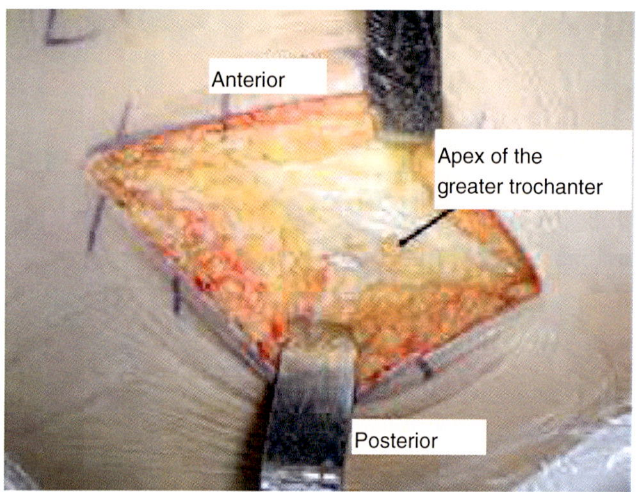

Fig. 10.2 Exposure to the fascia lata and the fascia of gluteus maximus

tighten the external rotation muscle group, expose the attachment point of the external rotation muscles (Fig. 10.3). Release off at the attachment point, and use the non-absorbable 2# ETHIBOND® suture (Polyester, Ethicon Inc.) to mark the piriformis tendon and conjoined obturator tendon of the external rotation muscles by figure 8 suturing (Fig. 10.4) for postoperative repair. Pay attention to the hemostasis of the blood vessels along the piriformis muscle and the terminal branch of the medial femoral circumflex artery in the quadratus femoris. Flip the external rotation muscles to the posterior side to protect the sciatic nerve. Bluntly dissect the gap between the gluteus minimus and the upper joint capsule, insert the Hoffman retractor and retract the gluteus medius and gluteus minimus upward for protection, fully expose the upper, posterior, and lower part of the joint capsule. And then make a "door" shaped incision along

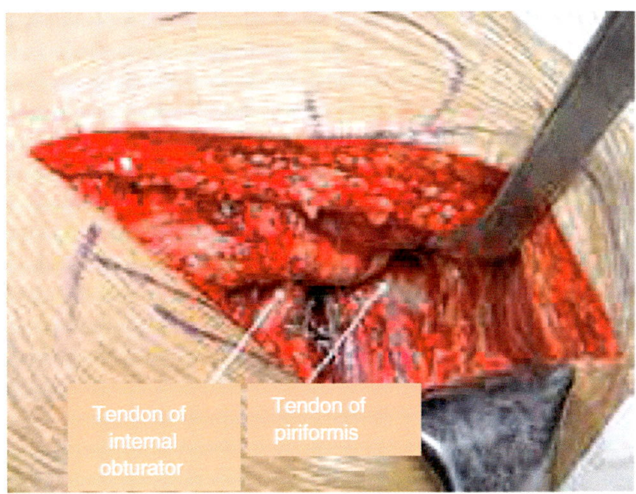

Fig. 10.3 Tendon attachment of external rotation muscles

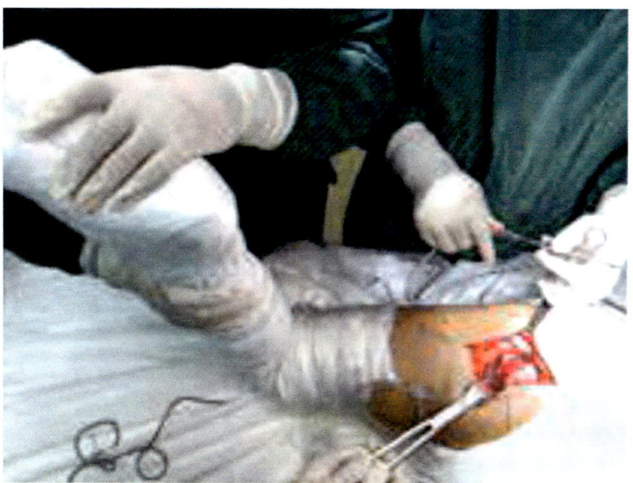

Fig. 10.5 Dislocate the hip joint by flexion, adduction, and internal rotation

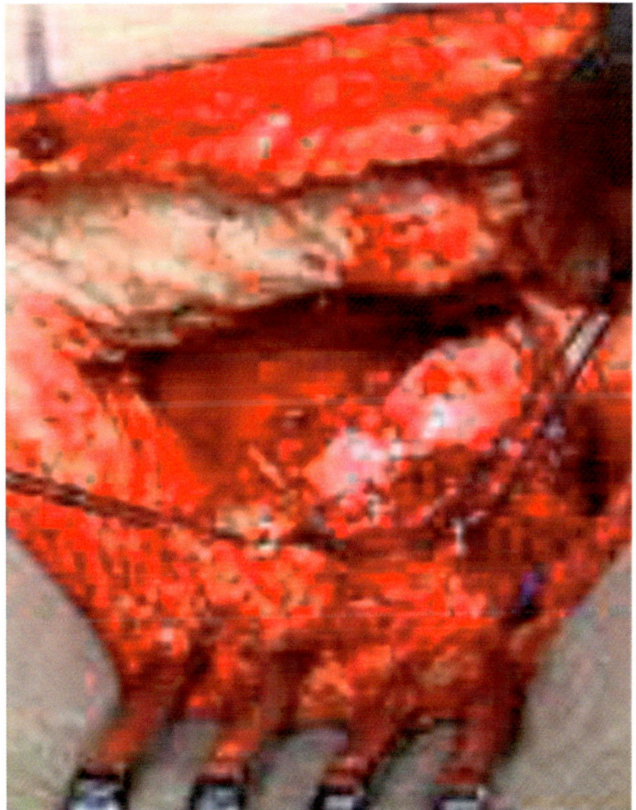

Fig. 10.4 Suture and mark the external rotation muscles for repair

the femoral attachment of the joint capsule, expose the glenoid labrum, retract the posterior joint capsule, clearly expose the femoral head, neck, and posterior wall of the acetabulum. Dislocate the hip joint by flexion, adduction, and internal rotation (Fig. 10.5).

10.1.1.2 Direct Lateral Approach (Modified Hardinge Approach)

The direct lateral approach was first advocated by Bauer et al., and then introduced by Hardinge et al. in 1982 and promoted to hip arthroplasty surgery. The direct lateral approach preserves the posterior joint capsule and reduces the risk of postoperative joint dislocation and sciatic nerve injury. The extension of the distal end of the incision can also clearly expose the femoral shaft, which is suitable for most hip joint surgeries. Later, this approach was perfected and became one of the commonly used direct lateral hip approaches—the modified Hardinge approach.

For the modified Hardinge approach, the patient is placed in a supine or lateral position, with the greater trochanter of the surgical hip as the center, and a longitudinal incision is made along the lateral side of the hip. The distal end of the incision extends in the direction of the femur, and the proximal end can be extended directly upwards, or curved slightly backward (Fig. 10.6). The total length is about 10–15 cm. For the obese patient, it can be extended appropriately. Incise the skin, subcutaneous tissue, and tensor fascia lata in turns (Fig. 10.7).

Retract the tensor fascia lata muscle to the anterior side and the gluteus maximus muscle posterior side to expose the insertion of the gluteus medius at the greater trochanter and the insertion of the vastus lateralis muscle (Fig. 10.8). Explore the gap between the two muscles, cut the anterior 1/3 attachment of the gluteus medius at the insertion of the greater trochanter from far to near, and pay attention to preserve the 3–4 mm tendon tissue at the femoral insertion point (Fig. 10.9) for postoperative gluteus medius repair. Flip the anterior tendinous insertion of the gluteus medius to expose the gluteal minor muscle, and cut its anterior insertion in the

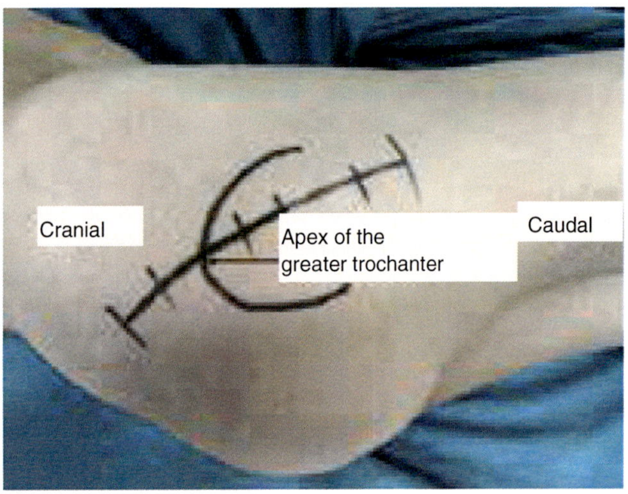

Fig. 10.6 Hip joint direct lateral approach incision in the lateral position

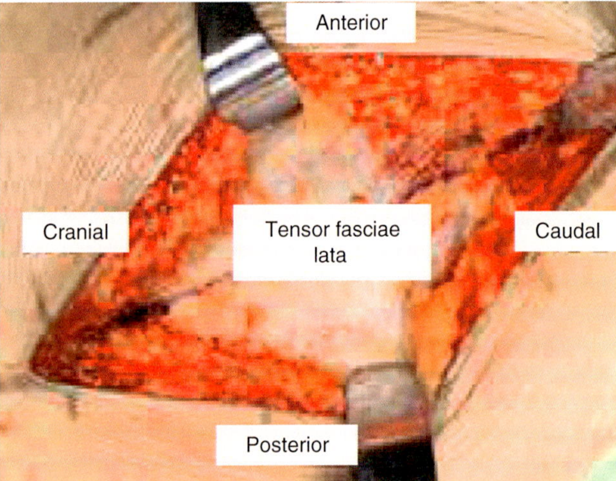

Fig. 10.7 Incision of the tensor fascia lata

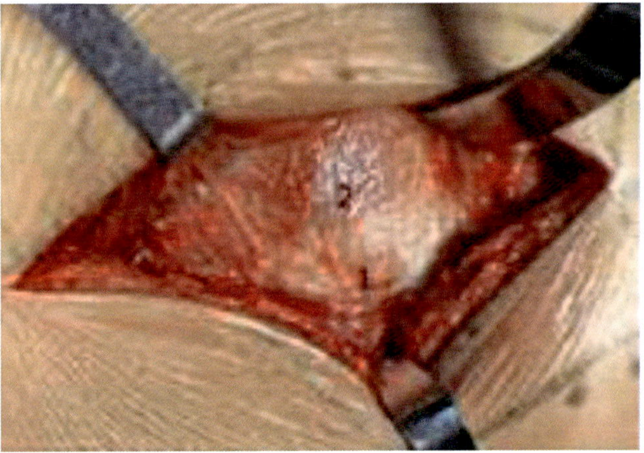

Fig. 10.8 Expose the greater trochanter, gluteus medius, and vastus lateralis muscle during the surgery

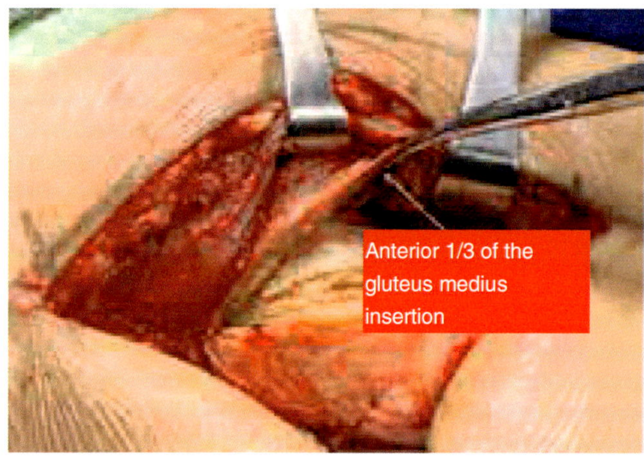

Fig. 10.9 Incise anterior 1/3 of the gluteus medius insertion, retain 3–4 mm tendon tissue at the insertion of the greater trochanter

same way. The caudal part of the gluteus medius and the gluteus minimus integrate into a joint tendon, and the intact joint tendon is good for gluteus minimus repair. It should be noted that the range of proximal splitting along the gluteus medius fibers should be controlled within a safe range of 4 cm above the upper rim of the acetabulum or within 5 cm from the apex of the greater trochanter to avoid injury to the superior gluteal nerve branch.

External rotation of the affected hip joint can expose the anterior part of the joint capsule. Place a Hoffmann retractor at the anterior rim of the acetabulum parallel to the midline of the longitudinal axis of the femoral neck to retract the abductor. Use the periosteum elevator for blunt dissection, and place the cautery at the surface of the joint capsule for dissection, fully expose the anterior part of the joint capsule. Then place two Hoffmann retractors above and below the joint capsule at the femoral neck, and cut open the anterior joint capsule in a T-shape or H-shape. First incise along the midline of the longitudinal axis of the femoral neck, and then cut the joint capsule along the intertrochanteric line about 1 cm medial to its femoral attachment, stay away from the base of the femoral neck as far as possible, so that the joint capsule is T-shaped or H-shaped cut open (Fig. 10.10). Retaining of the joint capsule which is still connected to the femoral side facilitates the reattachment of the gluteus minimus after surgery. Make one balance stitch at each side of the joint capsule as a mark in order to make apposition suture and repair the joint capsule. In case of joint capsule adhesion, hyperplasia, and hypertrophy, deformity and laxity or severe hip joint deformity, the anterior joint capsule can also be resected in order to expose the surgical field, soft tissues release, and subsequent procedures. After the anterior joint capsule is opened or resected, the femoral neck, femoral head, and acetabular rim can be exposed, dislocate the hip joint by adduction, flexion, and external rotation.

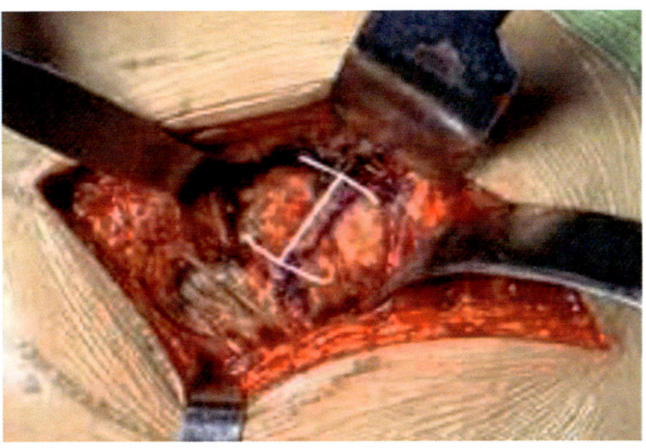

Fig. 10.10 H-shaped incision of the anterior joint capsule, exposing the hip joint

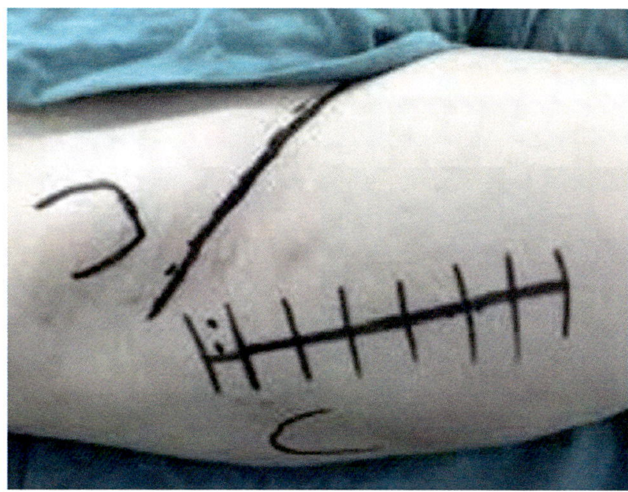

Fig. 10.11 DAA approach skin incision in the supine position

10.1.1.3 Direct Anterior Approach

The direct anterior approach (DAA) exposes to the hip joint through neuromuscular space and avoids damage to the external rotation muscles, which helps the patient rapid recovery after surgery. Moreover, the patient being placed in the supine position, it is easier to evaluate the stability of the hip joint and the lower limb discrepancy during the surgery. This approach was first introduced by Smith-Petersen in 1917 for the reduction of congenital hip dislocation and was promoted for hip arthroplasty surgery in 1949 [3]. In 1950, French doctor Judet modified the Smith-Petersen approach. A similar Hueter approach was used together with the Judet traction table for hip arthroplasty surgery. This approach included only the lower part of the Smith-Petersen approach. It enters the hip joint through the gap between the tensor fascia lata and the sartorius muscle, retaining the integrity of the muscle [3]. Coupled with the special minimally invasive surgical retractors and hooks, the incision can be reduced to 6–8 cm. Currently, DAA is one of the popular hip arthroplasty surgical approaches.

The patient is in the supine position in the conventional operating table, with the hips slightly elevated, and the anterior superior iliac spine is at the folding part of the operating table (appropriate folding of the operating table can make the hip joint in hyperextension, which helps the exposure of the femur and procedure). The incision starts from the point 3 cm from the distal end of the anterior superior iliac spine and 3 cm laterally, and extends to the fibular head (Fig. 10.11). The incision length is 8–10 cm. When necessary, the incision could be extended: the distal extension can increase the femur exposure, and the proximal extension can make the acetabulum exposed more thoroughly. Incise the skin and subcutaneous tissue layer by layer, and cut the fascia layer on the surface of the tensor fascia lata.

To avoid injury of the lateral femoral cutaneous nerve in the superficial layer of the sartorius muscle, longitudinally

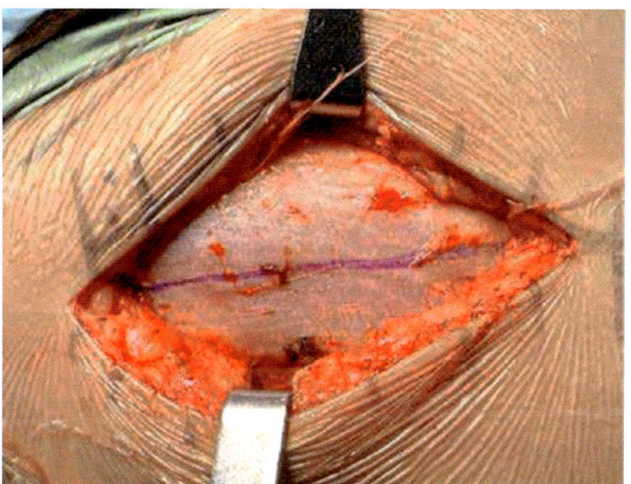

Fig. 10.12 Separate tensor fascia lata through the gap between tensor fascia lata and sartorius muscle

incise the fascia lata 1 cm lateral to the space between the tensor fascia lata and the sartorius muscle, bluntly dissect along the tensor fascia lata fibers downward (Fig. 10.12), retract the fascia lata muscle fibers to the lateral side and the sartorius muscle medial side to expose the deep fascia covering the rectus femoris and medial femoris muscles (Fig. 10.13). Carefully remove the fat tissue around the joint capsule, expose to the anterior joint capsule. Pay attention to protect and ligate the lateral femoral circumflex artery (Fig. 10.14).

Place blunt retractors under the femoral neck outside the joint capsule, and then separate proximally to expose the joint capsule, make a T-shaped incision on the joint capsule (Fig. 10.15), use non-absorbable 2# ETHIBOND® suture (Polyester, Ethicon Inc.) to make figure 8 suturing to mark the incised joint capsule and retract it backward (Fig. 10.16), release the joint capsule and expose to the femoral neck.

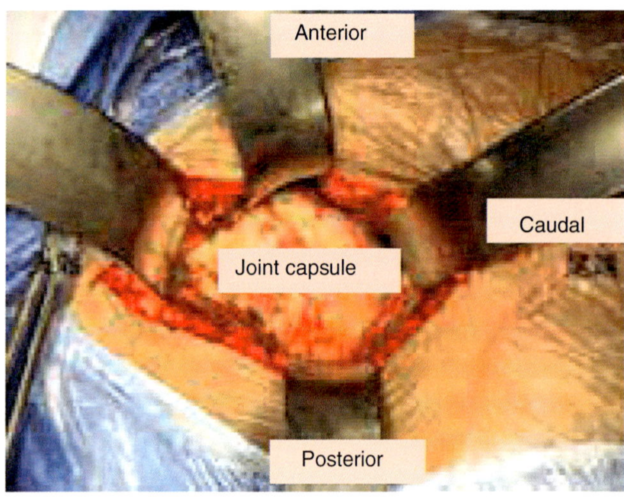

Fig. 10.13 Cut the deep fascia and remove the fat tissue around the joint capsule

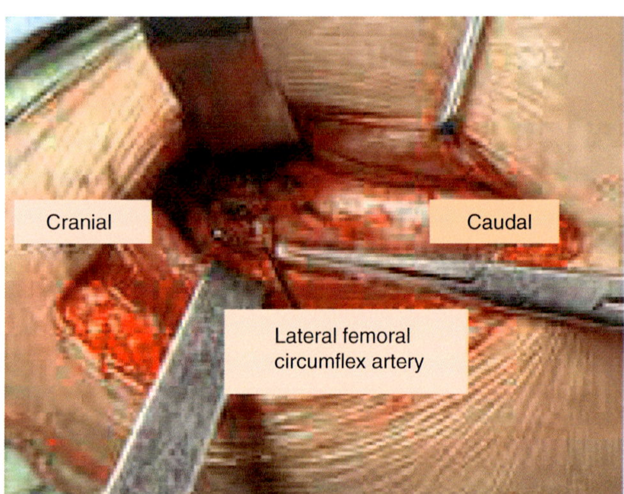

Fig. 10.14 Lateral femoral circumflex artery

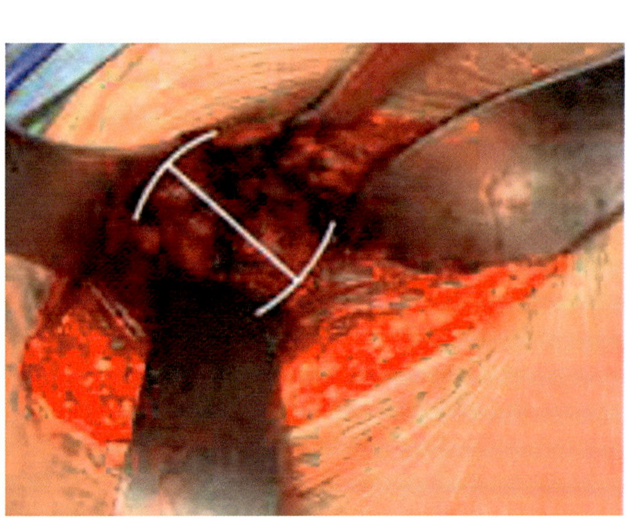

Fig. 10.15 T-shaped incision of the joint capsule

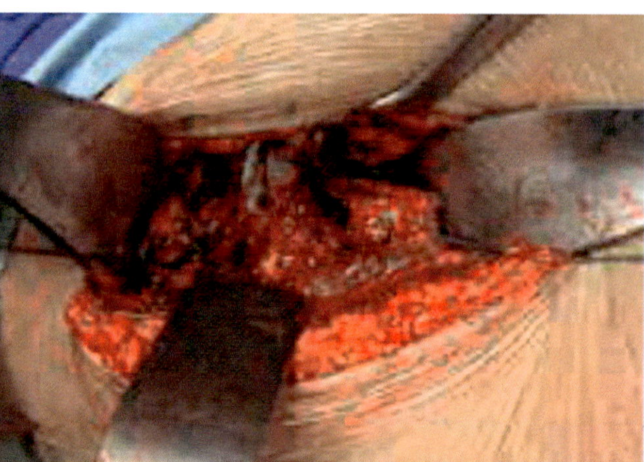

Fig. 10.16 Joint capsule suturing mark

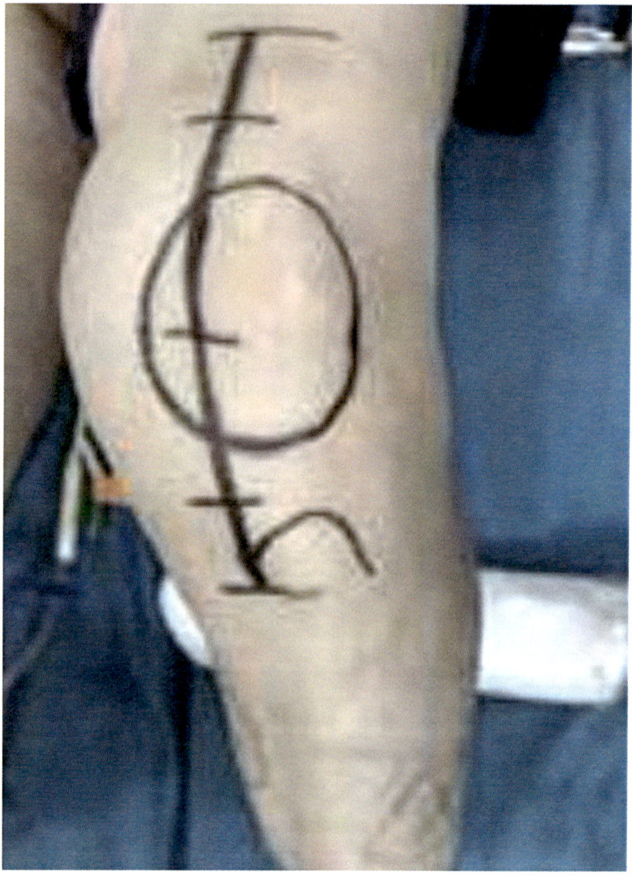

Fig. 10.17 Skin incision of the medial parapatellar approach

10.1.2 Knee Joint Replacement Surgical Approach

10.1.2.1 Medial Parapatellar Approach

Anterior median incision and medial parapatellar approach are often used for knee arthroplasty surgery (Fig. 10.17). The skin is cut longitudinally around the patella. The proximal

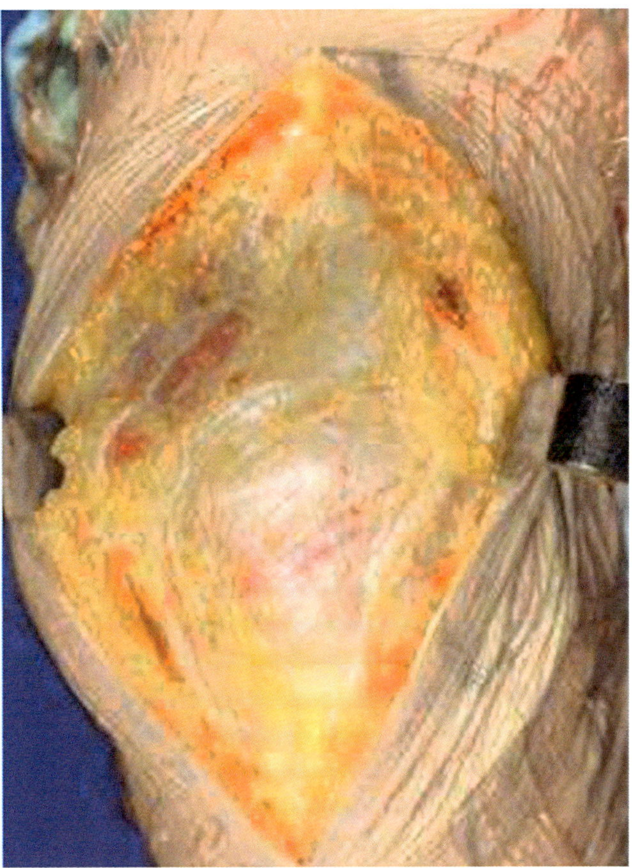

Fig. 10.18 Incise the joint capsule and synovium along the "red-white" junction of the medial vastus muscle and the inner edge of the quadriceps tendon

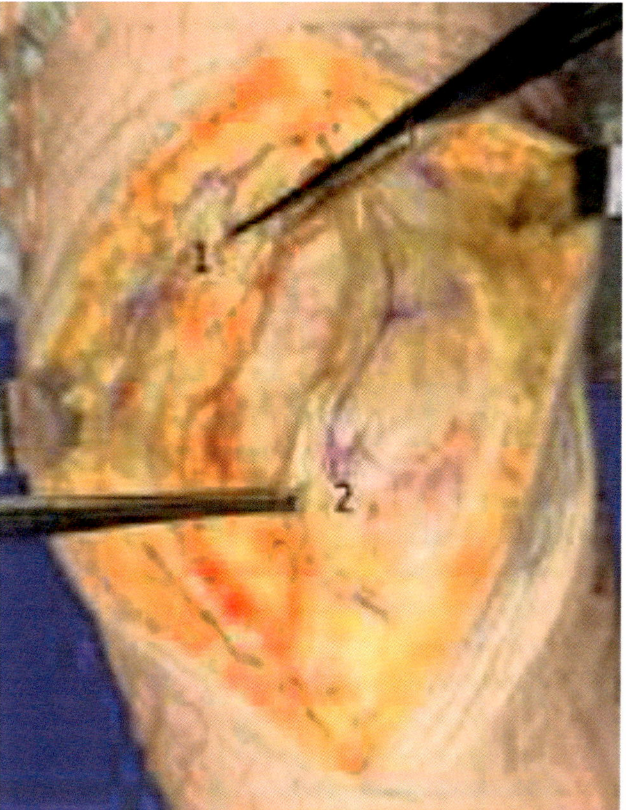

Fig. 10.19 Retain 5 mm of the tendon at the medial edge of the patella to facilitate the suturing after the surgery

end of the skin incision starts at 4–5 cm above the patella, and the distal end ends at the medial side of the tibial tubercle or the medial side of its distal end. The skin is usually cut with knee flexion. The skin incision should be long enough to avoid skin necrosis caused by excessive tension. Cut the subcutaneous tissue and pull it to both sides.

Then extend to incise the joint capsule and synovium along the "red-white" junction of the medial vastus muscle and the inner edge of the quadriceps tendon to the proximal end (Fig. 10.18). The methylene blue marking facilitates the incision balance. Retain the medial vastus muscle tendon 3–4 mm to facilitate the suturing after the surgery; at the medial side of the patella (retain 5 mm of the tendon at the medial edge of the patella to facilitate the suturing after the surgery) cut along the medial side of the patellar tendon to the medial edge of the tibial tubercle (Fig. 10.19).

10.1.2.2 Auxiliary Exposure Technique

For the initial arthroplasty or the revision of stiff knee joint, if it is difficult to expose using the standard medial parapatellar approach, some auxiliary exposure techniques are needed. (1) Insall's modified quadriceps oblique incision technique (Fig. 10.20), which extends from the top end of the standard medial parapatellar incision to the lateral superior side directly, passes through the quadriceps tendon and cuts the rectus femoris tendon, retains the whole vastus lateralis attachment, and the lateral superior genicular vessels; (2) Scott and Siliski modified VY-plasty (Fig. 10.21), which incises from the standard medial parapatellar side, extends proximally, then folds back, incises the quadriceps tendon in an inverted V shape to the lateral parapatellar retinaculum. Pay attention to protect the lateral superior genicular artery, change the V shape to Y shape when suturing, so that the patella and its attached quadriceps tendon move to the distal end. (3) Tibial tubercle osteotomy (TTO): this method was originally reported by Dolin, and later modified and promoted by Whiteside and Ohl. The specific procedure is to use an oscillating saw to cut an 8–10 cm bone block with tibial tubercle and part of the anterior tibial spine (Fig. 10.22). The depth of osteotomy is usually 1.5–2 cm behind the tibial tubercle. Pay attention to protect the periosteum and soft tissue attachment at the surface of the bone block. (4) Banana Peel: for patients with knee osseous or fibrous ankylosis, Windsor and Insall recommend the auxiliary exposure method of Banana Peel (Fig. 10.23), that is to peel the distal femur soft tissue, including the insertion of the collateral ligaments, from the femoral condyle [4].

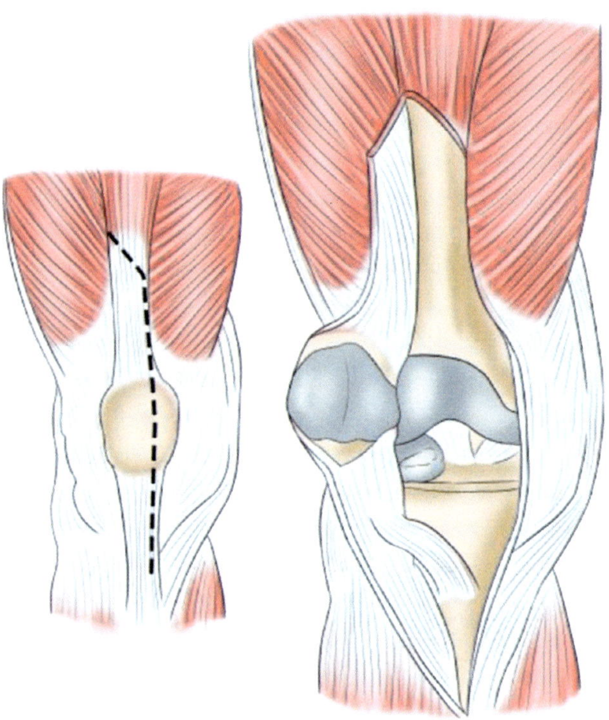

Fig. 10.20 Diagram of quadriceps oblique incision technique (the diagram needs to be redrawn) (lack of suturing diagram)

10.2 Incision Suturing Technique for Joint Replacement Surgeries

There are many incision suturing techniques for hip and knee arthroplasty surgeries, refer to Chap. 3 for details. The specific suturing techniques are as follows.

10.2.1 Incision Suturing of Hip Joint Replacement

10.2.1.1 Posterolateral Approach

1. *Preparation Before Incision Closure*: After the implantation of the artificial hip joint prosthesis, first soak in diluted iodophor for 3–4 min, rinse the wound with pulsed lavage for 3~5 min, soak the wound with tranexamic acid sodium chloride injection 100 ml (concentration 1 g/100 ml) for 3~5 min, dry the incision with clean gauze and start suturing. Carefully check for active bleeding. After confirming that there is no active bleeding, the drainage tube does not have to be placed.
2. *Repair of Joint Capsule and External Rotation Muscles*: Use absorbable 1# VICRYL® Plus suture (Polyglactin 910, Ethicon Inc.) or non-absorbable 2# ETHIBOND® suture (Polyester, Ethicon Inc.) to suture and rebuild joint capsule and external rotation muscle group, and drill two bone tunnels in the greater tuberosity, and use a needle suture to assist the external rotation muscle group marking suture to pass through the bone canal. Knot the mark-

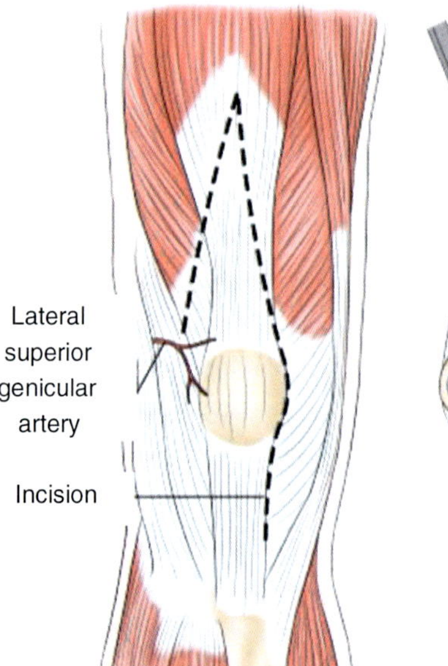

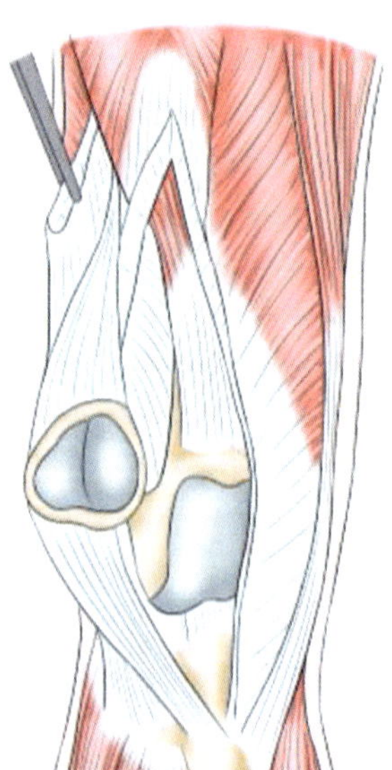

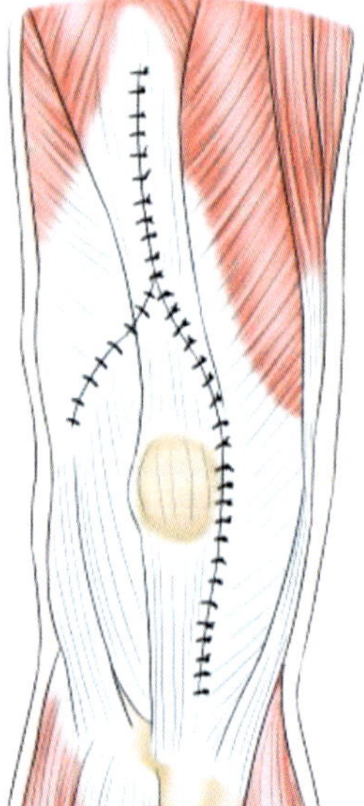

Fig. 10.21 Diagram of V-Y plasty (the diagram needs to be redrawn)

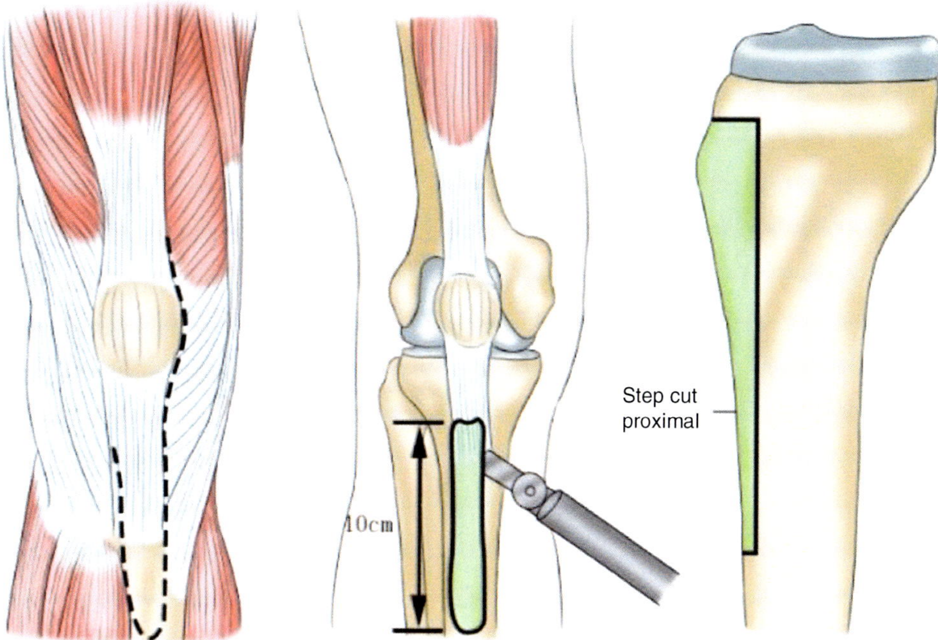

Fig. 10.22 Tibial tubercle osteotomy (diagram needed)

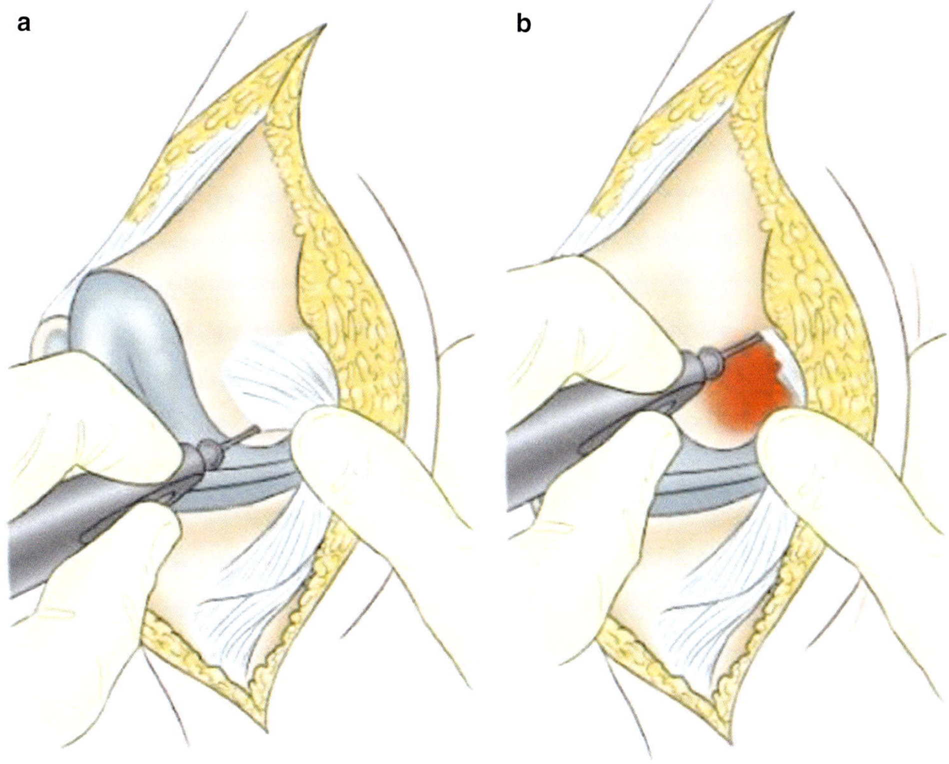

Fig. 10.23 (**a**, **b**) Femoral dissection. Banana peel (diagram needed)

ing suture of the proximal and distal ends of the joint capsule with at least six square knots, and knot the marking suture of the piriformis and external rotation brevis group to each other, with at least six square knots (Figs. 10.24, 10.25, 10.26 and 10.27).

3. *Suturing of Deep Fascia Layer*: After the reconstruction of the joint capsule and external rotation brevis group, position the affected limb in the hip flexion 30° and knee flexion 60°, and the hip joint is positioned in the abduction and external rotation position (Fig. 10.28). Conduct

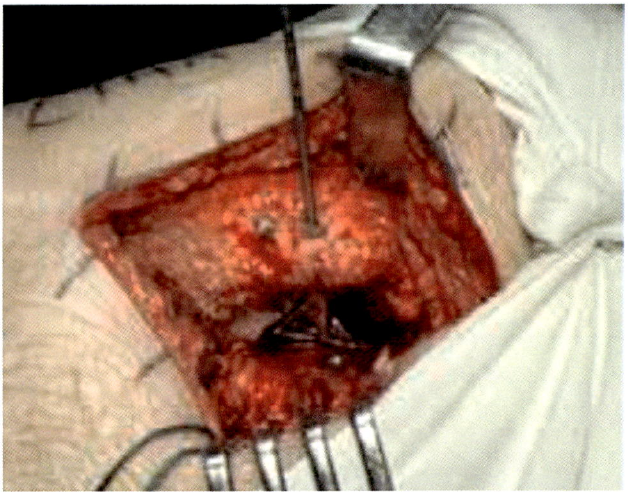

Fig. 10.24 Reconstruction point of fine drill hole

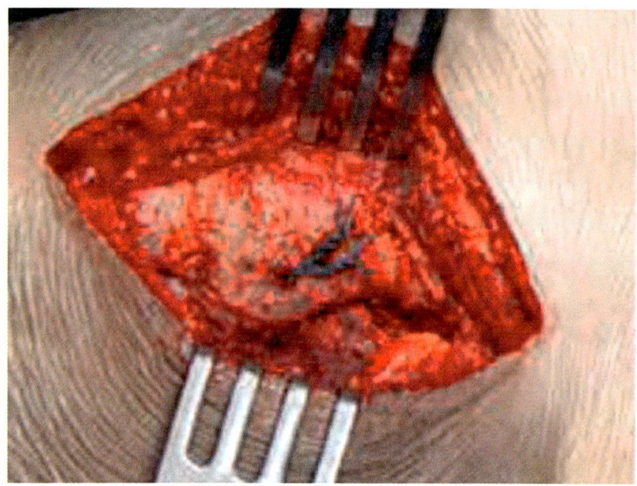

Fig. 10.27 The repaired external rotation muscle group

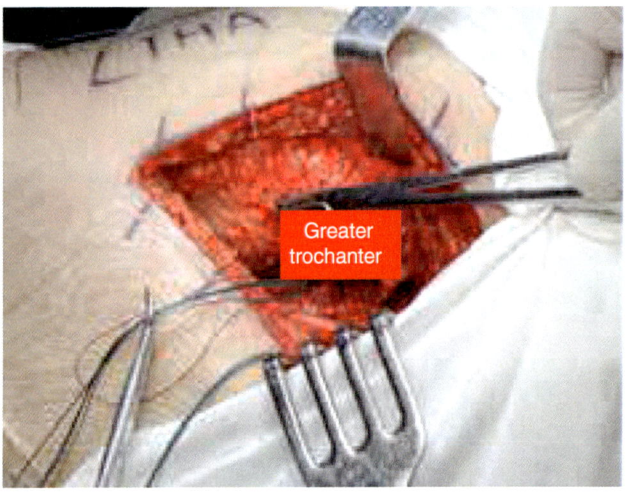

Fig. 10.25 Use a needle suture to bring the marking suture through the bone tunnel, step 1

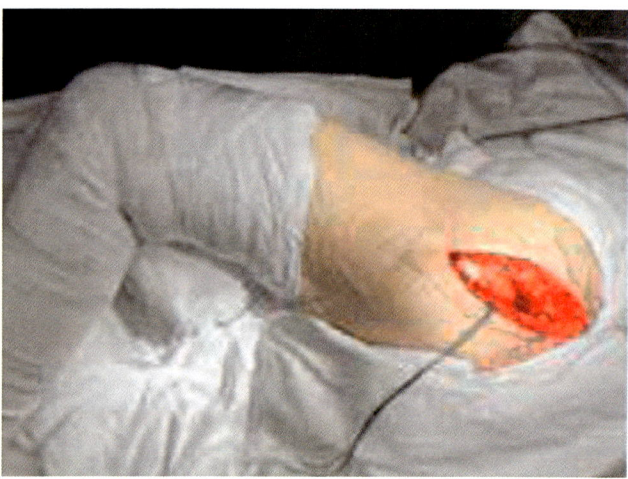

Fig. 10.28 Hip joint positioned in abduction and external rotation position

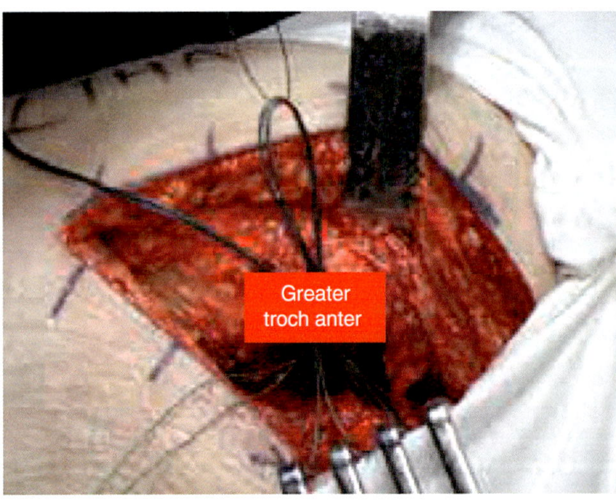

Fig. 10.26 Suture passing of needle suture, step 2

continuous suturing of the fascia lata with absorbable 1# STRATAFIX® Symmetric PDS PLUS knotless tissue control device (Polydioxanone, Ethicon Inc.) from the distal end of the incision to the proximal end (Fig. 10.29) or absorbable 1# STRATAFIX® Spiral PDO bidirectional knotless tissue control device (Polydioxanone, Ethicon Inc.) from the middle of the incision to both distal and proximal ends simultaneously (Fig. 10.30). The stitch distance is 5–8 mm. After the suturing is completed, check whether the suturing apposition is tight or not, and add suturing when necessary.

4. *Subcutaneous Tissue Suturing*: Remove the larger free fat particles in the subcutaneous tissue, and rinse the incision again with normal saline. Use absorbable 2-0 VICRYL® Plus control release suture (Polyglactin 910, Ethicon Inc.) to make simply interrupted suturing of the subcutaneous tissue (Fig. 10.31), or choose the absorbable 2-0

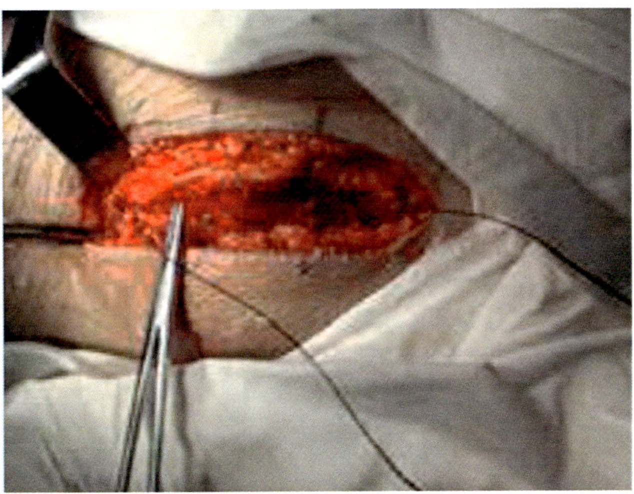

Fig. 10.29 Continuous suturing of the fascia lata from the distal end of the incision to the proximal end

STRATAFIX® Spiral PDO bidirectional knotless tissue control device (Polydioxanone, Ethicon Inc.) to continuously suture the subcutaneous tissue without knotting (Fig. 10.32). Simple interrupted suturing can reduce dead space and ensure good balance. Use inverting suture, the stitch distance is 5–8 mm, the suture knot should not be too large, otherwise, it could be easily touched under the skin, difficult to be absorbed, and induce knot reactions. It is also possible to use continuous knot-free suturing for the subcutaneous tissue to quickly complete the suturing, shorten the procedure, reduce the wound exposure time, and reduce the probability of infection. If the patient's subcutaneous tissue is thick, the suturing should be performed layer by layer to ensure that no residual cavity is left to avoid blood and fluid accumulation. After the suturing, check whether the suturing gap is tight, whether the tension is uniform, to avoid misalignment and

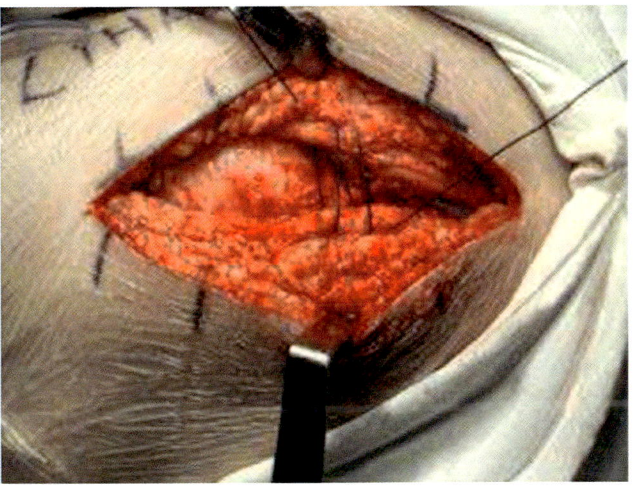

Fig. 10.30 Continuous suturing technique, from the center of the incision to both distal and proximal ends simultaneously to suture the fascia lata

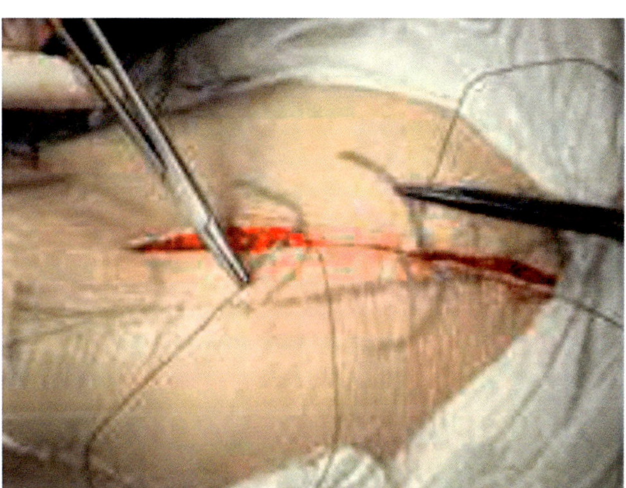

Fig. 10.32 Absorbable 2-0 STRATAFIX® Spiral PDO bidirectional knotless tissue control device (Polydioxanone, Ethicon Inc.) continuous suturing technique to suture the subcutaneous tissue

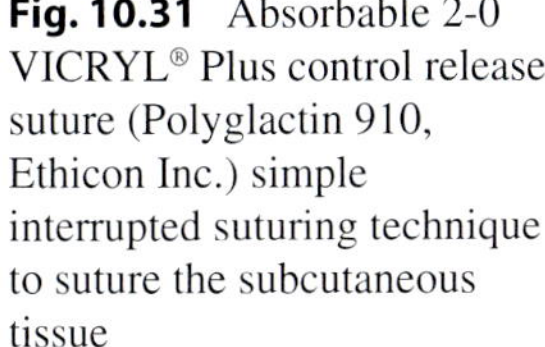

Fig. 10.31 Absorbable 2-0 VICRYL® Plus control release suture (Polyglactin 910, Ethicon Inc.) simple interrupted suturing technique to suture the subcutaneous tissue

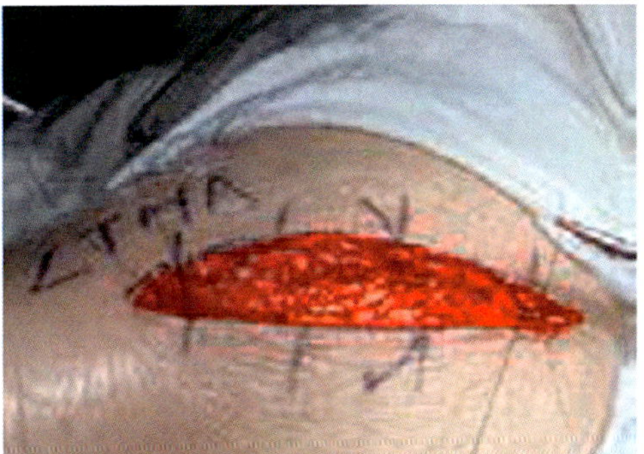

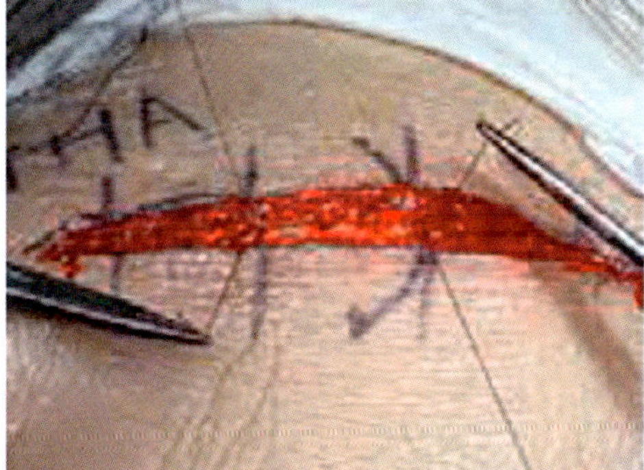

cross-layer suturing, as well as uneven skin margins. When necessary, additional suturing should be made or stitches removed for adjustment.

5. *Skin Suturing*: Tear off the antibacterial membrane within 5 cm around the incision, disinfect both sides of the skin with alcohol gauze, and use continuous intradermal suturing technique [e.g., Absorbable 4-0 STRATAFIX® Spiral PGA-PCL bidirectional knotless tissue control device (PGA-PCL, Ethicon Inc.) (Fig. 10.33) or Absorbable 4-0 STRATAFIX® Spiral PGA-PCL unidirectional knotless tissue control device (PGA-PCL, Ethicon Inc.) for skin suturing. Tissue glue [such as: medical skin tissue glue (Dermabond Prineo, 2-octyl cyanoacrylate, and self-adhesive mesh, Ethicon Inc.)] can also be used to seal the incision. After drying with sterile gauze, use the clean dressing to cover the incision (Fig. 10.34).

10.2.1.2 Direct Lateral Approach

1. *Preparation Before Closing the Incision*: Remove all bone debris, soft tissue fragments and blood clots around the acetabulum and femoral neck, recheck the tightness, stability, and range of motion of the implanted artificial hip joint, and confirm that no soft tissue is embedded in the joint. Soak the wound with diluted iodophor for 3–4 min, and use bulb syringe or pulsed lavage to repeatedly rinse with the saline for 3–5 min. Suck all the washing fluid, carefully check for active bleeding in the incision, and make through hemostasis. Decide whether to place a drainage tube according to the blood exudation. If the blood exudation is not obvious, no drainage is needed.
2. *Joint Capsule Abductor Repair*: for those whose joint capsule is not removed, use absorbable 1# VICRYL® Plus control release suture (Polyglactin 910, Ethicon Inc.) or non-absorbable 2# ETHIBOND® suture (Polyester, Ethicon Inc.) figure 8 suturing repair to enhance the stability of the anterior soft tissue of the hip joint (Fig. 10.35). Then, use non-absorbable suture [such as: use non-absorbable 5# ETHIBOND® suture (Polyester, Ethicon Inc.)] for figure 8 or knot-free continuous suturing for the junction of the incised gluteus medius tendon and the greater trochanter to ensure the tendon-tendon anastomosis (the gluteus medius can also be sutured to the bony structure of the greater trochanter insertion) (Fig. 10.36). The gluteus minimus tendon is attached to the gluteus medius and vastus lateralis muscle layer and is integrated

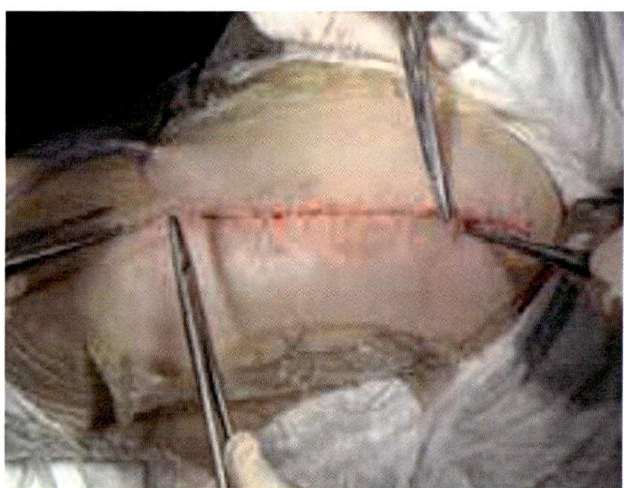

Fig. 10.33 Use Absorbable 4-0 STRATAFIX® Spiral PGA-PCL bidirectional knotless tissue control device (PGA-PCL, Ethicon Inc.) for continuous intradermal suturing technique to suture the skin

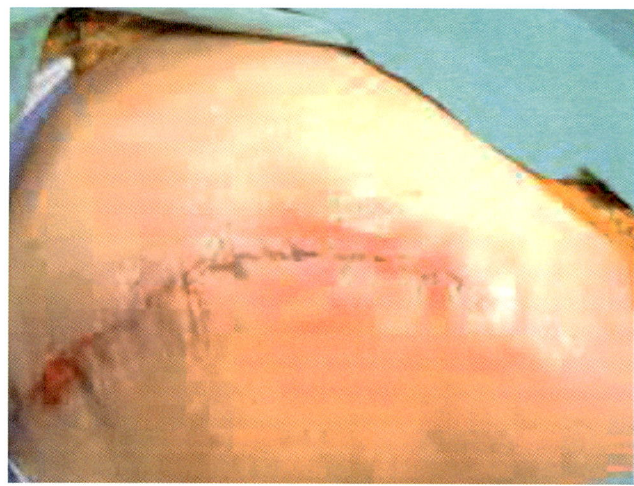

Fig. 10.34 Sealing incision with skin tissue glue

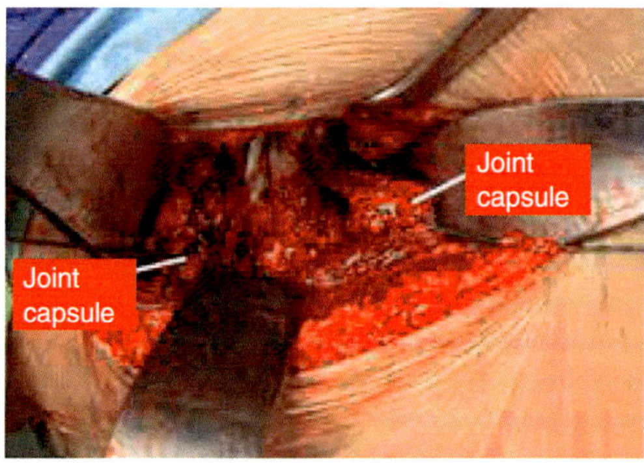

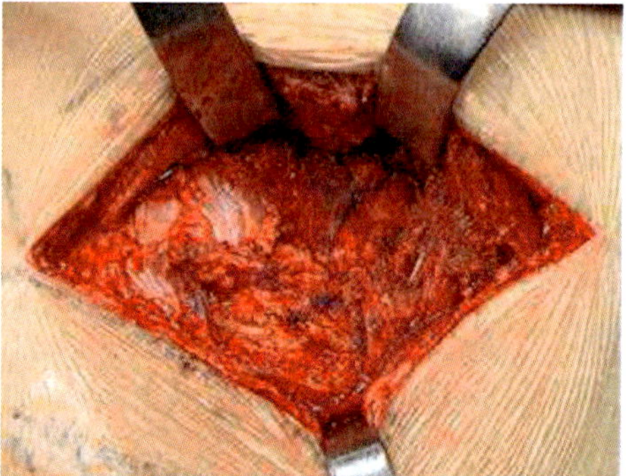

Fig. 10.35 Interrupted suturing of the anterior joint capsule after the balance

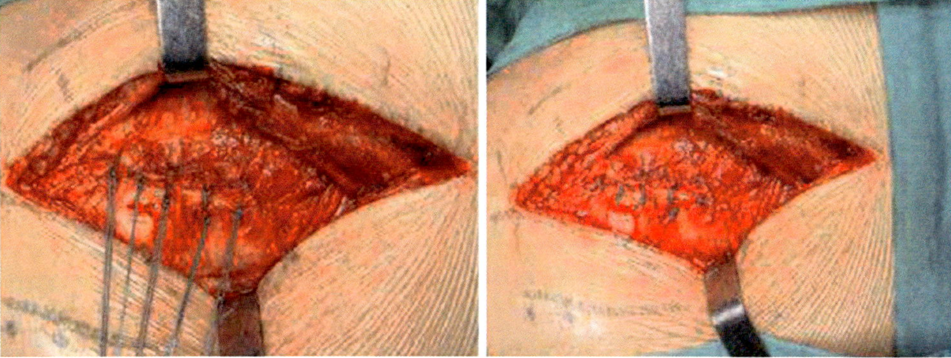

Fig. 10.36 Use non-absorbable 5# ETHIBOND® suture (Polyester, Ethicon Inc.) to repair the gluteus medius with figure 8 suturing technique

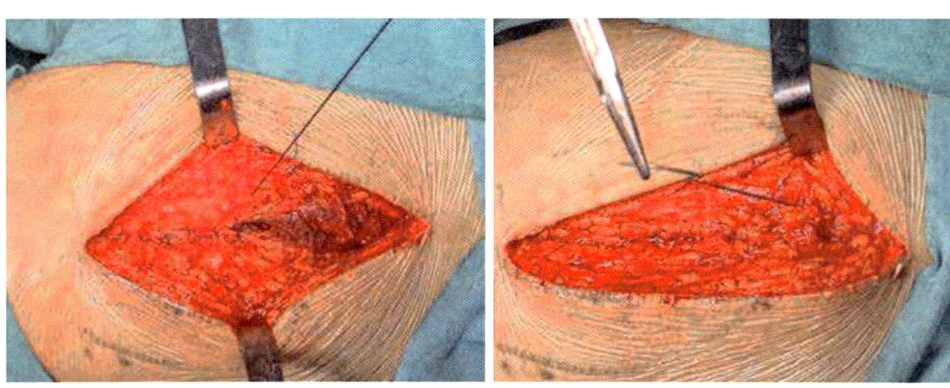

Fig. 10.37 Suture the tensor fascia lata by continuous suturing with absorbable STRATAFIX® Symmetric PDS PLUS knotless tissue control device (Polydioxanone, Ethicon Inc.)

with the caudal part of the gluteus medius into a joint tendon, no need to repair layer by layer. Gluteus medius repair is very important in lateral approach arthroplasty surgery. Unsatisfactory suturing will cause the abductor muscle insertion burst in a short period of time after surgery, especially when the patient is in the posture of external rotation of the affected limb, which will cause the abductor muscle tension reduction, claudication gait, and even affect the stability of the hip prosthesis. The advantage of figure 8 suturing is to ensure that the tissue will not be cut and torn due to the high tension of the tissue balancing, which is beneficial to healing. After the suturing, the femur should be slightly externally rotated. Observe if the repair is robust under direct vision, and add additional suturing when necessary.

3. Suturing of Tensor Fascia Lata: Slight abduction of the affected limb to reduce the incision tension and facilitate suturing. Use the absorbable 0# STRATAFIX® Symmetric PDS PLUS knotless tissue control device (Polydioxanone, Ethicon Inc.) or absorbable 1# STRATAFIX® Spiral PDO bidirectional knotless tissue control device (Polydioxanone, Ethicon Inc.) for continuous suturing of the tensor fascia lata with about 5–8 mm of stitch distance (Fig. 10.37). Pay attention not to involve or trap other subcutaneous tissue when suturing. The tension should be suitable, neither too tight nor too loose is good for healing. Cross suture 2–3 stitches retrogradely at the end, cut the suture close to the tissue to prevent the exposed suture tail from continuously irritating the soft tissue around. Knotless tissue control device is a new type of suturing, with enough tension support, and strong and even tissue purchase. It can be operated by one or two people by using Knotless tissue control device. Try to complete the suturing quickly, shorten the procedure time, reduce wound exposure time, and reduce the probability of infection. When suturing, also pay attention to avoid the trapping of the distal drainage tube. In addition, after the suturing, check whether the suturing gap is tight, especially whether there are leaks at both ends of the incision, otherwise, muscle hernia may occur. If necessary, add suturing. After the tensor fascia lata is sutured, tranexamic acid sodium chloride injection 1 g/100 ml could be injected into the joint cavity through direct puncture or drainage tube reversely, flex and extend the hip joint to check the suture tightness.
4. Subcutaneous tissue and skin suturing: the same as the posterolateral approach of the hip joint (Figs. 10.38 and 10.39).

10.2.1.3 Direct Anterior Approach

1. *Preparation Before Closing Incision*: The direct anterior approach is relatively simple and time-saving compared with the posterolateral approach. There is no need to reconstruct the external rotation muscle group, but the joint capsule needs to be reconstructed. The pre-suturing preparation is basically similar to the posterolateral approach. After the artificial hip prosthesis is implanted,

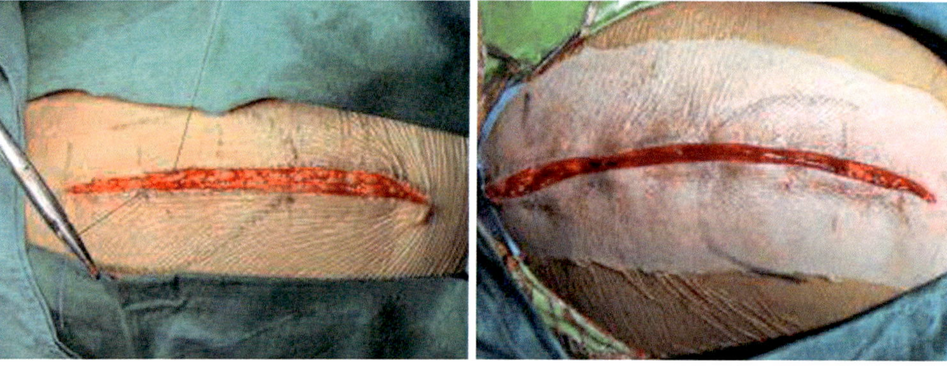

Fig. 10.38 Absorbable 2–0 VICRYL® Plus control release suture (Polyglactin 910, Ethicon Inc.) simple interrupted suturing technique to suture the subcutaneous tissue

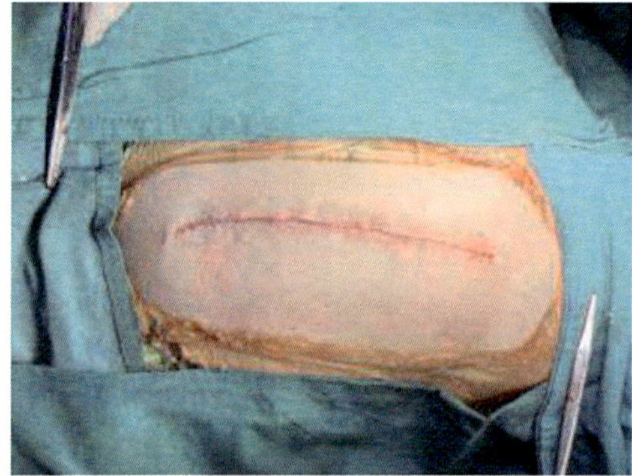

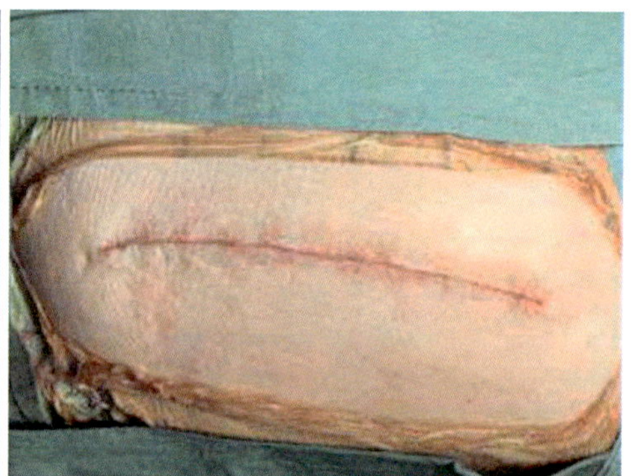

Fig. 10.39 Absorbable 4–0 STRATAFIX® Spiral PGA-PCL bidirectional knotless tissue control device (PGA-PCL, Ethicon Inc.) intracutaneous suturing for skin suturing

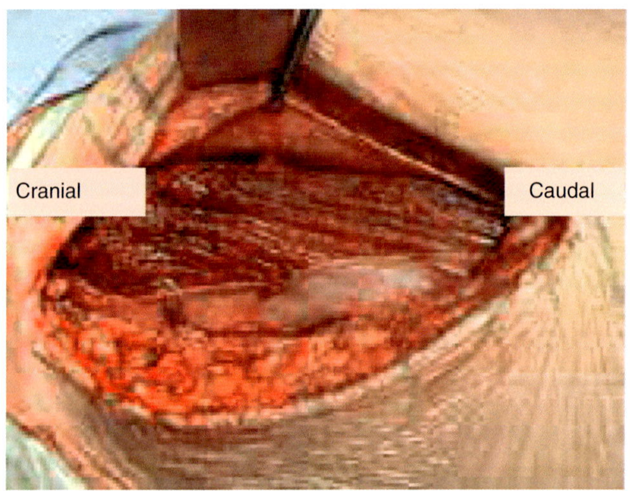

Fig. 10.40 Remove the injured tensor fascia lata fibers during the exposure process of the surgery

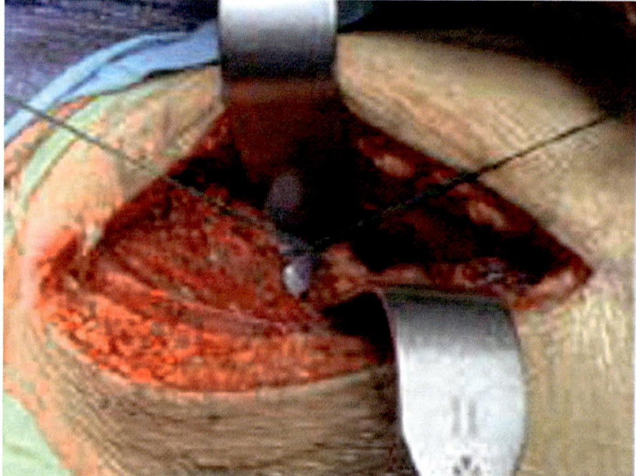

Fig. 10.41 Reconstruction of joint capsule 1

first soak the wound with diluted iodophor for 3–4 min, rinse the wound with pulsed lavage for 3~5 min, and soak the wound with 100 ml tranexamic acid sodium chloride injection (concentration 1 g/100 ml) for 3~5 min, evaluate the activity of the tensor fascia lata tissue, and remove the injured tensor fascia lata fibers during the exposure process of the surgery (Fig. 10.40). Dry the incision with clean gauze, carefully check for active bleeding (ascending branch of the lateral femoral circumflex artery). After confirming that there is no active bleeding, the drainage tube is generally not placed, and then reconstruct the joint capsule (sometimes the joint capsule is too thick and not retained) (Figs. 10.41 and 10.42).

2. *Suturing of Deep Fascia Layer*: After the joint capsule is reconstructed through the direct anterior approach, the continuous suturing is made for fascia lata with absorbable 1# STRATAFIX® Spiral PDO bidirectional knotless tissue control device (Polydioxanone, Ethicon Inc.) (only suture the muscle membrane on the surface of the tensor fascia lata, do not suture the muscle belly) (Fig. 10.43). The stitch distance is 5 mm. After the suturing is com-

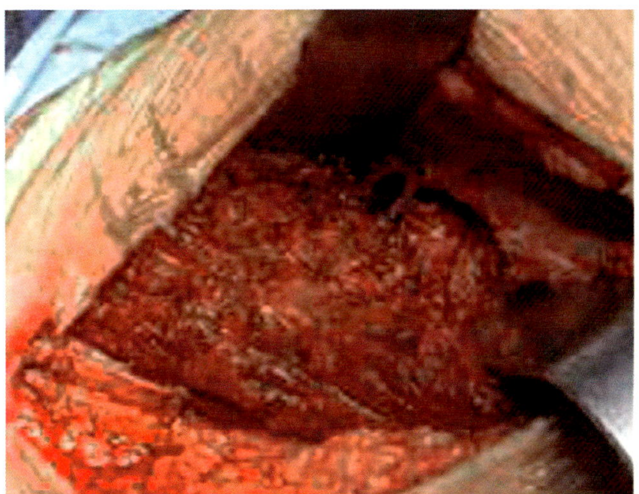

Fig. 10.42 Reconstruction of joint capsule 2

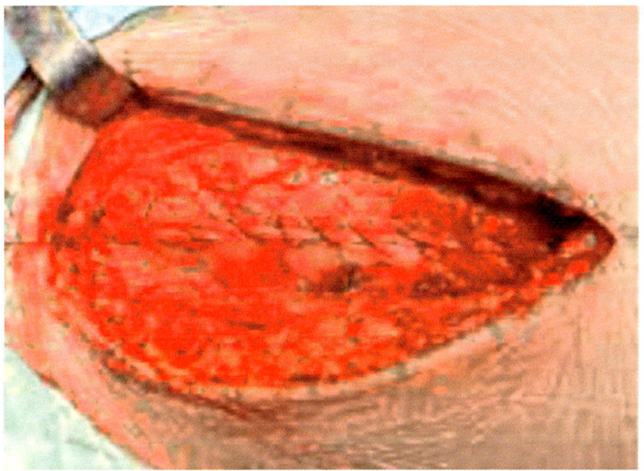

Fig. 10.43 Continuous suturing of the fascia lata with Absorbable STRATAFIX® knotless tissue control device

pleted, check whether the suturing apposition is tight or not, and add suturing when necessary.

3. *Subcutaneous Tissue and Skin Suturing*: The same as the posterolateral approach of the hip joint.

10.2.2 Incision Suturing of Knee Joint Replacement

1. *Preparation Before Incision Closure*: After the implantation of the artificial hip joint prosthesis, check if there is bone cement debris and bone debris. First soak in diluted iodophor for 3–4 min, rinse the wound with a pulse irrigation gun for 3~5 min, soak the wound with tranexamic acid sodium chloride injection 100 ml (concentration 1 g/100 ml) for 3~5 min, and dry the incision with clean

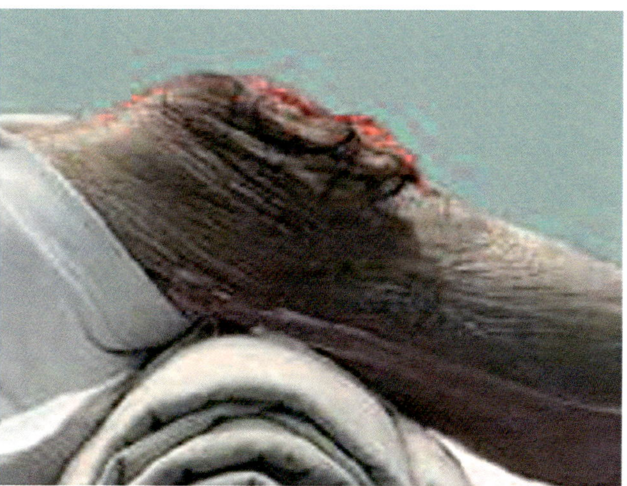

Fig. 10.44 The knee joint of the affected limb is flexed at 30°~60°, ready to suture the incision layer by layer

gauze. Flex the surgical knee joint for 30°~60°, and prepare to suture layer by layer (Fig. 10.44).

2. *Joint Capsule Suturing*: First use absorbable 1# VICRYL® Plus suture (Polyglactin 910, Ethicon Inc.) or non-absorbable 2# ETHIBOND® suture (Polyester, Ethicon Inc.) to perform preliminary balance suturing for 5–6 stitches of the deep incision according to the position marked by methylene blue (Fig. 10.45). Then use absorbable 1# STRATAFIX® Symmetric PDS PLUS knotless tissue control device (Polydioxanone, Ethicon Inc.) to continuously suture the joint capsule or use absorbable 1# STRATAFIX® Spiral PDO bidirectional knotless tissue control device (Polydioxanone, Ethicon Inc.) to suture the joint capsule from the incision center to the distal and proximal ends simultaneously (Figs. 10.46 and 10.47). The stitch distance is 5–8 mm. After the suturing is completed, inject 30–40 ml tranexamic acid sodium chloride injection into the joint cavity, and repeatedly flex and extend the knee joint to check whether the suturing gap is tight, and additional suturing should be added when necessary. The watertightness of joint cavity suturing is very important. Good watertightness can significantly reduce the risk of postoperative incision drainage, dehiscence, and other complications. After intra-articular injection of 30–40 ml tranexamic acid sodium chloride injection, the joint cavity with good watertightness maintains a certain tension, which can reduce bleeding from the bone surface and synovial soft tissue. At the same time, avoid the formation of the sinus communicating joint cavity and the skin.

3. *Subcutaneous Tissue Suturing*: Remove the large free fat particles in the subcutaneous tissue, rinse the subcutaneous tissue with pulsed lavage, use absorbable 2-0 VICRYL® Plus control release suture (Polyglactin 910, Ethicon Inc.) to suture the subcutaneous tissue with sim-

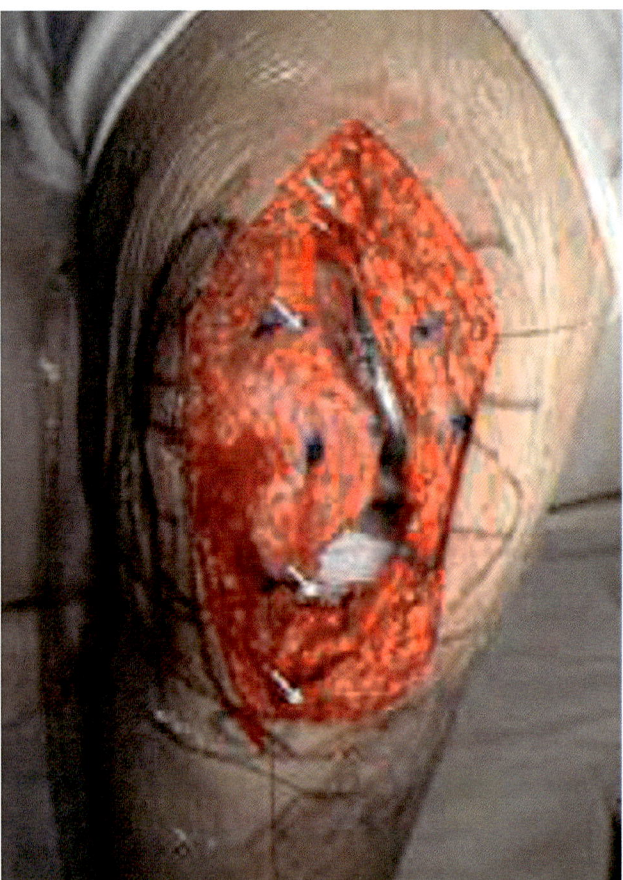

Fig. 10.45 Make 5–6 stitches at the upper and lower edges of the patella at the incision and the distal and proximal ends of the incision to balance the deep incision

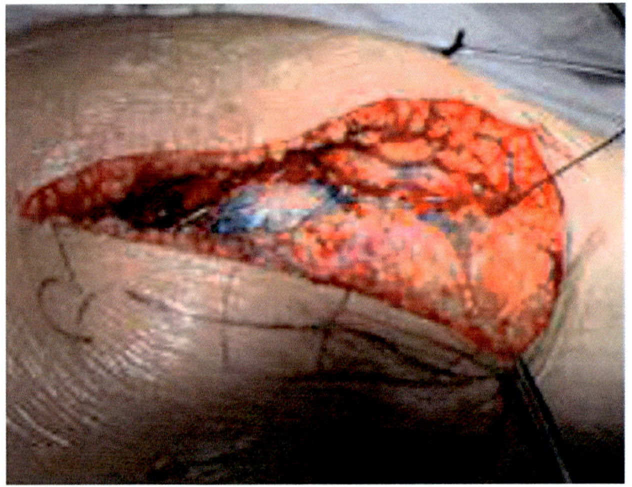

Fig. 10.46 Continuous suturing technique to suture the joint capsule from the distal end to the proximal end of the incision

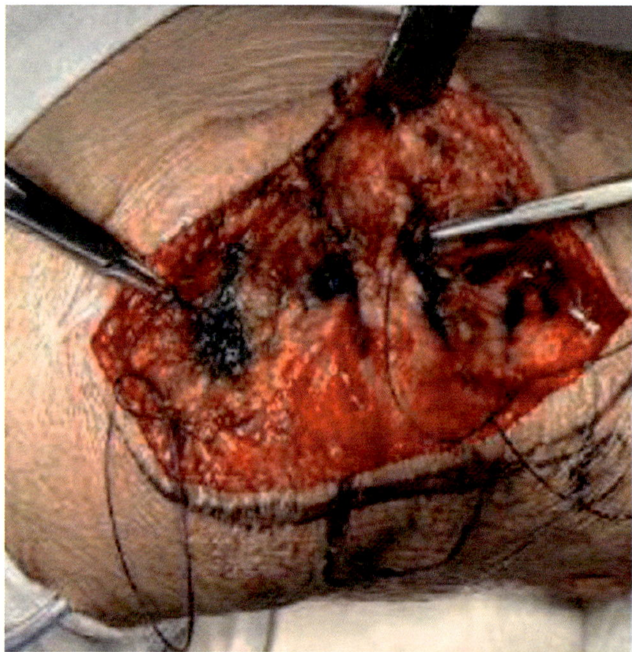

Fig. 10.47 Continuous suturing technique to suture the joint capsule from the center of the incision to both sides

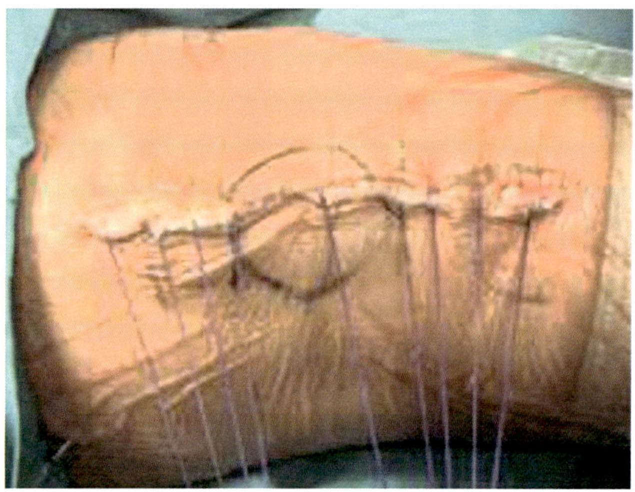

Fig. 10.48 Suture the subcutaneous tissue with simple interrupted suturing technique

ple interrupted suturing (Fig. 10.48), or use the absorbable 2-0 STRATAFIX® Spiral PDO bidirectional knotless tissue control device (Polydioxanone, Ethicon Inc.) for operation to quickly complete the suturing (Fig. 10.49), shorten the procedure and reduce wound exposure time to reduce the probability of infection. Simple interrupted suturing can reduce dead space and ensure good balance. The interval of interrupted suturing is 5 mm. After the suturing, check whether the suturing gap is tight and add suturing when necessary.

4. *Skin Suturing*: Tear off the antibacterial membrane within 5 cm around the incision, disinfect the skin with alcohol gauze, and use absorbable 4-0 STRATAFIX® Spiral PGA-

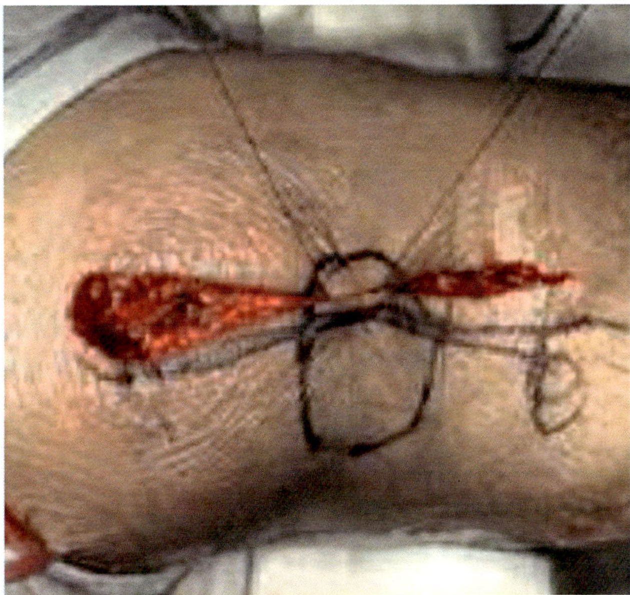

Fig. 10.49 Suture the subcutaneous tissue with knot-free continuous suturing technique

PCL bidirectional knotless tissue control device (PGA-PCL, Ethicon Inc.) to suture skin with continuous intradermal suturing technique (Fig. 10.50). Medical skin tissue glue (DERMABOND PRINEO™, 2-octyl cyanoacrylate, and self-adhesive mesh, Ethicon In.) to seal the incision (Fig. 10.51). Skin glue cannot be used when the subcutaneous tissue is too thin or the subcutaneous suture is not robust.

5. *Incision Dressing*: After the skin tissue glue is dry, wrap the incision with the sterile dressing.

10.3 Prevention and Treatment of Incision Complications

Periprosthetic joint infection (PJI) is a catastrophic complication of joint arthroplasty surgery. Once it occurs, debridement, prosthesis removal, revision, even amputation, and other treatments are required, which brings huge negative physical, psychological and financial effects to the patient. Therefore, joint surgeons have been working to reduce the incidence of PJI. Incision complication after hip and knee arthroplasty surgery is a high-risk factor for PJI. Therefore, it is necessary to prevent the incision complications that may occur after hip and knee arthroplasty surgery as soon as possible and to actively treat the existing incision complications as soon as possible. Incision complications that may cause PJI after hip and knee arthroplasty surgery include incision drainage, swelling, and ecchymosis around the incision, incision dehiscence, necrosis of the incisal margin, incision infection, etc.

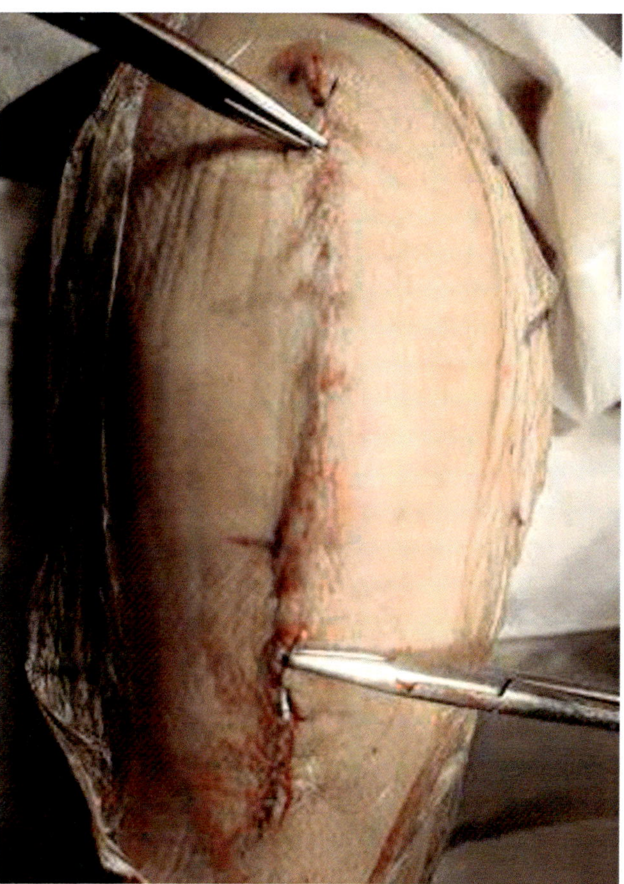

Fig. 10.50 Bidirectional knotless tissue control device continuous intradermal suturing technique for skin suturing

1. *Incision Drainage* (Fig. 10.52)
   (a) Definition: Incision drainage refers to the liquid that leaks from the incision after the surgery, which is the liquid component that leaks from the capillaries to the body tissue. It plays an important role in the healing of the incision, but the continuous exudation of the incision is not good for the incision healing. Persistent wound exudation refers to the post-op surgical site exudation with an area more than 2 cm × 2 cm and the exudation lasts for more than 72 h. The incidence of continuous exudation after joint arthroplasty surgery is high, up to 10% [5]. A small amount of early exudation is mostly related to the destruction of superficial capillaries by surgery, but a large amount or continuous exudation may indicate the risk of infection [6]. The literature results show that every additional day of incision drainage increases the risk of incision complications for hip and knee arthroplasty by 42% and 29% respectively [7].
   (b) Reasons: (1) Malnutrition: for elderly, weak patients, patients with immune system diseases, due to poor basic conditions, hypoproteinemia may occur during the perioperative period of joint arthroplasty, leading

to incision drainage; (2) Soft tissue injury: excessive intraoperative traction, non-standard use of cautery, thick fat layer, extensive exposure needed during surgery, dead space likely to occur, etc.; (3) Improper suturing: such as the suturing is not tight enough, water tightness is poor, too tight suturing causes tissue necrosis, etc.; (4) Use of anticoagulants: anticoagulation is routinely required after joint arthroplasty surgery, but excessive anticoagulation may cause incision drainage, effusion or hematoma, poor healing, etc.; (5) Acute incision infection.

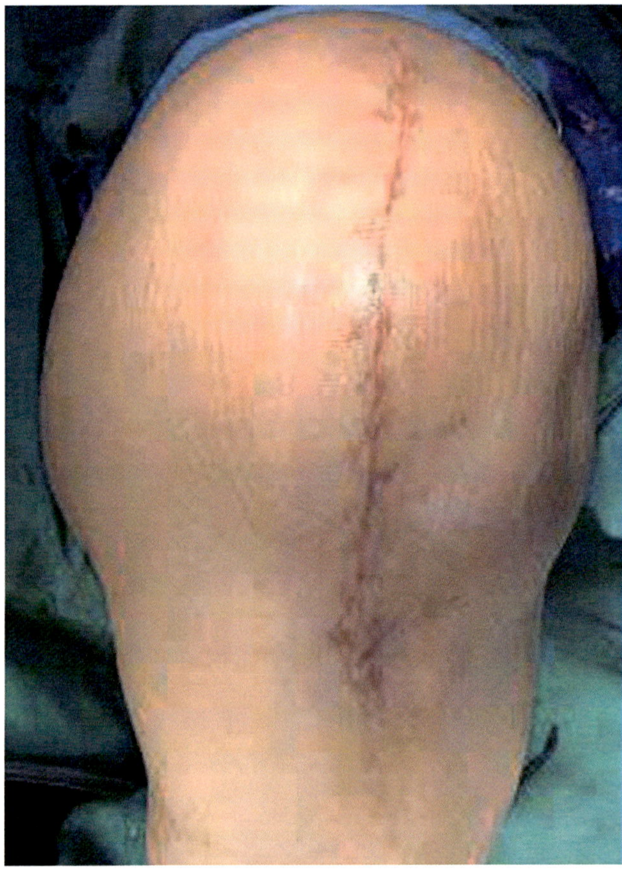

Fig. 10.51 Seal the incision with skin tissue glue

(c) Prevention: (1) Optimizing the patient's general condition before surgery, correcting malnutrition, treating underlying diseases, and discontinuing drugs that may affect the healing of the incision. If biological agents are being used, the patient needs to stop the drug for at least one cycle before surgery; (2) Intra-op soft tissue protection: avoid procedures that excessively damage soft tissues, such as excessive pulling of retractors, cautery used in large area, etc.; (3) Thorough hemostasis and use of tranexamic acid to reduce blood oozing in the incision; (4) Clear subcutaneous fat particles when suturing the incision so that the cutting edge is in the state of blood oozing, which is helpful for healing; (5) Pay attention to the incision suture technique and optimize the use of materials, so as to close the incision tightly without leakage, no dead space, and uniform tension, and reduce the suture damage to the tissue and the tissue rejection of the suture [8].

(d) Treatment: (1) Remove of the cause: correct anemia and hypoalbuminemia, and albumin correction to more than 35 g/L; (2) Reduce the dosage of anticoagulant drugs as appropriate after checking and ruling out deep vein thrombosis, and stop anticoagulation drugs for those with severe blood exudation, use tranexamic acid or antagonists for anticoagulant drugs (warfarin: antagonist vitamin K; unfractionated heparin, low molecular weight heparin: antagonist protamine; Xarelto: lack of antagonist); (3) Change dressing frequently and maintain adequate drainage. Incision dressings with negative pressure suction function can be used [9]. At the same time, activities should be restricted; (4) Conduct debridement in a sterile environment: international consensus on periprosthesis joint infection in 2018 [10] recommended that for patients with continuous incision exudation/drainage more than 3 days, close observation is

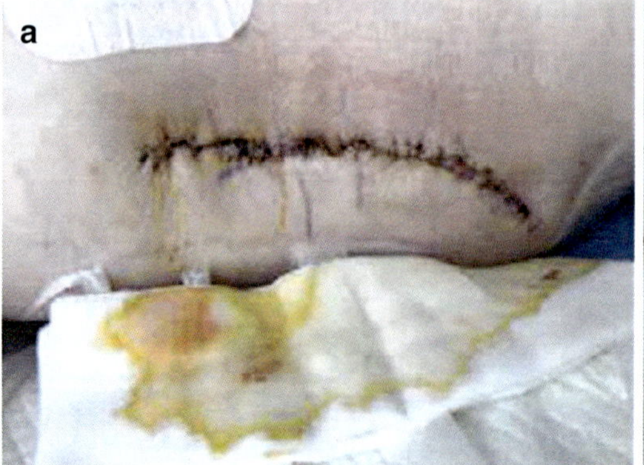

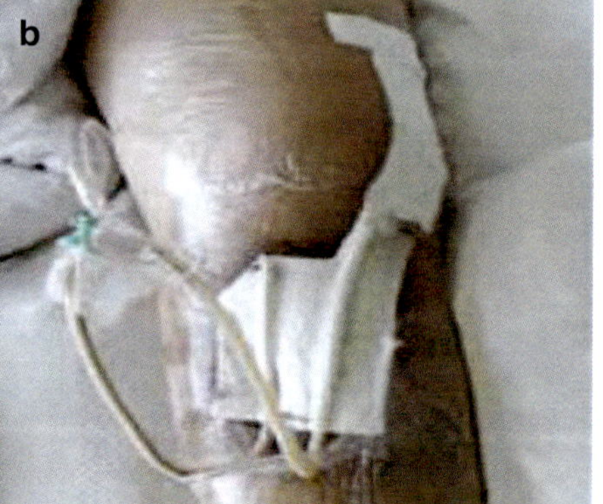

Fig. 10.52 (**a**) Incision drainage on the fourth day after the operation (no original image). (**b**) Continuous use of negative pressure suction material after surgery

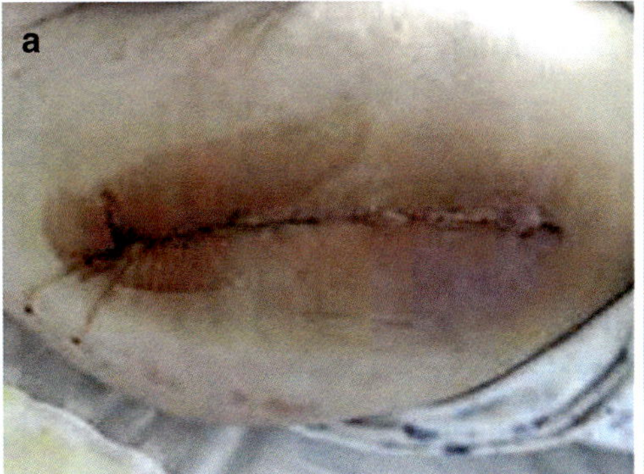

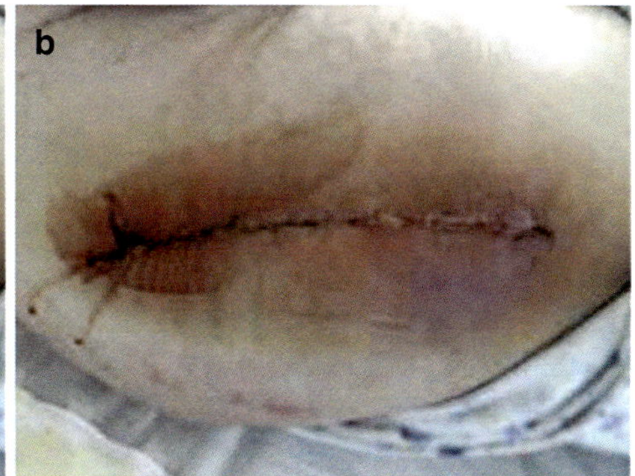

Fig. 10.53 (**a**) Swelling of the soft tissue around the incision. (**b**) Ecchymosis around the incision, black necrosis of the skin edge

needed, for more than 5–7 days, re-surgery is needed without delay; conservative dressing change or even gauze drainage treatment is not recommended; because bacterial culture results usually are skin resident bacteria, it is not recommended to take the exudation liquid directly for culture in the early stage, cause its diagnostic value is not high. (5) Treatment of incision infection: refer to "Incision infection" in this section for details.

Figure Continuous incision drainage after TJA

2. *Incision Swelling and Ecchymosis* (Fig. 10.53).
   (a) Definition: The soft tissue around the incision has increased volume, bruising, and ecchymosis due to edema, effusion, bleeding, inflammatory reaction, and other reasons. Swelling and ecchymosis can damage the skin barrier and increase the risk of deep infections.
   (b) Reasons: (1) Too long time in bed during the perioperative period; (2) The original vascular disease causing venous return disorder; (3) The surgical procedure causes soft tissue damage; (4) The tourniquet is used for too long time or excessive pressure causing ischemia reperfusion injury; (5) Early postoperative excessive activity or rehabilitation training, weight-bearing time is too long; (6) Anemia and hypoproteinemia; (7) Deep vein thrombosis of lower limbs; (8) Excessive use of anticoagulant causes a severe decrease in coagulation function.
   (c) Prevention: (1) Surgical operations should avoid excessive damage to soft tissues and rational use of minimally invasive techniques; (2) Optimize surgical procedures, reduce the time of surgery and tourniquet use, and tourniquet pressure should not exceed twice the systolic pressure or 250–350 mmHg; (3) Rational use of drainage devices, try to use it for patients with higher risk of postoperative bleeding to facilitate the drainage of intra-articular fluid; (4) Gradient compression bandaging or use of elastic stockings to promote blood return from the distal limbs; (5) Elevate the affected limb, use pneumatic blood circulation driver and other physical therapy methods to promote muscle contraction and blood return; (6) Encourage patients to start ankle pump exercise as soon as possible; (7) Apply local or all lower limb cold dressing; (8) Use anti-swelling drugs; (9) Balance anticoagulation and bleeding, and make targeted adjustments to the type of anticoagulant, timing of use, dosage, and time to stop.
   (d) Treatment: (1) Physiotherapy: elevate the affected limb, cold therapy, lower limb gradient compression bandaging/elastic stockings, ankle pump; (2) Choosing active or interactive dressings, such as water-absorbing gel, negative pressure dressing, etc. [5] (3) Nutritional support to correct anemia and hypoproteinemia; (4) Use drugs that promote swelling subsidence; (5) Reduce or stop using anticoagulant drugs after examination confirms that there is no deep vein thrombosis; (6) Reduce the intensity of rehabilitation training, limit the passive flexion angle;

Figure Incision swelling and ecchymosis after TJA

3. *Incision Dehiscence* (Fig. 10.54)
   (a) Definition: Refers to the formation of a cavity due to partial or complete discontinuity in the healing process of a tightly sutured incision.
   (b) Reasons: (1) Trauma: The most common cause of incision dehiscence after knee arthroplasty. It is caused by the shear or separation force formed in the incision by greater violence, which mostly occurs in the early postoperative period with weight-bearing walking when the limb sensation or muscle strength has not recovered, such as femoral nerve block or premature stop using walking aids or other auxiliary walking tools; (2) Delayed incision healing: the patient's underlying disease leads to weakened healing ability and slows incision healing. Suture removal at routine timing can cause the incision dehiscence; (3) Excessive

tissue tension, especially for complex joint arthroplasty or incisions in the areas of previous healed scars; (4) Suture technical factors, such as insufficient suture layers, unqualified knotting and suture breaks; (5) Inappropriate selection of sutures, the degradation time of sutures is earlier than the healing time of tissues; (6) Incision tissue necrosis; (7) Incision infection: long-term exudation can cause surgical site infection and even deep infection, affecting the healing of the incision and even the formation of the sinus.

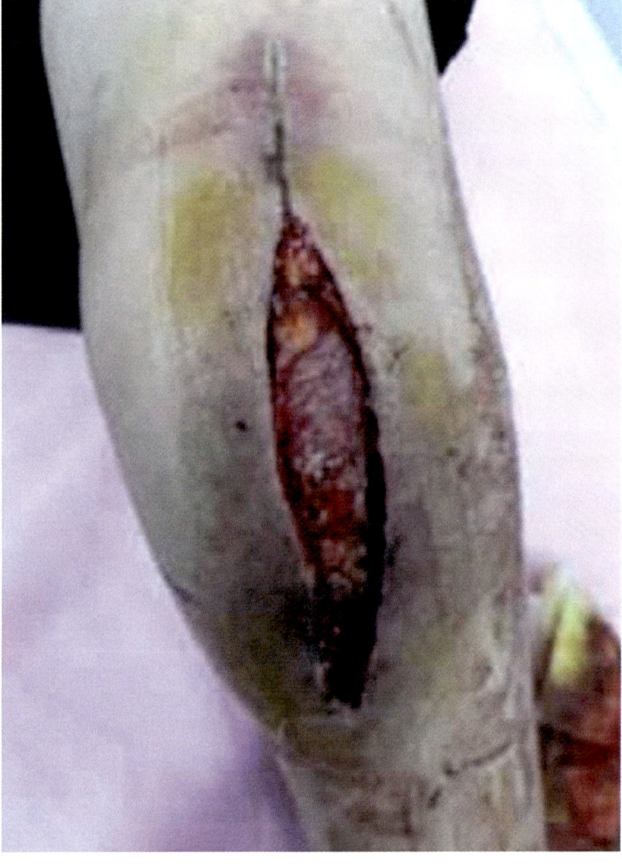

Fig. 10.54 Incision dehiscence after TKA (no original image)

(c) Prevention: (1) Treat underlying diseases, correct malnutrition, treat underlying diseases, discontinue drugs that may affect incision healing; (2) Reduce incision suturing tension, appropriately expand the range of release, and use continuous knot-free suturing, etc.; (3) Old scar incisions can be treated with the assistance of plastic surgery department. Preoperative skin expansion or intraoperative skin flaps to close the incision, negative pressure-assisted incision dressings can be used to maintain adequate drainage; (4) For patients with expected slow healing, delay the suture removal; (5) Choose appropriate suture materials to reduce the risk of suture breakage, and the risk of failure of continuous knot-free sutures is significantly lower than that of interrupted suturing [11]; (6) Improve interrupted suturing and knotting technique; (7) Avoid trauma: avoid using femoral nerve block, or start weight-bearing training after the block anesthesia has completely gone. After the surgery, the patient uses a walker or crutches to assist in walking until the muscle strength is basically normal. It is recommended for at least 6 weeks.

(d) Treatment: For the superficial incision dehiscence, debride then suture. The dehiscence of the deep fascia requires re-suturing in the operating room. Routinely take tissues and joint fluid during the surgery for culture. After the surgery, use antibiotics according to the results of bacterial culture and drug sensitivity test. The liner needs to be changed when necessary to facilitate more thorough debridement.

4. *Necrosis of Incisal Margin*

(a) Definition: the tissue around the surgical incision causes cell death and tissue inactivation due to ischemia, infection, or inflammatory reaction. The black necrotic tissue is formed by the necrosis and dehydration of healthy tissue, which is usually the result of local ischemia (Fig. 10.55).

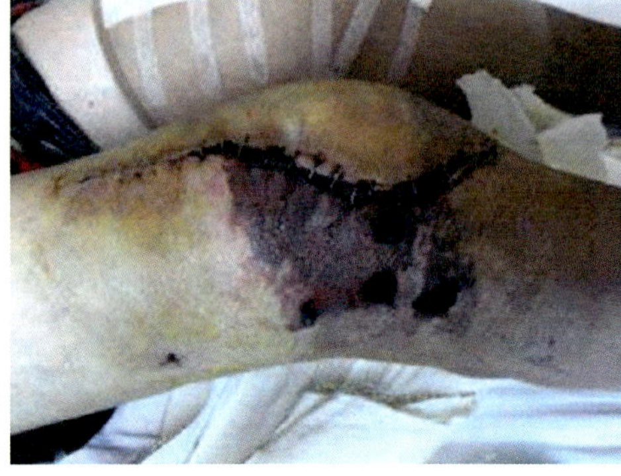

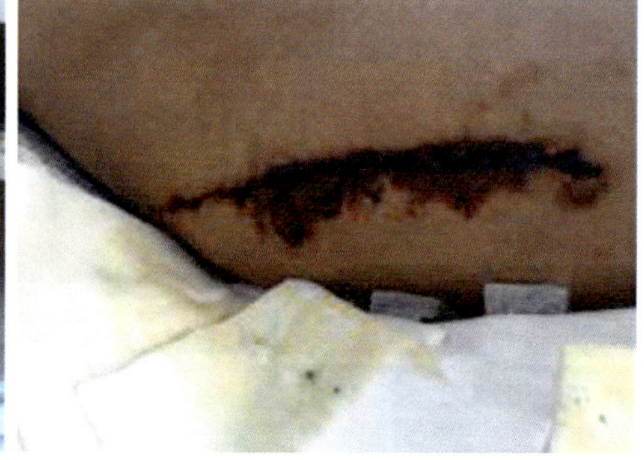

Fig. 10.55 Excessive stretching during the surgery causes necrosis of the skin margin

Incision Margin Skin Necrosis Repair after Total Knee Arthroplasty, China Repair and Reconstruction 201,408

(b) Reasons: (1) There was a previous surgical scar in the surgical area, and the new surgical incision of the knee joint is located at the medial side of the original incision, or lacking sufficient distance from the original incision; (2) Intraoperative excessive stretching, clamping or local skin compression: retractors causing the local tissue bear excessive tension, causing pressure ulcer; (3) The separation range of the fascia layer is too large, destroying the blood supply of the deep vascular network perforating branch artery to the superficial fascia and skin; (4) Cautery burns; (5) Density of sutures or skin staples or excessive tightening force during suturing cause ischemia of the skin margin; (6) Postoperative edema and hematoma lead to increased local tension of the incision; (7) Incision infection.

(c) Prevention: (1) Use the most lateral incision when there are multiple incisions at the knee joint, the new incision is perpendicular to the original incision or keep a certain distance between, and the long-wide ratio is about 2:1; (2) Avoid violent stretching of the incisal margin during the surgery. Use wide retractors to reduce local pressure; (3) Perform limited dissection of the superficial fascia, and place a drainage tube for larger range of dissection, which is good for the blood supply reconstruction of the superficial and deep fascia after surgery; (4) Use cautery appropriately, avoid patch of "scorched earth," spot hemostasis; (5) When suturing, tension-reduced suturing is required for subcutaneous tissue, the suturing tension of the suture or skin staples should be appropriate. Skin glue or zipper can be used to disperse the incision tension; (6) When suturing, avoid residual dead space causing hematoma, strengthen swelling treatment, elevate the affected limb, use elastic bandages or elastic stockings, use anti-swelling drugs; (7) Prevent infection.

(d) Treatment: Early intervention is required after necrosis of the incisal margin. (1) Remove the factors that may lead to necrosis. If the suture tension is too large, the stitches are removed intermittently to eliminate tension, elevate the affected limb for treating swelling, use hot lamps to promote local vascular expansion and improve blood supply; (2) Autolysis debridement: use the moist or semi-moist dressing to cover the necrotic tissue, use the wound fluid itself to decompose the necrotic tissue, promote the growth and arthroplasty of the deep granulation tissue, use various gel formulas to accelerate the decomposition of the necrotic tissue, or use debridement gel; (3) If the necrosis cannot be replaced by granulation, another surgery is required to remove the necrotic tissue, use negative pressure suction materials to promote granulation growth, and later use skin flap or skin graft to cover; (4) Use antibiotics to promote incision healing and prevent necrotic infection from invading the joint cavity.

5. *Incision Infection After Joint Arthroplasty Surgery* (Fig. 10.56a, b)
   (a) Definition: Refer to Sect. 3.1 for the definition and diagnostic criteria of surgical site infection. The key diagnosis point of incision infection after joint arthroplasty surgery is to determine whether the infection is communicated to the joint cavity.

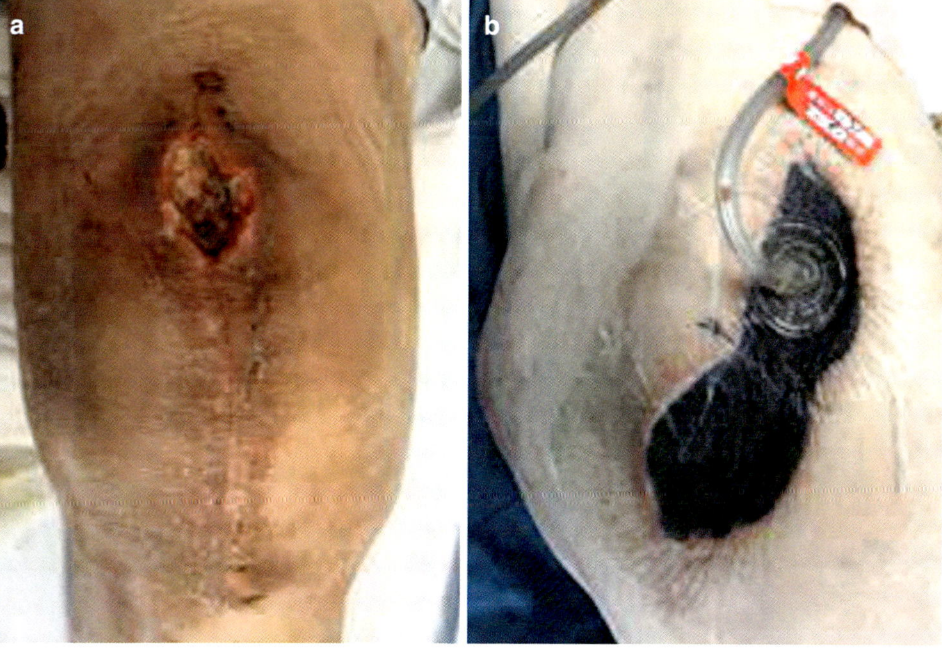

Fig. 10.56 (**a**) Infection of the proximal incision, deep fascia not involved. (**b**) Acute PJI after THA, debridement + continual negative pressure suction performed

(b) Reasons: (1) Patient factors: poor basic status, more comorbidities such as diabetes, malnutrition, immune system diseases, use of the hormone, skin injury diseases, etc.; (2) Surgical procedure factors: incomplete disinfection, non-standard aseptic operation, severe tissue stretching damage, extensive exposure of complicated surgery, long operation time, more bleeding, etc.; (3) Operating room environmental factors: too many personnel in and out, unqualified equipment disinfection, etc.; (4) With before-mentioned incision complications.

(c) Prevention: (1) Optimize the patient's systemic and local conditions, adjust the adjustable comorbidities to the best conditions [12, 13], such as quitting smoking before surgery, glycated hemoglobin not exceeding 7.5%–8% [13], stopping biological agents for one cycle, etc.; (2) Standard surgical procedure, strict aseptic operations, shorten the operation time, and avoid excessive tissue stretching; (3) Enhance the management of personnel flow in the operating room; (4) Choose suitable suture materials, such as sutures containing triclosan and knot-free sutures.

(d) The method for judging the communication between the infection and the deep joint cavity: under strict aseptic conditions, inject appropriate amount of normal saline into the joint cavity from normal skin, move the joints, and observe whether there is any fluid exudation from the superficial layer; add one ampule of methylene blue into 50 ml normal saline for better observation.

(e) Treatment: For infections confined to the skin and superficial fascia layer that do not communicate with the joint cavity, debride the wound under aseptic conditions, change dressings or sutures, extend the use of antibiotics, and adjust according to the culture results. If it communicates with the joint cavity, consider PJI, conduct thorough debridement in accordance with the treatment principles of acute PJI, and change the liner when necessary. There are different versions of PJI diagnostic criteria in different organizations, and the most used one was formulated by MSIS in 2011. In 2013, ICM launched the first version of PJI diagnosis and launched the second version after ICM re-voting in 2018. The 2013 version of the international consensus PJI diagnostic criteria for musculoskeletal system infection is shown in Table 10.1.

Figure Superficial incision infection after TJA
Figure Acute PJI after THA

Table 10.1 International consensus of PJI diagnostic criteria for musculoskeletal system infection in 2013

1. There is sinus communicating to the prosthesis, or.
2. The same pathogenic bacteria isolated by microbiological culture testing of at least two independent tissues or body fluid samples taken from the diseased joint prosthesis; or.
3. Three of the following five criteria
   (a) Increased erythrocyte sedimentation rate (ESR) and C-reactive protein (CRP).
   (b) Joint fluid white blood cell count increasing or white blood cell esterase test paper positive.
   (c) Increased percentage of neutrophils in joint fluid (PMN%).
   (d) The tissue samples around the prosthesis are tested with ×400 magnification times for histological examination, and the number of white blood cells in each 5 high power field exceeds 5.
   (e) Microbial culture of one tissue or body fluid sample around the prosthesis isolates microorganisms.

Diagnostic criteria	Acute PJI (<90 days)	Chronic PJI (>90 days)
ESR (mm/h)	Useless	30
CRP (mg/L)	100	10
Joint fluid white blood cell count (/μL)	10,000	3000
Joint fluid percentage of neutrophils	90	80
Leucocyte esterase	+ or ++	+ or ++
Pathology analysis	Neutrophil count >5 per high power field (×400)	The same as acute

References

1. Gibson A. Posterior exposure of the hip joint. J Bone Joint Surg (Br). 1950;32:183–6.
2. Moore AT. The Moore self-locking vitallium prosthesis in fresh femoral neck fractures: a new low posterior approach (the southern exposure). AAOS Instr Course Lect. 1959;16:309.
3. Smith-Petersen MN. Approach to and exposure of the hip joint for mold arthroplasty. J Bone Joint Surg Am. 1949;31A(1):40–6.
4. Lavernia C, Contreras Raygoza J, Alcerro J. The peel in total knee revision: exposure in the difficult knee. Clin Orthop Relat Res. 2011;469:146–53.
5. Weiss AP, Krackow KA. Persistent wound drainage after primary total knee arthroplasty. J Arthroplast. 1993;8(3):285–9.
6. Jaberi FM, et al. Procrastination of wound drainage and malnutrition affect the outcome of joint arthroplasty. Clin Orthop Relat Res. 2008;466(6):1368–71.
7. Al-Houraibi RK, et al. General assembly, prevention, wound management: proceedings of international consensus on orthopedic infections. J Arthroplast. 2019;34(2S):S157–68.
8. Hansen E, et al. Negative pressure wound therapy is associated with resolution of incisional drainage in most wounds after hip arthroplasty. Clin Orthop Relat Res. 2013;471(10):3230–6.
9. Galat DD, et al. Surgical treatment of early wound complications following primary total knee arthroplasty. J Bone Joint Surg Am. 2009;91(1):48–54.

10. Abdel Karim M, Andrawis J, Bengoa F, Bracho C, Compagnoni R, Cross M, et al. Hip and knee section, diagnosis, algorithm: proceedings of international consensus on orthopedic infections. J Arthroplasty. 2019;34(2S):S339–S50 (Proceedings of the International Consensus Meeting on Periprosthetic Joint Infection. Foreword. J Orthop Res. 2014;32 Suppl 1:S2–3).
11. Patel VP, et al. Factors associated with prolonged wound drainage after primary total hip and knee arthroplasty. J Bone Joint Surg Am. 2007;89(1):33–8.
12. Ares O, et al. General assembly, prevention, host related local: proceedings of international consensus on orthopedic infections. J Arthroplast. 2019;34(2S):S3–S12.
13. Shohat N, et al. Serum fructosamine: a simple and inexpensive test for assessing preoperative glycemic control. J Bone Joint Surg Am. 2017;99(22):1900–7.

Cosmetic Skin Suture and Irregular Skin Wound Suture

11

Yixin Zhang, Huifeng Song, Xin Wang, Maoguo Shu, Lianzhao Wang, Jiaping Zhang, Yangmin Xu, Heng Xu, and Tian Liu

Abstract

Skin scars cannot be avoided, but its degree is closely related to the shape of the incision, local tension, blood supply, and other factors. In this chapter, we focus on the structure of the skin and the concept of relaxed skin tension line (RSTL). Through a detailed discussion of the tissue structure involved in suturing and the local tension of the incision, we try to make readers understand: (1) Influence of different tissue structures on the appearance of the incision after suturing; (2) Characteristics of local blood supply; (3) The distribution of human skin tension, so as to design the surgical incision and adjust the shape of the wound edge in irregular wound suture.

In clinical practice, no matter well-designed surgical incisions or irregular wounds are seen in the ER, the cosmetic effect is the most concerned factor (sometimes the only factor) for the patients. Therefore, the demand for skin cosmetic suturing in modern surgery has been increasing. Skin cosmetic closure is achieved based on suturing principles, techniques, and suture selection. Although scarless cannot be achieved, flattering of the skin and the relative inconspicuity of the sear can be achieved. From a practical point of view, this section will sequentially describe the principles of skin cosmetic suture, suture techniques, suture techniques for irregular wounds, finally, the "Zhang's super relaxation suture" with the ultra-small scar.

Achieving clinical results of cosmetic skin closure requires not only familiarity with principles and mastery of suturing techniques, but also the application of appropriate surgical instruments and sutures. This is not to say that the smaller or the thinner the better, but to be familiar with the potential damage that different devices may cause to sutures and skin tissues. At the same time, different tissue reaction, absorption time, and strength of sutures of different materials will also affect the healing of the skin and the appearance of scars. In this chapter, we focus on the characteristics of commonly used surgical instruments and sutures and introduce in detail the suture selection experience of the Plastic Surgery Department, Shanghai Ninth People's Hospital, Shanghai Jiaotong University School of Medicine.

Keywords

Skin · Anatomy · Blood supply · Skin suture · Standard suture technique · Irregular wound · Device · Matching

Y. Zhang (✉) · H. Xu
Shanghai Ninth People's Hospital, Shanghai JiaoTong University School of Medicine, Shanghai, China

H. Song · T. Liu
Department of Burns and Plastic Surgery, The Fourth Medical Center of PLA General Hospital, Beijing, China

X. Wang
Ningbo No.6 Hospital, Zhejiang, China

M. Shu
The First Affiliated Hospital of Xi'an Jiaotong University, Xi'an, Shaanxi, China

L. Wang
Plastic Surgery Hospital, CAMS, Beijing, China

J. Zhang
The Southwest Hospital of AMU, Chongqing, China

Y. Xu
The First Affiliated Hospital, Sun Yat-sen University, Guangzhou, China

P. Tang et al. (eds.), *Tutorials in Suturing Techniques for Orthopedics*, https://doi.org/10.1007/978-981-33-6330-4_11

The history of cosmetic skin suture began in ancient times. The Greeks and Romans noticed the importance of cosmetic appearance in wound closure and first proposed a layered closure technique. Later, Liszt's antiseptic principle prompted cosmetic dermatologic surgery represented by aseptic wound closure technology to enter a modern stage [1, 2]. With the rapid development of skin suture materials, devices, and suture techniques, skin cosmetic suture technology has been constantly innovating, enabling the purpose of optimal scar morphology.

The primary goal of skin cosmetic suture is to close the wound with minimal esthetic loss. Ideally, the edges of the sutured wound should be as close as possible so that the tissue can close the skin through the formation of scar tissue. The scar formed after skin closure is located on the body surface, and its shape, color, size, and other attributes will accompany the patient for a lifetime. Poor morphology may impair the appearance of the patient, which in turn affects their self-confidence and quality of life.

Understanding the basic principles of cosmetic skin suture and established surgical techniques can help achieve the most predictable results. However, in some cases, even for experienced surgeons, unsatisfactory results may still occur. This is mainly due to individual differences between patients, furthermore, the dynamic processes involved in wound healing and scarring are only partially predictable.

Based on the above, this chapter introduces cosmetic skin suture in three aspects: skin anatomy, suture methods, and technique, and selection of device and suture, as well as current postoperative wound treatment methods in order to obtain the best cosmetic skin closure.

Rules and Techniques 1

1. Plan the suturing process comprehensively before each procedure, photographs may be helpful.
2. Considering the age of the patient, the surgical incision should be carefully designed in view of the high incidence of hypertrophic scars in children and adolescents.
3. The poor esthetic result is not necessarily the fault of the surgeon, so avoid giving in to the patient's blind dissatisfaction.

11.1 Skin Structure

Zhang Yixin, Song Huifeng, Shu Maoguo, Wang Lianzhao, Wang Xin, Zhang Jiaping, Xu Yangbin and Xu Heng

11.1.1 Skin Anatomy

Figure 11.1 depicts the anatomy of the skin, which consists of two layers: epidermis and dermis. The epidermis is composed of the stratum corneum (upper layer) and the non-stratum corneum (lower layer). The increase of melanocyte content makes the skin darker, and vice versa. The dermis is generally divided into papillary and reticular layers, which are directly nourished by blood vessels and

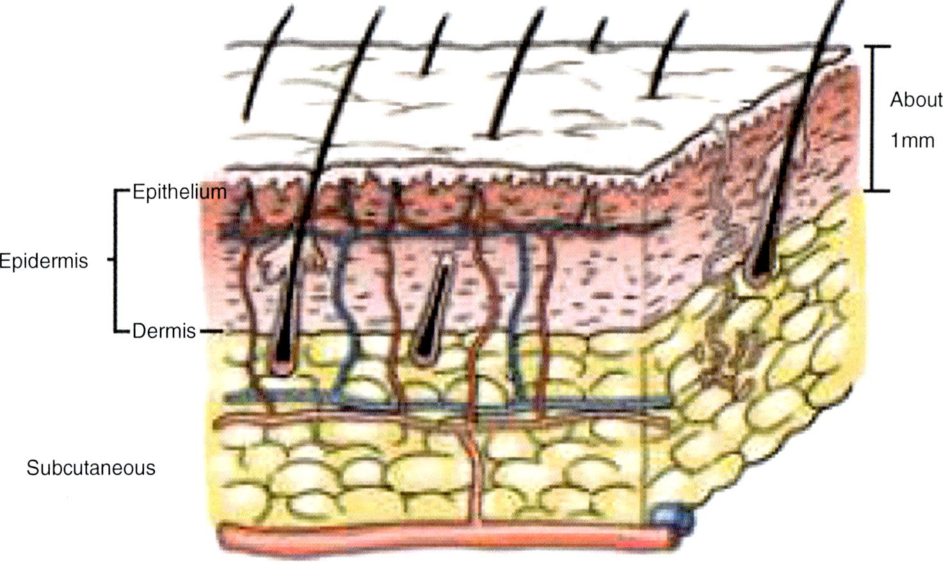

Fig. 11.1 Skin anatomy structure

nerves. Rich in elasticity and collagen fibers are responsible for skin elasticity and contractility.

The papillary dermis intersects the epidermis so that the two layers do not move horizontally from each other. Therefore, any movement of the skin always occurs at the level of the subcutaneous fat layer, which separates the skin from the underlying structural tissues (muscles, bones). The development of the dermis in different areas is different, that is, the thickness varies greatly, for example, the dermis of the back and the thighs are thicker, while the dermis of the eyelids and ears are thin [3, 4].

Hair, sebaceous glands, and sweat glands are mostly located in the skin as skin appendages, and a small part in the subcutaneous fat layer. In cosmetic skin closure, the focus is to understand that skin appendages run through the epidermis and dermis. Wound healing may be affected by the content of sebaceous glands in the skin. In areas rich in sebaceous glands (especially in the forehead, nose, back, and other parts of adolescents), significant scarring may occur around the suture line. This is due to the epithelialization of the scar after puncture injury of the injured gland.

The blood supply in the dermis is generally derived from two ways: The subcutaneous vascular plexus, which runs under the dermis; specific arteries (accompanied by veins). These arteries usually run parallel to the skin between muscles/surface and give rise to blood vessels perpendicular to the skin (except the blood vessels of the subcutaneous nerve plexus).

The amount of subcutaneous fat tissue varies depending on its distribution area. For example, the tissue of the eyelid is thinner, while the tissue of the abdominal subcutaneous fat layer is thicker. The blood supply is abundant but lacks reliable rules. A common issue during suturing is that the subcutaneous fat layer is liquefied due to electrocautery thermal injury, which affects the tissue healing. In addition, pay attention to trimming the fat tissue beneath the skin edge during suturing, otherwise, it will be embedded between the skin edges to affect their healing [5, 6].

11.1.2 Relaxed Skin Tension Line

The incision designed before the surgery should match the relaxed skin tension line (RSTL, Fig. 11.2) and skin wrinkles. The wrinkle lines are perpendicular to the direction of the muscle fibers, while RSTL refers to the place where the tension formed by collagen and elastic fibers in the skin is minimal. RSTL can correspond to the wrinkles formed spontaneously after skin laxity, so both are roughly the same. But they are different in some areas, such as the glabella and the nasal side. When the surgical incision corresponds to the direction of the RSTL, less tense wounds can be obtained, so that the wound heals the fastest and scars the least; when there are wrinkles, the principle of "hiding the scar in the skin wrinkle" should be followed, and the incision should be designed in the skin wrinkles [1, 2, 5].

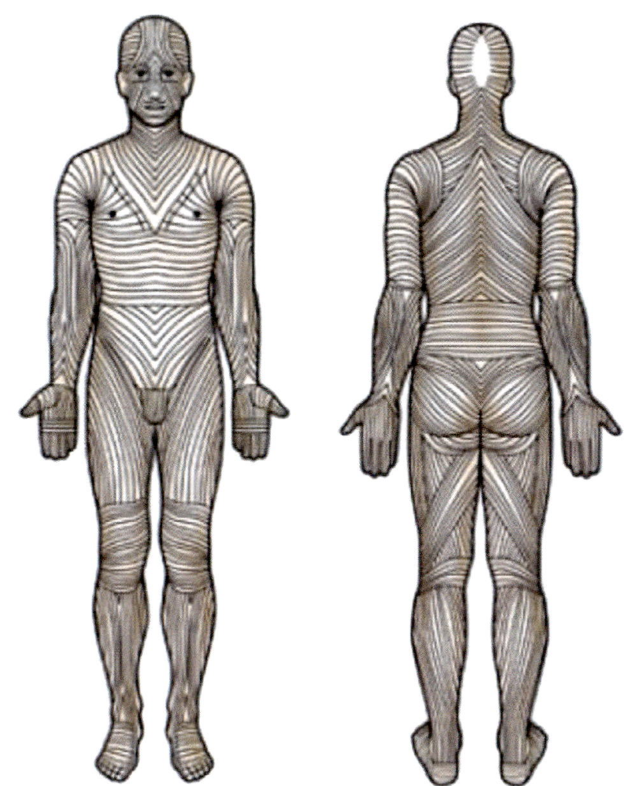

Fig. 11.2 Relaxed skin tension line

11.2 Skin Cosmetic Suture Methods and Techniques

11.2.1 The Principle of Cosmetic Skin Suture

After skin suture, the wound should be slightly averted, and the suture should be tense enough but not too tight. At the same time, knots should be buried deep in the tissue to reduce the irritation of the knots and avoid scarring.

The Hollander wound evaluation scale proposes that ideal wound healing should meet the following six key points:

1. No tissue dislocation.
2. The wound is aligned neatly.
3. The distance between wound alignment does not exceed 2 mm.
4. No skin edge inversion.
5. No excessive distortion of skin tissue.
6. Overall esthetics.

Reaching each of the above key point is scored 1 point, 6 points are the best wound healing.

11.2.2 Standard Suture Technique

Skin wound suture usually includes subcutaneous suture and skin suture (Fig. 11.3). Subcutaneous sutures are generally closed with Absorbable 2–0/3–0 Coated VICRYL® Plus Control Release Suture (Polyglactin 910, Ethicon Inc.) to reduce the tension on both sides of the wound with interrupted suturing technique, and leave the knot buried deep in the tissue (Fig. 11.3a). It should be noted that the subcutaneous tissue has low flexibility and cannot provide sufficient tension reduction effect, so a small amount of dermal tissue can be carried over the subcutaneous suture. In addition, the subcutaneous adipose tissue can be trimmed before suturing to prevent tissue accumulation affecting the alignment of the skin edges and inserting between the skin edges to affect the healing of the wound edges.

Use interrupted suture to reform skin edges for skin closure (Fig. 11.3b, c). It is generally believed that interrupted suturing could adjust local tension easily, and poor suturing effect and loose knots in a single site or other adverse events have little effect on the overall appearance. Therefore, the interrupted suture is the most commonly used and most effective suture technique for cosmetic skin suture [7–10].

However, it should be noted that more knots and more sutures are required. So the surgeon will spend more operating time and certain patience.

11.2.3 Suture Techniques for Irregular Wounds

1. For wounds with the length difference of the two sides less than 1 cm (Fig. 11.4a), first suture the middle part of the wound (Fig. 11.4b), then suture the middle parts of the wounds on both sides (Fig. 11.4c) and then continue to suture the middle part of each wound until the wound is completely closed, namely: middle-middle-middle.
2. When the length difference of two sides of the wound is less than 1 cm, in order to avoid small "cat ears" at both

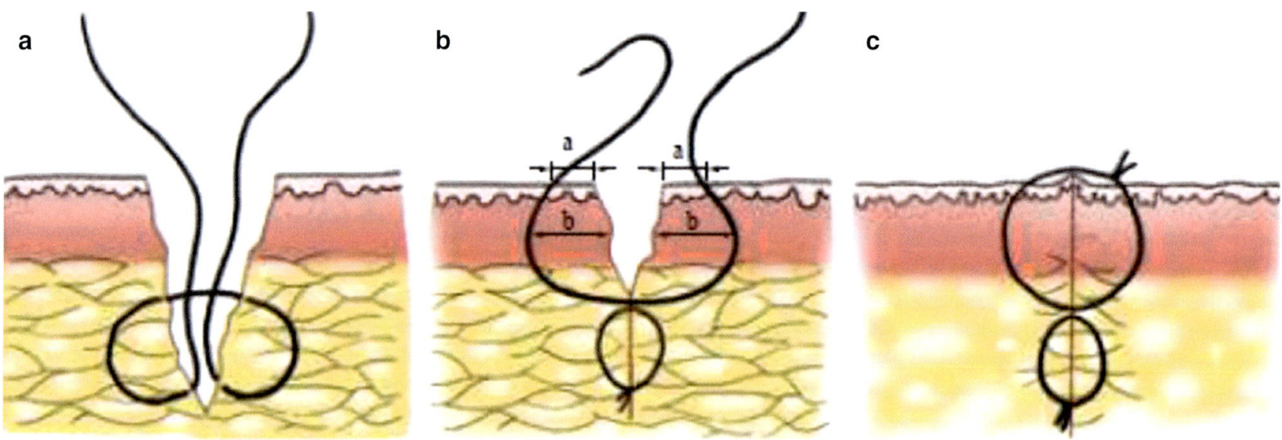

Fig. 11.3 Standard technique of skin suture. (**a**) Bury the suture knots deep in the tissue; (**b**) Interrupted skin suture, pay attention to avoiding dead space. During skin closure, the needle entry direction should be far away from the wound edge, (**c**) A small hill shape formed after tying the knot

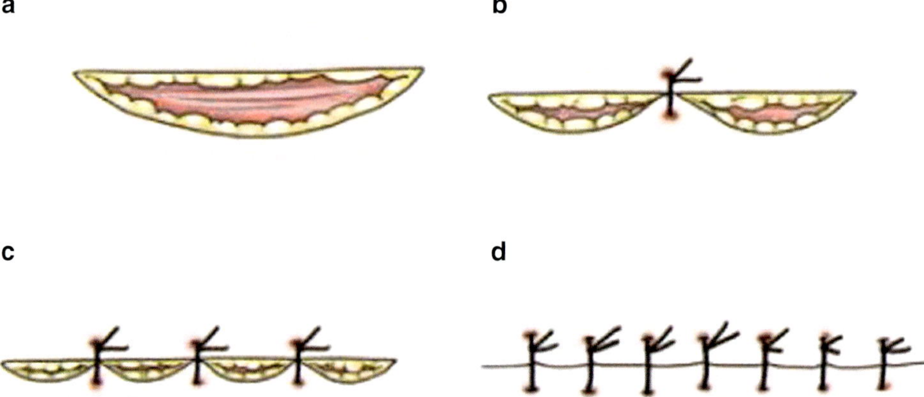

Fig. 11.4 The length difference between the two ends of the irregular wound is less than 1 cm. (**a**) When the wound is in a relaxed state, the lower edge is longer than the upper one; (**b**) Suture the middle part of the wound, (**c**) Then suture the middle parts of the wounds on both sides, (**d**) Close the wound

ends, after confirming both suturing ends are flat, and then follow tip 1 to close the wound, namely: both ends-middle-middle (Fig. 11.5).

3. The length difference between two sides of the wound is greater than 1 cm (Fig. 11.6a), and "cat ears" will inevitably appear. At this point, start suturing from one end of the wound (Fig. 11.6b), and "drive" the excessive skin at the longer edge to one end (Fig. 11.6b). Then make an oblique incision (1–2 cm, Fig. 11.6c), cut off the extra skin beyond the incision and suture (Fig. 11.6d)

Rules and Techniques 2

Appropriate suture results depend on:

1. The wound edges of the skin must be of similar length, otherwise "cat ears" will appear. The latter can be eliminated by trimming or other techniques (Figs. 11.4, 11.5 and 11.6).
2. Through skin excision and skin movement, the deep wound edges can reach the same level (Fig. 11.7).
3. The entrance and exit depth of the subcutaneous suture area must be equal (otherwise the wound edge will be deformed) (Fig. 11.7b).
4. When the skin is sutured, the knot should not be pulled too tight, otherwise, scar contraction will be formed (postoperative wound swelling must be considered).
5. The suture's ends must be left long enough for easy removal, but they must be cut short enough to prevent them from interfering with adjacent sutures.
6. The wound edges should be inspected after closure. The epithelium should not be turned inward but should be turned outward (Fig. 11.7c).

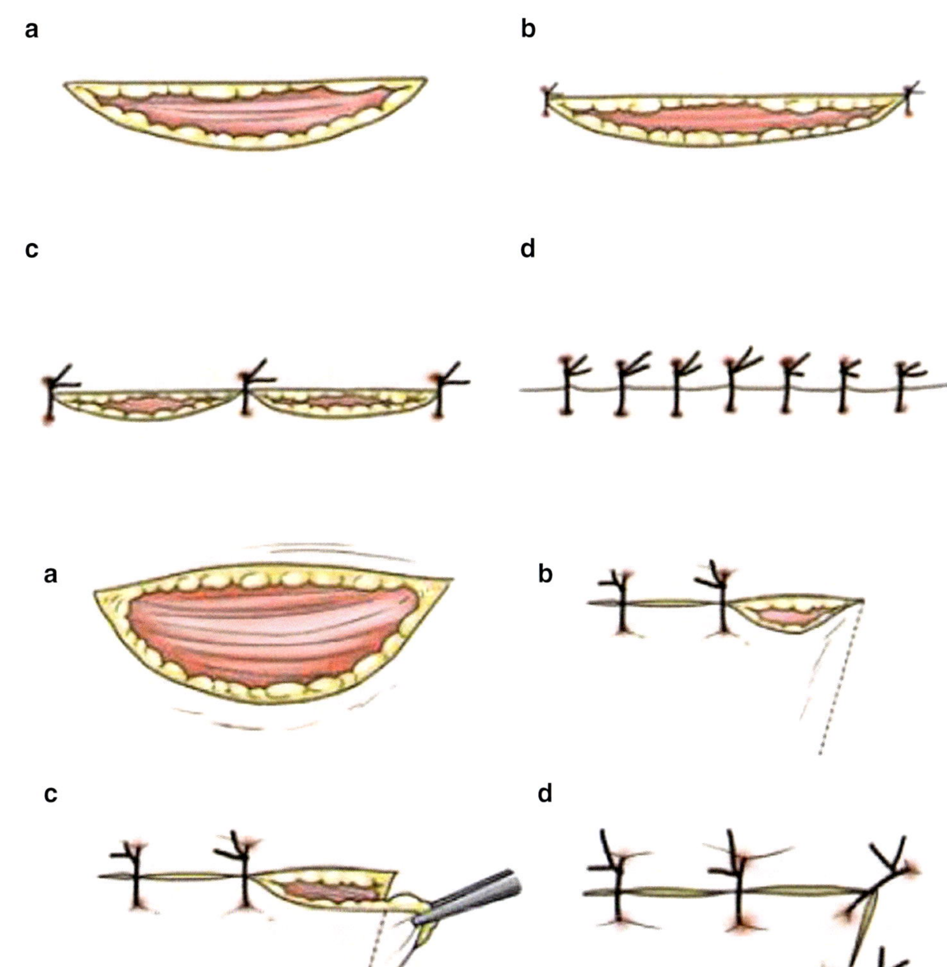

Fig. 11.5 (**a**) When the wound is relaxed, the lower margin is longer than the upper margin; Figure (**b**) First close both ends, then (**c**, **d**), close the wound in sequence

Fig. 11.6 The length difference between the two sides of the irregular wound is greater than 1 cm. (**a**) When the wound is in a relaxed state, the lower edge is longer than the upper one; (**b**) Start suturing from one end of the wound, and "drive" the excessive skin on the longer side edge to one end; (**c**) Then make an oblique incision (1–2 cm), unfold the excessive skin to identify the part to be removed; (**d**) Cut the extra skin beyond the incision then suture

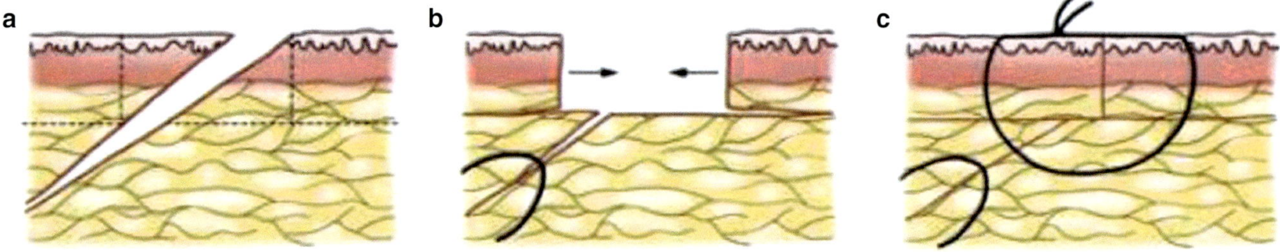

Fig. 11.7 Downward oblique incision. (**a**) Trim the skin edge (otherwise the skin edge is not easy to be aligned after suture, and soft tissue is accumulated); (**b**) After suturing the subcutaneous tissue, free the skin edge (free in the subcutaneous fat layer); (**c**) Suture the skin

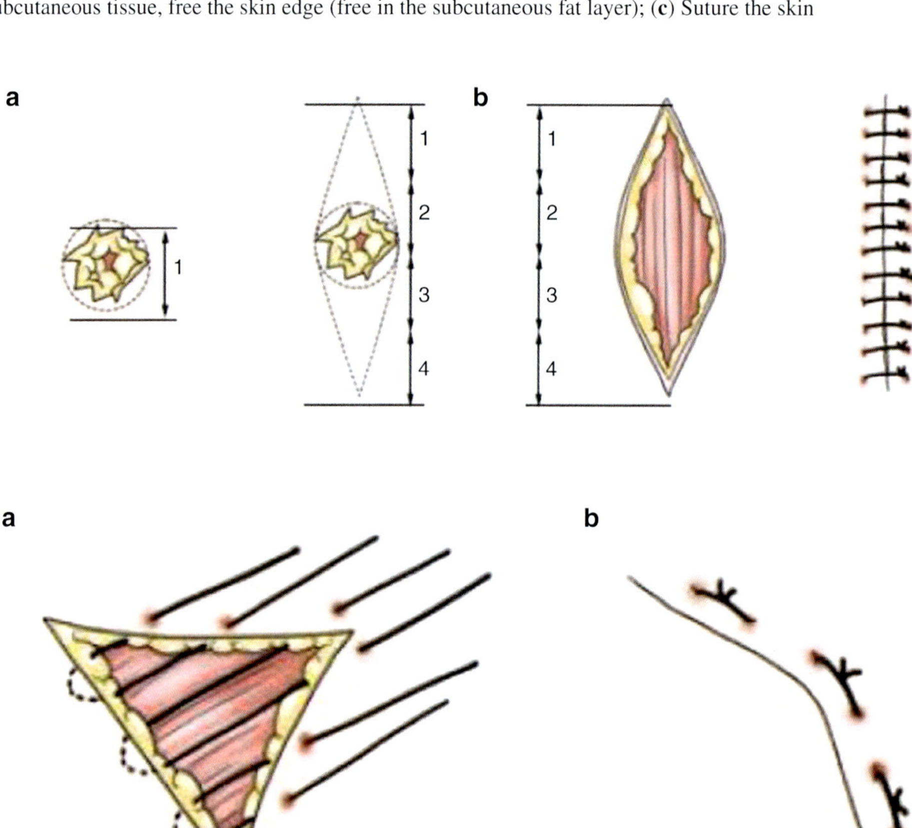

Fig. 11.8 Suturing of round-like irregular wounds. First identify the direction and length difference of the long and short axis, trim the wound into a fusiform, and then suture it. (**a**) round-like irregular wounds; (**b**) trim the wound into a fusiform

Fig. 11.9 Treatment of irregular triangle-like wounds. (**a**) After the wound is trimmed into an obtuse triangle; (**b**) The wound is sutured along the direction of obtuse angle

4. Round-Like Irregular Wound (Fig. 11.8).
   (a) If the long and short axes of the wound are equal, the wound can be trimmed into a fusiform and sutured along the relaxed skin tension line or perpendicular to the direction of greater skin tension.
   (b) If there is a big difference between the long and short axis of the wound, trim the wound into a fusiform in the direction of the extension axis and suture it.

   It should be noted that during the initial trimming of the wound, avoid removing a large amount of skin tissue. It can be trimmed according to the treatment method of the linear irregular wound when suturing and aligning.
5. Triangle-Like Irregular Wound (Fig. 11.9)
   (a) For an obtuse triangle or when the tension in a certain direction of the triangle is small, the wound can be trimmed into an obtuse triangle and then sutured into a line shape. The locally accumulated skin tissues are treated in the same way as linear irregular wounds.
   (b) For triangles cannot be trimmed or wounds tend to be triangles, triangular suturing can be used to treat the wounds, that is, the tips of the three sides are sutured

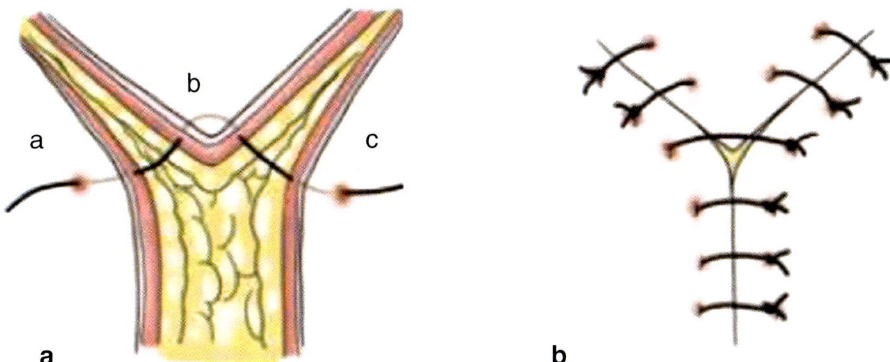

Fig. 11.10 Treatment of triangle-like irregular wounds. (**a**) Triangular suturing technique; (**b**) Tying knots after triangular suturing, and the rest is treated according to linear suturing technique

together, and the rest are treated as linear suturing. When suturing the tips of three sides, insert the needle from side a and carry the tip tissue on side b (note that tip necrosis may occur when less tissue is carried), and then draw the needle from side c and tie the knot [3, 11, 12] (Fig. 11.10).

Rules and Techniques 3

1. When suturing irregular wounds, try to orient the suture to the direction with the least skin tension.
2. Avoid removing too much skin tissue when trimming "cat ears." Smaller "cat ears" can improve over time.
3. Try to avoid using the suture technique in Fig. 11.10a, because it may cause avascular necrosis of the tip and poor healing at the triangular suturing site.

11.2.4 Special Suture Technique

11.2.4.1 Continuous Intradermal Suturing

1. Advantages. The advantage of this suturing technique is that usually only one entering hole and one exit hole are required. This avoids excessive epithelialization of too many puncture holes, especially in areas rich in sebaceous glands of the skin, which is beneficial to reduce postoperative scar formation.
2. Suture Technique (Fig. 11.11). The suture needle first enters the skin near one side of the wound and enters the wound intracutaneously. The suture is then passed through the other side of the wound to the distal end with exactly the same length in the plane of the dermis. Then the needle leaves the skin distal to the wound. Adjust the length of the wound edge by slightly pulling the suture, and finally fix the suture with "buttons," sterile surgical adhesive, and other tools to avoid unintentional removal [12–15].

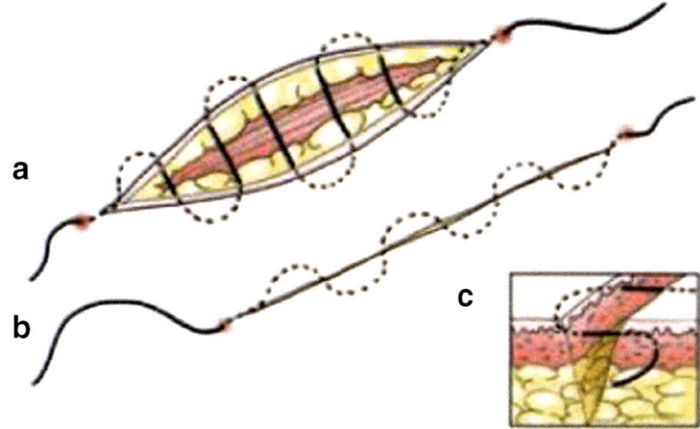

Fig. 11.11 Subcutaneous continuous suturing. (**a**) The entry and exit points of the skin are at both sides of the wound, 1 cm away from the incision edge, and run continuously in the skin at the same distance; (**b**) Close the incision after suturing, and pull the suture to adjust edges of the skin on both sides; (**c**) Section view of running suture

Rules and Techniques 4

Continuous subcutaneous suturing is only suitable for incisions with similar lengths of the skin edges on both sides

1. It is not suitable for suturing curved wounds because it will cause the distortion of the wound.
2. Absorbable 4–0 STRATAFIX Spiral PGA-PCL Knotless Tissue Control Device (Polyglycolicacid-Polycaprolactone, Ethicon Inc.) can be used to improve the suture stability.

11.2.4.2 Vertical Mattress Suture (Donati Suture)

1. Advantages. The advantage of vertical mattress suture is a safer reconstruction of incisions with large differences in depth, so that both sides of the skin edges are relatively flat. At the same time, the wound eversion helps to avoid the formation of groove scars, even epithelial inversion, or poor wound healing.
2. Suture Technique (Fig. 11.12). The insertion point is located approximately 4 mm at the edge of the incision, and then the needle exits at the same distance from the contralateral skin edge, then the needle is inserted at the edge of the incision about 1 mm to the same distance from the contralateral side. The knot can be slightly tightened to turn the edge of the incision outward.

Rules and Techniques 5

As an alternative, a half-buried vertical mattress suture can also be used (Fig. 11.13). The horizontal mattress suture can also evert the skin edges, but it is not as stable as the vertical mattress suture. However, each stitch of the mattress suture will produce four suturing marks, and it will affect the blood supply of the skin edge, so use with extreme caution [12–16].

11.2.4.3 Interrupted "Heart-Shaped" Subcutaneous Suturing

1. Advantages. The advantage of subcutaneous "heart-shaped" suturing is that more dermal tissue is carried on both sides of the incision edge, making the skin edge

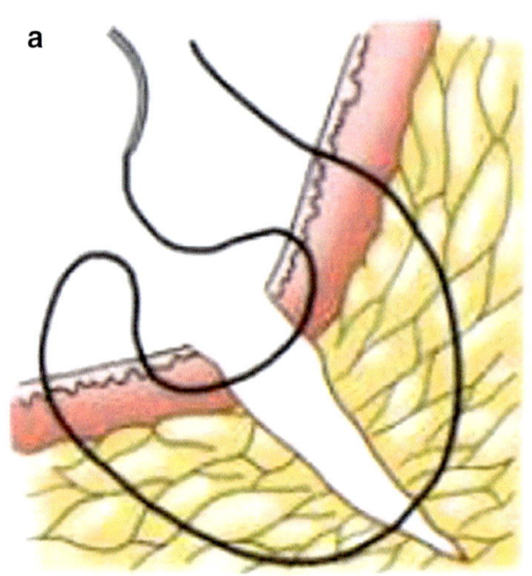

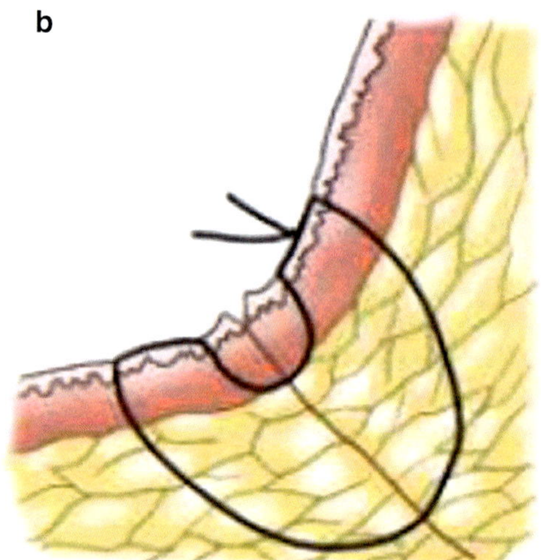

Fig. 11.12 The needle entry point is about 4 mm from the edge of the incision vertical mattress suturing. (**a**) The suture method shown is to avoid the formation of dead space. Before suturing, the skin edge can be trimmed to facilitate alignment; (**b**) The skin edge turns slightly outward after knotting

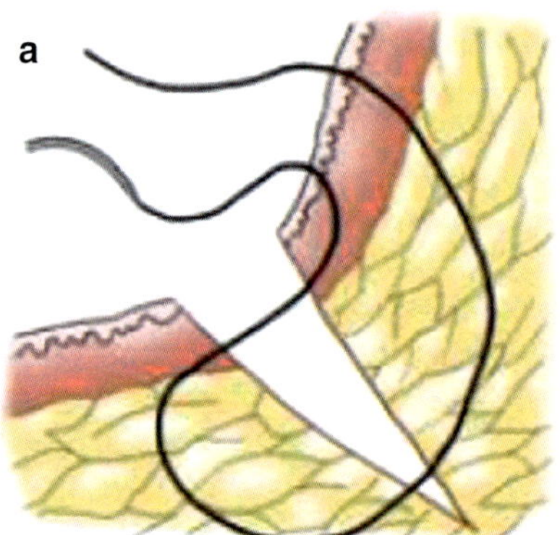

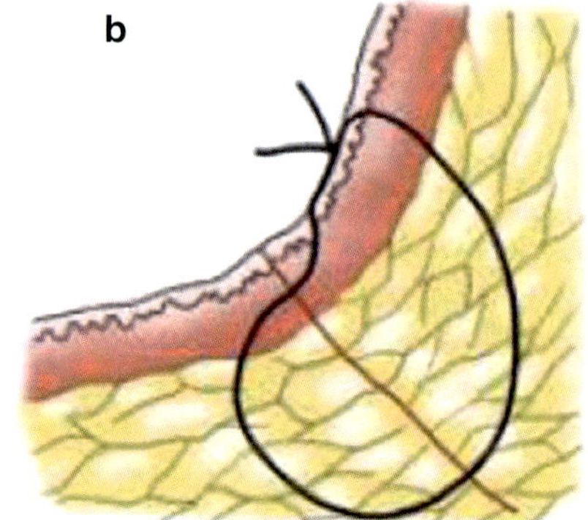

Fig. 11.13 Half-buried vertical mattress suture. (**a**) Suture the needle entry point, the needle does not exit from the opposite side, it exits from the same side after holding part of the dermal tissue; (**b**) Then close the incision with knots

extremely everted after knotting. The subsequent skin suturing can reduce the number of stitches and the tension of the knot. It is beneficial to improve the appearance of scars [15, 17].

2. Suturing Technique (Figs. 11.14 and 11.15). Heart-shaped suture needle handling steps (enter deep and exit shallow, for opposite side enter shallow and exit deep): Put the needle on the bottom layer of the dermis about 7 mm away from the edge of the incision. Handle the suture needle, gently attach the thumb to the needle holder (do not sink the thumb deep in the needle holder) penetrate the needle into the fat layer by rotating the wrist. Swap out the thumb and move it to the other side of the needle holder, so that the needle holder can be rotated in the hand to make the shortest distance from the upper epidermis (about 1 mm) at the position about 5 mm from the edge of the incision, and then exit the needle at the site which is 2 mm away from the upper epidermis. Use the same suture needle handling technique on the opposite side. Make sure that there is no difference in the thickness of the needle across the tissue, otherwise uneven skin approximation can occur. Knot and complete suturing.

In this way, when the skin has not been sutured, the edge of the skin has turned outward and the tension is

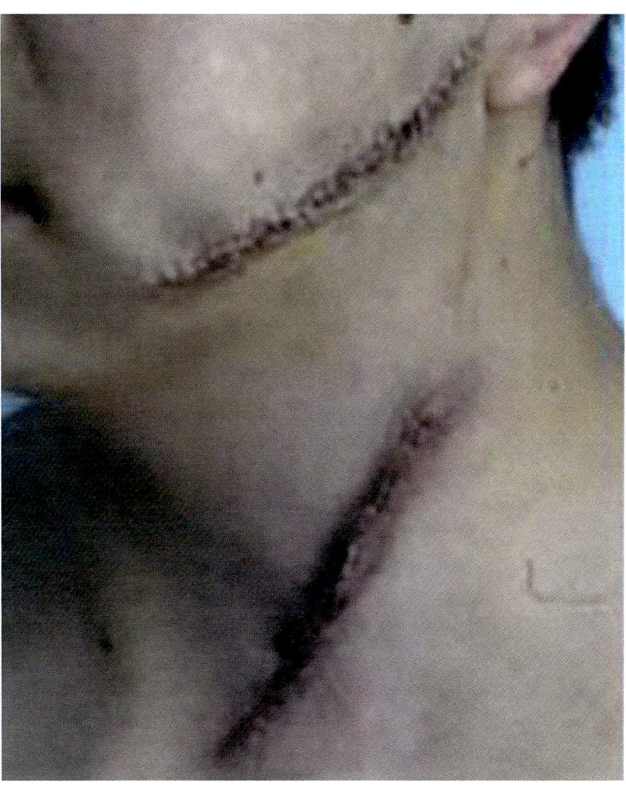

Fig. 11.15 Heart-shaped suturing effect diagram

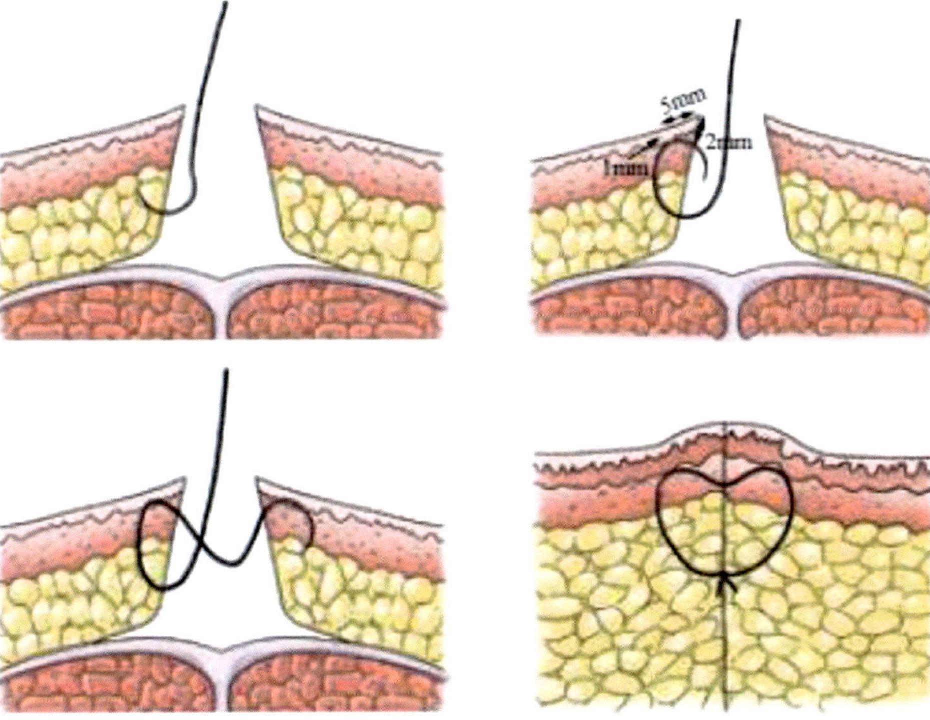

Fig. 11.14 Diagram of needle handling for heart-shaped suturing

small. After the skin is sutured, the cutting effect and tension of the suture on the tissue are correspondingly reduced, which is beneficial to reduce postoperative scars.

11.2.4.4 Zhang's Super Relaxation Suture

We divide the suture levels into the superficial layer, dermis layer, and deep layer. Full tension reduction of the three layers plus the alignment of superficial and dermal layer wound edges helps to achieve the esthetic appearance of scars. Current literature suggests that full tension reduction after the wound edge suturing, and even eversion can effectively reduce the volume of the scar after healing and improve its appearance (Level I) [18–20]. Based on the existing rationale and suturing technique as reference, Professor Zhang Yixin of the Department of Plastic Surgery, Shanghai Ninth People's Hospital, Shanghai Jiaotong University School of Medicine, proposed a new suture technique—the "Zhang's super relaxation suture."

1. The advantage of the "Zhang's super relaxation suture" is to use the laxity of the tissues on both sides of the incision edge to maximize the carrying of normal skin and subcutaneous tissue, so that the flaps on both sides of the incision edge are extremely everted, which requires less stitches to suture subcutaneous tissue under the incision and epidermis, and it can be aligned. After about 3 months, the extremely eversion flap tissue will gradually become flat, which is beneficial to obtain a less obvious prognosis of scarring. The "Zhang's super relaxation suture" plus interrupted suturing of the dermis and plus superficial skin suturing is the combination of suturing techniques to obtain the best skin suturing appearance.
2. Suturing method.
   (a) "Z" shape changes the direction of tension, so that the tension is distributed on both sides of the wound edge.
   (b) Continuous suturing, short time-consuming, and easy operation.
   (c) The needle enters 1 cm away from the wound edge, and carry part of the dermal tissue when entering and exiting the needle to improve the tissue friction and increase the strength of tension reduction.
   (d) Select Absorbable 3–0 STRATAFIX™ Spiral PGA-PCL Knotless Tissue Control Device (Polyglycolicacid-Polycaprolactone, Ethicon Inc.) + Absorbable 5–0 Coated VICRYL® Plus Suture (Polyglactin 910, Ethicon Inc.) + Non-absorbable 6–0 PROLENE® Suture (Polypropylene, Ethicon Inc.).

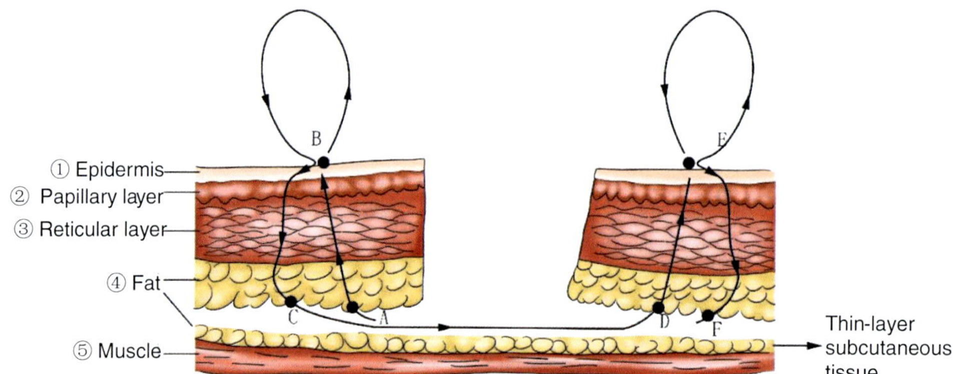

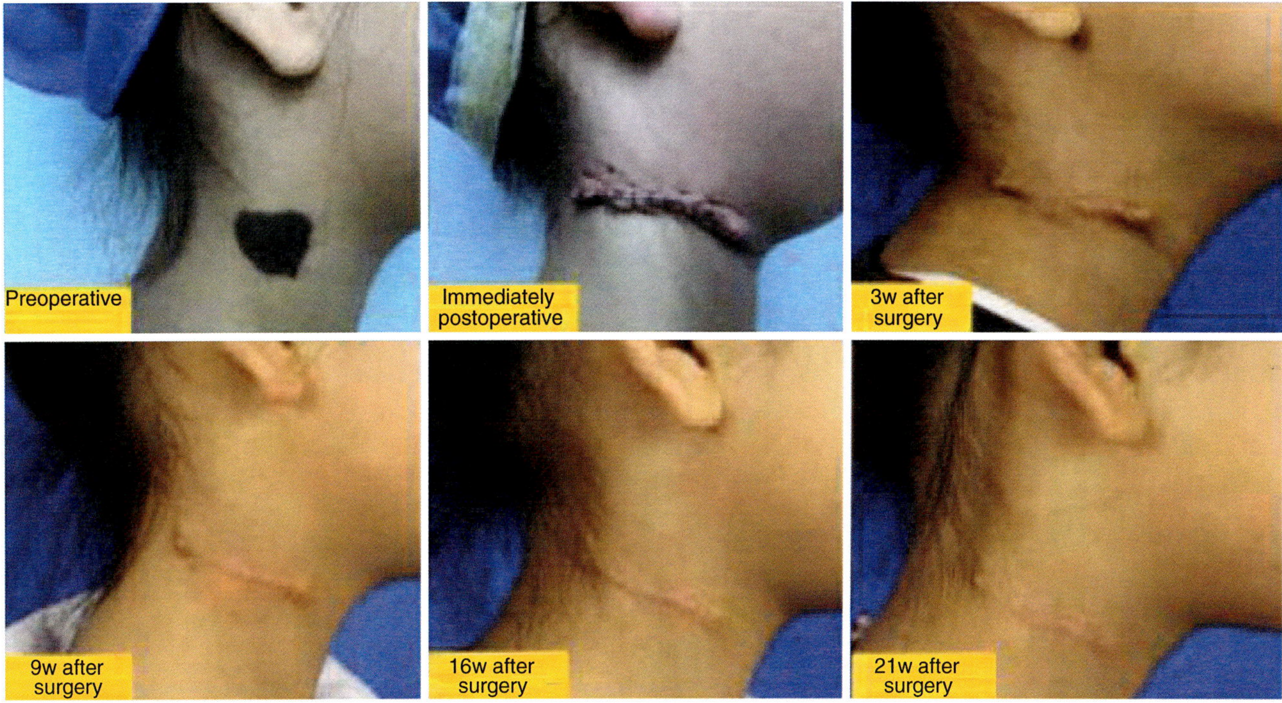

Enter the needle from point A under the skin, go vertically to point B and out of the skin, then enter point B, go vertically to point C and exit from the subcutaneous tissue, suture the contralateral side in the mirror way, the stitch path: A-B-C-F-E-D

11.3 Selection of Instruments and Sutures

11.3.1 Device Selection

The instrument must be suitable for the special requirements of skin cosmetic suturing. This means: avoid the use of vascular forceps, try to use forceps, and the tip or jaw of the forceps should be appropriately small [9, 13]. Current evidences prove:

1. The tip of the forceps or the jaws may damage the local integrity of the suture, resulting in weakening of the tensile strength of the suture when suturing or tying knots.
2. Too large tip or jaws of the forceps will increase tissue injury. If possible, we should only grasp subcutaneous tissue.

When cutting the suture, choose to use smaller round-tip scissors to avoid skin tissue damage. There is no clear requirement for surgical blades, but it is more convenient and accurate to use a sharp blade (No.11) when trimming "cat ears" and skin edges.

11.3.2 Suture Selection

For subcutaneous suturing, generally absorbable sutures made of Polyglactin 910 material is used, such as Absorbable Coated VICRYL® Plus Suture (Polyglactin 910, Ethicon Inc.). This type of suture is degraded by the self-hydrolysis process and does not need to rely on the cell activity around the suture. The final product formed in the body is water and carbon dioxide, so the tissue reaction is less.

Synthetic absorbable sutures have higher initial tension than silk and catgut sutures. Experiments have found that although the silk suture is a non-absorbable suture, after being implanted in the body, the tension of the silk suture is significantly reduced within 1 week after being implanted in the body due to its highly hydrophilic nature. Some synthetic absorbable sutures, Polyglactin 910 (such as Absorbable Coated VICRYL® Plus Suture), although the tension is uniformly reduced after being implanted in the body, can still provide an absolute tension higher than that of silk suture within 1–2 months. Studies have shown that the initial tension of Polyglactin 910 (such as Absorbable Coated VICRYL® Plus Suture) is twice that of silk suture. The effective wound support time is 30 days and the material absorption time is 56–70 days. On day 14, the remaining tension is 75%. On day 21, 50% of the tension remains.

Skin sutures generally use single-strand absorbable sutures made of poliglecaprone. For example, continuous intracutaneous suture with Absorbable MONOCRYL® Plus Suture (Poliglecaprone 25, Ethicon Inc.) can completely avoid skin edge wounds and obtain a better wound appearance. The Absorbable MONOCRYL® Plus Suture (Poliglecaprone 25, Ethicon Inc.) has high tensile strength and meets the tension demand of skin suturing. Compared with other sutures, the Absorbable MONOCRYL® Plus Suture (Poliglecaprone 25, Ethicon Inc.) has less tissue reaction and faster tissue repair. Studies have shown that after suturing the wound with Absorbable MONOCRYL® Plus Suture (Poliglecaprone 25, Ethicon Inc.), there is less inflammatory cell infiltration and less redness or swelling, which are beneficial to tissue repair (Figs. 11.16 and 11.17) [18, 21].

Compared with skin staples, the use of sutures can reduce the risk of surgical wound infection. According to the experience of our center (plastic surgery department of the Shanghai Ninth People's Hospital, Shanghai Jiaotong University School of Medicine), suture selection is generally (the smaller the coding number of the suture combination, the better the effect):

11.3.2.1 Incision with Less Tension (Subcutaneous Suturing + Skin Suturing)

1. Absorbable 5–0 Coated VICRYL®/Coated VICRYL® Plus Suture (Polyglactin 910, Ethicon Inc.) + Non-absorbable 6–0 PROLENE® Suture (Polypropylene, Ethicon Inc.)
2. Absorbable 5–0 Coated VICRYL®/Coated VICRYL® Plus Suture (Polyglactin 910, Ethicon Inc.) + Non-absorbable 4–0 Stainless Steel Suture
3. Absorbable 5–0 Coated VICRYL®/Coated VICRYL® Plus Suture (Polyglactin 910, Ethicon Inc.) + Absorbable 6–0 PDS® Plus Suture (Polydioxanone, Ethicon Inc.)
4. Absorbable 5–0 PDS® Plus Suture (Polydioxanone, Ethicon Inc.)

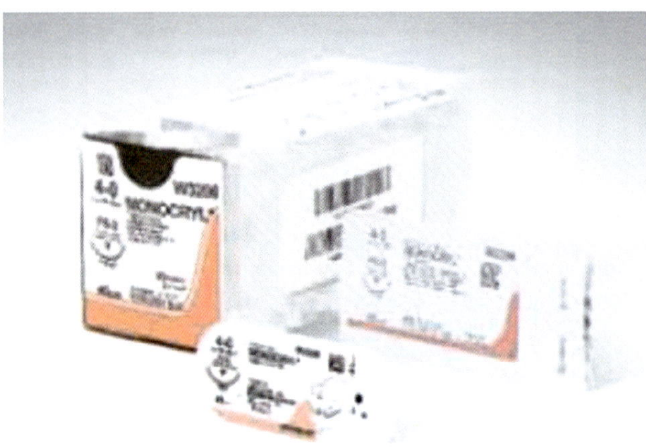

Fig. 11.16 Examples of Absorbable MONOCRYL® Plus Suture (Poliglecaprone 25, Ethicon Inc.) product

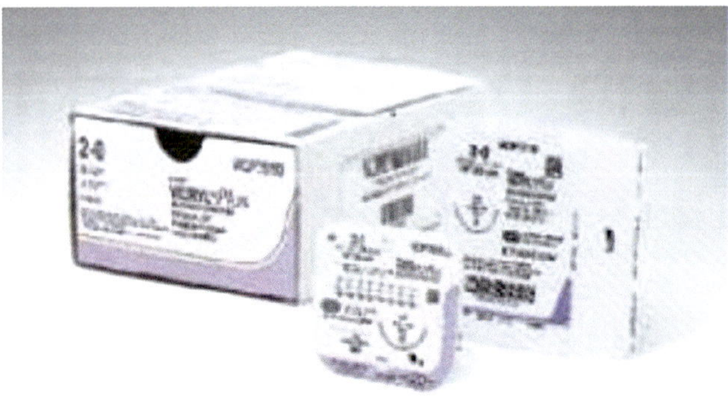

Fig. 11.17 Examples of Absorbable Coated VICRYL® Plus Suture (Polyglactin 910, Ethicon Inc.) product

11.3.2.2 Incision with Greater Tension

On the basis of (one), select the Absorbable 3–0 Coated VICRYL®/Coated VICRYL® Plus Suture (Polyglactin 910, Ethicon Inc.) for subcutaneous suturing with tension-reduced suturing (suture selection of subcutaneous tension-reduced suturing + subcutaneous suturing + skin suturing).

1. Absorbable 3–0 Coated VICRYL®/Coated VICRYL® Plus Suture (Polyglactin 910, Ethicon Inc.) + Absorbable 5–0 Coated VICRYL®/Coated VICRYL® Plus Suture (Polyglactin 910, Ethicon Inc.) + Non-absorbable 6–0 PROLENE® Suture (Polypropylene, Ethicon Inc.).
2. Absorbable 3–0 Coated VICRYL®/Coated VICRYL® Plus Suture (Polyglactin 910, Ethicon Inc.) + Absorbable 5–0 Coated VICRYL®/Coated VICRYL® Plus Suture (Polyglactin 910, Ethicon Inc.) + Non-absorbable 4–0 Stainless Steel Suture.
3. Absorbable 3–0 Coated VICRYL®/Coated VICRYL® Plus Suture (Polyglactin 910, Ethicon Inc.) + Absorbable 5–0 Coated VICRYL®/Coated VICRYL® Plus Suture (Polyglactin 910, Ethicon Inc.) + Absorbable 6–0 PDS® Plus Suture (Polydioxanone, Ethicon Inc.).
4. Absorbable 3–0 Coated VICRYL®/Coated VICRYL® Plus Suture (Polyglactin 910, Ethicon Inc.) + Absorbable 5–0 PDS® Plus Suture (Polydioxanone, Ethicon Inc.). When suturing orthopedic skin incisions, sutures with appropriate thickness can be selected according to the specific surgical site.

11.3.2.3 Needle Selection

Suture needles are used to penetrate tissues and place sutures to bring the wound/incision close together. Although there is no need for needles in the wound healing process, choosing the most suitable needle is of great significance for ensuring the wound alignment and reducing tissue damage.

The performance of the needle depends on its geometric structure and material. For example, the width and depth of the needle through the tissue are determined by the chord length and arc respectively; the diameter of the needle body and the cross-sectional design determine the stability of the needle; the bending resistance (strength) is determined by the design of the alloy and the needle tip and body; the alloy not only determines the strength of the needle, but also affects the ductility and sharpness of the needle. In addition, the sharpness is also affected by the coating and the design of the needle tip.

The minimally invasive concept requires that the needle selection be as thin as possible without sacrificing the strength and sharpness. At the same time, during the suturing process, the rigidity is sufficient to resist bending, and the flexibility is sufficient to resist fracture. Chord length and radian should be considered for needle type, and different needle types should be selected according to the depth of the part and the thickness of the tissue. In general, a fine reverse needle with a smaller puncture force [18–22] is recommended (such as Prime®, Fig. 11.18).

Rules and Techniques 6

1. For skin cosmetic suturing, the stitch distance (about 5 mm) and the stitch distance (5–10 mm) are small, so small needle holders and tweezers are needed, and more time and patience are required.
2. Small-size sutures can only close the skin and the superficial subcutaneous fat layer, so the deep tissue should be tightly closed to avoid the formation of dead spaces.
3. When the subcutaneous suture is finished, the two sides of the wound should be basically aligned, and the tension of the skin suture is small. Therefore, we should pay attention to aligning the skin edges when suturing the skin, and avoid tight knots, which may cause ischemia of the skin edge.

11.4 Wound Healing and New Wound Closure Products

Abstract: With the understanding of the pathophysiology of wound healing and the development of new technologies and new materials, more and more new wound closure techniques have been introduced into the clinical practice of surgery. These techniques not only totally change the traditional suturing techniques to a certain extent, but their convenience is also favored by more and more surgeons. But it needs to be emphasized that the reliability and application indications of these techniques still need further research and discussion. We briefly describe the application of skin tension reducer and skin tissue adhesive in this section

Keywords:Healing, Skin tension reducer, Skin tissue adhesive

11.4.1 Wound Healing

Epithelial cells are the only regenerative cells during wound healing. The wound surface is initially covered by fibrin mesh. After 24 h, the epidermis begins to close above the wound to prevent pathogens from invading. However, this epithelial layer has not yet provided any tensile strength to the wound, and stability can only be achieved after skin fibroblasts secrete collagen and form scars.

Cracking or high tension on the wound edge will induce skin fibroblasts to produce too much collagen, causing scar widening and thickening, resulting in unesthetic skin appearance, so it must be limited to a certain range through correct wound treatment [1–3].

11.4.2 New Wound Closure Products

After the skin is sutured, the surface is covered with Vaseline + gauze and cotton pad. If it is necessary to prevent hematoma in the deep wound, a drainage strip or drainage tube can be placed. As the wound edge cracks will cause the postoperative scar to widen and thicken, and the greater skin tension on both sides of the wound is often the main reason for the wound to crack. For the above two issues, skin tension reducer can be used on both sides of the wound to reduce skin tension.

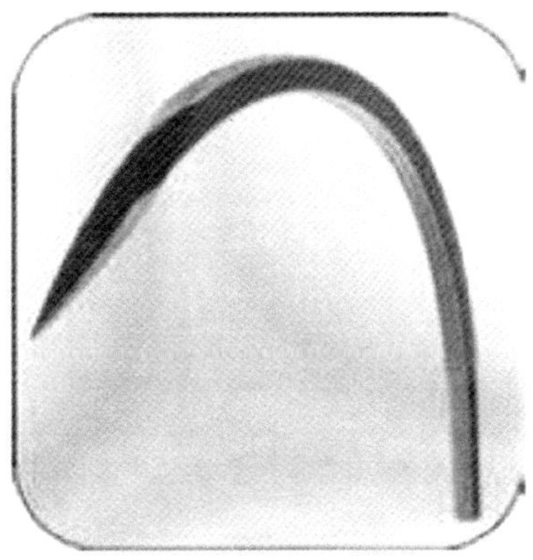
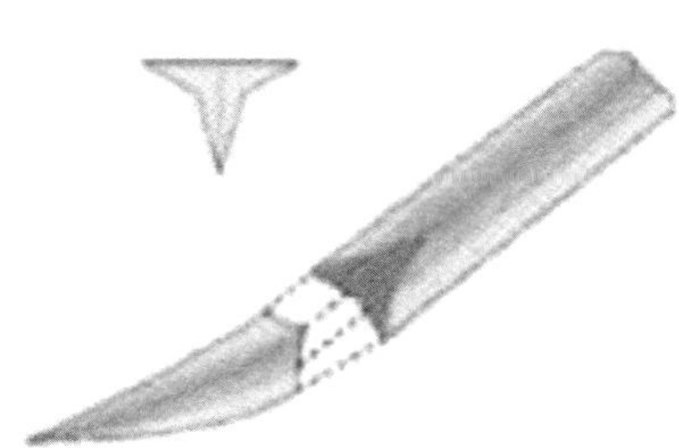

Fig. 11.18 Fine reverse needle

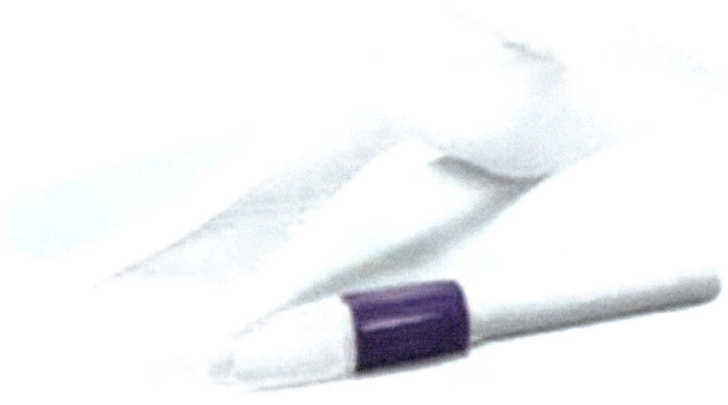

Fig. 11.19 Medical skin tissue adhesive

At present, a good skin tension reducer—Zipline has been proven in clinical trials to be able to effectively reduce the width and volume of postoperative scars, and the Vancouver Scar Score (VSS) has been significantly reduced [23].

Ideally, there should be no tension in the wound when the skin is sutured, and the tension should always be relieved by subcutaneous sutures. If in some cases, skin sutures need to reduce tension, it may cause obvious scar formation in appearance.

New wound closure products: with the development of skin closure technology, new wound closure techniques, and products emerge in endlessly. Medical skin tissue adhesive (such as DERMABOND™ PRINEO™ Skin Closure System (2-Octyl Cyanoacrylate, Ethicon Inc.)) is a new type of skin closure device that integrates additional tension support with waterproof and antibacterial protection [24, 25] (Fig. 11.19).

Studies have shown that compared with skin staples and sutures, medical skin tissue adhesive has better tensile strength and better tension distribution. The medical skin tissue adhesive is convenient for postoperative care, eliminating the need for dressing change, suture removal and staple removal. Patients can take a bath immediately after surgery. When the wound is fully healed, it is easier to remove the mesh tape with less pain.

Rules and Techniques 7

1. After using skin tissue adhesive to close the wound, occasionally moisten the wound briefly is allowed (such as showering), but do not soak or scrub the wound for a long time. Do not apply soap or shower gel on the adhesive layer. After bathing, please gently dry the wound with a towel.
2. Do not apply liquid medicine, ointment, or any medicine on the adhesive layer. These drugs may weaken the thin membrane formed by the skin tissue adhesive, causing the wound dehiscence.
3. There is no need to cover the adhesive layer with a dressing or bandage, but protective dry dressing could be used. Pay attention that the adhesive part of the dressing does not overlap the adhesive layer. So as not to affect the integrity of the adhesive layer during the dressing change process.

References

1. Neligan P. Plastic surgery: 6-volume set. 2012.
2. Murray DS. Grabb and Smith's plastic surgery. Br J Oral Maxillofac Surg. 1992;30(3):203–4.
3. Baker R. Local flaps in facial reconstruction (Expert consult – online and print).
4. Kaye BL. Plastic and reconstructive surgery of the face. Cosmetic Surg.
5. Siemionow MZ. Plastic and reconstructive surgery. ANZ J Surg. 2005;75(s1):A89–97.
6. Welshhans JL, Hom DB. Soft tissue principles to minimize scarring: an overview. Facial Plast Surg Clin North Am. 2017 Feb;25(1):1–13.
7. Papel I. Facial plastic and reconstructive surgery. In: Facial plastic and reconstructive surgery. New York: Thieme; 2009.
8. Pickrell KL. Reconstructive plastic surgery of the face. Clin Symp. 1967;19(3):71.
9. Petres J, Rompel R, Robins P. Basic surgical techniques. In: Dermatologic surgery. Berlin: Springer; 1996.
10. Moy RL, Lee A, Zalka A. Commonly used suturing techniques in skin surgery. Am Fam Physician. 1991;44(5):1625–34.
11. Tempest MN. Plastic and reconstructive surgery of the face: cosmetic surgery. British J Plastic Surg. 1982;
12. Papel ID, Frodel JL, Holt GR, et al. Facial plastic and reconstructive surgery | 30 cosmetic surgery of the asian face. 2016; https://doi.org/10.1055/b-004-135545.
13. Pickrell KL. Reconstructive plastic surgery of the face. Clin Symp. 1967;19(3):71.
14. Cannon B. Plastic and reconstructive surgery of the face and neck: cosmetic surgery, rehabilitative surgery. JAMA. 1972;96(4):393.
15. Lloyd JD, Marque MJ, Kacprowicz RF. Closure techniques. Emerg Med Clin North Am. 2007;25(1):73–81.
16. Regula CG, YagHoward C. Suture products and techniques: what to use, where, and why. Dermatol Surg. 2015;41(Suppl 10):S187.
17. Xi Z, Diao J-S, et al. Wedge-shaped excision and modified vertical mattress suture fully buried in a multilayered and tensioned wound closure. Cosmetic Plastic Surg. 2009;33(3):457–60.
18. Bloom BS, Goldberg DJ. Suture material in cosmetic cutaneous surgery. J Cosmet Laser Ther. 2007;9(1):41–5.
19. Khansa I, Bridget H, et al. Evidence-based scar management: how to improve results with technique and technology. Plastic Reconstr Surg. 2016;138(3 Suppl):165S–78S.
20. Alan M, Paul MD. Barbed sutures in cosmetic plastic surgery: evolution of thought and process. Cosmetic Surg J. 33(3_Suppl):17S–31S.
21. Moy RL, Waldman B, Hein DWA. Review of Sutures and suturing techniques. Dermatol Surg. 1992;18(9):785–95.

22. Sutures Y-HC. Needles, and tissue adhesives: a review for dermatologic surgery. Dermatol Surg. 2014;40(9):S3–S15.
23. Téot L, Boissière F, Bekara F, et al. Controle de la tension des berges cicatricielles après résection cutanée: un nouveau dispositif médical adhésif réglable. Revue Francophone De Cicatrisation. 2017;1(1):46–50.
24. Jenkins LE, Davis LS. Comprehensive review of tissue adhesives. Dermatol Surg. 2018;44(11):1.
25. Coulthard P, et al. Tissue adhesives for closure of surgical incisions. J Tissue Viability. 2004;(2):CD004287.

12 Microsurgical Reconstruction Suture Techniques

Yimin Chai, Yuqiang Sun, and Lei Xu

Abstract

Re-suture of blood vessels and peripheral nerves belongs to microsurgery category, i.e., it belongs to various surgical procedures performed by surgeons under the surgical microscope. In 1921, Swedish otologists Nylen and Holmagren first completed the operation on the inner ear using a microscope. Later, surgeons at home and abroad extended the microsurgery techniques to all fields of surgery, and the suture of blood vessels and peripheral nerves is the foundation and key to the success of most microsurgeries. This chapter will discuss, respectively, the technical requirements for microsurgery repair, the suture of blood vessels, and the nerve reconstruction suture separately.

Keywords

Microsurgery repair techniques · Vascular anastomosis · NERVE reconstruction suture

12.1 Training Requirements for Microsurgery Repair Techniques

Chai Yimin and Xu Lei

Fine tissues can be observed clearly and stereoscopically when operation is performed under a microscope, so precise dissection, dissociation, incision, and suture can be achieved, but there are also many inconveniences. ① The field of view (FOV) of the microscope is extremely narrow, so accurate and quick location of surgical field needs practice; ② The depth of field of the microscope is limited, and a slight movement may blur the FOV; ③ Under the microscope, even an imperceptible movement may be very noticeable, so the basic operation of microsurgery needs repeated training and an adaptation process. Some basic principles and norms are explained here first [1]:

1. The movement of hands should be gentle and steady to avoid shaking; keep the movement range as small as possible to avoid operating out of sight.
2. Incising, suturing, knotting, and suture cutting should be performed on one plane. Because the depth of field of the microscope is limited, a slight movement up and down can cause defocus. In order to avoid blur, all operations should be kept on a same plane as far as possible.
3. Synergic movement of the thumb, index finger, and wrist with the device is essential for proficient manipulation under a microscope. Therefore, the forearm should naturally rest on the operation table surface.
4. When the eyes keep leaving and returning to the eyepiece, the eye muscles need to re-focus, so it is practical to quickly reach and change instruments without moving eyes away from the eyepiece.
5. The microsurgery requires a tacit cooperation between the surgeon and the assistant.

Basically, practice until the operation under the surgical microscope can be as smooth and relax as under the naked eyes.

12.2 Suture of Blood Vessels

The situation that the blood vessels need to be sutured occurs when the blood vessels are lacerated or completely broken, and vascular repair or suture can be performed respectively [2].

Y. Chai · Y. Sun (✉)
Shanghai Sixth People's Hospital, Shanghai, China

L. Xu
Huashan Hospital, Fudan University, Shanghai, China

P. Tang et al. (eds.), *Tutorials in Suturing Techniques for Orthopedics*, https://doi.org/10.1007/978-981-33-6330-4_12

12.2.1 Vascular Repair

Simple and neat vascular laceration of large and medium blood vessels can be directly sutured; longitudinal suture can be used for transverse tear, and transverse suture can be used for longitudinal tear. For large laceration or vascular wall defect, the mesh method can be used. This method usually adopts autologous vein or artery wall, which is trimmed into defect shape and then sutured in situ (Fig. 12.1).

12.2.2 Angiorrhaphy

Commonly used vascular suture methods include end-to-end anastomosis, end-to-side anastomosis, disc-to-side anastomosis, disc-to-end anastomosis, and mosaic anastomosis.

12.2.2.1 End-to-End Anastomosis

1. **Adventitia dissection** The adventitia residue should be avoided at the anastomotic site. The adventitia should be pulled toward the broken end using forceps, and the pulled adventitia should be cut off using micro scissors, so that the media and intima naturally retract, and a smooth vessel wall will be exposed at this time (Fig. 12.2). The range of adventitia dissection should be 0.5 cm away from the broken end. However, the vein wall with outer diameter of less than 1 mm is thin, and it is difficult to identify the adventitia, the muscular layer of vessel may be damaged at dissection, so it is unnecessary to dissect the adventitia
2. **Dilation of blood vessels** If vasospasm exists, the spasm should be relieved, and mechanical expansion and hydraulic dilation can be adopted.
3. **Whole excision of broken ends of blood vessels** The broken ends of blood vessels are trimmed by straight scissors to make sections neat and make intima smooth and complete. The fibrous tissue on the section or broken end surface should be carefully removed for the blood vessels without adventitia dissection. For vessels with different calibers, the shape of anastomotic vessels can be trimmed properly to improve the quality of anastomosis (Figs. 12.3 and 12.4).

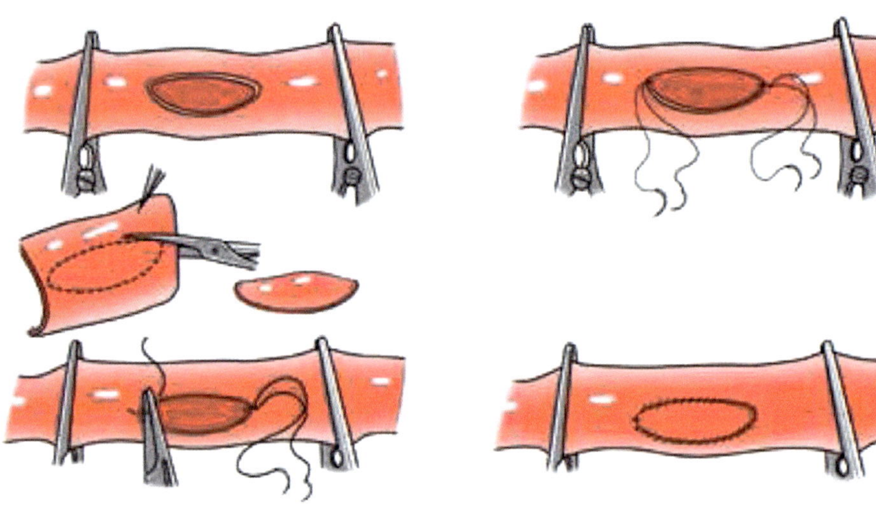

Fig. 12.1 Mesh repair of vascular defect with autologous vascular wall

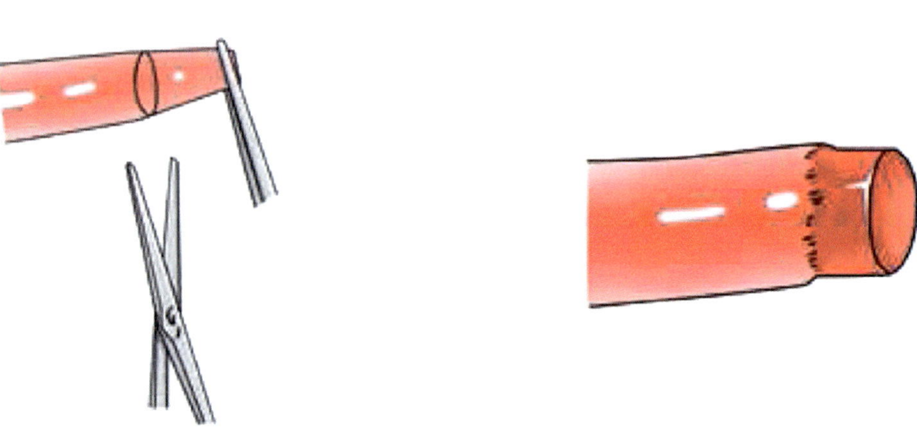

Fig. 12.2 The adventitia is pulled and cut off, and the adventitia retracts

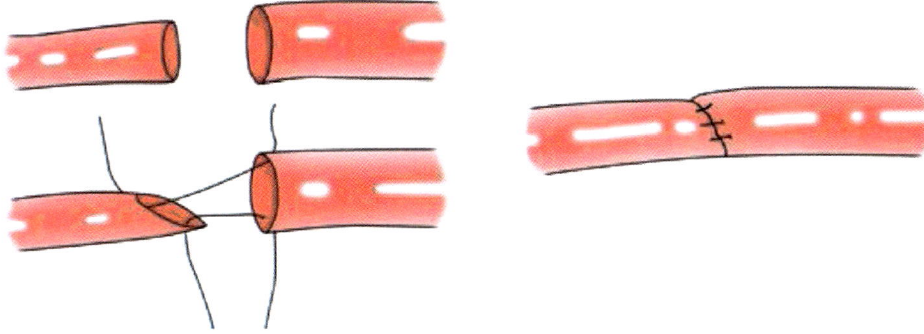

Fig. 12.3 The thin anastomotic vessel is trimmed into inclined planes and then sutured

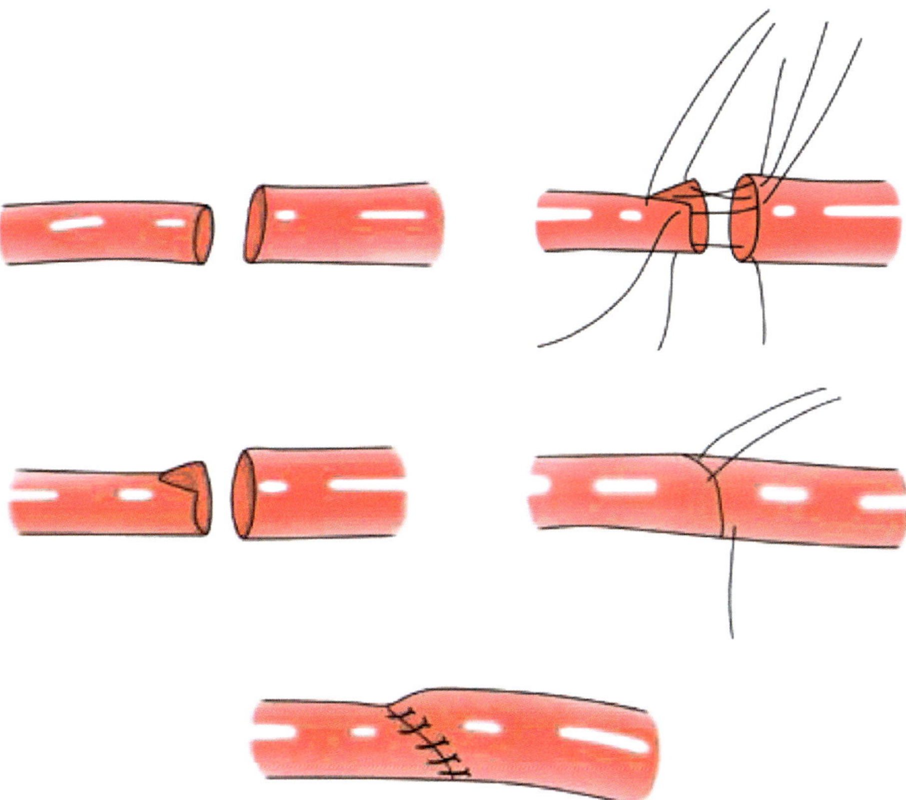

Fig. 12.4 Suturing after trimming the thin blood vessel into a V shape

4. **Margin and needle distance** Too wide or too narrow margin is not suitable, which will lead to varus and stenosis or anastomotic leak at the broken ends of blood vessels. When suturing arteries, the margin should be 1–2 times of the vessel wall, and the needle distance should be 2 times of the margin. When suturing visceral arteries and veins, the proportion can be slightly larger. Generally, blood vessels with a diameter of 2 mm are sutured for about 12 needles, and those with a diameter of 1 mm are sutured for 8 needles.
5. **Needle insertion** Check whether the blood vessels are distorted again before needle insertion, i.e., whether the blood vessels are aligned properly. Suture with 7-0 or 8-0 monofilament non-absorbable suture (such as PROLENE®). Have the needle to poke vertically through the whole layer of the blood vessel wall from the inner surface of the blood vessel wall. In order to keep the needle vertical, the assistant can use forceps to gently block and pressurize the vessel wall beside the needle, which can also stabilize the needle insertion position. If the poking is not vertical, the blood vessels may be inverted.
6. **Needle withdrawal** When withdrawing the needle, the assistant should gently block the vessel wall beside the needle with forceps, so as to avoid tearing the vessel wall. If the resistance is relatively large, it is necessary to pay attention to whether the adventitia or other tissues are brought into by the needle.
7. **Knotting** When knotting, a double knot is tied first, but should not be fastened. At this time, the assistant uses forceps to assist in coapting the two ends of the blood vessel

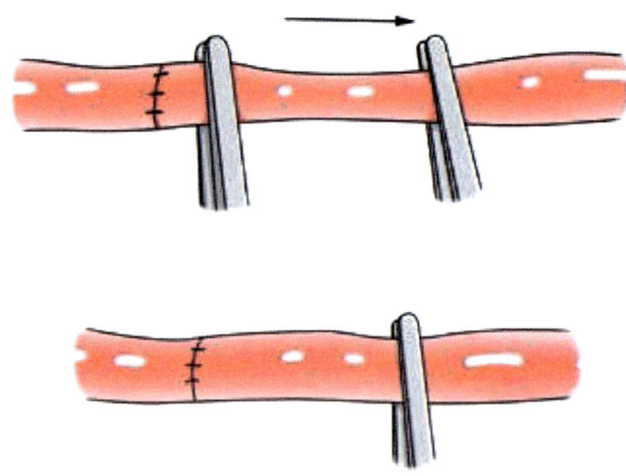

Fig. 12.5 Vascular patency test

to make the wall evert, and then tighten the double knot, and add another knot. It should be noted not to make the knot too tight use the strength just appropriately enough to couple up the ends of the two blood vessels. If the knot is too tight, the inner wall of the vascular lumen may wrinkle, affecting the lumen size and even damaging the blood vessel. The well-coapted broken ends of blood vessels should be everted properly, and the assistant can squeeze the blood vessel wall properly with forceps to help evert and suture.

8. **Needle sequence** Generally, the following needle sequence is adopted:

   ① Suture one needle of fixed point line on the wall at the broken ends of two blood vessels on the opposite side, and pull them together for coaptation; ② Suture one needle on the same side to bisect the vessel wall, and then pull the line away and fix it with a suture clamp; ③ Properly add needles between the two knots.
9. **Checking the quality of vascular suture** Block one end of blood vessel with a vascular clamp, inject normal saline at the other end, and check the anastomotic leak. If there is any leak, it is necessary to add a few more needles (Fig. 12.5)

12.2.2.2 End-to-Side Anastomosis

End-to-side anastomosis refers to the anastomosis at one end of one blood vessel with the side wall of another blood vessel, which is generally applicable to the case where the calibers of two blood vessels are quite different. Its basic principle is similar to that of end-to-end anastomosis (Fig. 12.6), and the basic steps are as follows:

First, a longitudinal incision is made on the side wall of the thicker blood vessel, which should be slightly larger than the inclined plane at the broken end of the thinner blood vessel, so as to avoid narrowing the anastomotic site. The design of incision is that the skew angle after anastomosis should be 30°–60°, the opening at the broken end of the thinner blood vessel should be inclined plane, and there are two ways to form the opening of the thicker blood vessel.

1. **Cut longitudinally with a straight scissor**

After the blood vessel is lifted with forceps, the blood vessel wall is opened first by using curved scissors or a suture needle, and then the straight scissors is extended into the lumen to cut the incision to an appropriate size.

2. **Cut ovally with curved scissors**

Cut off an oval directly on the vessel wall by using curved scissors, and pay attention to control the size to avoid lumen stenosis.

After the broken end is treated well, the blood vessel can be sutured: if the blood vessel is thick, the mattress suture can be used to make four fixed points first, and then continuously suture; if the blood vessel is thin, the interrupted suture can be used, and the suture method is the same as the anastomosis of the broken end (Fig. 12.7).

12.2.2.3 Disc-to-Side Anastomosis

If the calibers of blood vessels in the donor and recipient areas differ greatly, disc-to-side anastomosis can also be considered. The vascular disc refers to a discoid vascular wall structure with a diameter of about 5 mm which is cut at the root of the blood vessel when the blood vessel in the donor area is cut. Nutrient vessel should open in the center of vascular disc. There are two ways to make vascular disc: The oval vessel wall is cut off directly or the vessels at the upper and lower ends of the nutrient vessel origin are cut off, and then the vascular disc is constructed. The defect of vascular disc in the donor area can be repaired with vein wall. Refer to end-to-side anastomosis for vascular suture method (Fig. 12.8).

12.2.2.4 Disc-to-End Anastomosis

It is also suitable for the situation that the calibers of blood vessels in the donor and recipient areas differ greatly. In this anastomosis method, the vascular disc is round and directly anastomosed to the broken end of another blood vessel. This method is mostly suitable for vein suture (Fig. 12.9).

12.2.2.5 Mosaic Anastomosis

It is also suitable for the situation that the outer diameters of blood vessels differ greatly. When the blood vessels in the donor area are cut, 1–2 cm of the nutrient vessels are attached, and the nutrient vessels cut are directly embedded and anastomosed to the middle of the thick blood vessels in the donor area (Fig. 12.10).

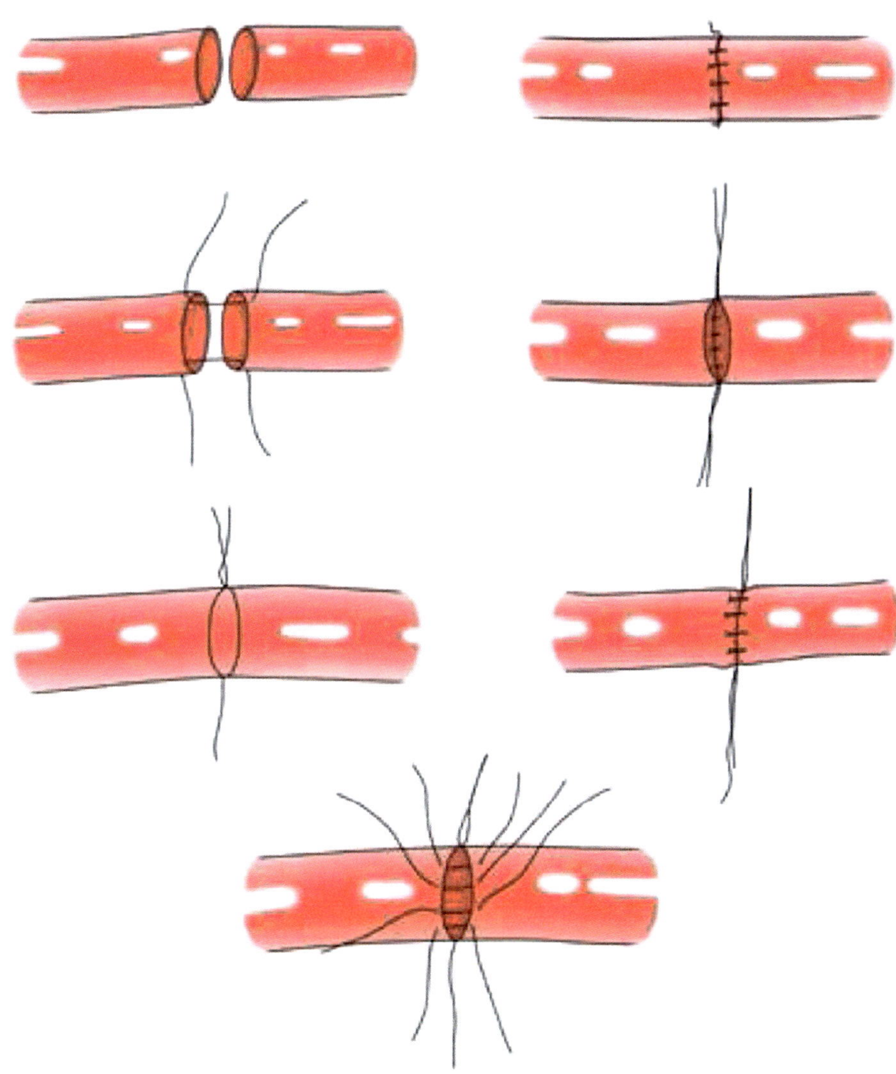

Fig. 12.6 End-to-end anastomosis

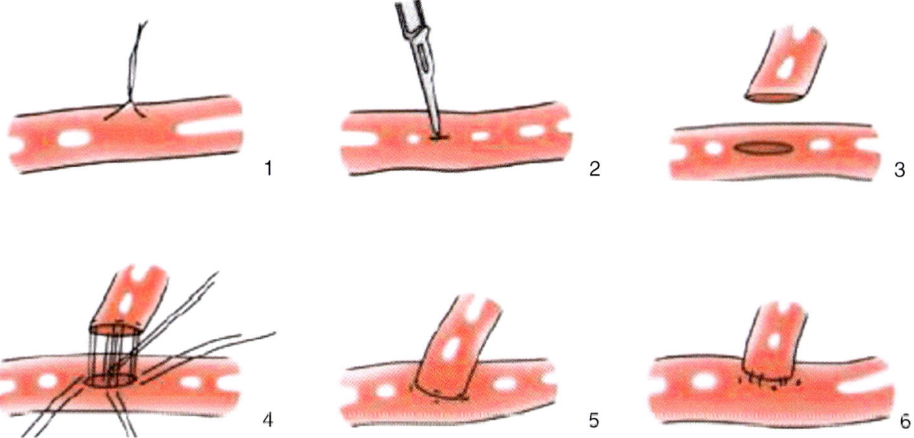

Fig. 12.7 End-to-side anastomosis

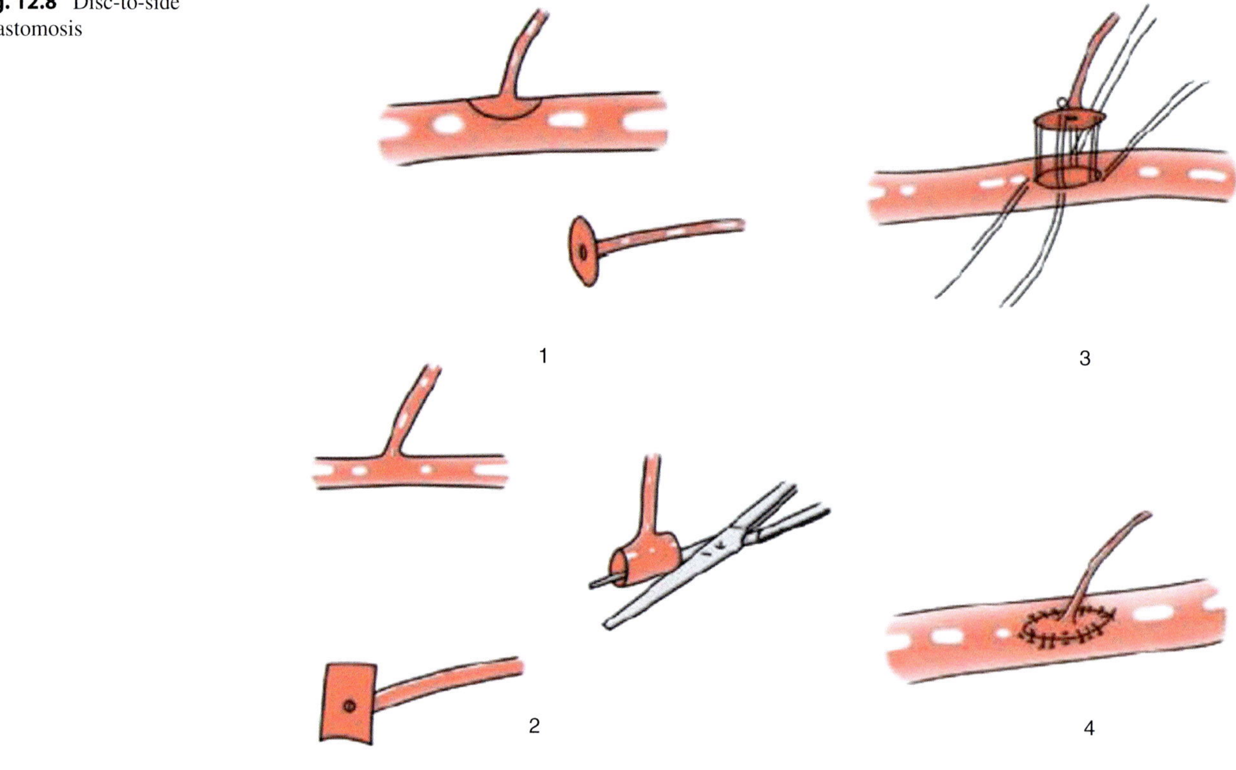

Fig. 12.8 Disc-to-side anastomosis

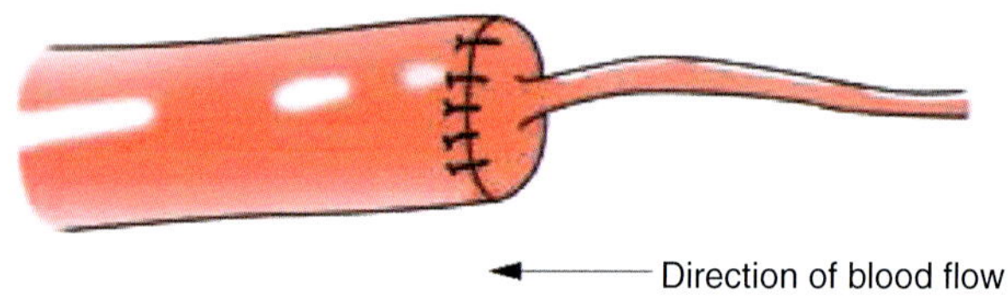

Fig. 12.9 Disc-to-end anastomosis

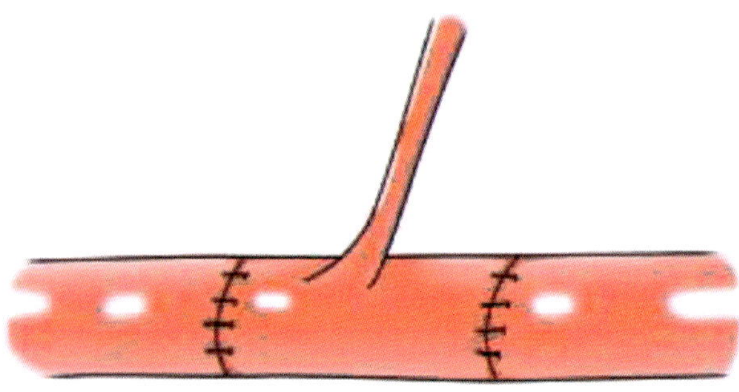

Fig. 12.10 Mosaic anastomosis method

12.3 Nerve Reconstruction Suture Techniques

12.3.1 Basic Principles to be Emphasized Before Nerve Suture

1. The closed suspicious complete nerve injury is not advocated to undergo exploration and repair in the first phase, which can be observed until 3 months after injury. If it still does not recover, surgical exploration can be performed.
2. Forceps with teeth or hemostats cannot be used for nerve holding, only fine forceps can be used to hold the interfascicular tissue between epineurium and nerve trunk; in order to avoid injury to the nerve axon, the needle should be avoided from entering the nerve bundle as much as possible during suture.
3. Neuroma often forms at the proximal end of injured nerve. Before suture, the neuroma and scar tissue should be gradually removed towards the proximal end until normal nerve tissue is observed.

4. Nerve coaptation emphasizes the precise coaptation of nerve bundles, so as to make the nerve fibers in the bundle cross the anastomotic sites as much as possible.
5. When it is difficult to separate the injured nerve, the normal nerve tissue near the distal end can be separated first and then the injured nerve can be separated.
6. After nerve anastomosis, it should be in a tension-free position; once tension occurs, the gap formed at the suture port is easy to form scar, which affects the passage of nerve fibers; in addition, the blood supply of nerves under tension becomes worse, and they also face the risk of avulsion at the anastomotic site.
7. The anastomotic site of the nerve should be placed in a good soft tissue bed, because the nutrition of the nerve at the anastomotic site mostly comes from the infiltration of the surrounding soft tissue. If there is no good soft tissue bed, the soft tissue can be reconstructed with skin flap or myocutaneous flap in the first stage and then the nerve anastomosis repair can be conducted in the second stage.
8. For nerve fracture caused by trauma, nerve suture should not be performed in the contaminated incision. If the wound is contaminated seriously, the broken end of nerve can be fixed on the adjacent healthy soft tissue after full debridement for surgical repair in the second stage.

12.3.2 Nerve Suture Methods [3]

Traditional nerve suture methods are divided into three types, including epineurial suture, perineurial suture, and combined epiperineurial suture. In addition, some special anastomosis methods can be selected for large differences in nerve calibers or some other special cases. Similarly, nerve suture should be performed under a microscope, and the requirements for needle insertion and needle withdrawal are basically the same as those of suturing blood vessels.

12.3.2.1 Epineurial Suture

1. **Nerve trimming**

Before suturing, the quality of the broken ends of two nerves to be sutured should be ensured, and the neuroma at the broken ends of nerves should be trimmed with a blade until the normal nerve bundle structure appears.

2. **Traction suture**

According to the nerve thickness, 8-0 or 9-0 monofilament non-absorbable suture (such as PROLENE®) is used to suture on each side of the broken end of nerve as the lead suture, so that the broken ends of nerves can be aligned accurately.

3. **Interrupted suture of anterior side**

The epineurium is sutured interruptedly between the positioned lead sutures, and attention should be paid not to bring the needle to the nerve tissue. The needle distance and margin should be such that the nerve bundle is not exposed and the epineurium is not inverted.

4. **Interrupted suture of posterior side**

The posterior part of the nerve is sutured in the same way after the nerve is turned over by 180° with the lead suture (Fig. 12.11).

12.3.2.2 Perineurial Suture

Perineurial suture method is to cut off the epineurium near the broken end of nerve and then directly perform perineurial anastomosis. The specific steps are as follows:

1. **Trimming nerves**
2. **Cutting off the epineurium**

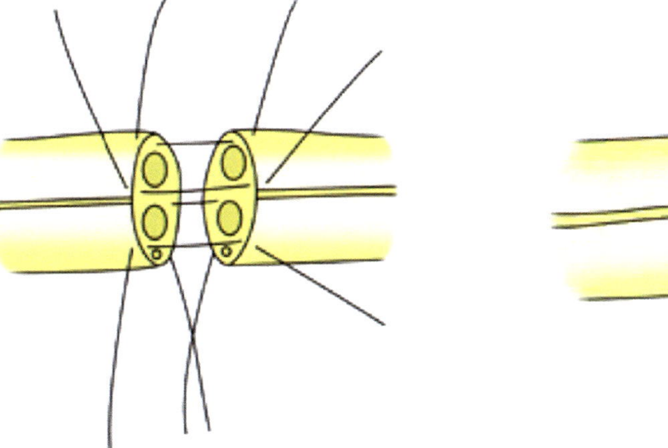

Fig. 12.11 Epineurial suture

Cut off the epineurium within 5 mm of the broken end of nerve, and expose the nerve bundle at this time.

3. **Suturing nerve bundle**

Stitch from outside of one side of the perineurium with 9–0 monofilament non-absorbable suture (such as PROLENE®), withdraw the needle under the perineurium to the other side, stitch from the perineurium, and withdraw the needle outside the perineurium, and gently tighten and knot the two bundles of nerves. Suture each nerve bundle with 1–2 needles, and suture the nerve bundle group with 2–3 needles, first superficial layer and then deep layer, suture in turn (Fig. 12.12).

12.3.2.3 Combined Epiperineurial Suture Method

The epineurium and the perineurium of the outer layer are sutured and aligned as a whole using this suture method, which is basically similar to the epineurial suture, except that the outermost perineurium is brought in at needle insertion and needle withdrawal.

12.3.2.4 End-to-Side Neurorrhaphy

Implanting the distal end of damaged nerve into the end side of accompanying normal nerve is called end-to-side neurorrhaphy. The perineurial fenestration may or may not be performed for the normal donor nerve. The fenestration method may refer to end-to-side suture fenestration of vascular anastomosis. A longitudinal incision is made on the side of nerve with a blade or micro scissors. The donor nerve is trimmed according to the diameter of the nerve to be repaired, and the elliptic epineurium is cut off; but the fenestration may not be performed. There are two ways of anastomosis.

1. **Direct anastomosis of epineurium**

Trim the broken end of the nerve to be repaired straight, and anastomose it to the side of donor nerve at right angle (Fig. 12.13).

2. **Spiral anastomosis of epineurium**

Trim the broken end of the nerve to be repaired in wedge shape, and perform diagonal model fenestration on the donor epineurium for spiral anastomosis (Fig. 12.14).

12.3.2.5 "Fish-Mouth Like" Suture

It is suitable for the situation that a relatively thick nerve is anastomosed with multiple thin nerves (for example, radial nerve/musculocutaneous nerve is anastomosed with multiple intercostal nerves), and two symmetrical V-shaped cuts can be made on the thick recipient epineurium, at this time, the

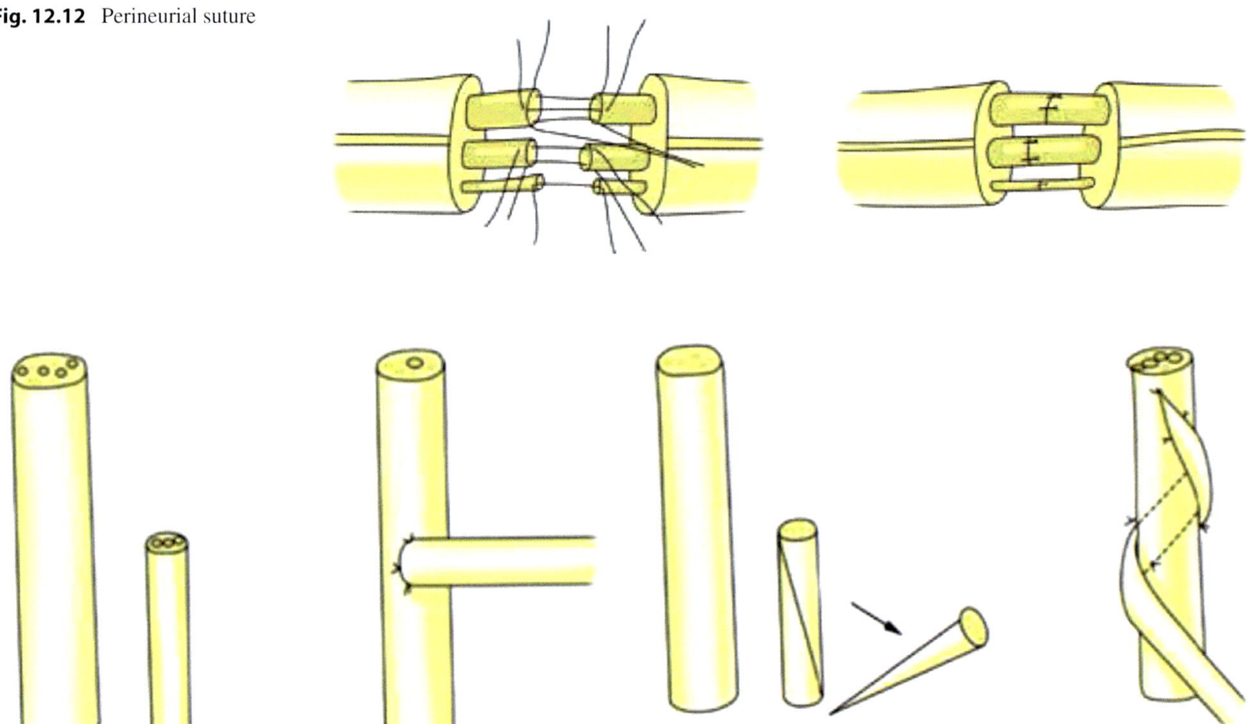

Fig. 12.12 Perineurial suture

Fig. 12.13 Direct end-to-side anastomosis of epineurium

Fig. 12.14 Spiral end-to-side anastomosis for increase of nerve contact area

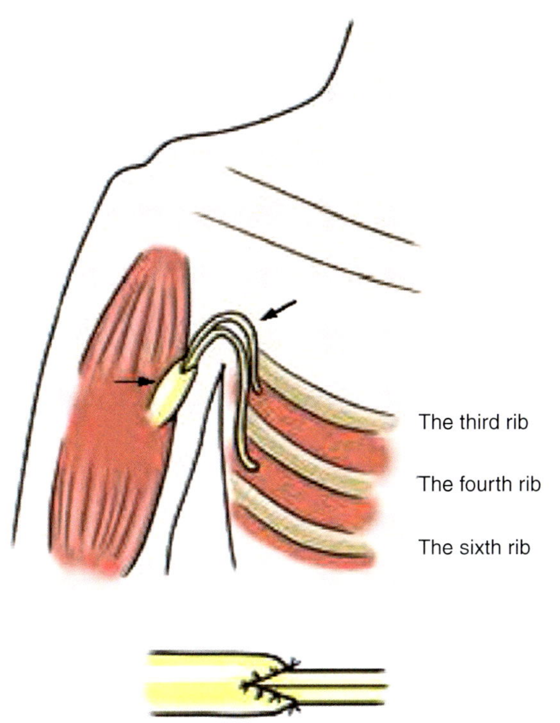

Fig. 12.15 "Fish mouth-like" suture, the intercostal nerve is anastomosed with two intercostal nerves

nerve is fish-mouth like, and the epineurium anastomosis is performed [2–3 needles for each nerve, with 9–0 or 10–0 monofilament non-absorbable suture (such as PROLENE®)] (Fig. 12.15).

12.3.3 Comparison of Epineurial Suture and Perineurial Suture

The two most commonly used suture methods of epineurial suture and perineurial suture have their own supporters. Some scholars think that accurate alignment of nerve bundles is difficult to achieve, so it is better to conduct loose epineurial suture to reduce the damage to nerve bundles; some scholars believe that epineurial suture can cause fibrosis of epineurium, so it is better to remove epineurium and conduct perineurial suture. But most clinical trials show that there is no difference between the two suture methods. Lundborg believes that the proximal nerve anatomy is complex and the nerve fibers have different functions, so accurate coaptation is difficult in perineurial suture; however, the anatomy in the distal nerve bundle is relatively clear, so perineurial suture can be attempted. The combination of the two suture methods is significant: perineurial suture can accurately align the nerve bundle which can identify alignment, while keeping part of the perineurial tissue and suturing the perineurium properly to ensure the strength and alignment of the whole nerve.

References

1. Yudong G. Basic theory and operation of microsurgery. Shanghai: Fudan University Press; 2011. p. 50–63.
2. Jianing W. Atlas of hand surgery of Wei Jianing. Beijing: People's Medical Publishing House; 2005. p. 687–701.
3. Wolfe SW. Green's operative hand surgery. Beijing: People's Military Medical Press; 2012. p. 972–7.

Suture Techniques for Spinal Soft Tissue Reconstruction

13

Weishi Li, Wenyuan Din, Tongwei Chu, Yu Jiang, Yang Liu, Min Qi, Zezhang Zhu, Jun Qiao, Bo Huang, and Lei Ma

Abstract

The surgical incision closure technique is an important and indispensable part of spinal surgery. It greatly affects the postoperative prognosis of spinal disease, and for certain diseases, it can even become a critical factor determining the success or failure of the treatment. By taking cervical, thoracic, and lumbar posterior median surgical approaches as examples, this section will focus on the closure techniques of spinal incisions, operating skills, and precautions for the reconstruction and closure of the soft tissue of surgical incisions.

Keywords

Cervical posterior approach · Thoracic posterior median approach · Lumbar posterior median approach Anatomical layer · Incision closure · Anterolateral cervical approach · Incision exposure · Incision closure Complication treatment · Scoliosis orthopedics · Incision exposure · Incision closure · Prevention and treatment for incision complications · Spinal surgery · Dural injury Dural suturing · Treatment of postoperative cerebrospinal fluid leakage · Anterior cervical surgery · Dural injury · Cerebrospinal fluid leakage · Dural suturing Thoracic surgery · Dural injury · Cerebrospinal fluid leakage · Dural suturing · Lumbar surgery · Dural injury Dural suturing · Cerebrospinal fluid leakage · Surgical site infection (SSI) · Spinal surgery · Complication Treatment

13.1 Suture Techniques for Posterior Spinal (Cervical, Thoracic, and Lumbar) Surgery

Li Weishi and Jiang Yu
Department of Orthopedics
Peking University Third Hospital
Beijing, China

More than 120 years ago, American doctor, W.F. Wilkins, treated a patient with T12/L1 fracture and dislocation by using silver wires for reduction and fixation, which was believed to be the first documented spinal internal fixation [1, 2]. His attempt was undoubtedly bold and creative. This pioneering work laid the theoretical foundation for spinal internal fixation and spinal fracture reduction. Its influence continues to this day. The rapid development of science and technology and emerging novel materials usher in a golden age for the development of spinal surgery over the past two decades. Brand-new surgical approaches and new surgical internal fixation instruments emerged one after another. Surgical approaches also have developed from traditional open surgery to the percutaneous endoscopic approach. Minimally invasive approaches and their concept have won a wide support. Take internal fixation and fusion of the lumbar spine as an example; in addition to the traditional and classic PLIF and TLIF approaches, spinal fusion can also be realized by ALIF, XLIF, OLIF, and other different surgical approaches. Some scholars have also tried spinal fusion under an endoscope.

No matter how the approaches and methods of spinal surgery have evolved, incision closure has always been a challenge for the spine surgeon. Surgical incision closure technique is an important and indispensable part of spinal surgery. It greatly affects the postoperative prognosis of spi-

W. Li (✉) · Y. Jiang
Peking University Third Hospital, Beijing, China

W. Din · L. Ma
The Third Hospital of Heibei Medical University, Shijiazhuang, Hebei, China

T. Chu · B. Huang
Xinqiao Hospital, Army Medical University, Chongqing, China

Y. Liu · M. Qi
Shanghai Changzheng Hospital, Shanghai, China

Z. Zhu · J. Qiao
Nanjing Drum Tower Hospital, Nanjing, Jiangsu, China
e-mail: zhuzezhang@nju.edu.cn

P. Tang et al. (eds.), *Tutorials in Suturing Techniques for Orthopedics*, https://doi.org/10.1007/978-981-33-6330-4_13

nal disease, and for certain diseases, it can even become a critical factor determining the success or failure of the treatment. The scientific closure and management of surgical incisions is an effective measure to prevent surgical incision complications, and reduce the incidence of incision-related complications, thereby avoiding a second operation due to poor healing of surgical incisions or incision infection [3]. A good healing of the surgical incision, on the one hand, can relieve the pain caused by surgical incision complications. On the other hand, it can smoothen the implementation of postoperative rehabilitation, shorten the postoperative LOS, reduce the hospitalization cost, improve bed occupancy rate and achieve the optimal utilization of medical resources [4, 5]. Incision closure is the key and systemically decisive factor in a surgery. This Chapter focuses on the closure of spinal incisions. By taking cervical, thoracic, and lumbar posterior median surgical approaches as examples, this section will focus on the closure techniques of spinal incisions, operating skills, and precautions for the reconstruction and closure of the soft tissue of surgical incisions.

13.1.1 Anatomical Features of Spinal Soft Tissue

The anatomical structure of the soft tissue on the spinal dorsal side is quite complex. As the spine is covered by multiple layers of muscles, it is difficult to get whole view of each muscle group via the spinal posterior median incision approach. One can only see where that the muscles of different levels attached to the spinous process. The posterior cervical muscle group is mainly a suboccipital group, also known as nuchae muscles, including rectus capitis posterior major, rectus capitis posterior minor, obliquus capitis superior and obliquus capitis inferior. These muscles enable the head to rotate and recline backward. The deep quadratus muscles include semispinalis capitis and semispinalis cervicis. The rectus capitis posterior minor, obliquus capitis superior, and obliquus capitis inferior form a triangular space, through which the occipital artery and the inferior occipital nerve pass. The posterior ramus of the second cervical nerve passes under the obliquus capitis inferior.

The soft tissues at the lower back are divided into the muscular layer, thoracolumbarfascia, subcutaneous tissue (fat layer), and skin from inside to outside.

1. **Muscular Layer** The superficial spine muscles include trapezius and latissimus dorsi as the first layer; levator scapula and rhomboid muscle as the second layer; serratus superior posterior and serratus inferior posterior as the third layer. The deep dorsal spinal muscles include splenius (splenius capitis and splenius cervicis) and erector spinae (iliocostalis, longissimus, and spinalis) as the first layer; transversospinales (semispinalis, musculi multifidi and musculi rotatores) as the second layer; suboccipital muscles (musculi rectus capitis anterior, rectus capitis lateralis, rectus capitis posterior major, rectus capitis posterior minor, obliquus capitis inferior and obliquus capitis superior), intertransversarii, and interspinalis as the third layer. The lower back muscles are important for maintaining the upright position and rotary movement of the trunk and therefore, they can be very strong.
2. **Thoracolumbar Fascia** The superficial layer of thoracolumbar fascia is the thickest, located on the deep side of the latissimus dorsi and serratus inferior posterior, and the surface of erector spinae. There is a gap between the thoracolumbar fascia and erector spinae, known as subthoracolumbar fascial space, housing the cutaneous nerve, fat and loose connective tissue. Normally, the superficial layer of the thoracolumbar fascia plays the role of limiting the erector spinae and strengthening its acting force, while the loose connective tissue under the thoracolumbar fascia acts as a lubricant between the thoracolumbar fascia and erector spinae. The middle layer of the thoracolumbar fascia is located between the erector spinae and quadratus lumborum. The medial side of it is attached to the lumbar transverse apex and the intertransverse ligament, and the lateral side is fused with deep stratum at the lateral edge of quadratus lumborum, forming the sheath of quadratus lumborum. The superficial layer, the middle layer of the thoracolumbar fascia, and the spinous and transverse processes of the lumbar spine form the lumbosacral osteofascial compartment, which houses the erector spinae, musculi transversospinales, and the posterior medial and lateral branches of lumbar nerve and nutrient vessels. The presence of this osteofascial compartment may be one of the anatomical bases for osphyalgia. The deep layer of the thoracolumbar fascia is located in front of quadratus lumborum, also known as quadratus lumborum fascia. It continuously connects with the anterior psoas major fascia, as a part of the intraabdominal fascia. The psoas major fascia and iliac fascia form the iliolumbar fascia, which covers the psoas major and iliacus, and extends down to the lesser trochanter of the femur. The three layers of fascia meet at the medial edge of the quadratus lumborum and become the starting point of the intraabdominal obliquus and musculus transversus abdominis.
3. **Subcutaneous Tissue (Fat Layer)** The subcutaneous fat at the lower back is relatively thick. This site is where adipose tissue tends to accumulate. The fat layer at this position is highly mobile. A cavity is likely to occur during incision closure. For obese patients, special attention should be paid to the closure of this level of the incision.
4. **Skin** Skin includes epidermis and dermis. Compared to other parts of the body, the skin on the lower back is thicker and has a higher tension than the skin on the ven-

tral side, especially in those patients who are thin with less subcutaneous fat. If the median incision in the lumbosacral area is selected for surgery, when incising the skin and subcutaneous tissue, the skin incisions are usually pulled to both sides of the body due to tension. Patients with less subcutaneous fat or strong back muscles have higher skin tension.

13.1.2 Characteristics of Dorsal Spinal Soft Tissue and Suture Requirements

An ideal method of surgical incision closure should consider the following four aspects: A. How to close the incisions in sequence according to different anatomical levels, ensuring accurate alignment of identical anatomical structures, leaving no cavity deep inside of the incision? B. How to close the incision quickly? What kind of suture and suture method should be chosen to shorten the entire operation time? C. How to suture the incisions tightly while preventing the suture from damaging the surrounding soft tissues that provides sufficient blood supply for the good healing of the incision edge? D. How to choose multifunctional sutures (antibacterial coating, knotless, barbed suture, etc.) that can provide sufficient tension for tissue healing according to the characteristics of anatomical tissue? [6, 7]. The composition, property, and fiber arrangement of the anatomical tissue determine its strength. The healing time of muscles, fascia, subcutaneous tissues, and skin are different after injury, and the tension supports provided by sutures that are required during the critical period of wound healing vary as well. If the above four questions are answered, our considerations on the scientific management of spinal soft tissues can be comprehensive. The characteristics of dorsal spinal soft tissue and suture requirements are as follows:

1. **Muscular Layer** Taking the lumbar muscles as an example, among the erector spinae, musculi multifidi, and spinalis are closest to the midline, and stop on both sides of the spinous process of lumbar, zygapophyseal joint, and processus transversus. In the process of surgical incision closure, if the spinous process of the lumbar is conserved, the attachment point of the muscle at the spinous process should be reconstructed. Interrupted suture can be used to make the suture pass through the muscles on both sides and the interspinous ligament as a closure of this anatomical layer. If total laminectomy for decompression is performed, the lamina and spinous process have been completely removed. The muscles on both sides should be pulled to the center and sutured together to fill in space where the original lamina and spinous process are previously located on the dorsal side to avoid cavity forming at the deep position of the thoracolumbar fascia. Meanwhile, the thoracolumbar fascia can be sutured to the supraspinous ligament to maintain the continuity of the deep quadratus muscular layer and prevent the deep muscles from "floating."
2. **Thoracolumbar Fascia** The healing of thoracolumbar fascia is slow, requiring about 6–8 weeks. Its tension can restore to 40% of the previous level 2 months after the operation. Good closure of thoracolumbar fascia can provide sufficient lumbar tension and reduce the leakage of deep tissue fluid into the subcutaneous tissue. Tight suture of the thoracolumbar fascia can reduce the incidence of postoperative complications such as CSF cyst and wound infection, especially when the dura mater is torn during the operation with cerebrospinal fluid leakage. In the process of incision closure, it is best to choose round needles to minimize fascia cutting by the needle and suture. In addition, the suture material should be strong enough and free of tissue reaction or foreign body residue. If absorbable sutures are chosen, make sure that the sutures can provide enough durability to ensure a good healing of the fascia layer during the normal absorption process.
3. **Subcutaneous Tissue (Fat Layer)** Subcutaneous adipose tissue is characterized by poor stability, high mobility, and blood supply there is not very rich. It may be easily burned by an electrotome and prolonged traction can easily cause fat cell rupture and adipose tissue liquefaction, which can generate subcutaneous soft tissue exudation after surgery and finally causing the formation of subcutaneous exudate, and increasing the risks of wound infection. Superficial surgical incision infection is mostly seen at this anatomical level. The fat layer tissues are difficult to align and easy to tear off when sutured. In view of these characteristics, it is essential to reduce dead space during the suture process to avoid wound infection. A well-closed incision with sufficient strength is the most effective way to reduce skin cracks; continuous suture method can be adopted to reduce the residual suture knots, avoid forming cavities around the knots, and reduce the incidence of wound infection and foreign body cyst caused by suture foreign body reaction [8, 9].
4. **Skin** The skin on the lower back usually takes 10–14 days to heal. In the process of surgical incision closure, after completing the suture of subcutaneous tissue, make sure that the edges of the skin can be neatly aligned without obvious tension. Sutures are used to hold the skin edges together rather than providing a great tension to pull the skin edges together. The greater tension the skin suture has to undertake at the edge, the greater possibility of scarring from the surgical incision after the operation can be seen. In the case that the skin may have excessive effusion or a great tension at the edge postoperatively, sutures with less damage to soft tissue and less tissue reactions should be selected for skin edge suturing.

13.1.3 Suture Techniques of Cervical Posterior Soft Tissues Reconstruction

The clinical practice of cervical posterior surgery has a long history. In 1985 and 1986, professor Cai Qinlin from the Department of Orthopedics of Peking University Third Hospital first carried out cervical posterior bilateral open-door expansive laminoplasty and cervical posterior unilateral open-door expansive laminoplasty in China. The surgical principle is to expand or directly remove the cervical posterior column structure. By expanding the spinal canal, posterior spinal compression can be directly relieved. Based on the bowstring principle, the anterior spinal compression can be indirectly relieved by the posterior displacement of the spinal cord. The indications of this surgery include developmental cervical spinal stenosis, spinal cord compression caused by multi-segment (≥3 segments) degenerative cervical spinal stenosis, continuous or mixed ossification of the posterior longitudinal ligament (OPLL). At present, posterior cervical surgery has been developed into multiple surgical methods including cervical posterior unilateral open-door expansive laminoplasty, bilateral open-door laminoplasty, and posterior cervical laminectomy. Since laminectomy can cause many complications such as trachelocyrtosis and neck stiffness, the applications of laminectomy are quite limited clinically. In some cases, it can be used as a remedy for laminoplasty.

During the surgery, the patient should be placed in the prone position. Incise the skin and subcutaneous tissues from C2 to T1. After reaching the muscular layer, use periosteum exfoliator and electrotome to perform paravertebral muscle detachment. It should be noted that in order to ensure the stability of cervical vertebrae postoperatively, the muscle attachment points on C2 should be conserved. Peel the muscles to the edges of the bilateral articular processes. The exposure can be completed after hemostasis. There is no important anatomical structure in posterior cervical soft tissues except for the posterior cervical muscle group. Pay attention to the depth of the electrotome during the peeling process, and always keep the electrotome head above the lamina. After the posterior decompression operation is completed, the following aspects need to be noted during soft tissue reconstruction.

1. **C2 Muscle Insertion Reconstruction** The posterior cervical muscle group plays an important role in maintaining the cervical lordosis and its sagittal mechanical equilibrium. After a cervical posterior surgery, due to stripping of the posterior extensor muscle group, it lacks an attachment point. In addition, some patients suffer from weakness of the posterior cervical muscle group due to postoperative cervicis brake muscle atrophy, which will result in a reduction of cervical lordosis. Furthermore, the posterior cervical muscle group will keep the head at the normal position by continuous contraction, resulting in neck stiffness and pain, etc. Among them, C2 spinous process is the main attachment point of the posterior cervical muscle ligament. The muscles attached to the C2 spinous process include rectus capitis posterior major, obliquus capitis inferior, semispinalis cervicis, musculi multifidi, interspinalis, etc. If the continuity of the C2 spinous process and muscles can be conserved as much as possible, postoperative cervical axial symptoms will be reduced to a certain extent. Therefore, some spine surgeons have made relevant improvements to the classic surgical procedures through continuous exploration, such as expansive conserving muscular ligament complex, C4-C6 single-opening or double-opening expansion surgery, or C3 laminectomy plus C4-C6 single-opening or double-opening surgery. These methods are designed to adequately decompress the spinal cord decompression and meanwhile conserve or rebuild the muscle attachment points, shorten the operation time and reduce the complications caused by muscle dissection. This shows the importance of wound closure in posterior cervical spine surgery, especially at the muscle level.

   This surgery was a C3-C7 unilateral open-door expansive laminoplasty and C2 muscle insertion reconstruction was administrated during surgical incision closure after the operation. Specifically, chisel off the attachment points of the muscle on both sides of the C2 spinous process along with partial bone with a narrow osteotome, and then make a hole at the C2 spinous process. Suture the C2 muscle insertion bone pieces separated on both sides back in situ. Suture with Absorbable 0# Vicryl Plus® Control Release Violet Sutures (Polyglactin 910, Ethicon.Inc). Make sure that the suture is firm enough to make bones contact and fix with each other. The peripheral fascia and tendinous tissues could be strengthened by Absorbable 2-0 Vicryl Plus® Control Release Eight Sutures (Polyglactin 910, Ethicon.Inc). In most cases, the muscle is cut off 1 cm from the attachment point during peeling. When closing the surgical incision, Absorbable 0# Vicryl Plus® Control Release Violet Sutures (Polyglactin 910, Ethicon.Inc) can be used directly to suture the muscle end in an 8-shaped manner or suture at the attachment point of the muscle (Fig. 13.1).
2. **Suture of Deep Muscular Layer and Ligamentum Nuchae** For posterior cervical deep muscles, including splenius capitis, semispinalis capitis, semispinalis cervicis, etc. Absorbable 0# Vicryl Plus® Control Release Violet Sutures (Polyglactin 910, Ethicon.Inc) can be used to suture discontinuously in figure-eight shape. Avoid

forming dead space when suturing. After the posterior cervical deep muscles are sutured, the ligamentum nuchae needs to be sutured. The ligamentum nuchae is an important fascial structure located between the muscles on both sides of the cervical spine. Since its attachment point is far away from the head's motor axis, the ligament nuchae plays an important mechanical role in antagonizing the anterior flexion of the head and neck. Absorbable 0# Vicryl Plus® Control Release Violet Sutures (Polyglactin 910, Ethicon.Inc) can be used for interrupted suturing (Fig. 13.2).

3. **Subcutaneous and Skin Suture** The posterior cervical skin and subcutaneous tissues are thicker than those of the anterior cervical skin. The incision is located at the back of the neck and cannot be seen easily. Therefore, the suturing is less difficult than that for the anterior cervical approach. Absorbable 2-0/3-0 Vicryl Plus® Control Release Violet Sutures (Polyglactin 910, Ethicon.Inc) can be used for interrupted suturing on subcutaneous tissues or Absorbable 2-0/3-0 Vicryl Plus® Control Release Violet Sutures (Polyglactin 910, Ethicon.Inc) for continuous suturing, and then Absorbable 4-0 Vicryl Plus® Control Release Violet Sutures (Polyglactin 910, Ethicon.Inc) can be used for intradermal suturing of skin (Fig. 13.3a, b).
4. **Cerebrospinal Fluid Leakage** Cerebrospinal fluid leakage is also a rare intraoperative and postoperative complication of posterior cervical spine surgery. Specific suture and repair are the same as those for cerebrospinal fluid leakage in anterior cervical spine surgery. Tightly closed suturing is

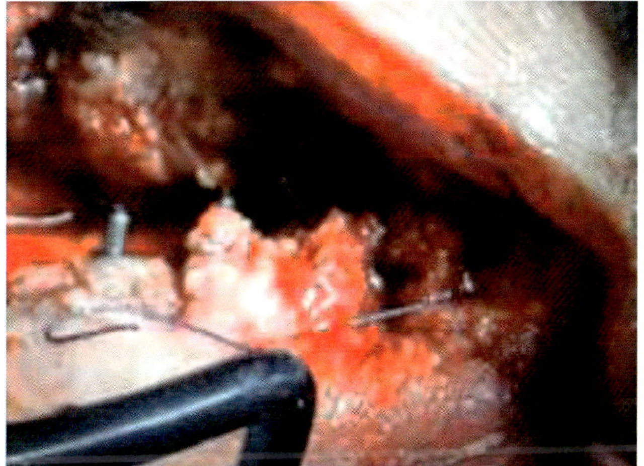

Fig. 13.1 C2 muscle insertion reconstruction

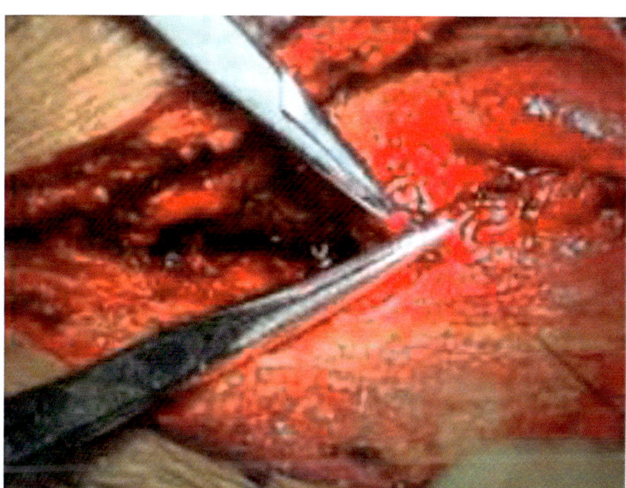

Fig. 13.2 Interrupted suturing of the posterior cervical deep muscles

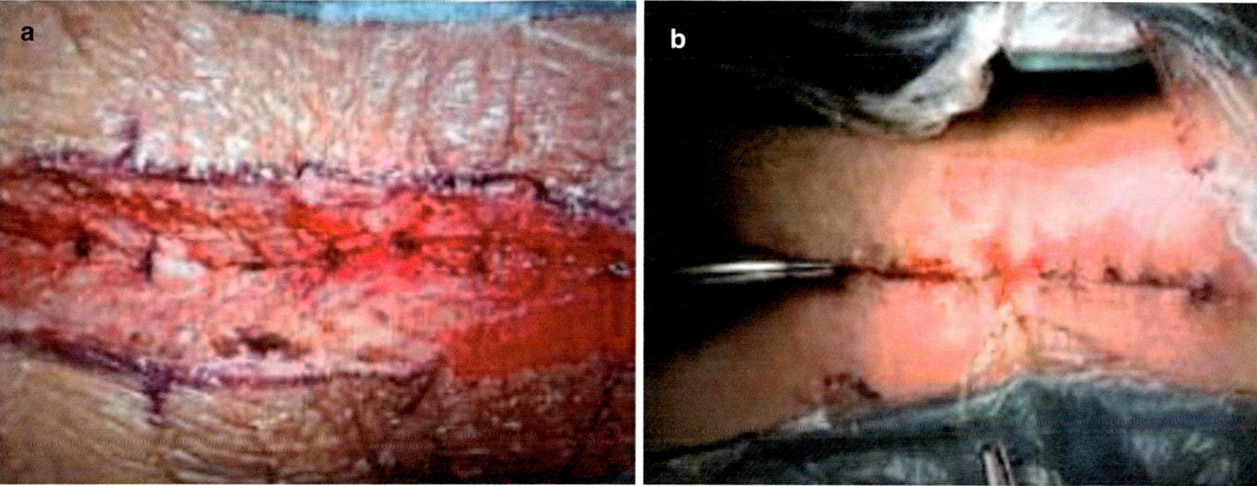

Fig. 13.3 (**a**) Interrupted subcutaneous suturing of the posterior cervical wound. (**b**) Intradermal suturing of the posterior cervical wound

the key basis for reducing the complications of cerebrospinal fluid leakage. For details on incision enclosure, please refer to the treatment of cerebrospinal fluid leakage during internal spinal-related surgery in this textbook.

13.1.4 Incision Closure Technique for Thoracolumbar Posterior Median Approach

1. **Muscular Layer** It is controversial among some scholars about whether or not to close the muscular layer tissues, because it depends on the size of the surgical incision and the surgeon's experience. The author believes that perfect closure of the muscular layer plays an important role in the management of soft tissue healing. If the posterior incision surgery preserves the spinous process (posterior median approach or Wiltse approach), and the length of the incision is less than two segments of muscle dissection, direct closure of the fascia layer can ensure the continuity of the underlying muscle tissues [10]. If the length of the incision is greater than two segments or total laminectomy is adopted, it is necessary to reconstruct the attachment point of the muscle at the median site and tightly close the muscular layer tissues, which can reduce the risk of deep effusion [11, 12].

Before closing the incision of thoracolumbar posterior median approach surgery, the surgical incision should be flushed with normal saline. The muscular layer can be closed by interrupted suturing with Absorbable 0# Vicryl Plus® Control Release Violet Sutures (Polyglactin 910, Ethicon. Inc), or "8-shaped" interrupted suturing, or continuous suturing. At the lumbar and thoracic level, the multifidus and spinous muscles are close to the lamina surface. The direction of the muscle fibers should be considered when suturing this anatomical layer. This requires the surgeon to bluntly peel off most of the muscle fibers on the spinous process and the lamina surface during incision exposure. The attachment points of the muscles on the spinous process and articular process need to be accurately and sharply peeled off in order to provide satisfactory soft tissue conditions for closing this anatomical layer. During the surgery, do not use a spreader at the same anatomical site for a long time since such operation will cause ischemia and inactivation of muscle tissues.

For thoracolumbar surgery by posterior median approach with the conservation of spinous processes, closing the fascia layer and sewing the muscle tissues to the interspinous ligament can avoid effusion space formation between the deep muscles and the lamina (Fig. 13.4). For total spine laminectomy, the muscle tissues on both sides should be accurately closed during the closing process, which provides a good foundation for the closure of thoracolumbar fascia in the next step. Muscle healing requires sufficient blood supply. During the suturing process, sutures should be used to pull the muscles on both sides together rather than cutting the muscle tissues by trying to tighten the sutures. The surgeon should particularly pay attention to cutting damage of the muscle or muscle necrosis due to poor perfusion caused by over-tightened sutures. During interrupted suturing, the suture needle should be 0.5 cm away from the edge of the muscle tissue. The distance between two interrupted stitches or "8-shaped" stitches is 2–3 cm. Each suturing should align the muscles in the incision and meet with each together instead of tightening them at one place. 1# sutures (Ethicon Vicryl Plus® Control Release Sutures) can be used for continuous suturing of the muscular layer. It should be noted that during the incision exposure, most of the paravertebral muscles and multifidus are exposed by blunt dissection. Continuous suturing is not a full-thickness suturing of the muscular layer. It is applied to ensure that adequate muscles are attached to the surface of the dura or lamina to reduce submuscular space.

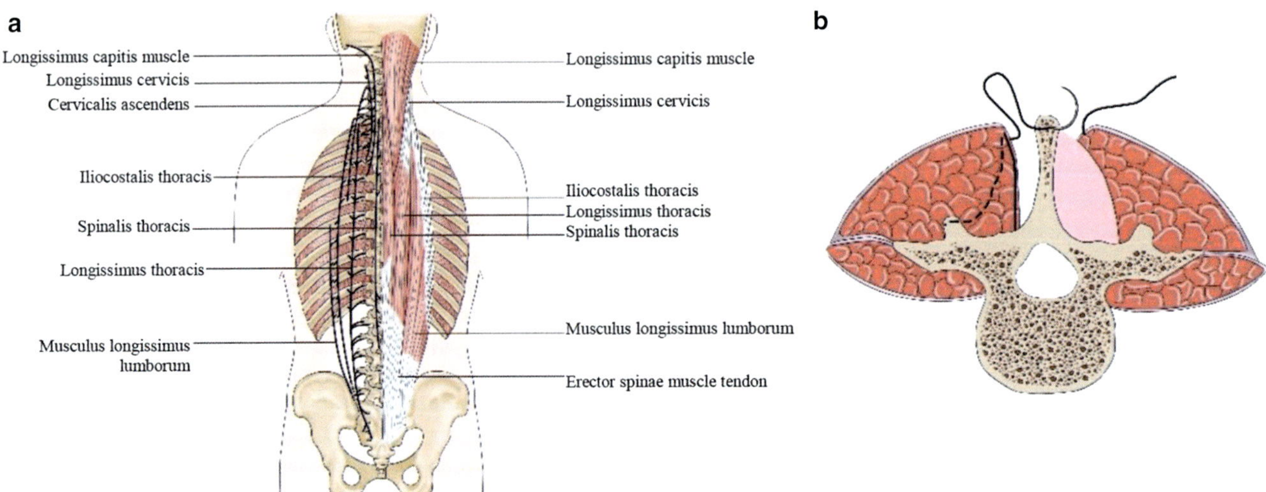

Fig. 13.4 (**a**) Anatomy of deep muscles at the lower back. (**b**) Schematic diagram of erector spinae muscle reconstruction

Regardless of whether intermittent or continuous suturing is used, the author does not recommend using barbed sutures for closure of this level. The following two reasons are mainly considered: Firstly, unlike other anatomical tissues, the barbs of the sutures will cause muscle incising damage when passing through the muscle fibers. Secondly, the barb is designed to reduce the relative displacement between the suture and tissue. During the suturing process, the suture can be tightened in an unhurried manner so as to reduce the suturing time and complete incision closure rapidly. However, for the muscular layer, using barbed sutures may cause over-tightening that leads to the poor blood supply to the muscles, resulting in avascular necrosis of the muscles, increasing the risk of deep soft tissue infection of the surgical incision. Based on the above two points, the average healing time of combined muscle tissues is about 2 weeks. Taper-point needle, smooth single-strand or multiple-strand absorbable sutures can be used to close the anatomical layer to provide sufficient tension, sutures can ensure that the muscle tissue can heal effectively with suture support.

Some surgeries (degenerative lumbar scoliosis correction surgery, thoracolumbar kyphosis correction surgery) have longer incisions. For example, scoliosis can lead to asymmetric development of muscles on both sides of the spine, or kyphosis can cause paravertebral muscles in a stretched state for a long time, muscle atrophy, and muscle volume decrease [10]. Special consideration should be given to the design of the surgical incision and the precautions in the suture process. The author will introduce the technique of surgical incision closure for spinal deformity in a separate section.

2. **Thoracolumbar Fascia** Thoracolumbar fascia provides strong support for the lower back muscles. It is characterized by high tension and slow healing. It can regain 40% of the original tension 2 months after the surgery. When selecting surgical incision sutures, the selected sutures should be of high material strength and low tissue reaction given the above characteristics. Absorbable 0# Vicryl Plus® Control Release Violet Sutures (Polyglactin 910, Ethicon. Inc) can be selected for interrupted suturing, or Absorbable 1# Vicryl Plus® Control Release Violet Sutures (Polyglactin 910, Ethicon.Inc) or Absorbable 1# Stratafix Symmetric PDS PLUS Knotless Tissue Control Device Sutures (PPDO, Ethicon.Inc) can be used for continuous suturing of fascia layer. During the suturing process, it should be noted that there should be no cavity at the head or end of the incision. No matter continuous suturing or interrupted suturing is adopted, it is necessary to explore whether there are residual cavities at both ends of the incision, which can be explored by fingertips or instruments at the end of suturing. According to the author's experience, if the starting and ending sections of some surgical incisions show poor healing or presence of exudation, it may be caused by poor closure of the fascia layer and residual cavities. Especially for small skin incision with bigger incision deep inside, pay more attention to the tight closure at both ends. If cerebrospinal fluid leakage occurs during spinal surgery, particular attention should be paid to the closure of the thoracolumbar fascia during incision closure. Tight suturing is an important barrier to reducing the flow of cerebrospinal fluid through this layer to subcutaneous tissues thus to avoid cerebrospinal fluid cyst formation and wound dehiscent.

Due to the great tension of the thoracolumbar fascia layer, the suggested needle space of continuous suturing is 0.8–1 cm. Keep the needle space consistent. The needle should be about 0.5 cm away from the fascia. All layers of the fascia are sutured. Sometimes due to the lengthening or exposure of the incision, the edge of the incised fascial layer may contract into the subcutaneous tissue due to the traction of the instrument or the skin tension. Pay attention to the distinction when suturing to ensure that the thoracolumbar fascia is closed at the correct anatomical level. In the posterior decompression surgery that preserves the spinous processes of the thoracolumbar vertebrae, sutures can be applied to the supraspinous ligament to continue the tension of the fascia. After the suturing, fingertips or instruments can be used again to detect for any residual cavities in the fascial layer to ensure tight suturing at this anatomical level. No matter interrupted suturing or continuous suturing is used, it should be noted that needle cutting of the fascia tissue should be minimized during the suturing process. The suture of PDS material can still have 60% tension at 6 weeks after the operation, and it is completely absorbed 182–238 days after the operation with no remained in the body. The author recommends the Absorbable 1# Stratafix Symmetric PDS PLUS Knotless Tissue Control Device Sutures (PPDO, Ethicon. Inc) to sew the thoracolumbar fascia. In addition to fast sewing to shorten the operation time, the anti-slip design, knot-free, and high tension of PDS material of the barbs on the suture provide sufficient effective tension for thoracolumbar fascia healing and ensure good healing at this layer.

3. **Subcutaneous Tissue (Fat Layer)** When closing the subcutaneous tissues, 2–0# Ethicon Absorbable Vicryl Plus® Control Release Sutures can be used for interrupted suturing or continuous suturing. The adipose tissue of this layer has a great mobility with loose soft tissues, and it is not prone to be traction by the suture needle. It is easy to be cut by the thread during stitching. During the suturing process, part of the fascia layer and subcutaneous dermis layer can be sutured appropriately to wrap the adipose tissue in it, thus to ensure complete closure at the anatomical level and avoid the accumulation of fluid in the incision. The author recommends continuous suturing to close the anatomical layer to reduce the number of knots left in the anatomical layer to form cavities in the adipose tissue. If 2–0# Vicryl Plus® Control Release

Violet Sutures (Polyglactin 910, Ethicon.Inc) is used for continuous suturing, Aberdeen knot can be used to ensure suture continuity while avoiding loosening of sutures in sutured tissues. In recent years, some scholars have also tried to use 2–0# Stratafix Symmetric PDS PLUS Knotless Tissue Control Device Sutures (PPDO, Ethicon.Inc) to close this layer, avoiding knotting and shortening the time of surgical incision closure. The surgeon needs to continuously improve the suturing technique thus to meet the suturing requirements.

4. **Skin** There are many suture methods and techniques for skin suturing. The suture techniques of plastic surgeons are worthy of our study and reference. It is recommended that 4–0# Stratafix Spiral Bidirectional PGA-PCL Knotless Tissue Control Device Sutures (PGA-PCL, Ethicon.Inc) and 4-0# Vicryl Plus® Control Release Violet Sutures (Polyglactin 910, Ethicon.Inc) are used for intradermal suturing. Literatures [13] show that compared to skin closing with skin nails, in the posterior open spinal incision, suturing skin with sutures can effectively reduce the incidence of incision SSI (11.8% versus 4.2%, $P = 0.017$). The medical skin tissue glue (Dermabond Prineo, 2-octyl cyanoacrylate and self-adhering mesh, Ethicon.Inc) can be used on the epidermis to reduce epidermal tension, with hydrocolloid wet dressing being more conducive to skin incision healing. Skin suturing needs tight closure of subcutaneous tissues (fat layer) to ensure that there is no obvious tension during skin closure; meanwhile, no broken ends or knots of the suture should be left on the skin surface so as to reduce the risk of scar formation.

The above summarized the characteristics of soft tissue anatomy, selection of sutures, and suture techniques in cervical, thoracolumbar, and lumbar posterolateral surgeries with the median incision. Some of the above contents are cited from literatures and reference books, and some are the 62-year clinical experience in spinal surgery that the Orthopedics Department, where the author works, has gained. Novel materials and the development of surgical instruments have brought more options for spine surgeons and hopes to the patients. While facing many choices, spine surgeons should focus on not only the improvement of nerve functions, reconstruction, and stability of spine functions, but also pay attention to suturing techniques of the surgical incision. Reconstruction of the functions of the incision soft tissues and beautifying suturing incision tissue should be deemed as one of the required basic skills for the spinal surgeons, helping more patients with their skills. Patients will benefit not only from the sophisticated spinal surgery, but obtain good functional reconstruction of spinal soft tissues and healing appearance.

The anatomical layers of the soft tissues at the waist include skin, subcutaneous tissues, fascia layer, and muscles (Figs. 13.5, 13.6, 13.7, 13.8, 13.9, 13.10, 13.11, 13.12, 13.13, 13.14, 13.15, 13.16 and 13.17).

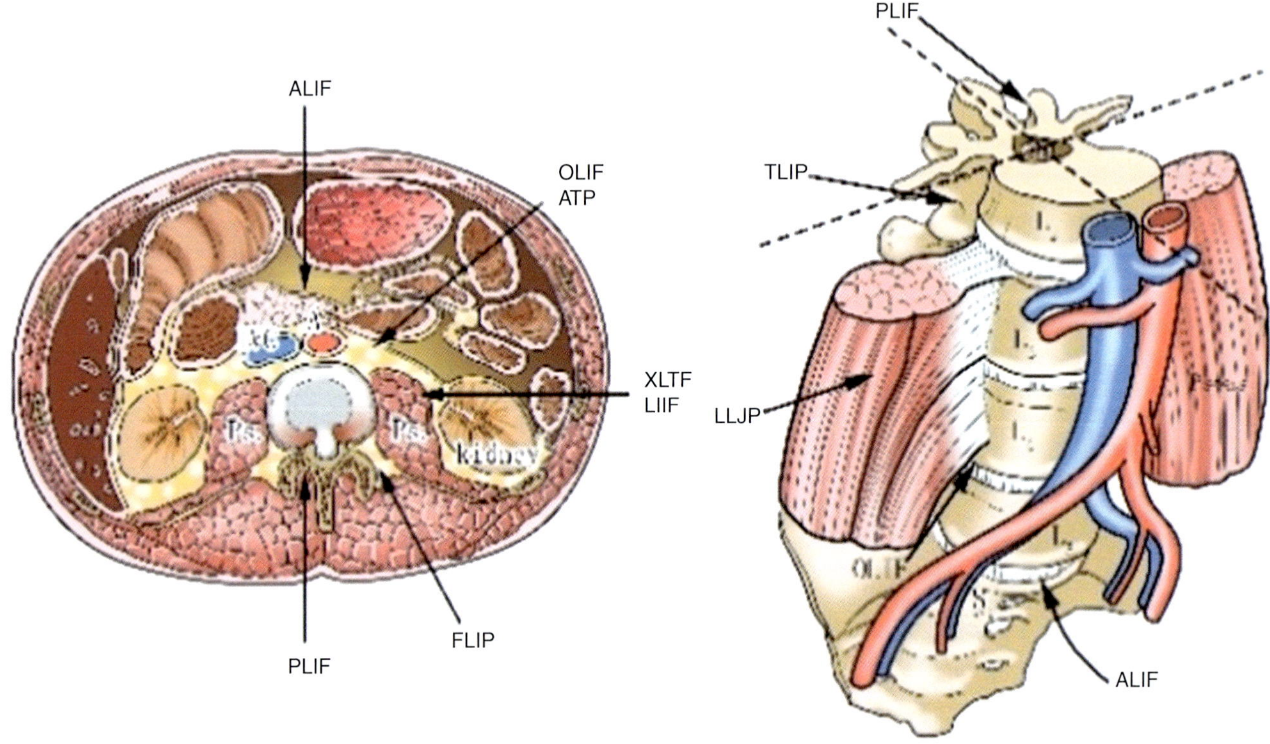

Fig. 13.5 Different surgical approaches for spinal surgery

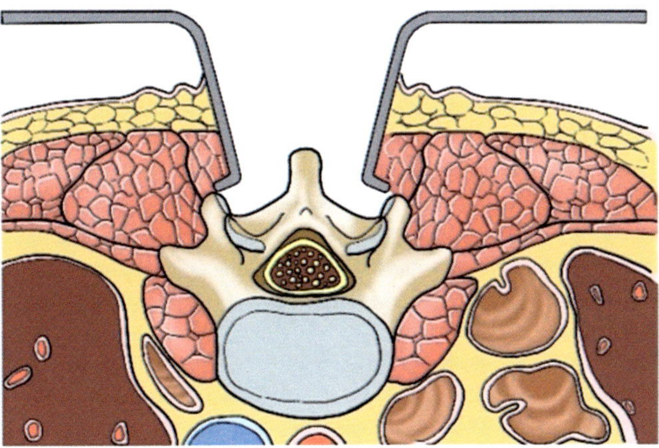

Fig. 13.6 PLIF surgical incision closure starts from the deep side and needs to complete the suturing of muscles, thoracolumbar fascia, subcutaneous tissues, and skin successively

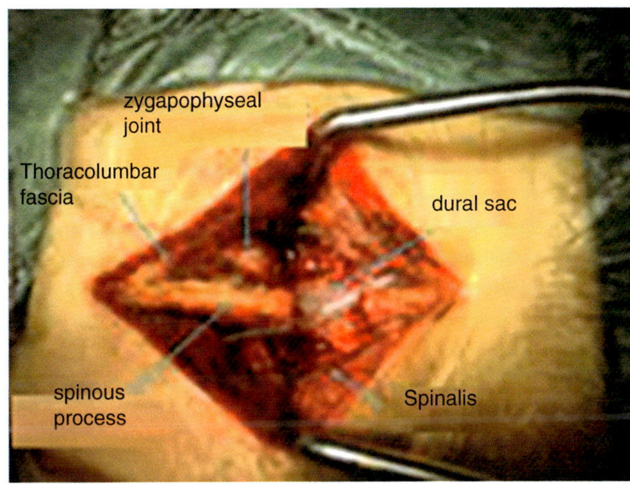

Fig. 13.7 Deep anatomical structure of the incision of the posterior median approach to the lumbar spine surgery

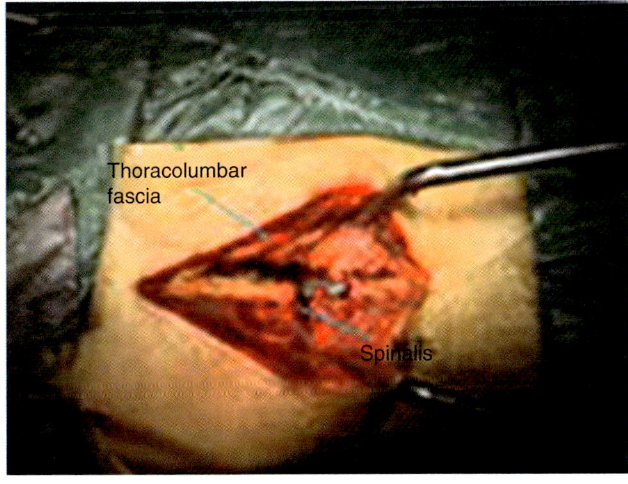

Fig. 13.8 Shallow anatomical structure of the incision of the posterior median approach to the lumbar spine surgery

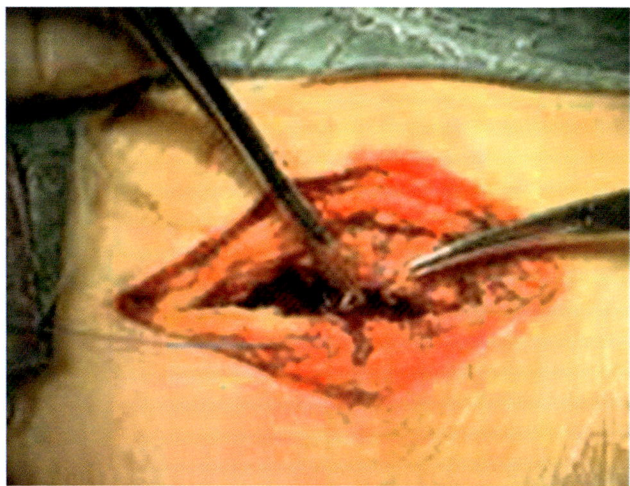

Fig. 13.9 "Fig. 8" suturing of the lumbar posterior paraspinal muscles

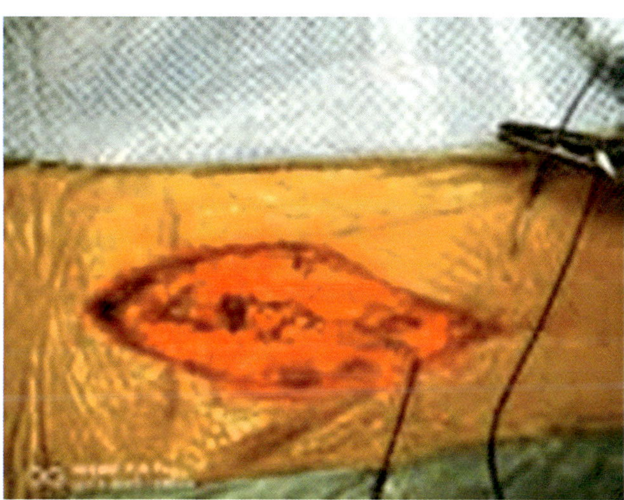

Fig. 13.10 Knot-free suturing of the posterior lumbar thoracolumbar fascia

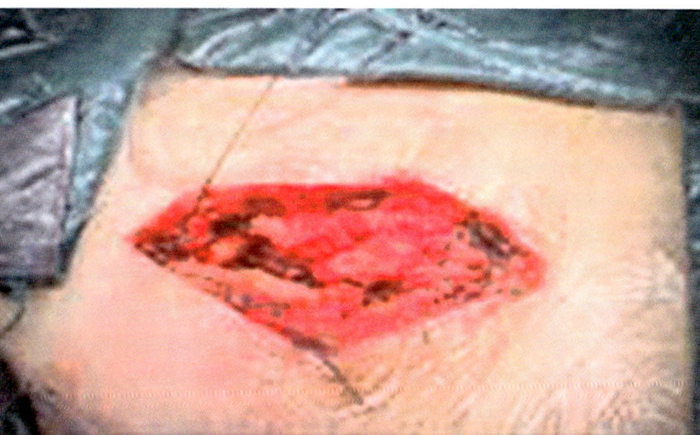

Fig. 13.11 Continuous suturing of the posterior lumbar thoracolumbar fascia

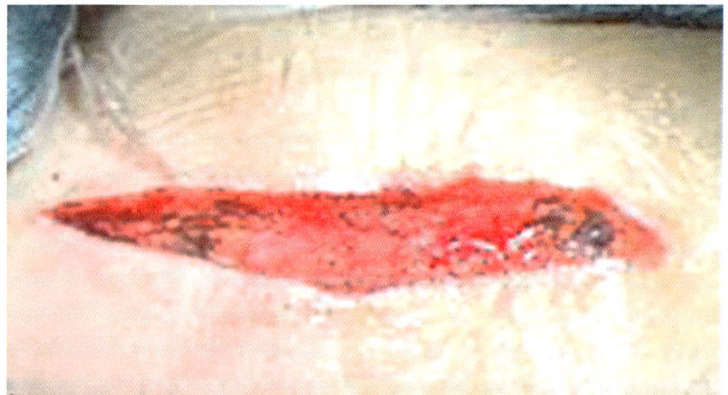

Fig. 13.12 Complete suturing of the posterior lumbar thoracolumbar fascia

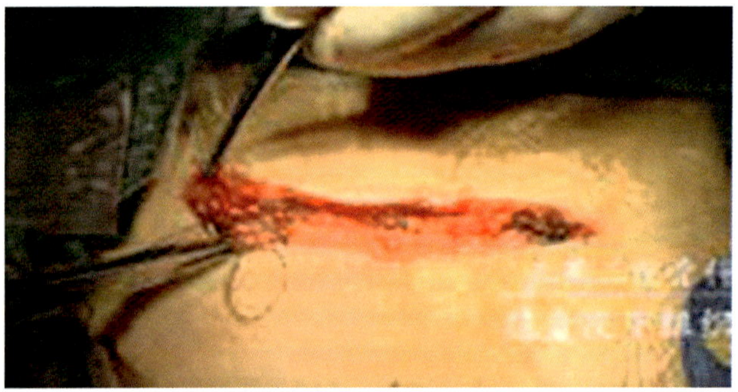

Fig. 13.13 Suturing of the posterior subcutaneous tissue of the lumbar spine

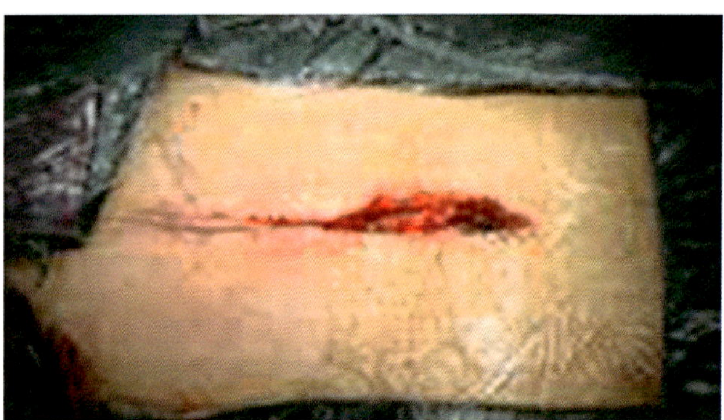

Fig. 13.14 Continuous suturing of the posterior subcutaneous tissue of the lumbar spine to ensure good skin closure

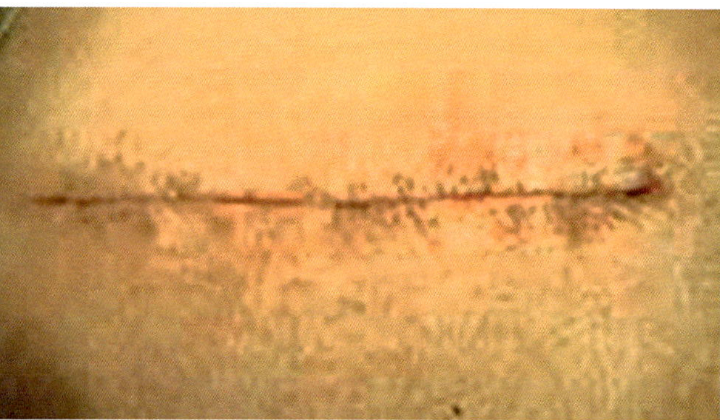

Fig. 13.15 Intradermal injection of local anesthetics to complete the suturing of the posterior subcutaneous tissues of the lumbar spine without tension on the skin edge

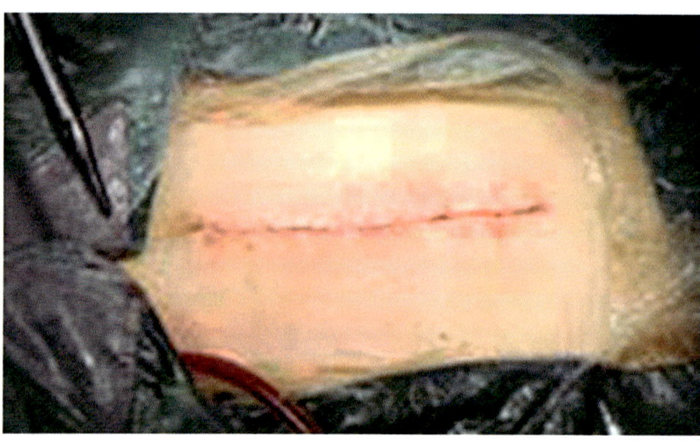

Fig. 13.16 Posterior lumbar intradermal suturing for cosmetic suturing

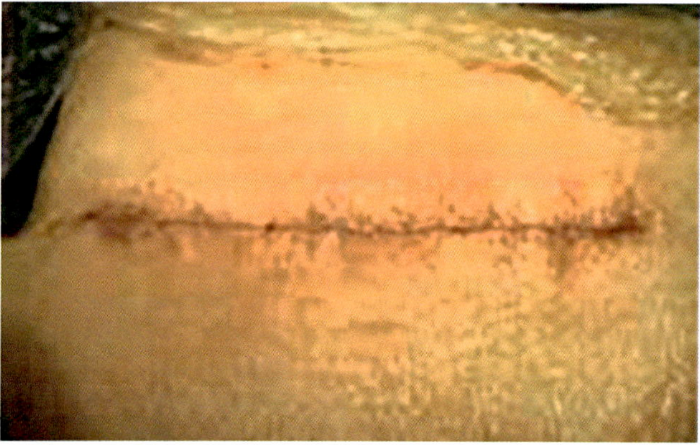

Fig. 13.17 Ending of closure of the posterior lumbar spine surgical incision

Postoperative incision closure process for one case of thoracic decompression surgery (Figs. 13.18, 13.19, 13.20, 13.21, 13.22, 13.23, 13.24, 13.25, 13.26, 13.27, 13.28, 13.29):

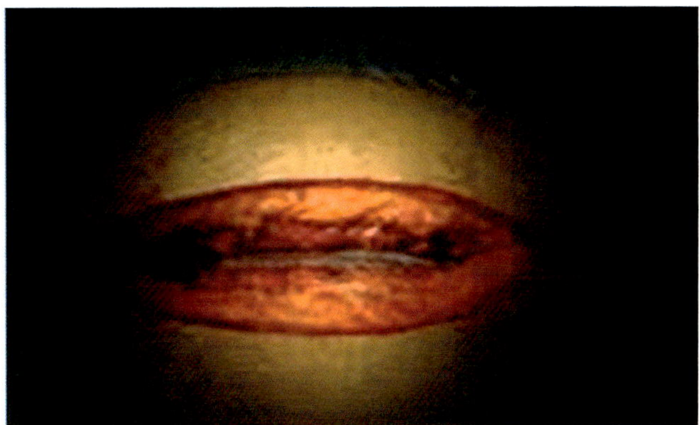

Fig. 13.18 Prepare to close thoracic surgical incision after completing the main steps of surgical incision and flushing the incision

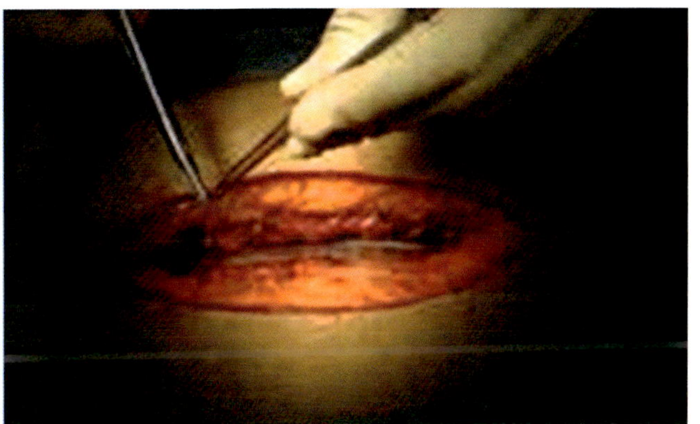

Fig. 13.19 Suture the posterior paravertebral muscles of the thoracic spine in "Fig. 8" shape

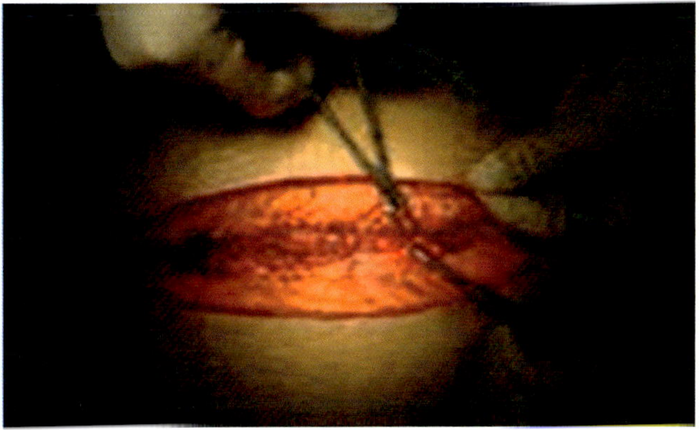

Fig. 13.20 Protect muscles during "Fig. 8" suturing of posterior paravertebral muscles of the thoracolumbar spine to avoid pulling too much

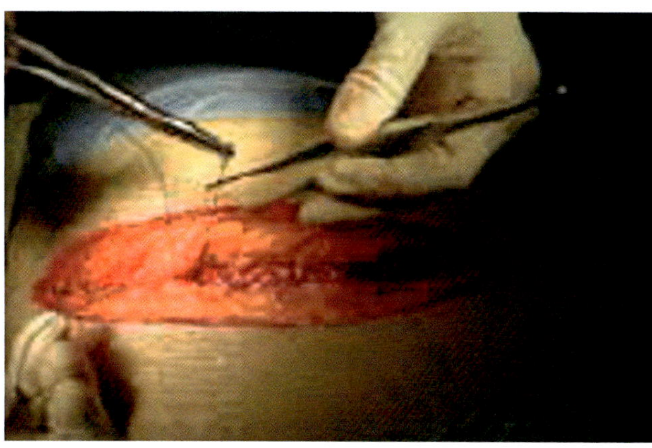

Fig. 13.21 Continuously suture the posterior thoracic thoracolumbar fascia

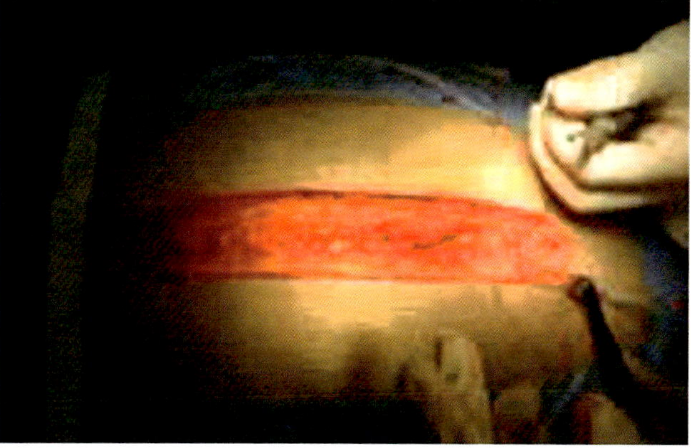

Fig. 13.22 Tightly suture the starting and end parts of the posterior thoracic fascia layer to avoid leaving a cavity

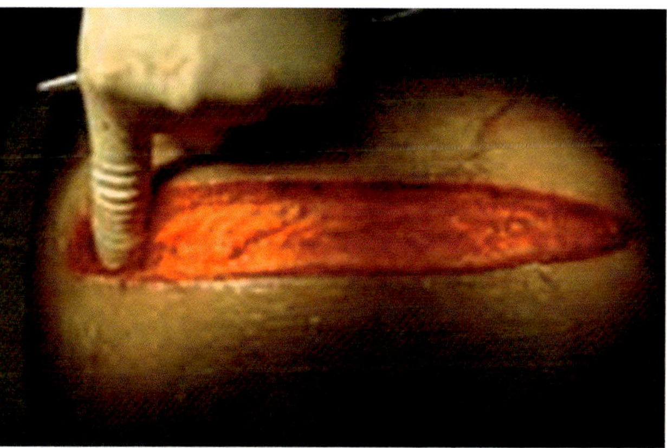

Fig. 13.23 Check the posterior thoracic fascia layer for any gaps missing during suturing

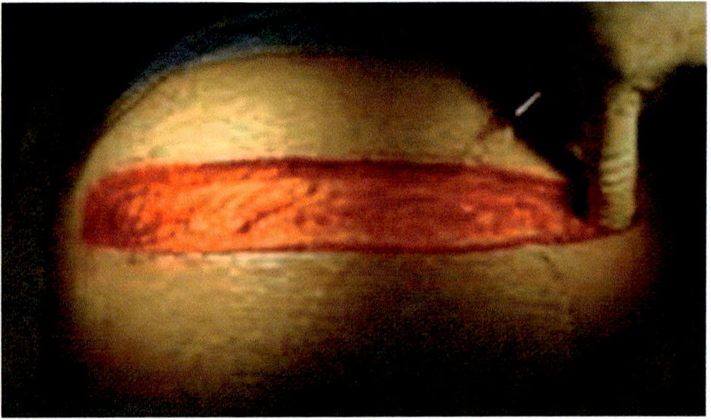

Fig. 13.24 Check the posterior thoracic fascia layer again for any gaps missing after suturing

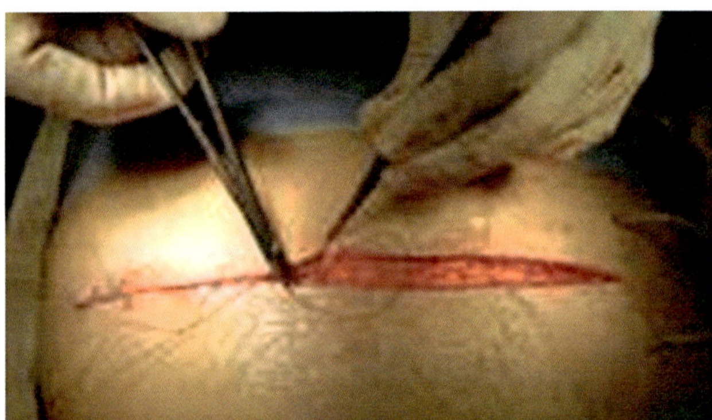

Fig. 13.25 Continuously suture the posterior thoracic subcutaneous tissue

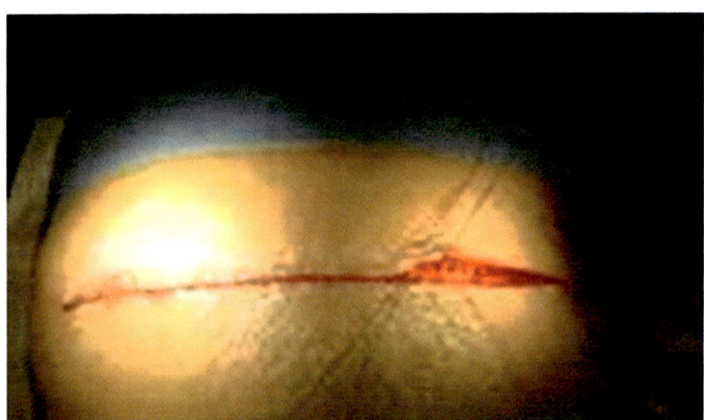

Fig. 13.26 Continuously suture the posterior thoracic subcutaneous tissues to reduce skin tension

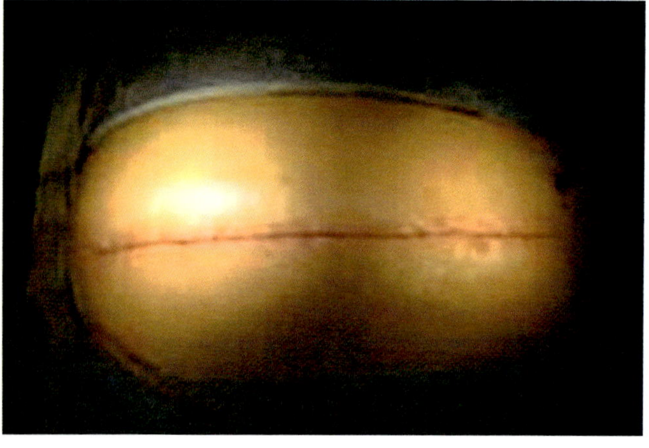

Fig. 13.27 Complete continuous suturing of the posterior thoracic subcutaneous tissues without tension at skin edges

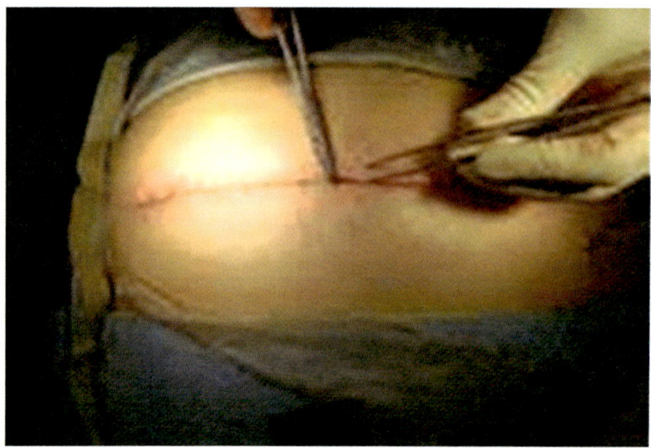

Fig. 13.28 Intradermal suturing of posterior thoracic inciseaneous layer

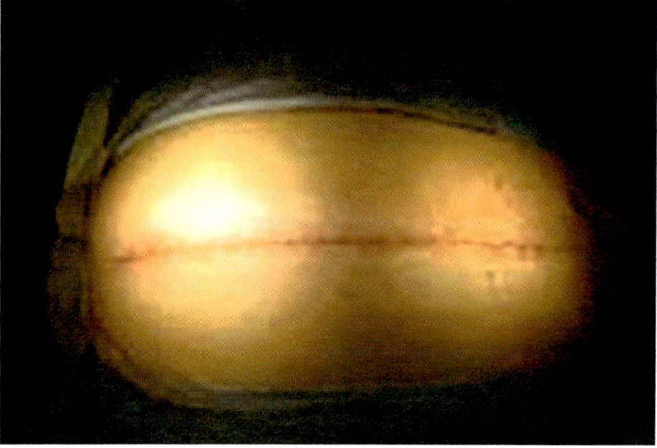

Fig. 13.29 Complete the posterior thoracic intradermal suturing to realize cosmetic suturing

13.2 Incision Closure Technique for Anterior Cervical Spine Surgery

Liu Yang and Qi Min
Department of Orthopedics, Changzheng Hospital
Shanghai China

Abstract
Anterior cervical spine surgery, as a common treatment method for cervical spine diseases, has been widely used in clinical practice. Due to anterior cervical lesions, such as disc herniation, posterior vertebral osteophytes, ossification of the posterior longitudinal ligament, etc., resulting in irritating the cervical spinal cord and nerve roots, anterior cervical surgery can directly and effectively relieve the compression, pain, neurological deficits, and other symptoms. This chapter describes in detail the exposure of surgical incisions for the anterolateral cervical approach, the closure techniques and material selection at each anatomical layer of the incision, and the treatment of postoperative incision complications.

Anterior cervical spine surgery, as a common treatment method for cervical spine diseases, has become more and more widely used in clinical practice. For compression from the anterior cervical spine, such as disc herniation, osteophytes on the posterior edge of the vertebral body, ossification of the posterior longitudinal ligament, etc., resulting in compression of the spinal cord and/or nerve roots, anterior cervical spine surgery can directly and effectively relieve the compression, pain, neurological deficits, and other symptoms.

Anterolateral cervical surgery, as the most common surgical procedure, applies to the region from the C2-C3 segment to the cervicothoracic junction.

13.2.1 Incision Selection

1. **C2–C3 Segment:** Anterior spine surgery involving C2 vertebrae is rare. For C2–3 intervertebral disc herniation, Hangman's fractures without obvious angulation or displacement, inflammation, and tumors, the anterior approach may be adopted. The incision can be selected from the right-side approach, horizontal oblique, and starts from a transverse finger below the mandibular angle for 1 mm forward, transverses toward the anterior inferior part in an oblique direction, and ends at a transverse finger above the thyroid cartilage, closing to the cervical median line. Incise the skin, subcutaneous tissues, and platysma in turn, carefully and bluntly separate the soft tissues under the platysma, from the lateral edge of the scapula hyoid muscle to the prevertebral fascia. In this process, protect the submandibular gland from iatrogenic injury. The blood vessels that cannot be pushed should be ligated or sewed. Reverse superior laryngeal nerve during the pulling process.
2. **C3-C6 Segment:** Since it is more convenient to operate with the right hand, most clinicians are accustomed to the right-side approach. In the cervical-thoracic junction, as the recurrent laryngeal nerve bifurcates into the visceral sheath on the right side at the C6–7 plane (Fig. 13.30), the right approach may cause injury to the recurrent laryngeal nerve due to traction. Therefore, the left approach is used in this area to reduce the possibility of recurrent laryngeal nerve injury. The patient should take the supine position, and keep the head slightly tilted back to make the cervical spine present the curvature of physiological lordosis. Do not tilt backward too much since such position will reduce the posterior intervertebral space, which is not conducive to decompression and increasing posterior facets load. Skin incisions are usually in the transverse form. A longitudinal incision can be made along the border of the sternocleidomastoid for a more extensile approach, such as in cases where multiple-segment (>3 segments) or revision surgery requires extensive exposure though it is much less cosmetic and rarely required. Two transverse incisions at distinct levels for long reconstruction constructs are also an option. The projection of the incision surface is generally marked by thyroid cartilage, which mostly corresponds to the C4–5 segment and the length of the incision varies from 3 to 5 cm according to the segment to be operated (Fig. 13.31a, b). Incise the skin and subcutaneous tissues to reach the platysma layer (Fig. 13.32). Incise the platysma and free the loose tissues under the platysma to reach the joint fascia (Fig. 13.33). Identify the medial edge of the sternocleidomastoid, and incise the joint fascia from the lateral or medial edge of the omohyoid according to surgical segments. Generally, the cross-plane projection of the omohyoid and sternocleidomastoid is directly facing the C5 vertebrae. If the surgical segment is C3-C6, it can be approached from the lateral edge of the omohyoid. If the surgical segment is C5-T1, it can be approached from the medial edge of the omohyoid (Fig. 13.34). After opening the deep cervical fascia, find the carotid pulse with the right index finger pulp to identify the position of the artery and ensure the safety of the blood vessel. Then bluntly separate the loose connective tissues between the visceral sheath and the vascular sheath to reach the anterior side of the vertebrae. Bluntly separate the intervertebral fascia and incise the anterior longitudinal ligament to reach the vertebrae and intervertebral disc. When exposed to C3–4 segment, there are often many vascular plexuses between the visceral sheath and the vascular sheath that will interfere with the expo-

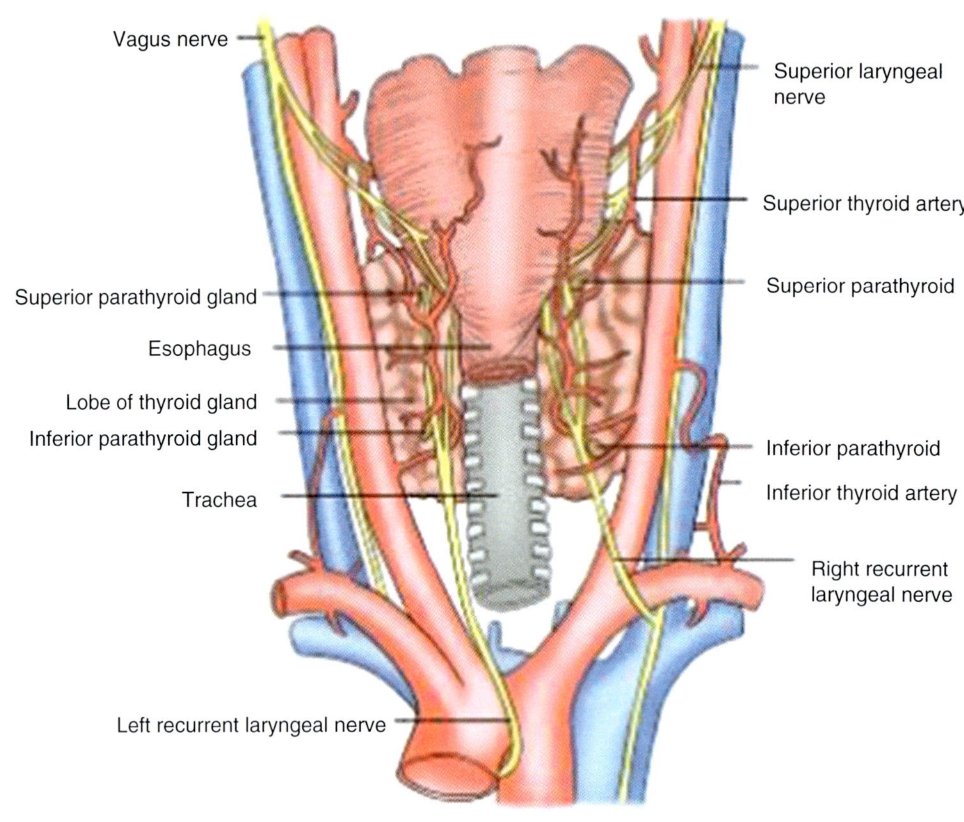

Fig. 13.30 Need to paint

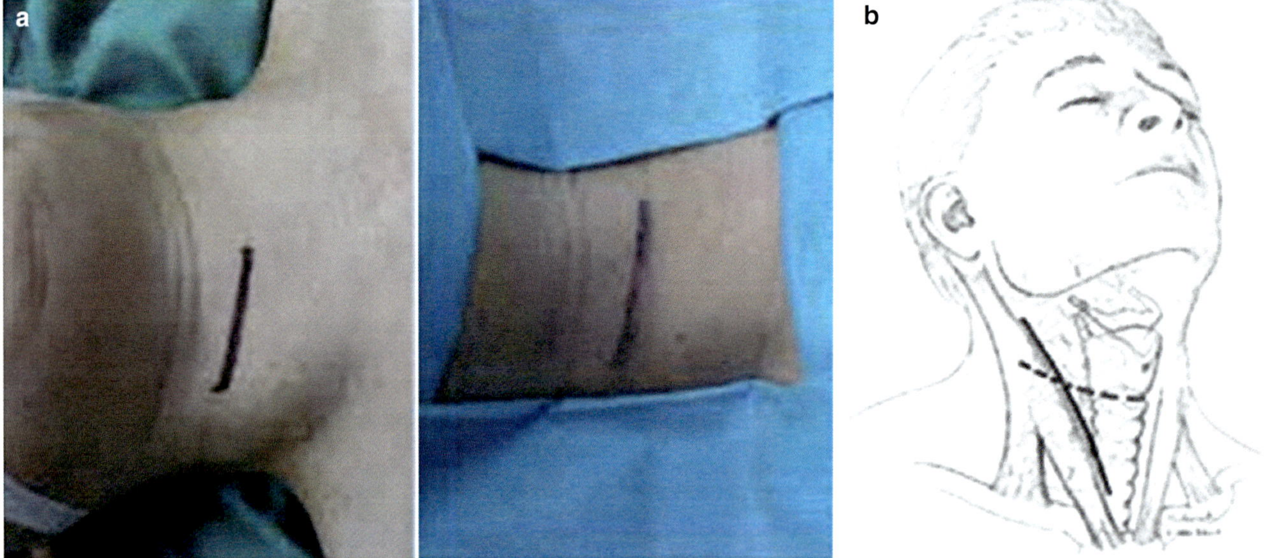

Fig. 13.31 (**a**) Skin incision. (**b**) Skin incision

sure. At this time, it should be carefully separated. Some thicker blood vessels should be ligated, and then bluntly separated to the front of the vertebral body. The musculus longus colli on both sides should be protected as much as possible. However, for some patients with insufficient decompression width of the intervertebral disc or vertebra due to hypertrophy of the musculus longus colli, the musculus longus colli can be separated to both sides as appropriate. Theoretically, there is no too much risk of postoperative Horner syndrome caused by injury of the sympathetic chain of the medial edge of the musculus longus colli. According to our experience, the incidence

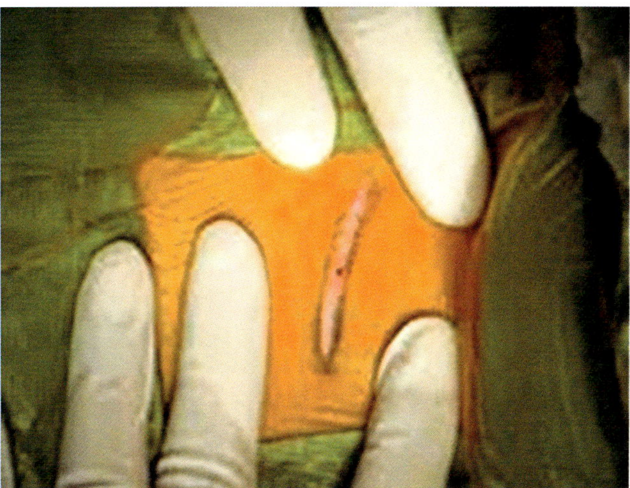

Fig. 13.32 Incise the skin

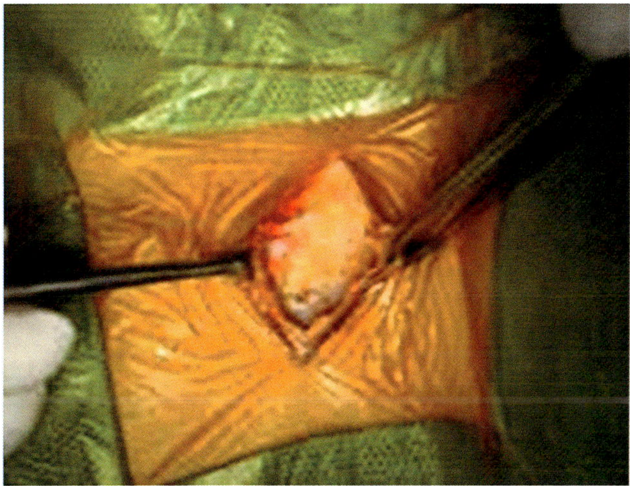

Fig. 13.33 Divide the deep layer of platysma

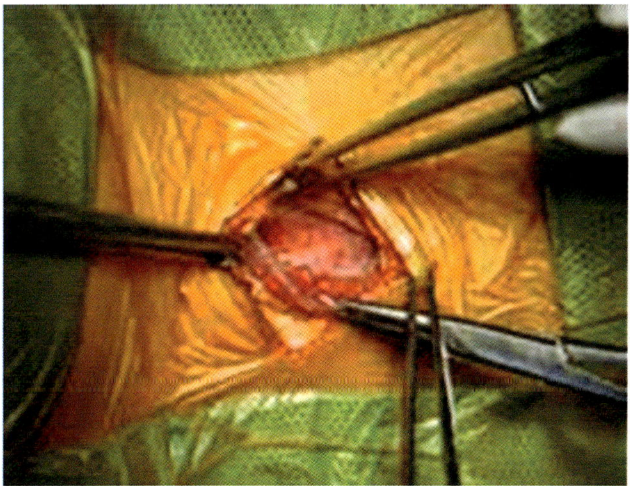

Fig. 13.34 Medial edge of omohyoid

of Horner syndrome after surgery is very low after hemostasis by bipolar coagulation to both ends with an electrotome or incision of musculus longus colli.

3. **Revision Surgery:** The same approach is generally chosen for revision surgery. Namely, if the right approach is adopted for the first surgery, it is not necessary to choose the left approach to avoid postoperative scars; instead, the right approach should still be chosen, which can avoid the serious postoperative complications caused by the possibility that the recurrent laryngeal nerve may be damaged by the first surgery and then the contralateral recurrent laryngeal nerve be damaged by the second surgery. If it is a revision surgery of adjacent segment degeneration and if the surgical segment is adjacent to the original surgical segment by ≥ 2 segments, a transverse finger incision should be made beside the original surgical incision to effectively avoid the influence of scar tissue on the process influences. If the revision surgery has a long segment and a large range, a longitudinal oblique incision should be selected, which is conducive to a wider range of safe exposure and surgery.

Anterior cervical surgery can be classified into fusion surgery and non-fusion surgery. Fusion surgery is considered to be the gold standard for the treatment of such diseases. The commonly used types include simple bone graft, internal fixation with autologous iliac bone graft, internal fixation with titanium mesh and titanium plate, intervertebral fusion cage, and zero-notch intervertebral fusion. Non-fusion surgery generally refers to cervical artificial disc replacement surgery, with the purpose to preserve the mobility of surgical segments and avoid the degeneration of adjacent joints. It has more stringent indications. After vertebral screw positioning, intervertebral disc and osteophyte resection and decompression, internal fixation and implantation, and other surgical operations start closing the wound.

13.2.2 Incision Closure

Cervical soft tissue reconstruction usually consists of three layers: joint aponeurosis layer, platysma layer as well as skin and subcutaneous layer.

1. **Joint fascia layer**

Deep cervical fascia is the fascia tissue between the carotid sheath and the visceral sheath. During anterior cervical surgical exposure, the deep cervical fascia needs to be incised. When the wound is closed in anterior cervical surgery, interrupted suturing with Absorbable 2-0 or 3-0 Vicryl Plus® Control Release Violet Sutures (Polyglactin 910, Ethicon.Inc) can be applied for deep cervical fascia suturing.

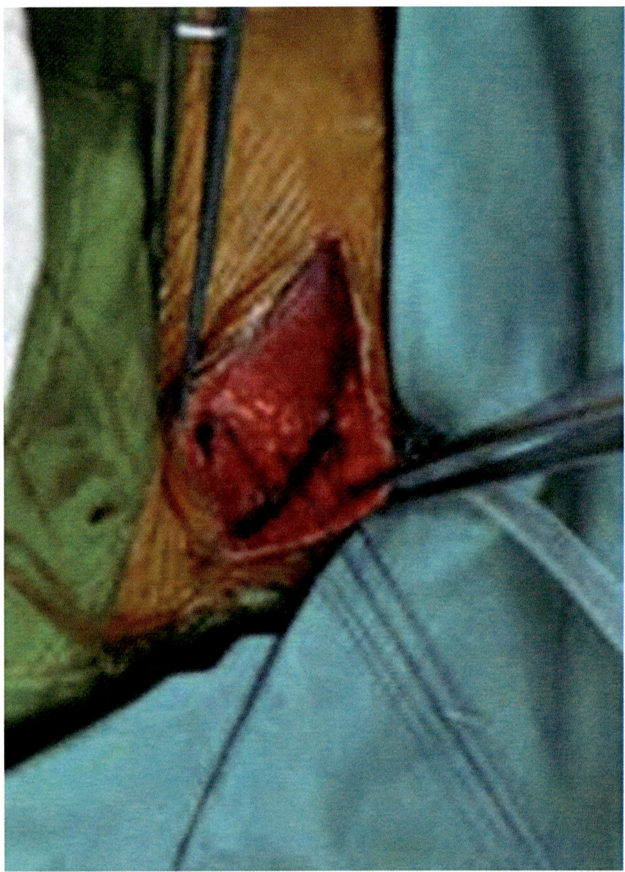

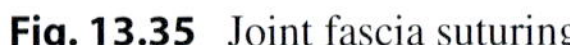
Fig. 13.35 Joint fascia suturing

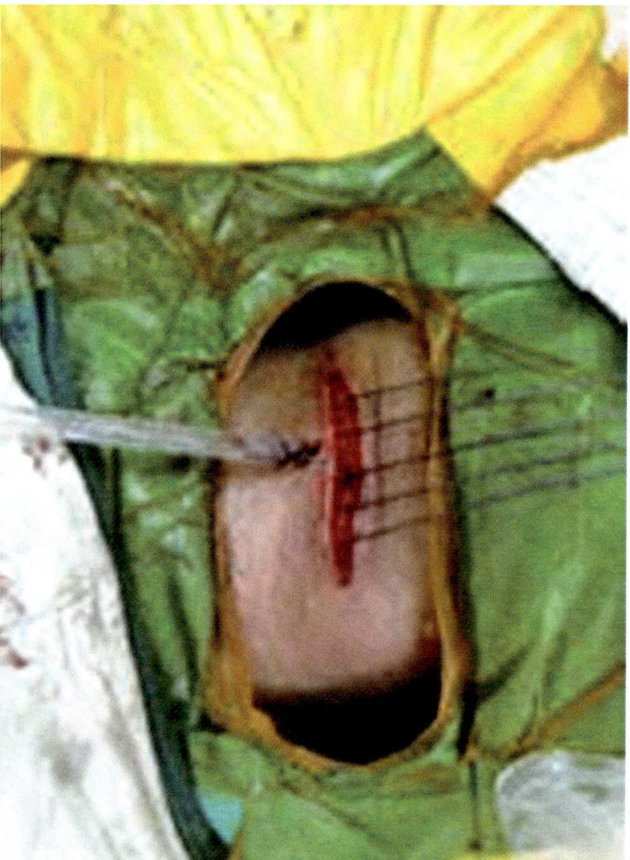

Fig. 13.36 Platysma suturing

It is not advisable to suture too tightly, usually 2–3 stitches, so as not to affect the smooth drainage; however, unstitching is generally not recommended since it may cause the possibility of negative pressure loss in the drainage tube (Fig. 13.35).

2. **Platysma**

The platysma and its fascia layer are located in the superficial cervical fascia on either side of the anterior cervical. They are thin and wide. Each piece is like an inverted fan, starting from the deep fascia on the surface of the pectoralis major and deltoids and ending upward at the mouth corner, which is innervated by the facial nerve. It can pull the mouth corner down and help open the mouth downward, and cause wrinkles in the neck. Because the skin and subcutaneous tissues of the anterior cervical skin are very thin, if the suturing of this layer of muscle is not smooth, it will affect the suturing of the skin layer, causing postoperative scar enlargement and widening. Interrupted suturing with Absorbable 3-0 Vicryl® Plus Control Release Suture (Polyglactin 910, Ethicon Inc.) can be applied for 4–5 stitches (Fig. 13.36). Bury the knots deeply. Or use a knot-free suturing device: Absorbable 3-0 Stratafix® Spiral PGA-PCL Knotless Tissue Control Device Sutures (PGA-PCL, Ethicon Inc.) can be used for continuous suturing. The Knotless Tissue Control Device is a new type of suturing material. A special "barb" suture is used to support sufficient tension, which provides strong and uniform grip on the tissue. It can be operated by an individual person to complete suturing quickly. Pay attention to the tightness of the suture. Please note not to suture too tightly and cross back 2 stitches at the end. Cut the suture close to the tissue to prevent local tissue damage at the end of the suture.

3. **Skin and subcutaneous layer**

Since transverse incision along the dermatoglyph is employed for anterior cervical surgery in most cases, if intradermal suturing is carried out after the surgery, the surgical incision can hardly be seen after healing. Absorbable 3-0 Vicryl Plus® Control Release Violet Sutures (Polyglactin 910, Ethicon.Inc) can be used to suture subcutaneous tissues for 3–4 stitches to fully reduce the tension, and then use Absorbable 4-0 Vicryl Plus® Control Release Violet Sutures (Polyglactin 910, Ethicon.Inc) or Absorbable 4-0 Stratafix Spiral Unidirectional PGA-PCL Knotless Tissue Control Device Sutures (PGA-PCL, Ethicon.Inc) for continuous intradermal suturing of skin layer (Figs. 13.37 and 13.38). Suturing depth shall be consistent during intradermal sutur-

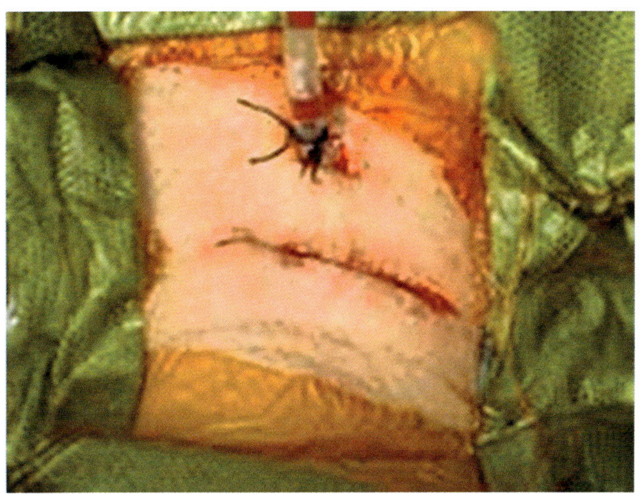

Fig. 13.37 Subcutaneous suturing

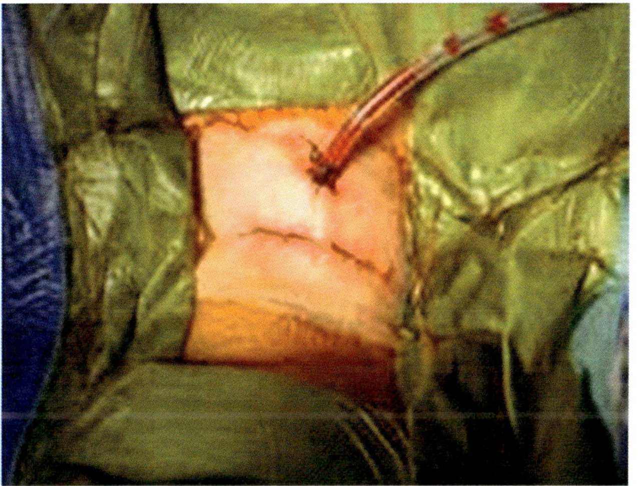

Fig. 13.38 Intradermal suturing

ing. The edges should be aligned neatly to ensure good healing effect. Postoperative incision scar can be almost invisible (Fig. 13.39).

13.2.3 Cerebrospinal Fluid Leakage

Cerebrospinal fluid leakage is quite rare during and after anterior cervical surgery. If not properly treated, secondary wound infection may occur and the leakage may enter the cerebrospinal fluid along the spinal dura mater leakage port. In serious cases, it may lead to central nervous system infection such as purulent meningitis. If spinal dura mater rupture with cerebrospinal fluid leakage is detected, it cannot be directly repaired if the leakage port is too small (<0.2 cm). Instead, the rupture should be covered with adipose or fascia tissues and spray fibrin glue locally. If the area of the spinal

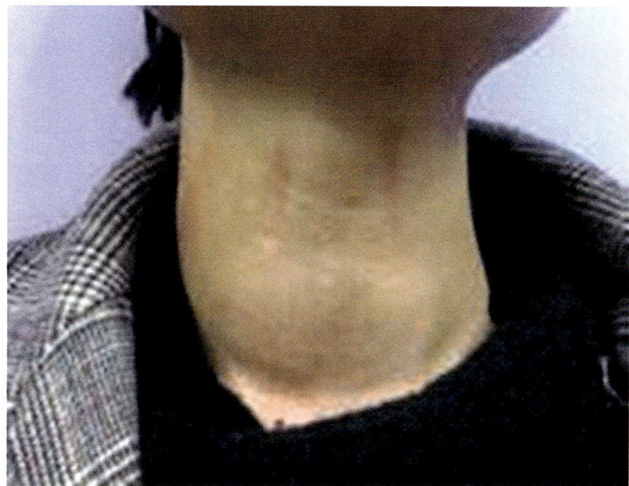

Fig. 13.39 1 year after surgery

dura mater rupture is greater than 0.5 cm × 0.5 cm, the lower back fascia, adipose tissue, or artificial spinal dura patch larger than the defect can be used to cover the defect, suture with unabsorbable 5-0 or 6-0 Prolene Suture (Polypropylene, Ethicon.Inc) and place drainage tubes. After the surgery, the Trendelenburg position, broad-spectrum antibiotics application to prevent infection, compression dressing, and other methods shall be used to avoid infection and promote the healing of the spinal dura mater leakage port. It should be noted that since there are many important vascular nerves in the anterior cervical region, excessive blockage and pressure will easily lead to poor drainage, affecting swallowing and breathing; the compression of the carotid sinus can lead to abnormal changes in blood pressure, heart rate, and oxygen saturation.

13.2.4 Esophagus Fistula

Esophageal fistula is not common in anterior cervical spine surgery. However, once it occurs, it is relatively difficult to treat. It can cause serious consequences if it is discovered or not handled in time. Esophageal fistula is generally divided into two categories. One is direct intraoperative injury: the common cause of direct injury is insufficient experience of the surgeon, unclear local tissues during the operation, and accidental damage to the equipment. Secondly, the retractor exerts a heavier traction and compression on the trachea and esophagus for a long time. Severe local compression leads to esophageal injury. Furthermore, accidental loosening of the assistant's retractor during the operation may cause the esophagus to be exposed to the surgeon's field of vision abnormally, which may cause accidental injury of the instrument. Therefore, the cooperation and concentration of intraoperative assistants are very important. The second category is postoperative injury. The reasons include internal fixation loosening, (plate screw displacement) leading to local esophageal tissue damage; local infection.

Once the esophagus is injured during the operation, it should be sutured immediately. Firstly, Absorbable 3-0 Vicryl® Plus Control Release Violet Suture (Polyglactin 910, Ethicon Inc.) to suture the mucosal layer, and then the muscular layer intermittently. After suturing, draw back the gastric tube above the fistula and clamp the esophagus with oval forceps below the fistula. Inject melanin liquid into the nasogastric tube. If there is no leakage of melanin liquid, complete closure of the anastomosis can be proved. Then loosen the oval forceps and reinsert the stomach tube into the stomach. Place negative pressure drainage tubes or half tubes around the repair site.

If an esophageal fistula is found after surgery, measures such as fasting, indwelling a gastric tube, anti-infection, enhanced dressing, close observation, etc. should be taken immediately, and the esophageal fistula should be confirmed as healed by esophageal barium swallowing or angiography, esophagoscopy, etc. 2–4 weeks later before eating normally.

If delayed postoperative esophageal fistula (several months or even 1–2 years), local infection or internal plant loosening occurs, the local internal fixation should be removed by reoperation and the esophagus repaired. For implant complications, the implant should be removed, the aggressive anti-infective therapy, intensive nourishment should be administered and the spacer was placed; the secondary surgery should be considered according to the local condition. The esophageal repair and suturing should be completed in corporation with thoracic surgeon: first clean up the abscess around the esophageal fistula, rinse with sufficient disinfectant, trim the necrotic esophagus, and suture the mucous layer and then the muscular layer intermittently with Absorbable 3-0 Vicryl® Plus Control Release Violet Sutures (Polyglactin 910, Ethicon Inc.). Finally, place negative pressure drainage tubes around the repair site (Figs. 13.40, 13.41, 13.42, 13.43 and 13.44 Typical cases).

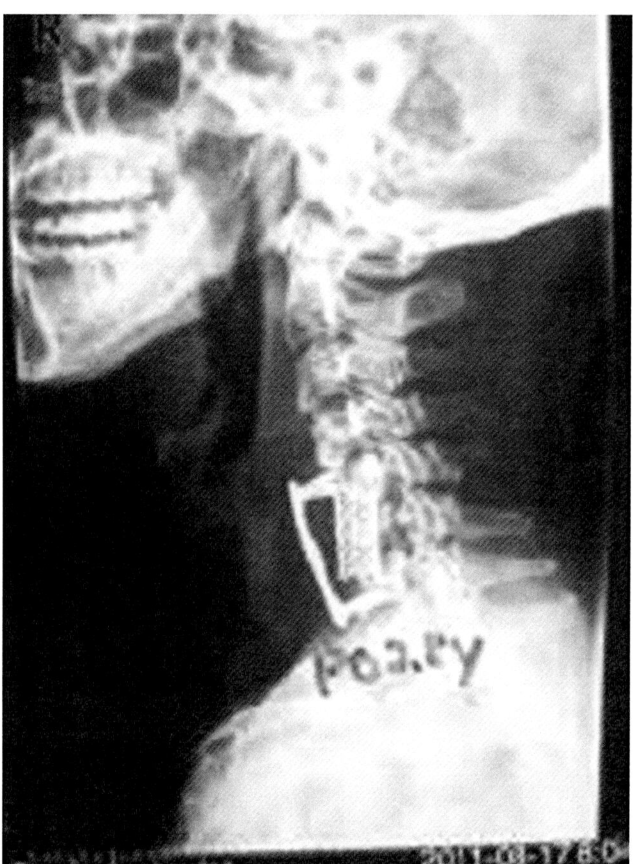

Fig. 13.40 2.5 years after operation

13.3 Incision Closure Technique for Scoliosis Orthopedics

Zhu Zezhang and Qiao Jun
Nanjing Gulou Hospital
Nanjing Jiangsu, China

Abstract
Scoliosis refers to a three-dimensional spinal deformity in which one or several segments of the spine are bent sideways with the rotation of the vertebrae. Scoliosis orthopedics is characterized by long incision, large exposure area, large amount of bleeding, and high incidence of postoperative incision infection. This chapter describes in detail the exposure of scoliosis orthopedic surgical incisions, the standardized incision suturing, and the prevention and treatment of incision-related complications.

Scoliosis refers to a three-dimensional spinal deformity in which one or several segments of the spine are bent laterally with the rotation of the vertebrae. Scoliosis Research Society (SRS) defines scoliosis as follows: The Cobb method is used to measure the lateral curvature of the spine in the standing orthographic X-ray image; if the angle is greater than 10°, it is scoliosis. Scoliosis is usually accompanied by rotation of the spine in the transverse position and increase or decrease of kyphosis or lordosis on the sagittal plane. It is a symptom or X-ray sign that can be caused by a variety of diseases [14].

Surgical treatment should be performed for scoliosis that has a large degree, rapid progress, or seriously affects the patient's quality of life. Scoliosis orthopedics is characterized by long incision, large exposure area, the large amount of bleeding, and high incidence of postoperative incision infection, ranging from 4.4% to 85% as reported [15–17]. There are certain differences in the incidence of incision infections after different types of scoliosis orthopedics. A review of case data involving 1347 patients undergoing scoliosis orthopedics showed that the incidence of incision infections after neuromuscular scoliosis orthopedics was as high as 9.2%, syndrome scoliosis followed by 8.4%; and then adolescent

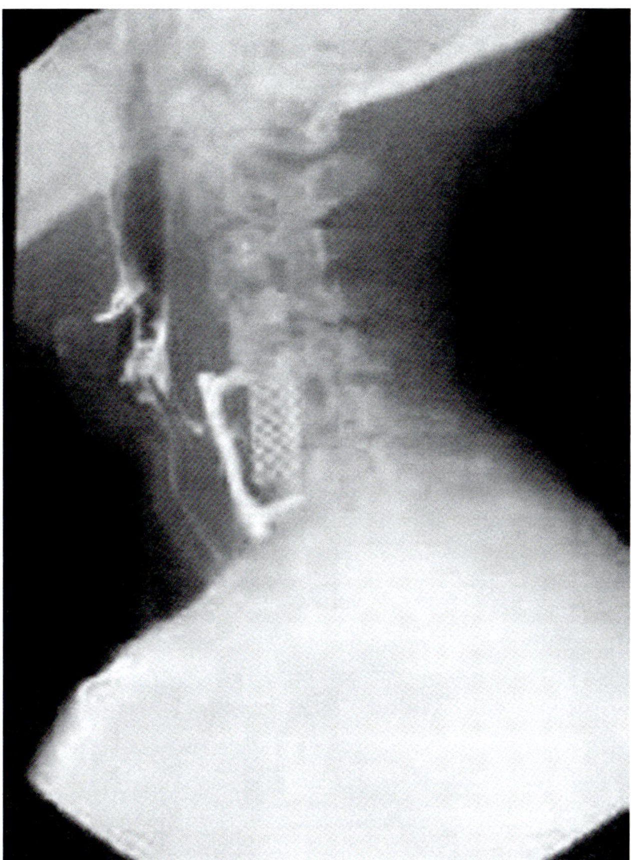

Fig. 13.41 Esophagogram

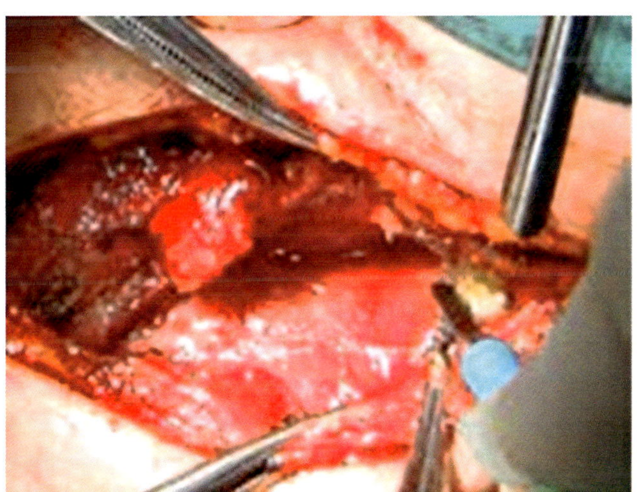

Fig. 13.42 Esophageal rupture

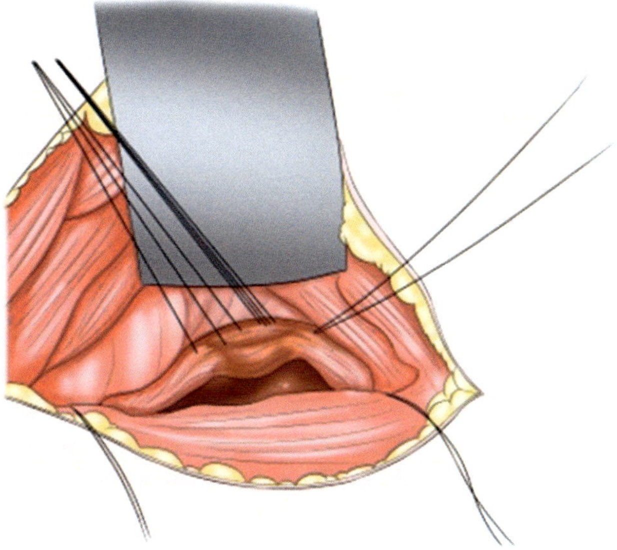

Fig. 13.43 Suturing of the esophageal mucosa (needs to be painted)

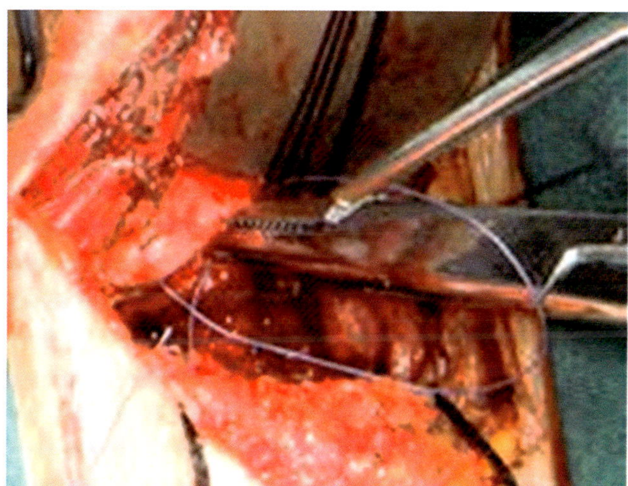

Fig. 13.44 Suturing of esophageal muscle

idiopathic scoliosis, 2.6% [18]. Neuromuscular scoliosis often needs to be fixed to the pelvis, and pelvic fixation is one of the risk factors for postoperative incision infection, with the incidence of being as high as 13.7%. Large amount of pelvic fixation soft tissue peeling, large cavities under postoperative soft tissues, and poor drainage are all risk factors for infection. In addition, revision surgery is characterized by large soft tissue damage and poor healing of the scar. The incidence of infection is also higher than the first surgery. For different types of scoliosis orthopedics, using different suturing strategies can promote tissue healing and effectively reduce the incidence of infection.

13.3.1 Anatomy by Posterior Approach

In patients with scoliosis, due to the rotation of the vertebrae, the muscle volume on both of the concave and convex sides is asymmetric; the muscle volume on the concave side is relatively small, and the volume on the convex side is relatively large (Fig. 13.45) [19]. The muscle tension on the concave side is low and it is easier to stretch when exposed, while the muscle tension on the convex side is high and it is

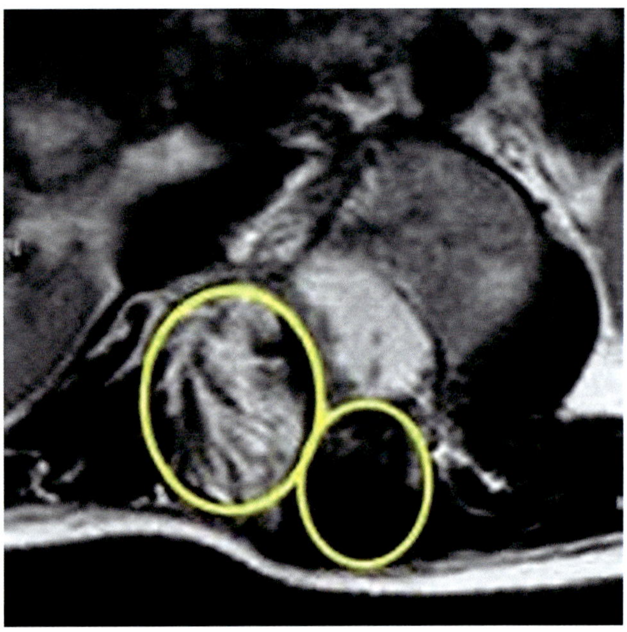

Fig. 13.45 The volume of paraspinal muscles on the convex side of the patient with scoliosis is significantly larger than that on the concave side. The patient is 28 years old, and the convex side muscles have started to show fat infiltration

difficult to stretch when exposed. Generally, when scoliosis is exposed, the concave side is exposed first, and then the convex side is exposed with the assistance of a spreader, which can reduce the difficulty of convex side exposure.

The back muscles are divided into three layers. The superficial layer is the upper limb girdle, including the superficial trapezius, latissimus dorsi, as well as large and small rhomboid muscles at the deep surface. The middle layer is the auxiliary respiratory muscles, including the serratus inferior superior and posterior. The deep layer is the musculus propria at the back, including the erector spinae on the superficial longitudinal direction and the semispinous, musculi multifidi, and musculi rotatores on the deep oblique (Fig. 13.46).

The muscles of the thoracic spine and lumbar spine show different directions and distribution, and the ranges of stripping are also different. In the thoracic spine, the muscles need to be stripped to the outside of the transverse process. The muscles that need to be stripped are spinalis, semispinalis, musculi multifidi, and musculi rotatores (Fig. 13.47). In the lumbar spine, the muscles need to be stripped to the lateral edge of the facet joints, and the muscles that need to be

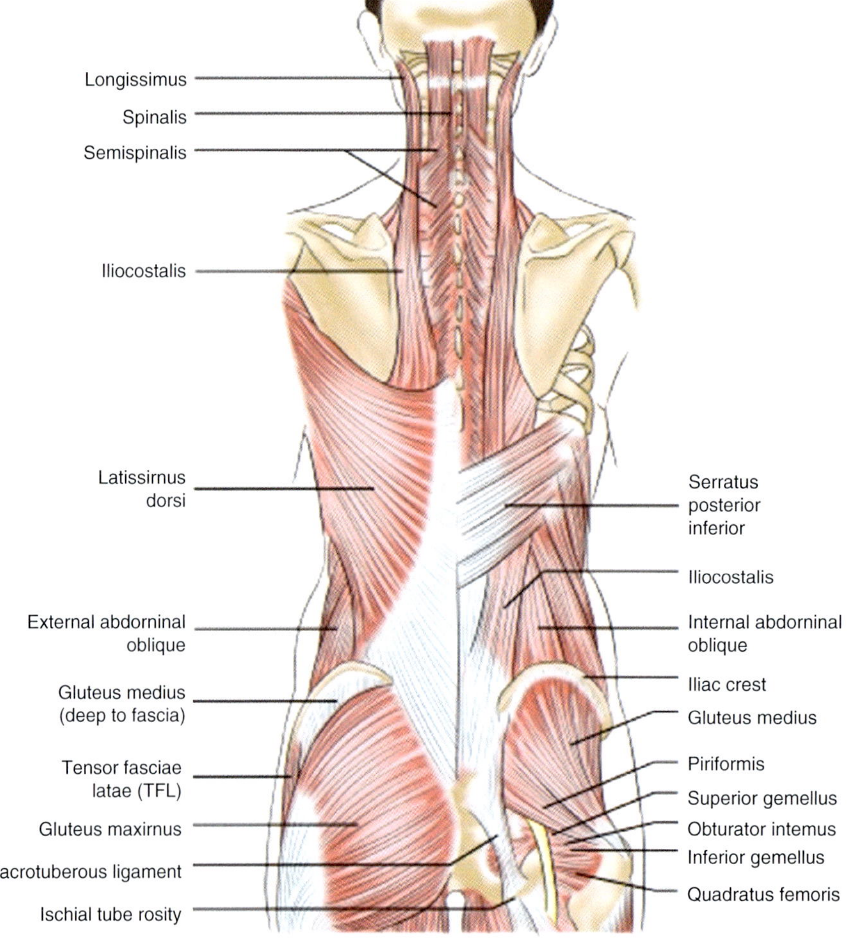

Fig. 13.46 Anatomy of different layers of muscles around the spine vertebra

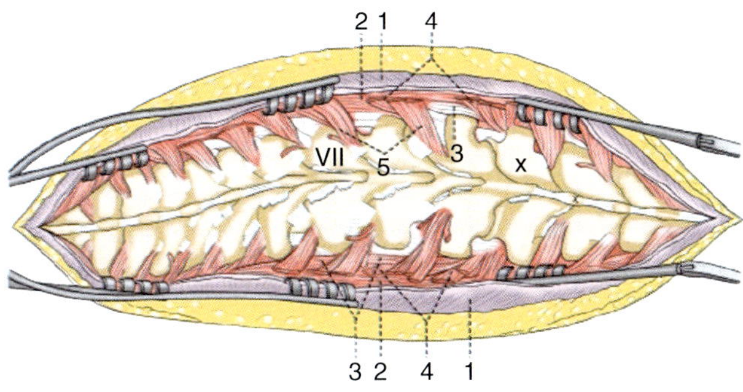

Fig. 13.47 Expose the rear structure of the thoracic spine. 1. Trapezius 2. Spinalis 3. Semispinalis 4. Musculi multifidi 5. Musculi rotatores VII, X: seventh and tenth thoracic spine

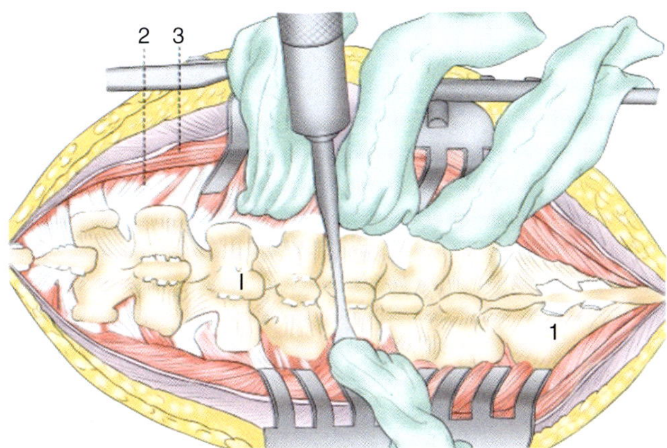

Fig. 13.48 Expose the rear structure of the lumbar spine. 1. Sacrum 2. Musculi multifidi 3. Longissimus I: Lumbar 1 spinous process

stripped are musculi multifidi and some longissimus (Fig. 13.48). If three-column osteotomy or posterolateral fusion is required, the transverse process of the lumbar spine needs to be stripped out so that it can be intermittent during osteotomy or used as a bone graft bed for posterolateral bone grafting. Otherwise, peeling should not exceed this range. Excessive exposure of the lateral thoracic spine can easily damage the pleura and cause pneumothorax; excessive stripping of the transverse process of the lumbar spine can easily lead to bleeding. The segmental arteries include the posterior intercostal artery and the lumbar artery, the dorsal branch of which is accompanied by the posterior branch of the spinal nerve and passes through the bony fiber foramen between the roots of the transverse process to the paraspinal muscles (Fig. 13.49) [20]. When the transverse process is exposed, it is easy to lose this artery and cause bleeding. Because the branches of different segments of the artery form a rich vascular network in the muscle, cauterizing and ligating the artery will not affect the blood supply of the muscle. The segmental artery directly originates from the aorta, and the pressure is high. Once bleeding, it should be completely stopped.

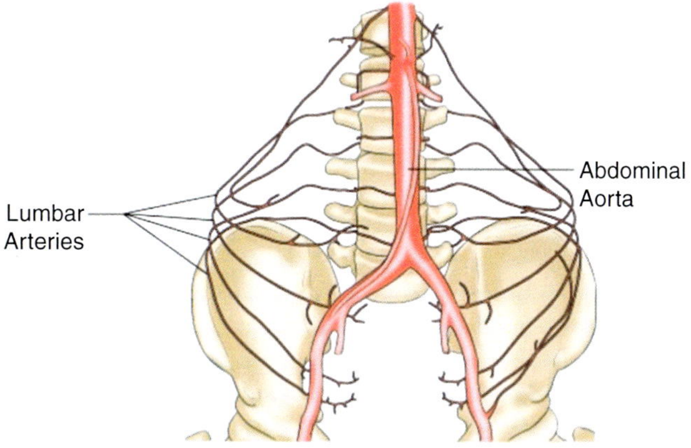

Fig. 13.49 The segmental arteries include the posterior intercostal artery and the lumbar artery, the dorsal branch of which is accompanied by the posterior branch of the spinal nerve, and passes through the bony fiber foramen between the roots of the transverse process to the paraspinal muscles

13.3.2 Exposure by Posterior Approach

1. The scoliosis vertebral body deviates from the midline, and the connecting line of spinous processes curves in an arc. After determining the upper and lower vertebrae, mark the incision in advance with a marker. We recommend a straight incision along the midline, which is more esthetic after the operation (Fig. 13.50). Some scholars also believe that a curve incision should be made along the connecting line of the spinous processes (Fig. 13.51). For patients with large degree of scoliosis and stiffness, the correction rate is limited. The spinous process cannot return to the midline completely after the surgery, and the curved incision cannot be straightened after the surgery, which is not in good appearance. It should be noted that some special types of scoliosis, such as scar contracture scoliosis show high skin tension on the contracture side (concave side). If a straight incision is used, after the scoliosis is corrected, the scar continues to be pulled, which may make the incision arc to the concave side. In this case, a curved incision can be considered to ensure the good appearance of the postoperative incision to the greatest extent (Fig. 13.52).
2. Incise the skin, subcutaneous tissues, superficial fascia, and back fascia to the spinous process in the thoracic spine. Incise the musculus sacrospinalis attached to the spinous process on both sides of the spinous process, and peel off the musculus sacrospinalis on both sides from the distal end to the proximal end under the periosteum to expose the transverse process of the lamina and the facet joints (Fig. 13.53). The thoracic spine is exposed to the tip of the transverse process, and dry gauze is packed to stop bleeding. Pull out the gauze strip and place the automatic

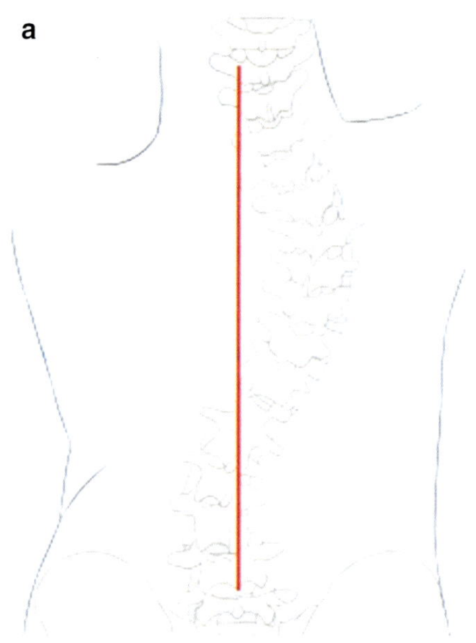

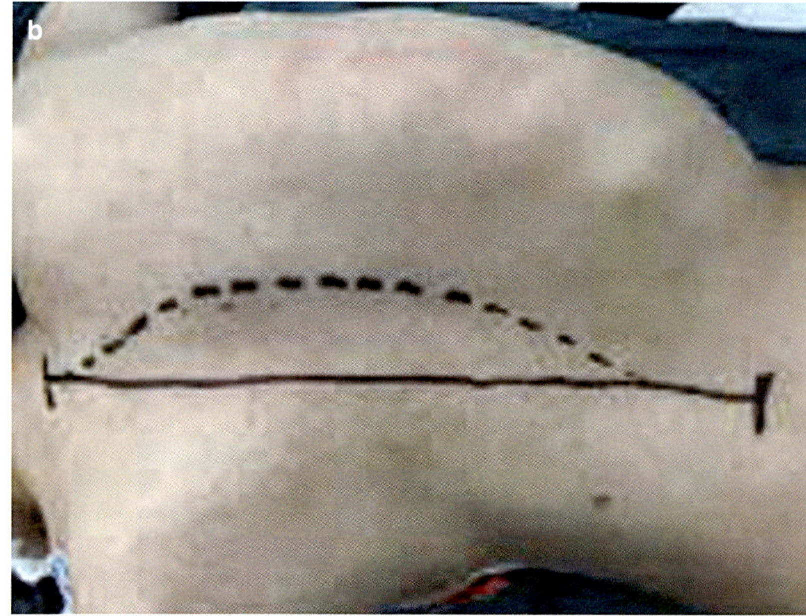

Fig. 13.50 (**a**, **b**) Straight incision diagram

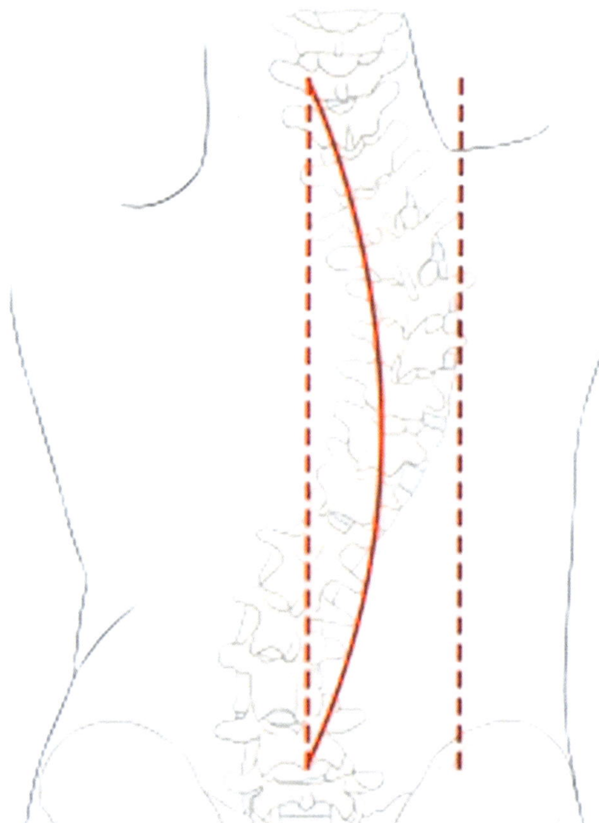

Fig. 13.51 Curved incision

retractor to retract the muscles on both sides, which can clearly expose the spinous process, lamina, articular process, and transverse process (Fig. 13.54).

3. Incise the skin and subcutaneous tissue in the lumbar spine to expose the spinous process and back fascia. Use a cauterizer to incise the fascia and spinous process periosteum close to the midline of the spinous process from the distal to the proximal end. Perform periosteum peeling close to the process and lamina with a Cobb detacher, and push the musculus sacrospinalis to the lateral side in turn, until to the lateral edge of the facet joint, and compress it with gauze with marking lines. The sacrospinous muscle is retracted outward with a lamina retractor to expose the lamina. Then use a periosteal dissector to further remove the spinous process, the lamina, and the residual tissue on the joint capsule. To expose both sides of the spine, use the same method to expose the contralateral structure (Fig. 13.54).
4. When performing sacral fixation, the S1 segment needs to be exposed to the lateral edge of the S1 facet joint; the S2 segment needs to be exposed to the lateral edge of the sacral foramen (Fig. 13.55). Be careful not to penetrate into the sacral foramen during exposure since there are a lot of blood vessels in the sacral foramen, which may cause bleeding. At this time, bipolar coagulation should be used to cauterize carefully. If the blood vessel cannot be burnt off, gel sponge can be used to stop bleeding.

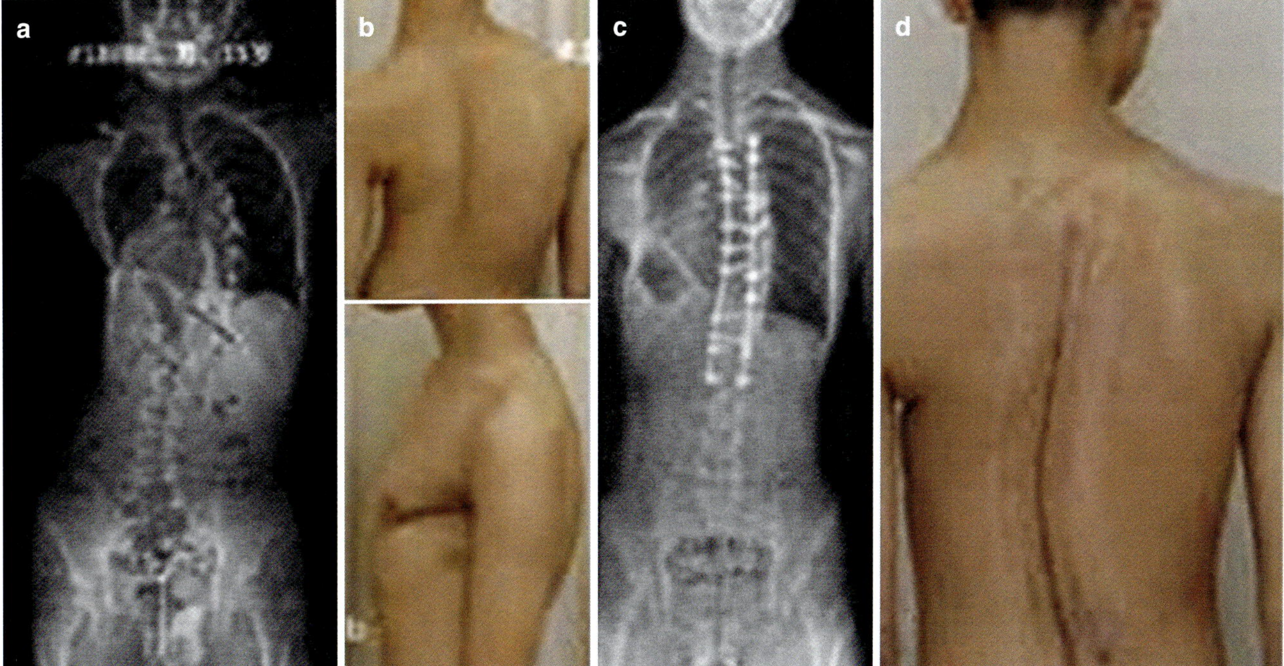

Fig. 13.52 #18988, A 15-year-old male patient who had ever undergone thoracotomy for scar contracture scoliosis (**a**). The scar was located on the concave side of scoliosis (**b**), underwent T4-L3 posterior orthopedic internal fixation, with a straight incision used during the surgery (**c**). After the surgery, the incision was curved to the concave side due to scar traction (**d**)

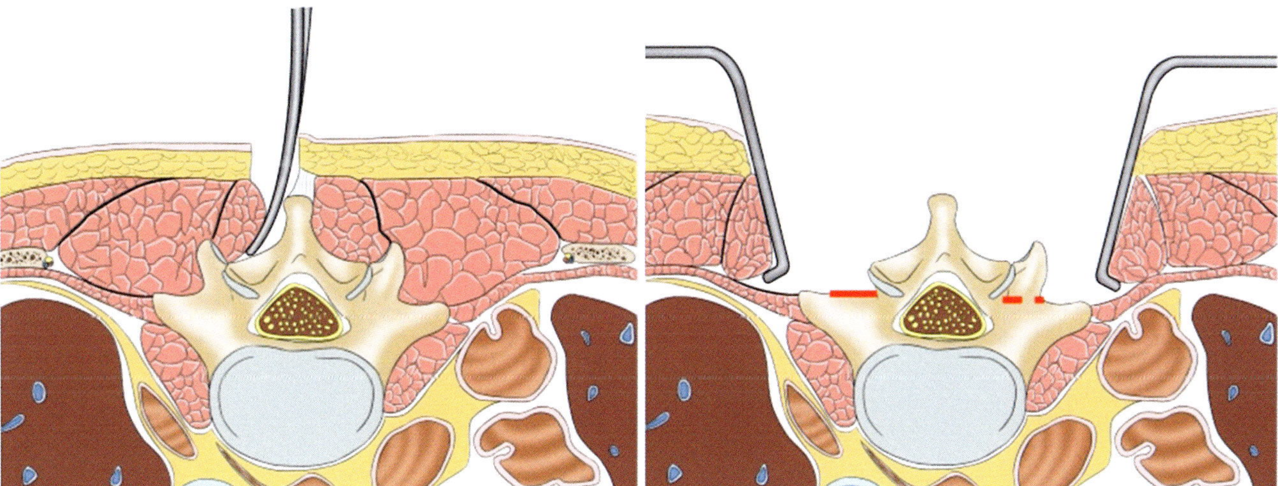

Fig. 13.53 Exposure method of the thoracic spine

13.3.3 Closure Method of Posterior Incision

The residual dead space of scoliosis is large. If the drainage is not smooth, it is easy to cause postoperative blood and fluid accumulation, leading to fever and even infection. For patients with long incision, it is recommended to place a drainage tube in the superior and inferior segments respectively. Incision closure is mainly divided into four layers: muscular layer, fascia layer, subcutaneous layer, and skin layer.

1. Muscular layer

The suturing of the muscular layer is controversial. Some scholars do not recommend suturing the muscular layer; they believe that the suturing of the muscular layer may affect the blood supply of the muscle and easily cause muscle ischemic necrosis, which may increase the incidence of infection. We, however, believe that patients with scoliosis have long incisions, large dead space, and asymmetrical muscle tension on both sides, if the muscular layer is not sutured, asymmetric muscles may not be able to align completely, resulting in dead space. It is recommended to suture the muscle intermittently with Absorbable 0# VICRYL® Plus control release suture (Polyglactin 910, Ethicon Inc.) in "8 shape." The two "8 shaped" stitches are 2–3 cm apart and 0.5 cm from the muscle edge. When suturing, pay attention to the correct alignment of the muscles on both sides. When tying the knot, gather the muscles on both sides without tightening, so as not to affect the blood supply of the muscles (Fig. 13.56).

2. Fascia layer

The fascia layer is the key to suturing. This layer has high tension and should be watertight sutured to prevent cerebrospinal fluid and tissue fluid from penetrating through the gap of deep fascia to subcutaneous tissue and skin, causing incision-related complications. Absorbable 0# PDS® II Antibacterial Sutures (PPDO, Ethicon.Inc) can be selected for interrupted suturing, or Absorbable 1# Stratafix Symmetric PDS PLUS Knotless Tissue Control Device (Polydioxanone, Ethicon Inc.) for continuous suturing. The stitch length of the suturing is 1 cm, 0.5 cm from the edge of the fascia. The stitch pitch is consistent, without dead angles remained at the start and end. When using barbed sutures, Absorbable 0# VICRYL® Plus control release suture (Polyglactin 910, Ethicon Inc.) can be used to suture 1–2 stitches in advance on the head and tail side to avoid dead angles during continuous suturing thus resulting loos suturing (Fig. 13.57a, b). Symmetric PDS PLUS suture is a new type of suturing device. The author believed that it presents strong tensile strength in the practice of suturing for scoliosis-corrected long incisions. It is free of traction, which eliminates the problem of cutting metacarpal and phalangeal joints with common PDS sutures during pulling or knotting; it is knot-free thus saving a lot of suturing time.

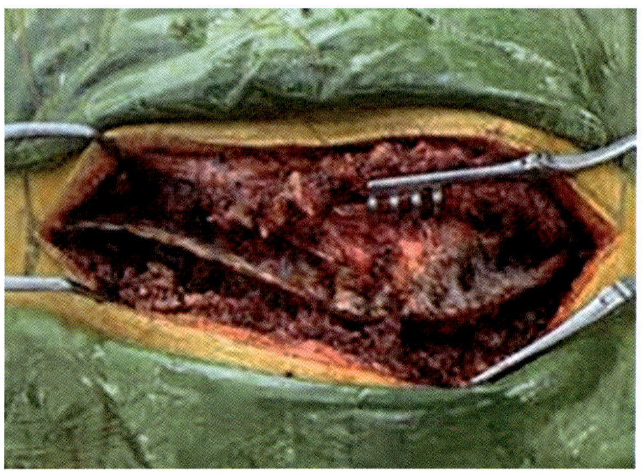

Fig. 13.54 Clearly reveal the articular process, transverse process, and lamina after exposure

3. Subcutaneous tissue

The subcutaneous tissue mainly refers to the fat layer. For patients with thin fat layer, we do not recommend suturing the fat layer too tightly. On the one hand, the fat layer has large mobility and is easily cut through by sutures; on the other hand, too tight fat layer suturing may easily cause fat necrosis. It is recommended to use Absorbable 2-0 VICRYL® Plus control release suture (Polyglactin 910, Ethicon Inc.) for interrupted suturing. During the suturing process, the deep fascia can be covered to the shallow layer to eliminate the dead cavity of the deep fat layer. Applying suturing at the fat superficial layer can be accompanied with some dermis layer, which is conducive to the alignment of the dermis

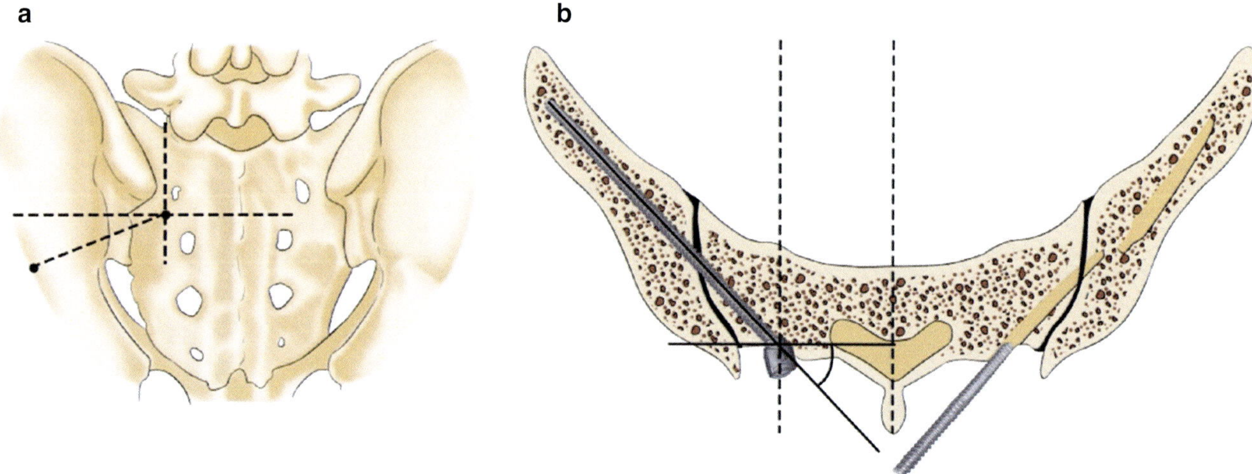

Fig. 13.55 Applying position of S2AI screw. The soft tissue shall be peeled to the lateral edge of the sacral foramen

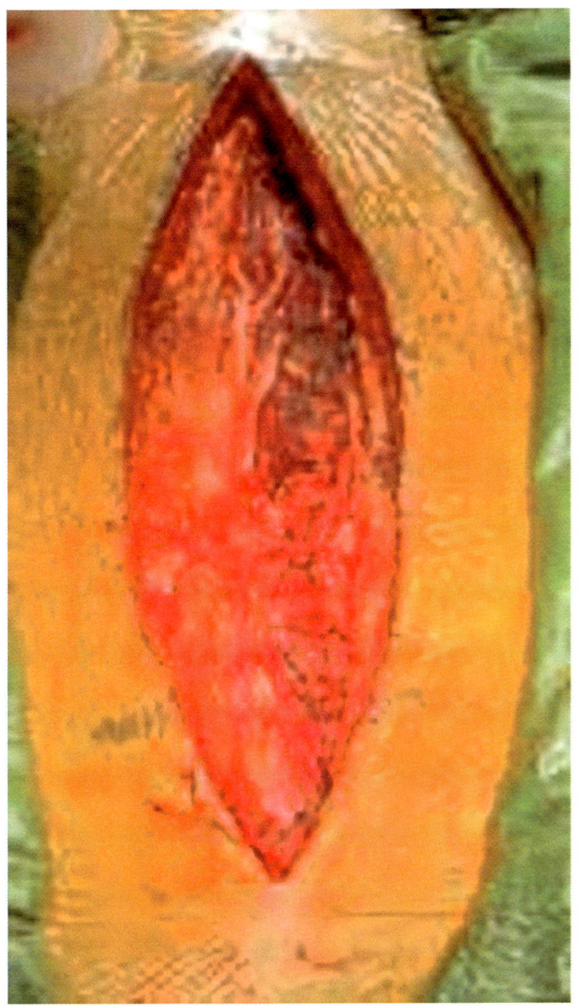

Fig. 13.56 "8 shaped" intermittent suturing in muscular layer

layer. Absorbable 2-0# STRATAFIX® Spiral PDO bidirectional knotless tissue control device (Polydioxanone, Ethicon Inc.) can be used on this layer. If the fat layer is too thick, Absorbable 2-0 VICRYL® Plus control release suture (Polyglactin 910, Ethicon Inc.) can be used for interrupted suturing of the deep fat layer. Be careful not to sew too tightly. The stitch length is generally 2 cm to achieve the initial effect of reducing tension. After the deep fat layer is sutured, the superficial fat layer is sutured routinely. It is worth noting that the subcutaneous layer should be sutured to reduce tension as far as possible to share the tension of the skin layer, creating a tension-free environment for suturing the skin layer and reducing the generation of skin scars (Fig. 13.58).

4. Skin

In addition to debridement surgery after infection, all scoliosis correction surgery should adopt intradermal suturing. Due to the long incision for scoliosis, traditional interrupted suturing will cause obvious scars, which will affect the patient's appearance and mental health (Fig. 13.59). Absorbable 4-0 VICRYL® Plus control release suture (Polyglactin 910, Ethicon Inc.) or Absorbable 4-0 STRATAFIX® Spiral PGA-PCL bidirectional knotless tissue control device (PGA-PCL, Ethicon Inc.) may be used for continuous suturing. The suturing pitch is 0.5 cm and the skin edges should be aligned perfectly. The needle should go through the dermis as much as possible. If it penetrates into the dermis layer, it will easily cause eversion of the skin edge, which will affect appearance (Fig. 13.60).

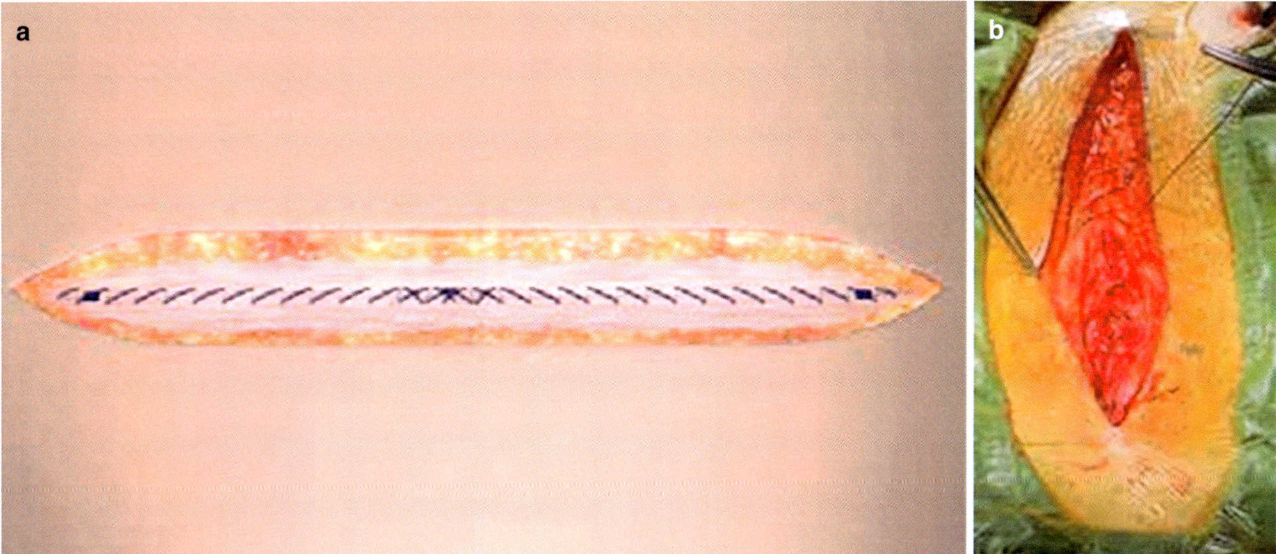

Fig. 13.57 (**a**) Schematic diagram of knot-free suturing fascia layer, (**b**) The fascia layer is sutured continuously with Symmetric PDS PLUS suture

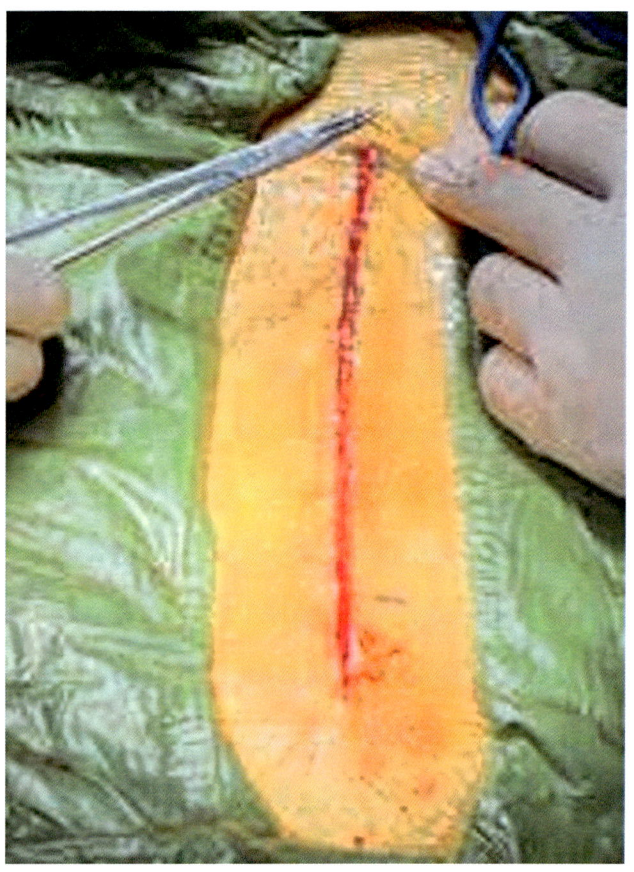

Fig. 13.58 Sufficient tension-reduced suturing of subcutaneous tissue, convenient for dermal suturing

For debridement after infection, it is recommended to suture the skin intermittently with Absorbable 2-0# VICRYL® Plus control release suture (Polyglactin 910, Ethicon Inc.). All layers of subcutaneous tissues and skin may be sutured in a mattress type.

In some special cases, such as Marfan syndrome and Aidan syndrome, the soft tissue development of the patient is abnormal, and the soft tissue coverage is poor after infection. It is necessary to invite a plastic surgeon to evaluate incision healing and even adopt skin flap coverage (Fig. 13.61).

13.3.4 Risk Factors and Prevention of Incision-Related Complications

Previous studies have identified multiple risk factors for incision-related complications. Incision complications of neuromuscular scoliosis are significantly higher than those of other types of scoliosis. Ramo et al. found that the incidence of neuromuscular scoliosis incisional infection was as high as 20.3% from 1980 to 1989, and dropped to 8.4% in 2009. They found that patients with spina bifida had the highest infection rate, up to 21.5%. BMI greater than 25 and constipation is also risk factors for infection. Other risk factors include insufficient antibiotic dosage, long incisions, long hospital stays, and preoperative anemia; and the use of drainage can reduce the incidence of infection [21]. A review by Subramanyam et al. found that irregular use of antibiot-

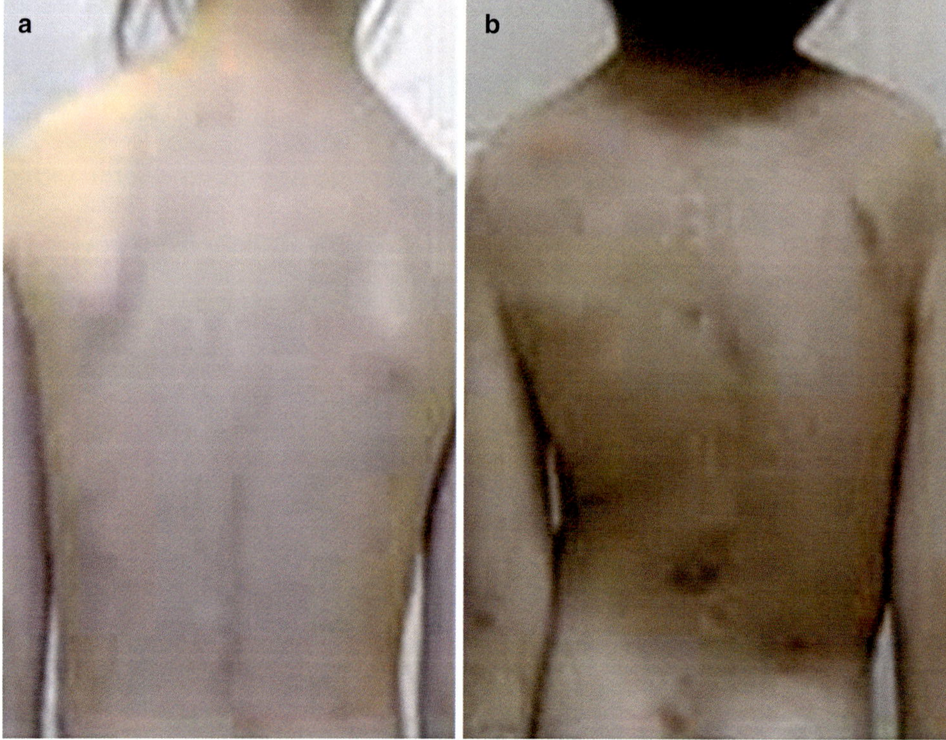

Fig. 13.59 Intradermal cosmetic suture. (**a**) and interrupted suturing (**b**) incision scar comparison

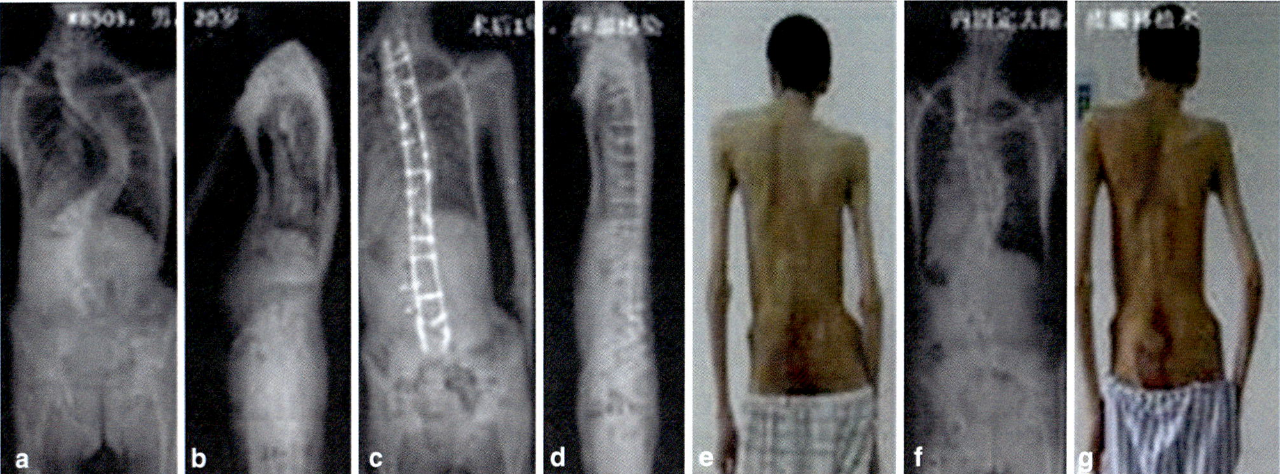

Fig. 13.60 Continuous intradermal suturing. (**a–d**) One year after surgery, deep infection. (**e–g**) Removal of internal fixation and transplantation of skin flap

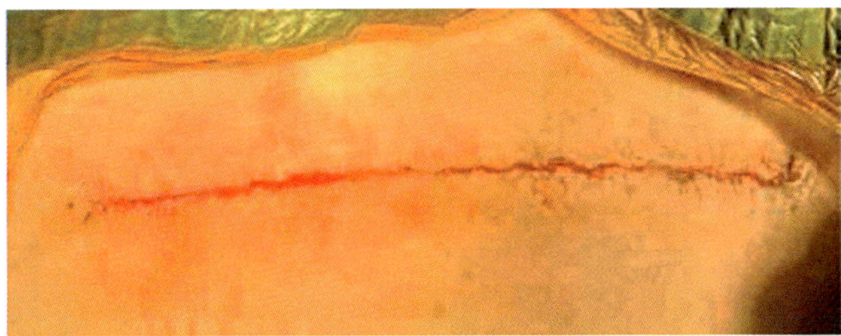

Fig. 13.61 #8503, a 20-year-old male patient with Marfan syndrome and scoliosis

ics, neuromuscular scoliosis, use of internal fixation, long hospital stay, and large residual degree of postoperative scoliosis are high-risk factors for incision infection [22]. Vitale et al. [23] proposed a consensus on the prevention of wound infection in children's spinal orthopedic surgery, including 14 opinions: (1) Patients should receive skin disinfection one day before surgery; (2) Patients should receive urine culture after surgery; (3) Patients should accept health education before surgery; (4) Nutritional assessment of the patient should be carried out before the surgery; (5) The hair should be cut short when preparing the skin. There is no need to shave with a razor, otherwise, the skin will be lost; (6) Patients should be injected with antibiotics in the perioperative period; (7) Anti-Gram-negative bacilli antibiotics should be infused intravenously to the patient in the perioperative period; (8) Strictly monitor the standard use of antibiotics; (9) Limit the number of surgical visitors; (10) It is not necessary to disinfect the operating room with ultraviolet light (11) Patients should receive incision lavage during surgery; (12) Vancomycin powder can be used to prevent infections on bone grafts or surgical incisions; (13) Impermeable dressings should be used after surgery; (14) Minimize the frequency of dressing replacement after surgery.

13.4 Repair and Suturing of Spinal Dura Mater and the Prevention and Treatment of Postoperative Cerebrospinal Fluid Leakage

Chu Tongwei and Huang Bo
Department of Orthopedics
Second Affiliated Hospital of Army Military Medical University
Beijing, China

Abstract
Rupture of the spinal dura mater is mostly caused by damage to the spinal dura mater during surgery without timely repair or insufficient repair. Direct suturing and repair is the most effective method to deal with the accidental injury of the spinal dura mater during surgery. When it is difficult to separate the dura mater, direct suturing can hardly be carried out. The dural repair graft material may be used in combination with gelatin sponge and bio-glue for coverage and seal. For postoperative cerebrospinal fluid caused by dura mater rupture, comprehensive conservative treatments such as body position adjustment, leak area compression bandaging, and lumbar cistern drainage may be used to achieve the purpose of healing.

The dura mater is composed of thick and hard dense connective tissues, and the spinal cord is protected and supported by the dura mater. Dural injury is a common complication in spinal surgeries, with an incidence of about 1–17% [24]. Cerebrospinal fluid leakage after spinal surgery is often caused by intraoperative tearing of the dura mater without proper treatment, which in turn affects postoperative wound healing, leading to secondary incision infections and even central nervous system infections. At present, the incidence of dural injury is increasing with the increase of patients with dural adhesions. It has been showed in the literatures that the incidence of cerebrospinal fluid leakage in spinal surgery dural injury is about 2–15.8% [25]. The risk factors include spinal fracture, dislocation and other direct trauma, adhesion factors between dura mater and surrounding tissues as well as iatrogenic injury.

The repair methods of ruptured dura mater include suturing and repair and non-suturing and repair. Suturing and repair can adopt direct suturing or graft patch repair; non-suturing and repair mainly adopt biological glue to seal the rupture. In recent years, dural repair by the suturing, patch, gelatin sponge + fibrin glue has achieved good clinical results. However, currently, there is no unified international standard for how to suture the ruptured dura mater during surgery and how to use suture materials.

It is very important to treat cerebrospinal fluid leakage timely to reduce postoperative complications and promote disease recovery. According to the postoperative cerebrospinal fluid leakage caused by different surgical sites and different surgical approaches, methods such as sealing, compression bandaging, body position adjustment, and lumbar cistern drainage can be used.

This chapter focuses on dural injury and cerebrospinal fluid leakage. Taking anterior cervical, posterior thoracic, and posterior lumbar spine surgery as examples, we introduce the suturing and repair of intraoperative dural injury and the treatment of postoperative cerebrospinal fluid leakage.

13.4.1 Understand Dural Suturing Repair and Postoperative Cerebrospinal Fluid Leakage

1. **Causes and High-Risk Factors of Dural Injury**

There are many reasons for the occurrence of dural rupture, most of which are caused by the injury of the dura mater during the operation without timely repair or insufficient repair. The common causes include: Spinal fracture, spondylolisthesis and other direct damages to the spinal dura mater; The dura mater and surrounding tissues form adhesions, such as ossified posterior longitudinal ligament of the cervical spine, ossified ligamentum flavum of the thoracic spine, severe lumbar spinal stenosis, secondary spinal surgery, etc.; the dura mater can be easily damaged during surgery; Iatrogenic injuries, such as surgeon's lack of operation skills and experience.

Among them, the adhesion between the dura mater and the surrounding tissues is the most important factor of intraoperative dural injury, because dura mater adhesion is a common symptom of patients with clinical spinal diseases. Any reason, as long as it can cause adhesion between the dura mater and tissues, can be classified as a high-risk factor for dural injury.

Other factors, such as older patients, longer operation time, larger surgical scope, poor neurological function, and secondary revision surgery are also important risk factors for dural rupture.

2. **Basic principles of dural suturing and repairing**

Direct suturing and repair is the most effective method to deal with the injury of the spinal dura mater during surgery.

When the dural injury occurs during the surgery, the defects with a better exposure and moderate crack should be sutured and repaired immediately in principle. Non-absorbable 4/0–7/0 PROLENE® Sutures (polypropylene, Ethicon.Inc) can be used for suturing. Hemoseal can be used if possible to reduce leakage through needle eyes (Figs. 13.62 and 13.63).

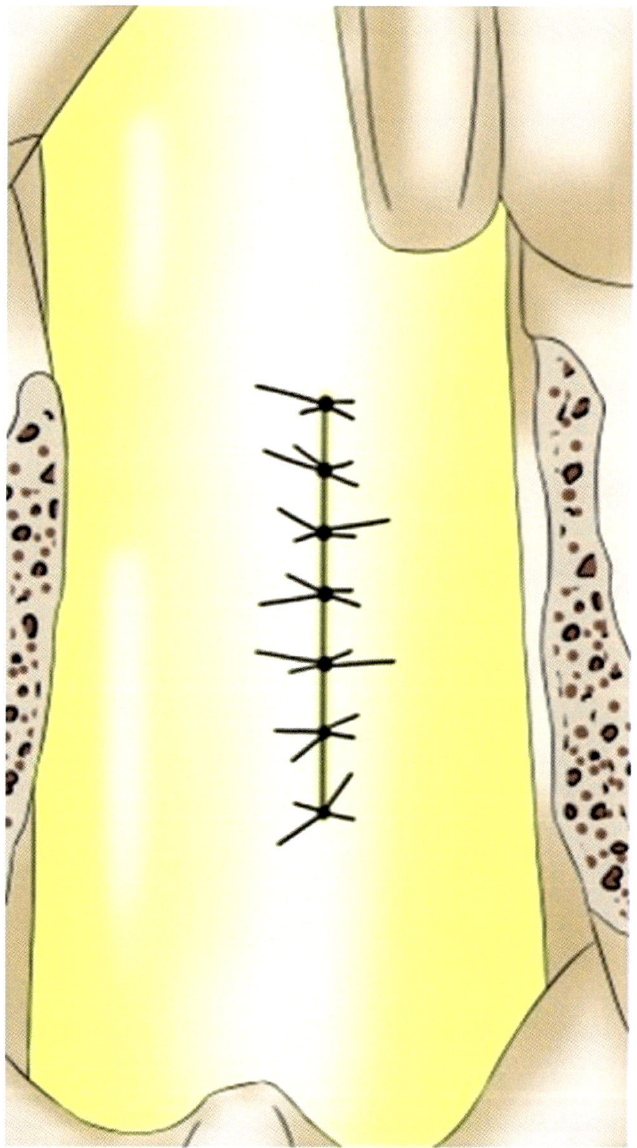

Fig. 13.62 Simple interrupted suturing of the spinal dura mater

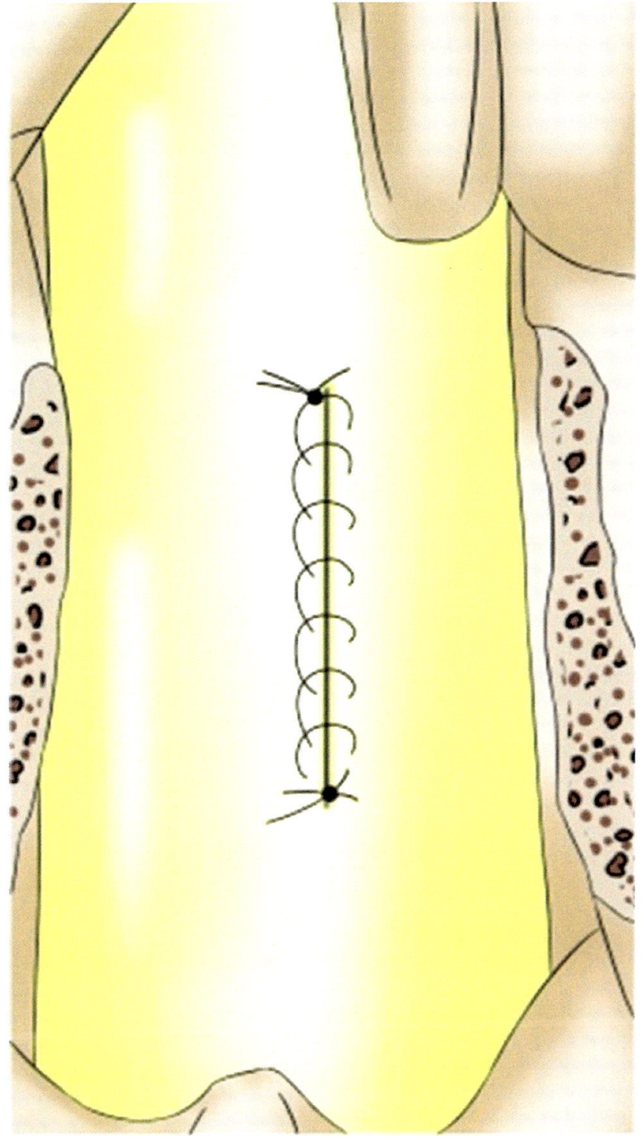

Fig. 13.63 Simple continuous suturing of the spinal dura mater

For surgical approaches with limited (such as anterior cervical surgery), or when the ossified spinal dura mater adheres to the soft tissues, the separation of the dura mater becomes very difficult, and direct suture is difficult to perform. Under such circumstances, dural repair graft materials can be used, such as autografts (autologous fascia, adipose tissue, muscle tissue, etc.), allografts (such as bovine pericardium) and artificial repair materials (such as gelatin sponge, non-bovine pericardium), and chemical sealants (such as fibrin glue, hydrogel) to enhance the tightness of the dural rupture (Fig. 13.64). According to the literature [26], intraoperative dural repair using gelatin sponge for coverage and suturing and repair can effectively reduce the incidence of postoperative cerebrospinal fluid leakage. For graft suturing and repair, non-absorbable 4/0–7/0 PROLENE® Sutures (polypropylene, Ethicon.Inc) combined with fibrin glue can be used to effectively improve the water tightness of the spinal dura mater.

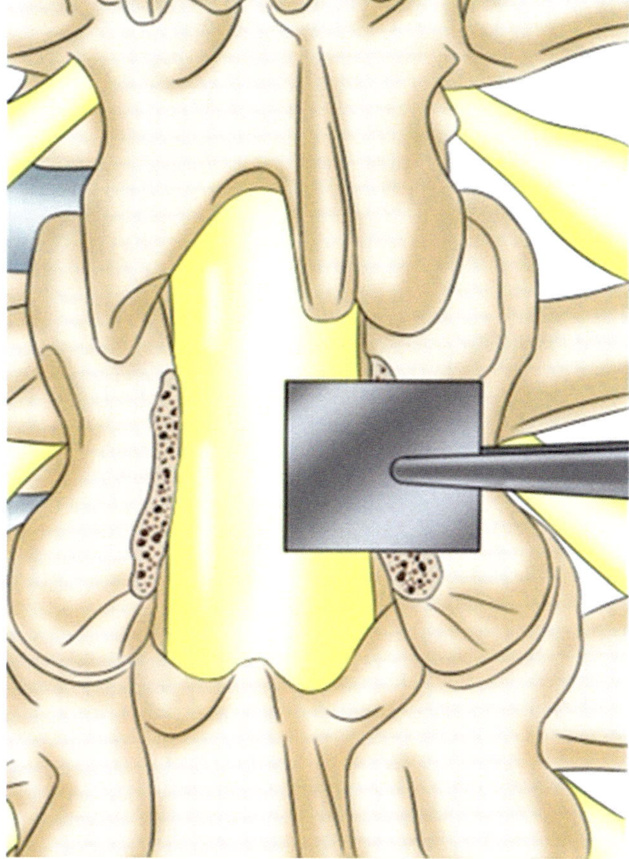

Fig. 13.64 Fat, muscle, artificial dura mater and other "patches" are used to repair the spinal dura mater

Valsalva (increased intrasaccular pressure) is often used to check the tightness of dural rupture after dural repair.

After dural suturing and repairing, the wound should be closed tightly in principle. Tight suturing increases the pressure of the external tissue on the dural rupture can promote its healing. However, for anterior cervical surgery, there are more important vascular nerves and organs in front of the cervical spine, and the soft tissues are relatively less than those of the posterior approach. Appropriate loosening suture can be used which is conducive to adequate drainage and can avoid the oppression of important organs such as trachea and esophagus caused by poor drainage.

In summary, when the spinal dura mater is accidentally injured during the operation, the repair method should be flexibly selected according to the actual injury. Direct suture repair is the most important and effective method (non-absorbable 4/0–7/0 PROLENE® Sutures (polypropylene, Ethicon.Inc) can be used). However, as being affected by factors such as suturing proficiency, surgical habits, and the degree of dural injury, there are many differences in the methods of dural repair by surgeons at present. As early as 1981, Eismont et al. [27] proposed some principles for dural repair. Later, Papavero et al. [28] proposed a ten-step closure principle for the emergency treatment of dural rupture. However, these principles of treatment do not form into normative standards and are still in constant updating and improvement.

3. **Postoperative cerebrospinal fluid leakage and its prevention and treatment**

Cerebrospinal fluid leakage means the cerebrospinal fluid flows into the nearby soft tissues and even the incision surface through the rupture when the spinal dura mater is damaged. (Fig. 13.65) Cerebrospinal fluid leakage is a common complication of spinal surgery. The literature shows that the incidence of cerebrospinal fluid leakage after spinal surgery is about 2.31–9.37% [29]. If it is not treated in time or properly, it can cause secondary wound infection, intraspinal infection, and even purulent meningitis, which are life-threatening. Complications related to cerebrospinal fluid leakage such as pseudodural bulge, incision infection, meningitis, cerebrospinal fluid fistula, and adhesive arachnoiditis also severely affect postoperative recovery. According to the literature, tightly closing the muscular layer and fascia layer can increase the pressure of epidural penetration, promote dural repair, and effectively prevent and slow down cerebrospinal fluid leakage [30]. It is recommended to close the muscular layer normally to eliminate deep dead spaces. Absorbable VICRYL® Plus control release suture (Polyglactin 910, Ethicon Inc.) can be used for interrupted suturing in "8" shape. For deep fascia layer suturing, 1# Stratafix Symmetric PDS PLUS Knotless Tissue Control Device (Polydioxanone, Ethicon Inc.) can be used for continuous suturing of fascia layer. The literature shows [31] that suturing the deep fascia layer with Stratafix Symmetric PDS PLUS sutures can achieve better water tightness to prevent cerebrospinal fluid, blood, and tissue fluid from penetrating into subcutaneous space through the deep fascial space and reduce the incidence of related incision complications.

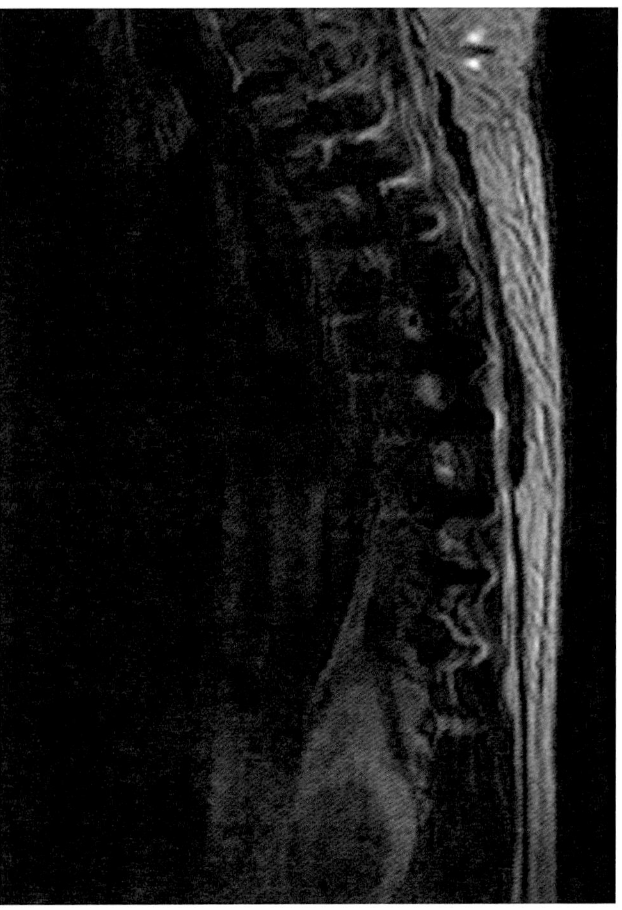

Fig. 13.65 Postoperative MRI of a patient with ossification of the thoracic ligamentum flavum indicates cerebrospinal fluid leakage

For the treatment of postoperative cerebrospinal fluid leakage, according to different parts of the neck, chest, and waist, methods such as body position adjustment, pressure bandaging of the leakage area, and lumbar cistern drainage are generally adopted.

Most spinal dura mater will generate clear fluid outflow when it ruptures during surgery, so it can be found during surgery. If the dural injury is not detected in time or the suturing and repair is not tight enough after being detected, the patient will experience postural headache, dizziness, blurred vision, tinnitus, and other symptoms due to the loss of craniocerebrospinal fluid. For postoperative cerebrospinal fluid leakage, it is usually recommended that patients stay in bed and take different positions according to different parts. Patients with cerebrospinal fluid leakage after cervical spine surgery should be placed in a supine position or Trendelenburg position with the head of the bed slightly elevated; for patients with cerebrospinal fluid leakage after thoracolumbar surgery, a prone position or trendelenburg position should be adopted [32].

In addition, postoperative drainage tube management and local compression bandage for wound are also effective adjuvant treatment methods. In principle, the drainage tube after the surgery should be pulled out as soon as possible after adequate drainage. In spinal surgery, the drainage tube can generally be removed about 3–4 days after the surgery. If the patient is accompanied with cerebrospinal fluid leakage, it is recommended to extend the drainage time appropriately, and at the same time, the drainage tube can be intermittently clamped. Closely observe the healing of the incision, and the drainage tube should be removed immediately when the drainage volume decreases. According to the guideline [32], early removal of the drainage tube with pressure bandaging and delayed removal of the drainage tube can effectively treat cerebrospinal fluid leakage. There is no significant difference between the two in terms of efficacy and complications. Regarding whether the drainage tube should be used for normal pressure drainage or negative pressure drainage, this research group recommends normal pressure drainage. Since the oozing blood and cerebrospinal fluid in the operation area after dilution are not likely to form blood clots and block the drainage tube, there is no need for negative pressure suction. In addition, negative pressure drainage will cause a large loss of cerebrospinal fluid, which is not conducive to the repair of dural damage. Pressure bandaging will not cause the cerebrospinal fluid to leak to the surrounding tissues, since the wound has been healed and the drainage tube has been wrapped by fibers to form a fistula. Keep the patient in the prone position, and then cover the dural rupture and soft tissues with sandbags thus effectively alleviate the postoperative cerebrospinal fluid leakage. For patients undergoing thoracolumbar surgery, thick pillows can be used to cushion the patient's chest or hips to reduce abdominal pressure and facilitate the sealing and repair of leaks.

If the above treatment cannot effectively alleviate the cerebrospinal fluid leakage, lumbar cistern drainage can be used. The lumbar cistern drainage can smoothly drain the leaked cerebrospinal fluid out of the wound, reducing the local pressure formed by the cerebrospinal fluid, facilitating the closure of the rupture, and effectively reducing postoperative incision complications, which has been widely used in clinical applications.

The principle of epidural blood filling (Maycock method) is to fill the autologous blood outside the dura mater to achieve the effect of blocking the dural leak, which can usually be operated under ultrasound guidance. However, the autologous blood-filled outside the dura mater may form a hematoma and compress the dural sac.

In addition, bacterial culture and drug sensitivity tests should be carried out on the drained cerebrospinal fluid. Antibiotics should be selected and applied reasonably (intrathecal injection is possible). Patients with headache can be infused with normal saline quickly. It is necessary to always pay attention to the patient's electrolyte changes.

For very serious postoperative cerebrospinal fluid leakage, if the above methods are ineffective, secondary surgery should be taken immediately to repair the dura mater. However, the above methods are mostly effective. Delayed cerebrospinal fluid leakage sometimes presents cerebrospinal fluid pseudocysts. Small non-communicating cerebrospinal fluid cysts do not need to be treated; pay attention to observe the conditions; larger non-communicating cysts or communicating cysts, once diagnosed by imaging examination, require surgical treatment as soon as possible.

In summary, the various treatment methods for postoperative cerebrospinal fluid leakage should be reasonably selected in combination with the patient's condition. Generally, it can be cured through active and effective comprehensive conservative treatment.

13.4.2 Dural Repair by Suturing and Treatment of Postoperative Cerebrospinal Fluid Leakage in Anterior Cervical Surgery

Abstract
The dural injury usually occurs when the ossified posterior longitudinal ligament is removed intraoperatively in the anterior cervical surgery. For minor dural tears or defects, direct suturing for dural repair is still the most effective way. If it is not allowed, fat, muscle, and fascial graft or gelatin sponge can be used to strengthen the closure, which is called "patch suturing." Patients with cerebrospinal fluid leakage after anterior cervical surgery should be strictly confined to bed, supplemented with position adjustment, pressure dressing, and lumbar cistern drainage in the early stage, which can achieve satisfactory therapeutic effects.

1. **Causes and risk factors of spinal dural injury in cervical spine surgery**

Dural injury accounts for a large proportion of all the common intraoperative complications of cervical spine surgery. According to the literature, the incidence of dural injury in anterior cervical surgery is about 0.5–3% [33], which generally occurs when the ossified posterior longitudinal ligament is removed in anterior cervical surgery. The adhesion between the spinal dura mater and the ossified posterior longitudinal ligament is hard to dissect, which renders the patients more vulnerable to dural injury during the operation.

The common causes and risk factors of dural injury in cervical spine surgery are as the following: Cervical spine trauma, such as spinal fractures, dislocations, etc. where the dura is directly injured; Cervical degenerative diseases, such as cervical disc herniation, ossification of the posterior longitudinal ligament, ossification of the ligamentum flavum, cervical canal stenosis, etc.; where there is a higher risk of the dural injury during the surgery; Cervical spine tumors, such as subdural extramedullary tumor, for which the spinal dura mater in adhesion to the tumor wall needs to be incised or removed during the surgery. Reoperation of the cervical spine, during which severe adhesion between the surgical scar tissue and the dura is observed; Iatrogenic injury, such as those caused by the poor experience and skill of the operator.

In addition, corpectomy, prolonged operation time, aged patients, and underlying diseases are also high-risk factors for dural injury in anterior cervical surgery.

2. **Anterior cervical dural repair by suturing**

Ossification of the posterior longitudinal ligament (OPLL) is taken as an example in the section. Currently, there are many surgical approaches for the treatment of OPLL, such as anterior surgery, posterior surgery, as well as combined anterior and posterior surgery. The ossified posterior longitudinal ligament can be directly resected in anterior surgery, but with the drawbacks that the surgery is riskier and challenging. During the operation of the posterior longitudinal ligament resection, it is easy to cause spinal dural injury, resulting in postoperative cerebrospinal fluid leakage.

For minor dural tears or defects, direct suturing is still the most effective method under good visualization of the surgical field. Non-absorbable 5/0–6/0 PROLENE® Sutures (polypropylene, Ethicon.Inc) can be used for suturing. Leakage-proof needle (Hemoseal) can be used if available to reduce needle hole leakage. The intermittent or continuous suturing is applied with a needle pitch <3 mm and edge distance <2 mm. Some studies [34] have shown that there is no significant difference among interrupted suturing, conventional continuous suturing, and continuous lockstitch suturing for dural repair.

However, in most cases, direct suturing cannot be applied through the window of discectomy. Especially when the anterior cervical spine surgery is performed for treating ossification of the posterior longitudinal ligament, the dura mater is usually not fully exposed, and the adhesion of the spinal dura mater during ossification to the posterior longitudinal ligament also make direct suturing much more challenging.

When direct suturing for dural repair is not allowed, fat, muscle, and fascial graft or gelatin sponge can be used to strengthen the closure, which is called "patch suturing." There are many methods of patch stitching, such as "sandwich technique," [28] inlay technique [35], and lateral patch technique [36]. They can be used in conjunction with each other in different situations (Fig. 13.66).

After the dural repair is completed, chemical sealant fibrin glue or hydrogel is sprayed on the suture for seal. Chemical sealants can significantly improve the sealing effect of the spinal dura mater. Fibrin glue and other sealants can increase the pressure being withstand by the repaired spinal dura mater after the operation, and can also be used to reduce cerebrospinal fluid leakage at the needle hole.

After suturing for dural repair, Valsalva is performed routinely to check the suture tightness of the dural tear.

Usually, effectively closing the dead space of the muscular layer, suturing the fascia layer tightly, and good approximation of the skin play an important role in the closure of the dural tear. However, closure of incision in anterior cervical surgery presents its particularity. Due to the complex anatomy of the anterior cervical approach involving the major organs (esophagus and trachea), aorta, and nerves, overtight suturing will inevitably cause poor drainage postoperatively, which then compress major neck structures. It can be sutured with appropriate relaxation to facilitate adequate drainage to avoid pressure on major organs such as the trachea and esophagus.

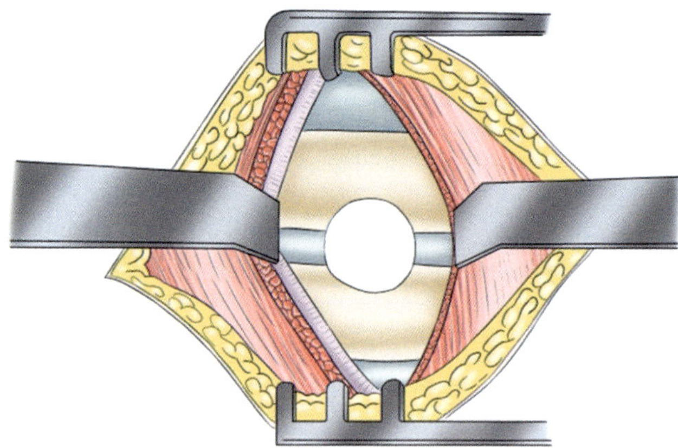

Fig. 13.66 Direct suturing is more challenging in anterior cervical surgery, instead "patch" is often used for repair

3. **Prevention of cerebrospinal fluid leakage in anterior cervical surgery**

For anterior cervical surgery, clinicians should review the images carefully before surgery. If the dural ossification is detected preoperatively, the risk of dural injury during surgery can be greatly reduced.

Intraoperative operation should be performed carefully. The safety of the surgery can be improved with the anterior floating method. The anterior floating method for lateral decompression of the posterior longitudinal ligament can effectively reduce the incidence and extent of dural injury [37], thereby theoretically reducing the incidence of cerebrospinal fluid leakage.

As mentioned above, tight suturing of muscle fascia and skin layer is helpful to prevent cerebrospinal fluid leakage. However, closure of incision in anterior cervical surgery presents its particularity. It can be sutured with appropriate relaxation to facilitate adequate drainage and protect important organs. For suturing of the anterior cervical fascia layer, platysma layer, and subcutaneous skin layer, the chapter of anterior cervical incision closure may be referenced.

Patients should be instructed to avoid severe cough. Systemic supportive treatment for patients should be strengthened. Anti-infection and nutrition supplements should be administered as necessary, and water/electrolyte balance should be maintained.

4. **Treatment of cerebrospinal fluid leakage after anterior cervical surgery**

For patients diagnosed with postoperative cerebrospinal fluid leakage, the body position should be adjusted routinely. For cervical cerebrospinal fluid leakage, it is recommended to take a supine position or Trendelenburg position with the upper section of the bed slightly elevated. It is recommended to use an elastic bandage to wrap around the neck, which can effectively compress the wound, reduce the leakage of cerebrospinal fluid, and facilitate dural closure. It should be noted that since there are many major vascular nerves in the anterior cervical region, excessive blockage and pressure will easily lead to unsmooth drainage and swelling of the intervertebral space, affecting swallowing and breathing; the compression of the carotid sinus can lead to abnormal changes in blood pressure, heart rate, and blood oxygen. For care of postoperative drainage tube, the drainage tube can be intermittently clamped under normal pressure. The retention time of the drainage tube can be appropriately extended.

Postoperative lumbar cistern drainage catheterization is suitable for patients with large postoperative drainage and large dural defects. Lumbar cistern drainage can promote the healing of dural tear by reducing the pressure difference of the cerebrospinal fluid at the rupture. For patients with lumbar cistern drainage after cerebrospinal fluid leakage, aggressive rehydration should be administered to maintain normal intracranial pressure and water/electrolyte balance to avoid symptoms of low intracranial pressure. If cerebrospinal fluid culture shows positive result for infection, antibiotics with good blood-brain barrier permeability should be used (intrathecal injection is acceptable).

As appropriate, epidural autologous blood injection or secondary surgery should be adopted for direct dural repair. However, generally the above methods can work.

In summary, the dural injury found during cervical spine surgery should be treated promptly and carefully. Patients should be strictly confined to bed postoperatively, supplemented with position adjustment, pressure dressing, and lumbar cistern drainage in early stage to achieve satisfactory therapeutic effects. If the above treatment is ineffective, secondary surgery for dural repair has to be performed.

13.4.3 Dural Repair and Treatment of Postoperative Cerebrospinal Fluid Leakage in Posterior Thoracic Surgery

Abstract
Thoracic dural injury often occurs in the surgery for treatment of thoracic ossification of ligamentum flavum. In most cases, direct suturing is challenging. The dural patch, fat, muscle fascia, and other tissue can be sutured together with the dura mater, covered with gelatin sponge, and sealed with biological glue. Tight closure of the incision plays an important role in preventing cerebrospinal fluid leakage after dural tear. Currently, for patients with large cerebrospinal fluid leakage after thoracic surgery, continuous lumbar cistern drainage is generally applied to reduce the cerebrospinal fluid pressure at the thoracic spinal dural tear and promote incision healing.

1. **Causes and risk factors of dural injury in posterior thoracic surgery**

Dural injury is one of the common complications in posterior thoracic surgery. The overall incidence of the dural tear in thoracic spine surgery is 3.8–50.0% [38], which is higher than that of cervical and lumbar surgery. Most dural injuries occur in the surgery for treatment of thoracic ossification of ligamentum flavum, which greatly increases the risk of postoperative cerebrospinal fluid leakage and seriously affects the outcome of surgical patients.

The common causes and risk factors of dural injury during thoracic surgery are as the following: Thoracic spine trauma, such as thoracic spine fracture, dislocation, and other direct injuries; Thoracic spine degenerative diseases, including thoracic spinal canal stenosis, thoracic ossification of ligamentum flavum, thoracic ossification of the posterior longitudinal ligament, etc., where there is an extreme possibility of dural injury during the surgery; Multiple-level thoracic spine surgery increases the probability of dural adhesion, and extended operation time affects the surgical efficiency of the surgeon; During thoracic spine revision surgery, dense adhesion between the spinal dura mater and surrounding scar tissues is observed; Iatrogenic injuries.

In addition, just like the anterior cervical surgery, the patient's nerve function, elderly age, and operation time are also high-risk factors for dural injury in posterior thoracic surgery.

2. **Dural suturing for dural repair in posterior thoracic surgery**

The thoracic ossification of ligamentum flavum with thoracic spinal stenosis is taken as an example. For dural tear in posterior surgery, direct suturing is still the gold standard for dural repair. If the dural tear is found in time during surgery, non-absorbable 5/0–7/0 PROLENE® Sutures (polypropylene, Ethicon.Inc), and Hemoseal (if available) can be used for intermittent or continuous suturing with a needle pitch <3 mm and edge distance <2 mm (Fig. 13.67).

However, due to the serious dural injury being often caused in the surgery for treating ossification of ligamentum flavum with thoracic spinal stenosis, dural fibrosis, and high tension which make direct suturing of dura impossible, direct

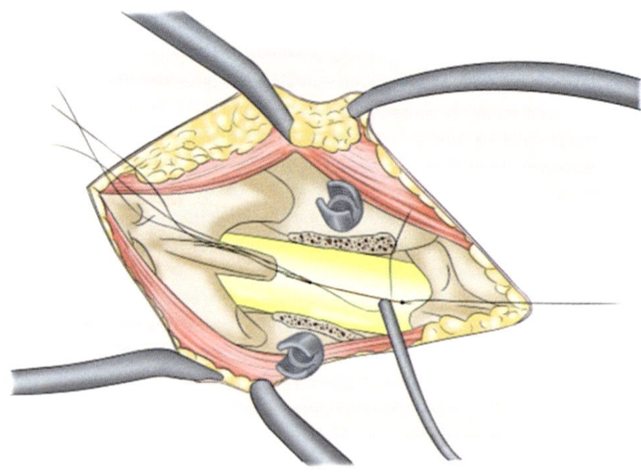

Fig. 13.67 Posterior thoracic surgery dural mater suturing by single intermittent suturing

suturing is not applicable in most cases. Under such circumstances, dural patch, fat, muscle fascia, and other tissue can be sutured together with the dura mater, with gelatin sponge applied subsequently. After suturing, fibrin glue is applied for the seal. Valsalva maneuver is performed to check the leakage from the closure, with the principle of tight closure being followed for the closure of the muscular layer, fascia layer, and skin layer.

3. **Prevention of cerebrospinal fluid leakage in posterior thoracic surgery**

The medical history and images should be reviewed and analyzed carefully and comprehensively before surgery to see if there are dural adhesion and calcification. For patients with a history of thoracic surgery and revision surgery, the prior surgery should be fully reviewed, such as surgical approach and extent of decompression. During the operation, the dissection of adhesion should be done carefully. Before the laminar rongeur is used to bite and remove the lamina and ligamentum flavum, etc., the dura mater and the overlying lamina and ligamentum should be carefully dissected to avoid dural injury as far as possible. Before the closure of incision for the surgery, it is required to carefully confirm whether there is dural injury, and if it is found, it should be sutured immediately. Finally, tight closure of the incision is an important measure to prevent cerebrospinal fluid leakage after dural tear.

4. **Treatment of cerebrospinal fluid leakage in posterior thoracic surgery**

Tight suturing of muscles, fascia, and skin can fill and compress the rupture; a reasonable posture is also conducive to healing of the dural tear. For patients who undergo posterior thoracic surgery, the prone position or alternate prone and semi-prone positions can be adopted; immediate dressing and pressure dressing of the incision will promote incision healing and reduce cavity formation. The posterior thoracolumbar spine is usually coated and covered with a large amount of soft tissues, so pressure dressing is an effective measure to treat cerebrospinal fluid leakage.

Currently, for patients with large cerebrospinal fluid leakage after thoracic spine surgery, continuous lumbar cistern drainage is generally adopted to reduce the cerebrospinal fluid pressure at the thoracic spinal dural tear and promote incision healing. Take care to prevent intraspinal infection caused by lumbar cistern drainage.

Properly extending the drainage tube indwelling time can lower the pressure of the cerebrospinal fluid and reduce postoperative incision complications. It is recommended that after the drainage tube is removed, use Absorbable 3–0# Vicryl Plus® Control Release Violet Sutures (Polyglactin 910, Ethicon.Inc) to sew the drainage tube for 1–2 stitches. Finally, maintaining the water and electrolyte balance, appropriate protein supplementation, and anti-infection are also important measures to promote the healing of the dural injury.

13.4.4 Dural Repair and Treatment of Postoperative Cerebrospinal Fluid Leakage of Posterior Lumbar Surgery

Abstract
Dural injury is the most common complication of lumbar spine surgery. During the surgery for treatment of degenerative lumbar diseases, direct suturing is not applicable to ossified dural injuries. Free fascia or fat graft can be trimmed into a patch of appropriate size for peripheral repair by suturing. Upon closure of the incision, tight suturing of lumbar dorsal fascia layer, subcutaneous tissue, and skin is required. For patients with cerebrospinal fluid leakage after lumbar posterior surgery, Trendelenburg position should be taken after the surgery. For other measures, please refer to the first three sections of this chapter.

1. **Causes and risk factors of dural injury in posterior lumbar surgery**

Dural injury is the most common complication of lumbar surgery. It is reported that the incidence of dural injury in lumbar surgery is 1.8–17.4% [39], accounting for about 15% of postoperative complications [40]. Severe cerebrospinal fluid leakage may occur if treatment is not administered in time.

The primary causes for the dural injury and cerebrospinal fluid leakage after lumbar surgery are as the following: During the reduction of lumbar fracture dislocation, the displacement of the bone fragment leads to the puncture and scratch of the spinal dura mater. For degenerative lumbar diseases, with varying degrees of ossification of the intervertebral disc, ligamentum flavum ossification, or severe lumbar spinal canal stenosis, the dural injury occurs more easily when biting off the lamina and ligamentum flavum with a rongeur. Lumbar decompression and placement of internal fixation cause dural tear. Iatrogenic factors such as the anatomical structure of the spinal canal being not well understood, rough operation, or insufficient preoperative preparation.

In addition, the extent of surgery, revision surgery, and comorbidities such as osteoporosis and diabetes are all risk factors for dural injury during lumbar surgery.

2. **Dural suturing and repair in posterior lumbar surgery**

In cases of minor dural tear and no obvious defect, the dural repair can be achieved with direct suturing. For suturing method, please refer to dural suturing in posterior thoracic surgery (Fig. 13.68).

For surgery for the treatment of degenerative lumbar disease, the ossified spinal dura mater or the dura mater in adhesion to the surrounding tissues are often injured extensively and not suitable for direct suturing. Free fascia or fat graft can be trimmed into a patch of appropriate size for peripheral repair by suturing (If the artificial spinal dura mater can be used for multiple injuries) with gelatin sponge covered. After suturing, fibrin glue is applied for the seal.

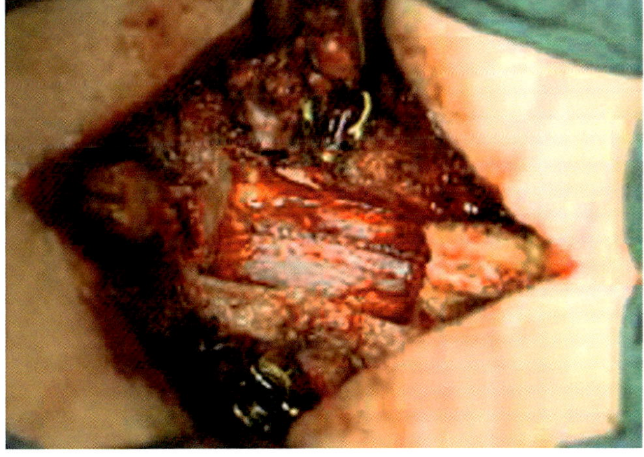

Fig. 13.68 Simple continuous suturing of spinal dura mater in posterior lumbar surgery

Valsalva maneuver should be performed to check the water tightness of the spinal dura mater and flush the surgical site with normal saline. Re-confirm that there is no dural sac leakage or nerve root injury.

The incision should be tightly sutured layer by layer, with dead space eliminated and tissue approximation achieved. The plasma drainage tube is then placed.

3. **Prevention of cerebrospinal fluid leakage in posterior lumbar surgery**

The surgery is planned after the images are reviewed carefully before surgery to evaluate the degree of ossification of the dura mater and its adhesion to surrounding tissues.

The operation should be performed carefully under direct visualization, with a clear surgical field being maintained throughout the surgery. For patients with severe lumbar spinal stenosis, lamina hyperplasia and sclerosis, ligamentum flavum hypertrophy, loss of epidural fat compression and other factors result in tight adhesion between the dura mater and lamina. The adhesiolysis and removal of laminar should be carefully performed by the surgeon. For patients with ossification of the posterior longitudinal ligament, ossified mass floating should be taken to avoid injury to the dural sac caused by excision.

The erector spinae muscle should be sutured to eliminate the deep dead space, the lumbar dorsal fascia layer should be tightly sutured, and the subcutaneous and skin layers should be sutured carefully as well. If the tightness of closure is not reached during the surgery, the lumbar cistern drainage should be applied at the end of the surgery. In cases where other treatments are ineffective, lumbar cistern drainage can be used as an alternative treatment for revision surgery9.

4. **Treatment of cerebrospinal fluid leakage in posterior lumbar surgery**

For patients with cerebrospinal fluid leakage after posterior lumbar surgery, the Trendelenburg position should be taken in combination with lateral decubitus position or prone position after the surgery to reduce the local pressure on dural tear. Lumbar cistern drainage should be placed as early as possible. If no improvement is shown, secondary surgical repair is considered. For other measures, please refer to the first three sections of this chapter.

13.5 Prevention of Spinal SSI and Treatment of Infected Incisions

Ding Wenyuan and Ma Lei
Department of Orthopedics
Third Hospital of Hebei Medical University
Shijiazhuang, China

Abstract
Spinal surgical site infection (SSI) is one of the common clinical complications after spinal surgery. Once not treated in time, it will lead to mounts of serious clinical outcomes. This chapter will introduce the related types of SSI after spinal surgery, discuss the suturing and related measurements of infected incisions, and provide relevant methods to prevent SSI in detail.

13.5.1 Background

Spinal surgical site infection (SSI) is one of the common clinical complications after spinal surgery. Once not treated in time, it will lead to mounts of serious clinical outcomes, such as delayed wound healing, pain, sepsis, and death [41, 42]. The incidence of SSI after spinal surgery fluctuated from 0.2% to 16.1% [43]. SSI can lead to prolonged hospitalization or rehospitalization with poor prognosis, followed by wound debridement or implant removal, which might unnecessarily increase the burden both on the patients and physicians. By the way, spinal SSI is considered to be multifactorial and can be effectively prevented. Inadequate preoperative preparation, poor sterile principle, improper postoperative infection prevention, and dressing replacement can all lead to postoperative infection. Prevention, diagnosis, and risk assessment are especially essential to reduce SSI after spinal surgery.

Studies have clarified that the risk factors of SSI after spinal surgery mainly include old age, obesity, smoking history, diabetes, immunosuppression, improper intraoperative aseptic operation, poor postoperative nutrition, previous history of infection, long duration of operation, or heavy intraoperative blood loss [44, 45]. In a series of 1629 patients undergoing spinal surgery, Fang et al. found that 61 cases (4.4%) showed incision infections [46]. A retrospective case-control study was conducted and concluded that age over 60 years, smoking, diabetes, previous history of incision infection, overweight, alcohol abuse, and combined anterior and posterior surgery were risk factors for increased incision infection after spinal surgery. When spinal SSI occurs, infection control and wound closure can be achieved by immediately and sufficient irrigation, drainage, clearance of necrotic tissue, and long-term patient wound management.

Due to the destruction of the immune barrier during the operation, intraoperative blood loss and fluid loss wound opening, and the application of large doses of hormones and antibiotics during and after the operation, it might lead to the invasion and infection of exogenous and endogenous pathogenic bacteria. The blood culture of wound secretions was mainly composed of *Escherichia coli*, enterococcus, methicillin-resistant *Staphylococcus aureus*, *Staphylococcus epidermidis*, *Enterobacter cloacae,* and other bacteria, among which *Staphylococcus aureus* was more common [47, 48]. Therefore, intraoperative aseptic operation and accurate suture are very important to prevent postoperative wound infection.

SSI after spinal surgery can be divided into early infection and late infection according to the occurrence time, superficial infection, and deep infection according to the location [49, 50]. However, there is no ideal surgical management guideline and no consensus on the management principal.

Superficial infection is usually manifested by redness, swelling, heat, and pain at the wound. Patients often recover after multiple wound dressing changes and antibiotic treatment. However, deep infection is difficult to diagnose with poor prognosis due to insignificant symptoms, atypical signs, inaccurate laboratory tests, and low positive bacterial culture rates (Figs. 13.69a, b and 13.70a, b). With the increasing proportion of internal fixation implants in spinal surgery, postoperative deep incision infection is gradually attracting the attention of surgeons. According to the occurrence time, the infection can be divided into early infection and late infection. How to define early infection and late infection is still controversial. Swimmer et al. [51] referred to infection occurring within 20 weeks after surgery as early infection, and infection occurring after 20 weeks as delayed infection. Ji Jianguo et al. [52] set 3 months as the dividing line between early and late infection.

Early deep infection mostly occurred within 1 week after surgery with increasing body temperature of >38.5 °C, wound pain, and inflammatory exudation. Few present with open wounds, redness, swelling, and fluctuating sensation. Laboratory inflammation indicators, such as white blood cell count, CRP and ESR, are helpful in the diagnosis of early infection [47]. Symptoms of the delayed infection are insidiously manifested with the normal wound healing. After several months, pain and discomfort appear at the original incision, followed by sinus tract and pus. Most patients have no systemic symptoms such as fever or poor appetite. Most of them have normal white blood cell count, which may easily lead to delayed diagnosis [53].

Early infection mainly caused by staphylococcus aureus and Escherichia coli. Due to the poor resistance-infection of the patients, SSI often caused by intraoperative contamination, blood-borne spread of bacteria in other body parts, or

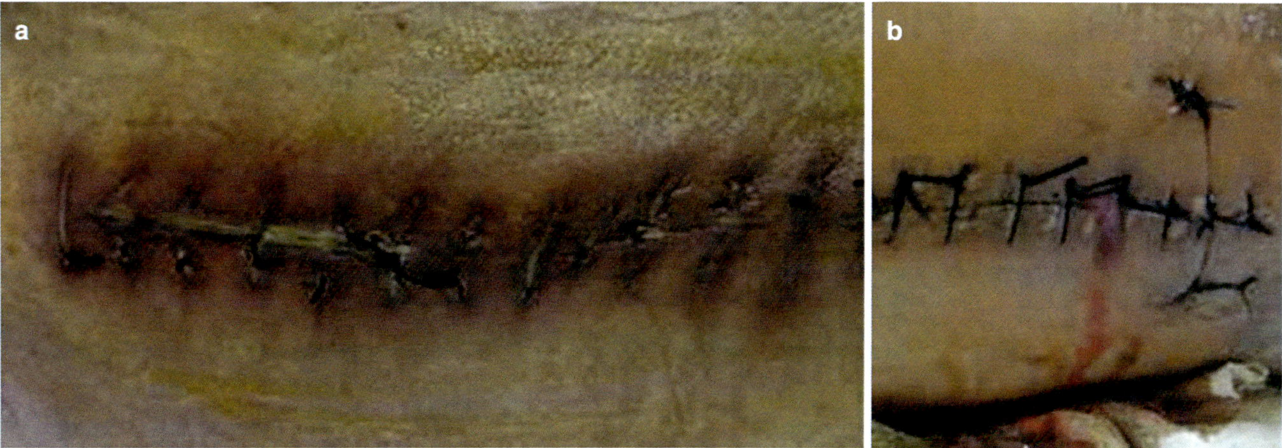

Fig. 13.69 (**a**) Superficial infection. (**b**) Superficial infection

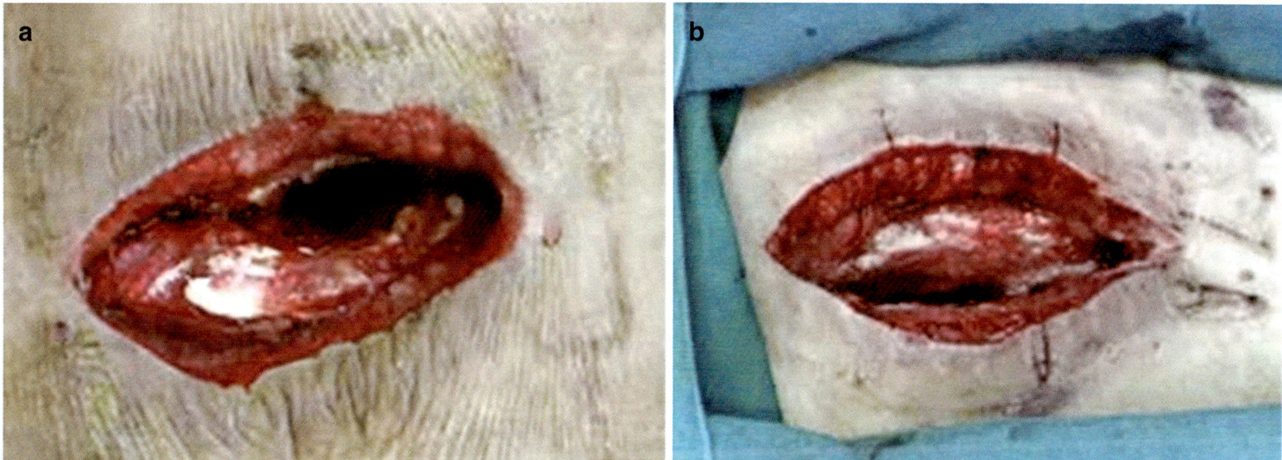

Fig. 13.70 (**a**) Deep infection. (**b**) Deep infection

migration of intestinal bacteria [52]. In deep infection, the bacteria can secrete more extracellular matrix, adhere to the surface of the internal fixator, then form a biofilm, which can escape the immune system and antibacterial drugs, resulting in persistent infection, and making it difficult to cure with conventional bacterial culture methods [54]. If fusion and stability have achieved, removal of internal fixation can completely eliminate the infected granulation tissue, thereby promoting blood supply and increasing the concentration of antibiotics in local tissues, killing the remaining bacteria [52, 53].

13.5.1.1 Early Superficial Infection

At present, the definitions of early infection and delayed infection after spinal surgery have not been unified. Some scholars refer to the infection over 30 days after surgery as delayed infection [55], while others consider the infection occurring 3, 6, or 12 months after surgery as delayed infection [56, 57]. Superficial infection refers to the infection located in the skin and subcutaneous superficial fascia, which is often manifested as pain, swelling, elevated skin temperature around the surgical incision, with or without exudation, and generally without systemic symptoms [58]. The treatment principle of early superficial infection is immediately diagnosis and intervention to prevent the infection from spreading to the deep tissue with incision dressing change combined with the application of sensitive antibiotics [59].

13.5.1.2 Early Deep Infection

Deep infection refers to the infection located under the deep fascia, with atypical early clinical manifestations, or just low back pain. Fever is the most common systemic symptom, and local incisions may show tenderness or exudation [60]. The treatment principle of early deep infection is still immediately diagnosis and intervention, surgical debridement combined with the application of sensitive antibiotics, but whether to retain the internal fixation device after surgery is controversial. Although the removal of internal fixation is conducive to complete debridement, postoperative spinal instability, loss of orthopedic angle and intervertebral height, fusion failure, and pseudarthrogenesis may occur [61, 62]. With the deepening understanding of SSI, there have been more reports on the retention of internal fixation devices after debridement in recent years. According to whether the infection spreads to the intervertebral space and whether the internal fixation is loose or not, you can choose debridement and drainage with internal fixation or with internal fixation removed. In the early stage of infection, the inflammation does not affect the intervertebral space, the internal fixation is stable, and the surrounding pseudomembrane is not yet formed or immature. The internal fixation device can be retained with thorough debridement during the operation, especially the removal of inflammatory granulation tissue around the internal fixation. Adequate lavage and drainage is needed, supplemented by sensitive antibiotic treatment [58, 61]. If the infection involves the intervertebral space, it is necessary to remove the intervertebral fusion cage, bone graft, and replace the internal fixation device [61]. If the internal fixation is loose, bacterial strong-resistance medicinal properties (such as MRSA), multiple debridements cannot control the infection, the internal fixation device should be removed [58, 61] (Figs. 13.71a–f and 13.72).

13.5.1.3 Delayed Deep Infection

It is often accompanied by systemic manifestations such as fever and local signs such as tenderness and exudation around the incision. The treatment principle of late-onset deep infection is also surgical debridement combined with

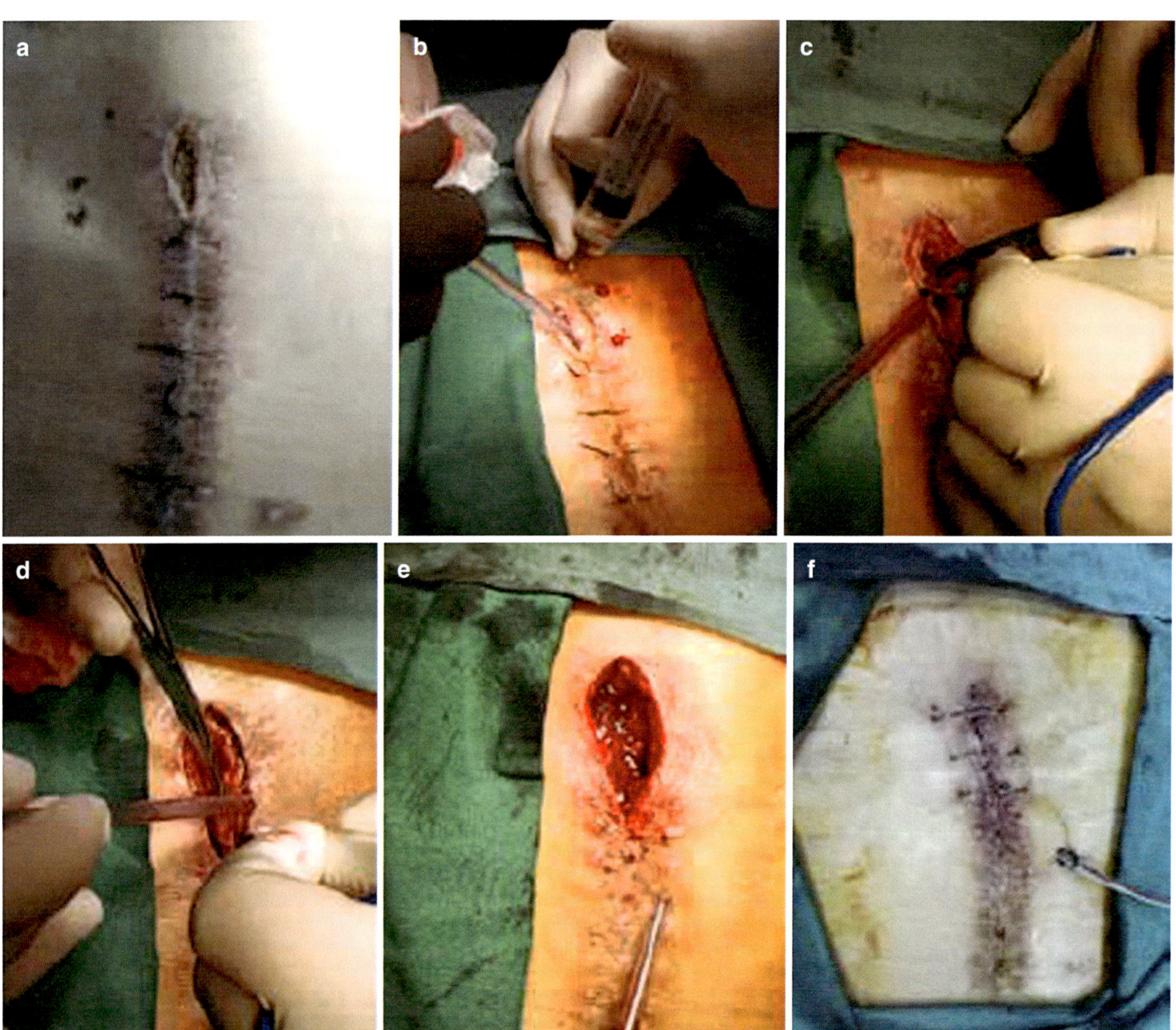

Fig. 13.71 (**a–f**) Debridement and suturing

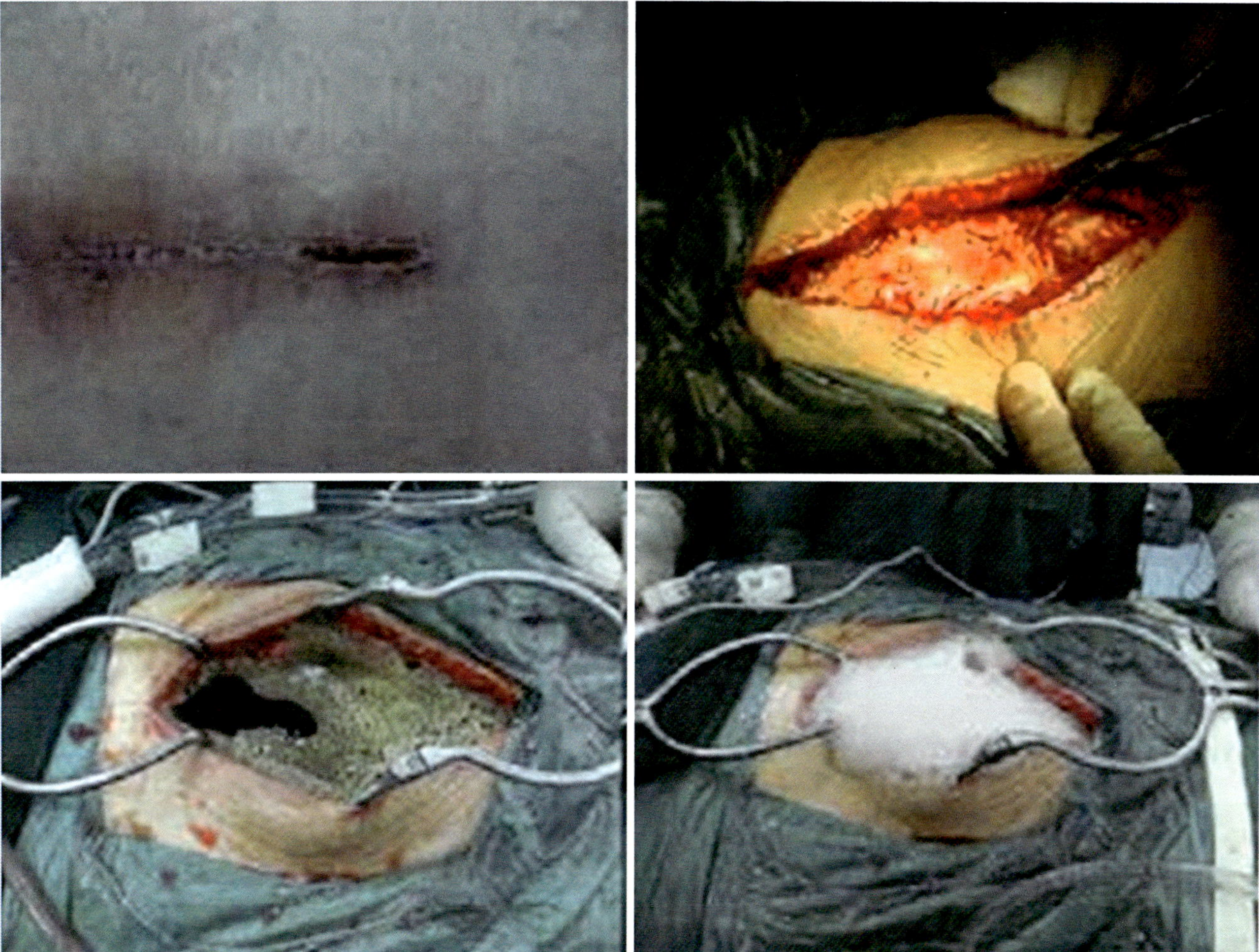

Fig. 13.72 Intraoperative flushing

sensitive antibiotics after immediately diagnosis, and there is also controversy about whether to retain internal fixation devices after surgery. If there is no loosening of the internal fixation, the surrounding pseudomembrane is immature, the infection does not involve the intervertebral space, and the intervertebral fusion is not sufficient, you should consider retaining the internal fixation device after debridement and closed drainage, and delay closing the incision, supplemented by sensitivity Antibiotic therapy [62]. If the pseudomembrane has been formed around the internal fixation device or the internal fixation has been loosened with the infection involving the intervertebral space, it is recommended to remove the internal fixation device to achieve complete debridement. Then make sure that postoperative closed lavage, drainage, delayed closure of the incision, and supplemented with sensitive antibiotic treatment [61, 63].

In summary, there is no consensus on the treatment principles of SSI after spinal surgery. Treatment needs to consider the wound condition, pathogenic bacteria, and patient factors. Early detection, early diagnosis, and early intervention are essential.

13.5.2 Spinal Surgery Infection Prevention and Infected Wound Suturing Technique

1. **Anterior cervical surgery**

Spinal surgery is usually to be aseptic surgery, but most of them are reconstructive surgery, which require implantation and internal fixation with the greater risk of infection after surgery. Once the infection occurs, it can affect wound healing and increase the number of hospitalization days. Of the worst, it can cause loosening of internal fixation, even reoperation, which might bring a great psychological and

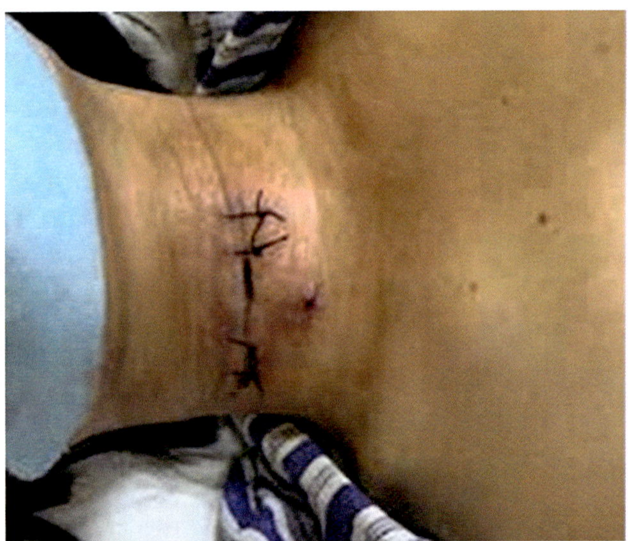

Fig. 13.73 Anterior cervical infection

economic burden to the patient and their family. It is reported that the incidence of incision infection after spinal internal fixation fluctuates from 0.2% to 16.1% [64, 65]. It is of great significance to prevent spinal surgery infection and ensure medical safety (Fig. 13.73).

For anterior cervical surgery, in order to prevent infection, patients are instructed to stop smoking 1 week before surgery and routinely inject antibiotics 20 min ~ 1 h before surgery. If the surgery time is longer than 3 h or intraoperative bleeding is greater than 1.5 L, the intraoperative antibiotics will be added [66]. Then you can use the 10% povidone-iodine solution and 3% hydrogen peroxide before closing the incision [67].

If the incision infection occurs after anterior cervical surgery, because the blunt separation and the clear anatomy, it can be rinsed repeatedly with sterile normal saline and given intravenous antibiotics. When the incision is ineffective with empirical anti-infective treatment or incision purulent discharge, it means that the drug alone cannot effectively control the infection. At this time, debridement is required. You should observe the sterility principle, explore layer by layer, thoroughly remove necrotic and inactivated tissue, and debride the wound to the deepest part of the infection. When suturing, because of the thin subcutaneous fat, the suturing should not be too dense. Generally, only part of the incision is sutured first, drainage strips are placed to drain blood and fluid, and the dressing should be changed daily. After the fresh granulation tissue has been grown and the aseptic growth is continuously cultured, the drainage strip might be taken out and the remaining wound can be sutured.

2. **Posterior cervical surgery**

The posterior cervical approach is common for the surgical treatment of cervical spinal stenosis. The surgical methods include single-door spinal canal expansion, double-door spinal canal expansion, and lateral mass screw laminectomy. The posterior cervical approach has its special anatomical structure which have the greater postoperative range of motion, the loose neck skin, the tough fascia layer, and the abundant muscles. Therefore, during the process of intraoperative suture, strict sterility principle should be observed. You can choose to use triclosan-absorbable antibacterial Vicryl suture (glycan lactic acid 910, Ethicon), layered suture of muscle, fascia, subcutaneous tissue, and skin, and continuous suture of the fascia layer. Studies have shown that diabetes, preoperative antibiotics, intraoperative use of internal fixation, and operation time are the main risk factors that affect the incision infection after the cervical spine posterior single-opening surgery [68]. The surgical incision of the cervical spine is deep, and the treatment of deep infection is often very difficult. Gong Feipeng et al. [69] used the method of inserting drainage tube into the wound and continuous suction for patients with superficial infection after cervical spine surgery. For deep infection spreading to the bone surface, they used gentamicin saline irrigation and drainage. When the drainage fluid is clear, the washing speed can be slowed down. When the patient's systemic and local symptoms disappear with the blood culture is negative two times, the drainage tube can be removed.

There are different treatment methods for early cervical incision infection. Closed negative pressure drainage is often used. The incision dressing should be changed once a day to ensure that the incision dressing is dry. Six to eight days after the negative pressure drainage, observing the drainage <20 ml and related laboratory results, the incision should be sutured in phase II. During the process of closing the incision, the muscle tissue and deep fascia must be tightly sutured, making sure that there is no dead space in the incision. A vacuum negative pressure drainage tube should be used in the incision, and the vacuum negative pressure drainage is connected externally. If the drainage <20 ml, you can remove the negative pressure drainage tube in 2–3 days [70–72].

Regarding whether to remove the internal fixation after infection, studies demonstrated that because the posterior cervical surgery often requires extensive dissection, the stability of the spine is significantly weaker than the preoperation. If the internal fixation is removed, it will further aggravate the instability of the cervical spine and aggravate cervical deformity. At the same time, it will cause neurological dysfunction [68–70]. So, we do not recommend to remove the internal fixation. Gong Feipeng et al. [69] have tried to wound irrigation, adequate drainage, and effective antibiotic treatment on 5 patients with postoperative cervical infection. The infection was completely controlled without removing the internal fixation.

3. **Posterior thoracolumbar surgery**

The incidence of postoperative infection after thoracolumbar surgery fluctuates from 0.7% to 11.9% which will seriously affect the fusion rate and patient's recovery. Therefore, during the operation, you can use the antibacterial Vicryl (glycan lactate 910, Ethicon) to suture containing triclosan to prevent wound infections. Before the surgery, it is necessary to correct the patient's malnutrition and supplement a high-protein diet. In the patients who might be severe hypoalbuminemia, consider combining intravenous albumin supplementation to make the concentration reach 35 g/L before performing surgery. By the way, intraoperative tissue traction should be reduced and shorten the operation time [73].

If the wound is infected and requires debridement, the corresponding treatment can be carried out according to the infection. Patients with infection are often accompanied by poor wound healing. In debridement and suture, you can choose to cut the incision fusiform and suture it. Observe the wound condition closely after the operation to prevent re-infection. The continuous exudation, redness, and pain of the wound gradually increased, suggesting that there may be a deep infection with multiple bacterial infections. Repeated postoperative infections are often accompanied by the anatomical disorder. Deep muscle tissue infections are mostly manifested as damage to the muscle tissue and dark brown with pus attachment. Deep infections, repeated infections, and delayed infections may cause bacteria to adhere to the surface of the internal fixation. Therefore, you can choose to remove all infected necrotic tissues and obviously infected grafts. If necessary, the loose internal fixation must be removed [74]. Moreover, early treatment is conducive to retaining the internal fixation, and it is also possible to choose a large bone graft to facilitate fusion [75, 76]. Suture the wound should be artificially layered. Continue closed lavage and drainage after surgery, and actively seek out the cause of repeated infections while paying close attention to the preoperational wound changes. When the drainage fluid is clear with no necrosis, the patient's body temperature is normal, the white blood cell count, ESR, CRP are normal, you can first pull out the lavage tube. Two days later or drainage <50 mL/d, you can pull out the drainage tube. Vacuum sealing drainage (VSD) can be placed. You can choose a suitable size of VSD vacuum suction foam material and place it in the wound surface so that the foam material is in the entire cavity fully in contact with the wound inside. Meanwhile, you can choose the absorbable antibacterial Vicryl suture (glycan lactic acid 910, Ethicon) to suture several stitches to fix the foam material to the skin. The suction tube of the foam material is connected to the negative pressure drainage, visible VSD foam material depression. (Figs. 13.74 and 13.75) After the

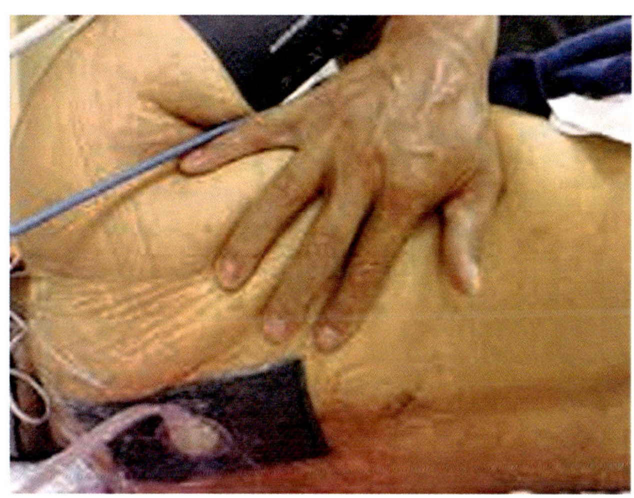

Fig. 13.74 VSD

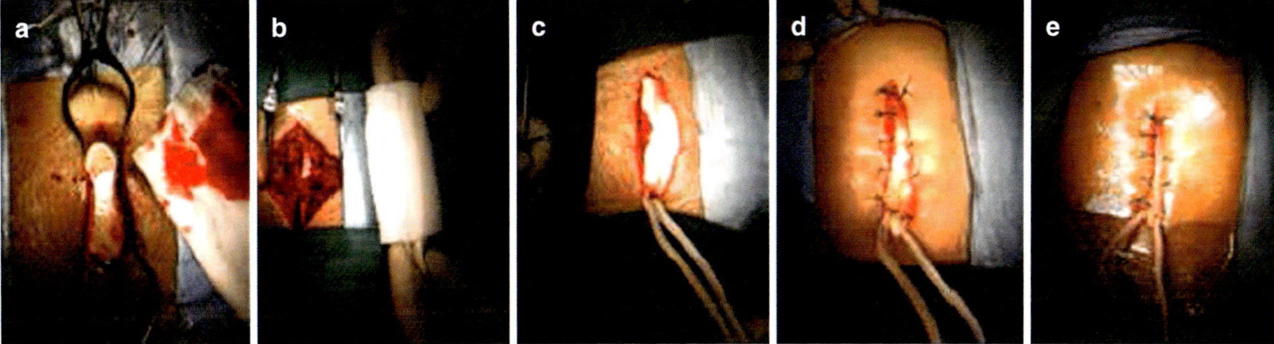

Fig. 13.75 A-E

operation, saline should be used for continuous lavage and negative pressure closed drainage. Generally, after continuous lavage for 30–60 min, the lavage and irrigation tube can be closed to maintain the state of negative pressure closed suction and drainage. According to the drainage fluid and wound condition, the continuous lavage can be repeated every 6–12 hours. The first 3 days choose rapid irrigation and then slow irrigation, and gradually reduce the volume of lavage fluid after the drainage is clear. When the symptoms and systemic inflammatory reactions disappear and the results of consecutive bacterial cultures in the drainage fluid are negative, the lavage can be stopped and the pressure closed drainage still should be continued. It should be closely observed whether the negative pressure closed suction device continues to be effective. After 7–10 days, take it out and directly use triclosan-absorbable antibacterial Vicryl suture (glycan lactic acid 910, Ethicon) to close the wound. If there are still secretions in the wound, place a new negative pressure suction device and set it on 7–10 days, choose to close the wound or replace the VSD depending on the situation [77, 78].

4. **Special population infection**

In clinical work, patients with obesity and infectious diseases are often encountered. Such people have poor immunity and decreased tissue repairment ability after surgery. The occurrence of fat liquefaction in surgical incisions is further increased. Liquefaction will cause secondary infections and even full-thickness dehiscence, which will prolong the healing time of the incision and bring pain to the patients [79].

For such patients, although the traditional incision suture method is conducive to local hemostasis and skin-marginal conjugation, it also has disadvantages, such as excessive sutures, increasing foreign body reactions, resulting in poor local blood supply, aggravating fat cell damage, and resulting fat liquefaction. Meanwhile, the incision should be trimmed appropriately before sutures. Patients with infectious diseases can choose to remove part of the inactivated tissue, and then use the special method to suture the skin and subcutaneous fat tissue with triclosan Antibacterial Vicryl suture (glycan lactic acid 910, Ethicon). It is inserted from the skin on one side of the surgeon's incision to the upper 1/3 of the subcutaneous fat, and the needle is inverted, then the needle is inserted from the upper 1/3 of the subcutaneous fat on the other side, pass through the lower 2/3 of the subcutaneous fat and the anterior sheath to the opposite side, suture the lower 2/3 to the upper 1/3 of the subcutaneous fat of the opposite side and exit the needle. And the last two sides of the skin are sutured at 4 points [80] (Fig. 13.76). This method can effectively prevent postoperative fat liquefaction and postoperative SSI. For patients with excessive incision tension, the needle insertion site should be kept away from the

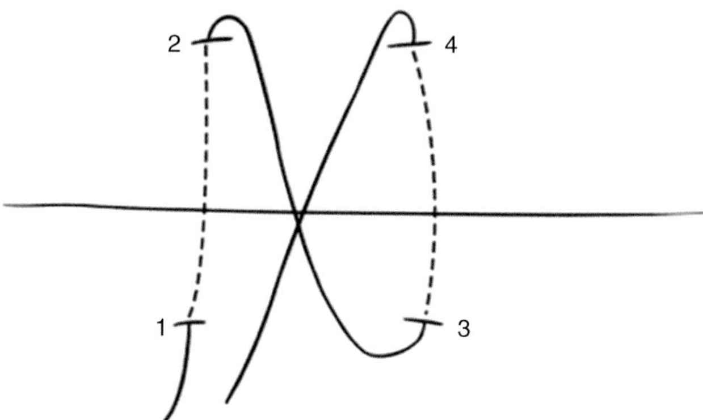

Fig. 13.76 Fig. 8 suturing needs to be painted

incision, and the needle distance should be appropriately widened, so as to help to reduce the margin pressure, which might ultimately accelerate the incision healing.

For special patients with infectious diseases (spinal tuberculosis, brucellosis), according to the guidelines of the US Centers for Disease Control and Prevention, it is recommended that the dose of antibacterial drugs should be double-used before surgery, and targeted antibacterial drugs can be applied around the incision, such as streptomycin, which can effectively reduce the infection rate of postoperative incisions.

5. **Precautions for suturing**

Thoracolumbar posterior surgery is difficult because of the deep anatomical location if the infection spreading to deep tissues. At this time, the deep infected tissue should be fully removed, and the sacral spinal muscles on both sides should be appropriately freed. It is recommended to use absorbable 2-0 antibacterial Vicryl suture (glycan lactic acid 910, Ethicon) interrupted suture to fully eliminate the death Cavity (Fig. 13.77). In addition, because the subcutaneous tissue has been infected with edema and poor blood supply, it is not recommended to suture the subcutaneous tissue separately. You can choose to use absorbable antibacterial Vicryl suture (glycan lactic acid 910, Ethicon) to suture the skin and subcutaneous tissue under full tension with moderate trimming. Make sure that keep an adequate blood supply to the skin edge to accelerate wound healing (Fig. 13.78a, b).

6. **Prevention of infection**

You should pay attention to assess the patient's own condition. For patients with high risk of infection such as immunosuppression and poor nutrition, risk factors related to preoperative infection should be strictly controlled. The patient's own condition should be adjusted before the surgery. The sterility principle should be strictly observed dur-

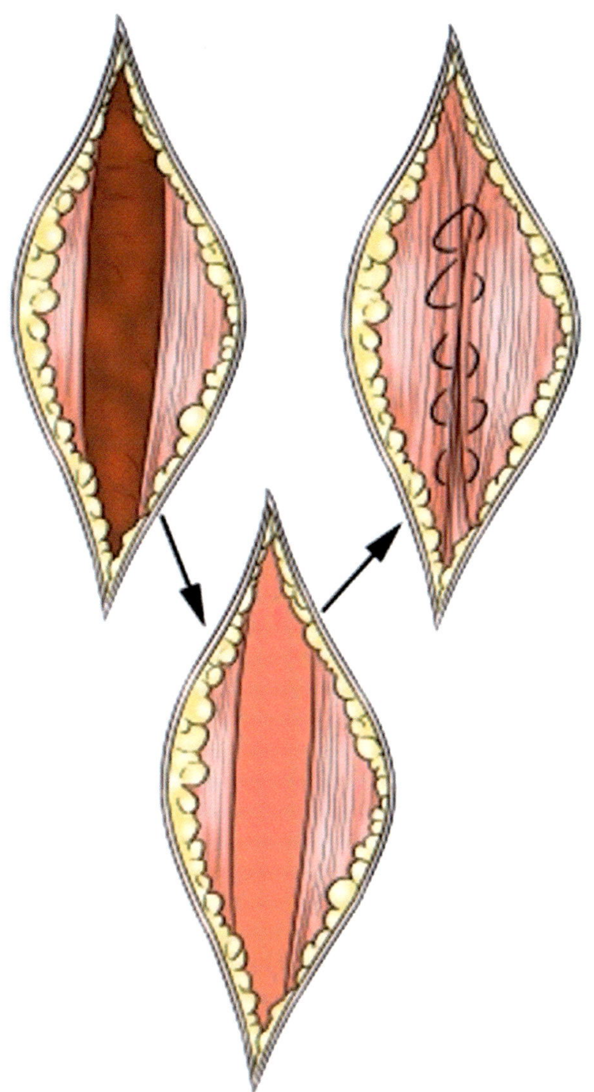

Fig. 13.77 Dead space closure requires painting

ing the operation. Many SSI prevention guidelines including WHO [81–84], all recommend the use of triclosan-absorbable antibacterial Vicryl suture (glycan lactic acid 910, Ethicon) to reduce the incidence of postoperative SSI. Masaki Ueno et al. [85] confirmed that compared with ordinary sutures, triclosan-coated antibacterial sutures can certainly reduce the occurrence of SSI (0.5% versus 3.9%, P = 0.020) by observing whether the wounds of 405 patients were infected or dehisced after spinal surgery. Another literature showed that compared with skin nailing, the use of sutures can effectively reduce the incidence of incision SSI (11.8% versus 4.2%, P = 0.017) [86]. If postoperative infection occurs, you should apply adequate sensitive antibiotics immediately. If there is no drug sensitivity result, choose broad-spectrum, high-efficiency, and adequate antibiotics. The patient's body temperature changes and wound conditions should be closely monitored. If the wound continues to leak, debridement and drainage should be performed [87]. When performing debridement and suture for SSI after spinal surgery, appropriate suture techniques should be adopted according to the preoperative evaluation and intraoperative situation. It is recommended to choose the eight-needle suture (glycan lactate 910, Ethicon). If the continuous suture is required, use absorbable No. 0 antibacterial Vicryl suture (Glycan Lactic Acid 910, Ethicon) to find out the cause of infection and try to avoid postoperative SSI.

In short, prevent infection is always the key point. After making sufficient preoperative preparations, strictly observing the sterility principle during the operation, it is important to adopt the correct suture method. After the operation, make sure to watch out for the wound and the patient's general condition. If the infection occurs, different treatment methods should be adopted in time according to the type, location of the infection to minimize the pain, accelerating the wound healing.

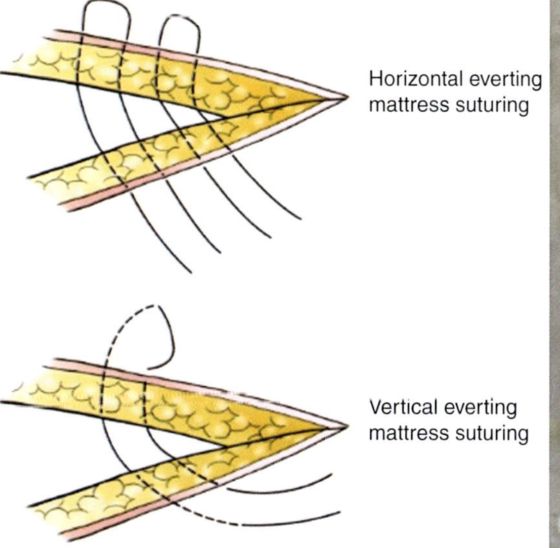

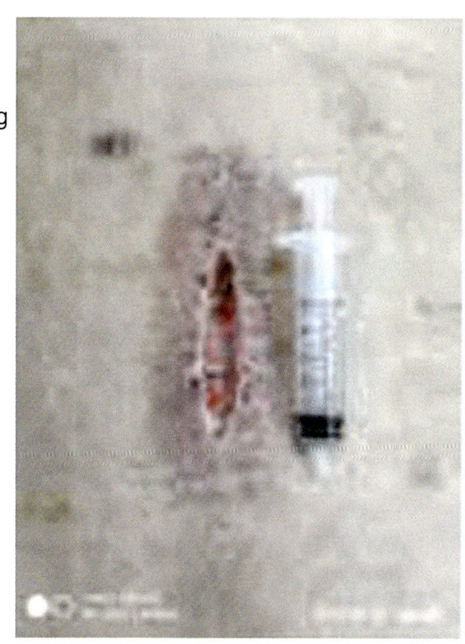

Fig. 13.78 (**a** and **b**) Tension-reduced suturing requires painting

References

1. Albee FH. Transplantation of a portion of the tibia into the spine for Pott's disease. JAMA. 1911;57:885.
2. Hibbs RH. An operation for progressive spinal deformities NY. J Med. 1911;93:1013.
3. Gililland JM, Anderson LA, Barney JK, Ross HL, Pelt CE, Peters C. Barbed versus standard sutures for closure in Total knee arthroplasty: a multicenter prospective randomized trial. J Arthroplast. 2014;29(Suppl. 2):135–8.
4. Borzio RW, Piveci R, Kapadian BH, Jauregui JJ, Maheshwari AV. Barbed sutures in total hip and knee arthroplasty: what is the evidence? A meta-analysis. Int Orthopaedics (SICOT). 2016;40:225–31.
5. Ting NT, Moric MM, Della Valle CJ, Levine BR. Use of knot-less suture for closure of Total hip and knee arthroplasties a prospective, randomized clinical trial. J Arthoplasty. 2012;27(10):1783–8.
6. Smith EL, DiSegna ST, Shukla PY, Matzkin EG. Barbed versus traditional sutures: closure time, cost, and wound related outcome in Total joint arthroplasty. J Arthroplast. 2014;29:283–7.
7. Gililland JM, Anderson LA, Sun G, Ericksoo JA, Peters CL. Perioperative closure-related complication rates and cost analysis of barbed suture for closure in TKA. Clin Orthop Relat Res. 2012;470:125–9.
8. Namba RS, Inacio MC, Paxton EW. Risk factors associated with deep surgical site infections after primary total knee arthroplasty: an analysis of 56,216 knees. J Bone Joint Surg Am. 2013 May 1;95(9):775–82.
9. Fowler JR, Perkins TA, Buttaro BA, Truant AL. Bacteria adhere less to barbed monofilament than braided sutures in a contaminated wound model. Clin Orthop Relat Res. 2013;471:665–71.
10. Mansour A, Ballard R, Garg S, Baulesh D, Erickson M. The use of barbed sutures during scoliosis fusion wound closure: a quality improvement analysis. J Pediatr Orthop. 2013;33:786–90. PMID: 24213622
11. Parikh PM, Davison SP, Higgins JP. Barbed suture tenorrhaphy: an ex vivo biomechanical analysis. Plast Reconstr Surg. 2009;124:1551–8.
12. Wu YJ, et al. Repositioning suture of the erector spinae muscle for lumbar spine surgery via the posterior approach: a prospective randomized study. Cell Biochem Biophys. 2014;69(1):75–80.
13. Shani A, Poliansky V, et al. Nylon skin sutures carry a lower risk of post-operative infection than metal Staples in open posterior spine surgery: a retrospective case-control study of 270 patients. Surgical infections. Published online December 31, 2019.
14. Shakil H, Iqbal ZA, Al-Ghadir AH. Scoliosis: review of types of curves, etiological theories and conservative treatment. J Back Musculoskelet Rehabil. 2014;27(2):111–5.
15. McLeod L, Flynn J, Erickson M, Miller N, Keren R, Dormans J. Variation in 60-day readmission for surgical-site infections (SSIs) and reoperation following spinal fusion operations for neuromuscular scoliosis. J Pediatr Orthop. 2016;36(6):634–9.
16. Mackenzie WG, Matsumoto H, Williams BA, et al. Surgical site infection following spinal instrumentation for scoliosis: a multicenter analysis of rates, risk factors, and pathogens. J Bone Joint Surg Am. 2013;95(9):800–S2.
17. Subramanyam R, Schaffzin J, Cudilo EM, Rao MB, Varughese AM. Systematic review of risk factors for surgical site infection in pediatric scoliosis surgery. Spine J. 2015;15(6):1422–31.
18. Sullivan BT, Abousamra O, Puvanesarajah V, et al. Deep infections after pediatric spinal arthrodesis: differences exist with idiopathic, neuromuscular, or genetic and syndromic cause of deformity. J Bone Joint Surg Am. 2019;101(24):2219–25.
19. Yagi M, Hosogane N, Watanabe K, Asazuma T, Matsumoto M. Keio spine research group. The paravertebral muscle and psoas for the maintenance of global spinal alignment in patient with degenerative lumbar scoliosis. Spine J. 2016;16(4):451–8.
20. Akhaddar A, Alaoui M, Turgut M, Hall W. Iatrogenic vascular laceration during posterior lumbar disc surgery: a literature review [published online ahead of print, 2020 May 12]. Neurosurg Rev. 2020; https://doi.org/10.1007/s10143-020-01311-5.
21. Mange TR, Sucato DJ, Poppino KF, Jo CH, Ramo BR. The incidence and risk factors for perioperative allogeneic blood transfusion in primary idiopathic scoliosis surgery [published online ahead of print, 2020 Mar 9]. Spine Deform. 2020; https://doi.org/10.1007/s43390-020-00093-6.
22. Subramanyam R, Schaffzin J, Cudilo EM, Rao MB, Varughese AM. Systematic review of risk factors for surgical site infection in pediatric scoliosis surgery. Spine J. 2015;15(6):1422–31.
23. Vitale MG, Riedel MD, Glotzbecker MP, et al. Building consensus: development of a best practice guideline (BPG) for surgical site infection (SSI) prevention in high-risk pediatric spine surgery. J Pediatr Orthop. 2013;33(5):471–8.
24. Kalevski SK, Peev NA, Haritonov DG. Incidental Dural tears in lumbar decompressive surgery: incidence, causes, treatment, results. Asian J Neurosurg. 2010;5(1):54–9.
25. AH S, G C, D S, et al. Predictive factors for dural tear and cerebrospinal fluid leakage in patients undergoing lumbar. Surgery. 2006;5(3):224–7.
26. Shengsheng C, Minjie R, Yuhong Q, et al. Clinical efficacy of medical glue combined with gelatin sponge in preventing cerebrospinal fluid leakage after spinal dural suture. J Chin Medical Guide. 2015;13(21):4–6.
27. Eismont FJ, Wiesel SW, Rothman RH. Treatment of dural tears associated with spinal surgery. J Bone Joint Surg American. 1981;63(7):1132–6.
28. Papavero L, Engler N, Kothe R. Incidental durotomy in spine surgery: first aid in ten steps. Eur Spine J: official publication of the European Spine Society tESDS. 2015;24(9):2077–84.
29. Strömqvist F, Jönsson B, Strömqvist B, et al. Dural lesions in lumbar disc herniation surgery: incidence, risk factors, and outcome. Eur Spine J. 2010;19(3):439–42.
30. Fang Z, Tian R, Jia Y-T, et al. Treatment of cerebrospinal fluid leak after spine surgery. Chin J traumatol = Zhonghua chuang shang za zhi. 2017;20(2):81–3.
31. Qi S. A randomized controlled study of suturing deep fascia during lumbar posterior short-segment decompression and fusion with barb-free sutures. Chin Tissue Eng Res. 2020;24(10):1585–90.
32. Zixiang W. Guidelines for evidence-based clinical diagnosis and treatment of orthopedics of the orthopedics branch of the Chinese medical doctor association: evidence-based clinical diagnosis and treatment guidelines for spinal dural tear and postoperative cerebrospinal fluid leakage. J Chin J Surgery. 2017;55(02):86–9.
33. Hida K, Yano S, Iwasaki Y. Considerations in the treatment of cervical ossification of the posterior longitudinal ligament. Chin Neurosurg. 2008;55:126–32.
34. Bosacco SJ, Gardner MJ, Guille JT, et al. Evaluation and treatment of dural tears in lumbar spine surgery: a review. Clin Orthop Relat Res. 2001;389:238–47.
35. Black P. Cerebrospinal fluid leaks following spinal surgery: use of fat grafts for prevention and repair. Technical note. J Neurosurg. 2002;96:250–2.
36. Narotam PK, Jose S, Nathoo N, et al. Collagen matrix (DuraGen) in dural repair: analysis of a new modified technique. Spine. 2004;29(24):2861–7.
37. Matsuoka T, Yamaura I, Kurosa Y, et al. Long-term results of the anterior floating method for cervical myelopathy caused by ossifi-

cation of the posterior longitudinal ligament. Spine (Phila Pa 1976). 2001;26(3):241–8.
38. Hu P, Yu M, Liu X, et al. Cerebrospinal fluid leakage after surgeries on the thoracic spine: a review of 362 cases. Asian Spine J. 2016;10(3):472–9.
39. Khan MH, Rihn J, Steele G, et al. Postoperative management protocol for incidental dural tears during degenerative lumbar spine surgery: a review of 3,183 consecutive degenerative lumbar cases. Spine (Phila Pa 1976). 2006;31(22):2609–13.
40. Gandhi J, DiMatteo A, Joshi G, et al. Cerebrospinal fluid leaks secondary to dural tears: a review of etiology, clinical evaluation, and management. Int J Neurosci. 2020;13:1–13.
41. Vaccaro AR. What is new in the diagnosis and prevention of spine surgical site infections. Spine J. 2015;15(2):336–47.
42. Ma L. Treatment of early infection after posterior spinal internal fixation with closed lavage and drainage. Sichuan Med. 2015;4
43. Samuel AM. CORR insights®: incidence of surgical site infection after spine surgery: what is the impact of the definition of infection. Clin Orthop Related Res. 2015;473(5):1620–1.
44. Anderson PA. An update on modifiable factors to reduce the risk of surgical site infections. Spine J Official J North American Spine Soc. 2013;13(9):1017–29.
45. Deyu C. Risk factors of incision infection after spinal surgery. Chin J Spine Spinal Cord. 3:77–80.
46. Bradford DS. Risk factors for infection after spinal surgery. Spine (Phila Pa 1976). 2005;30(12):1460–5.
47. Fangcai L. Clinical features and treatment of early deep infection after spinal internal fixation. Zhejiang J Traumatic Surg. 024(004): 739–741.
48. Hu SS. Clinical outcome of deep wound infection after instrumented posterior spinal fusion. Spine (Phila Pa 1976). 2009;34(6):578–83.
49. Patel R. A biofilm approach to detect bacteria on removed spinal implants. Spine (Phila Pa 1976). 2010;35(12):1218–24.
50. Kaye KS. Strategies to prevent surgical site infections in acute care hospitals: 2014 update. Infect Control Hosp Epidemiol. 2014;35(S2):S66–88.
51. Gluch H. Management of postoperative wound infection in posterior spinal fusion with instrumentation. J Spinal Disord. 1996;9(6):505–8.
52. Shugang L. Treatment of infection after posterior scoliosis orthopedic fusion. Chinese Journal of Orthopaedics. 21(8): 453–456.
53. Zhongjun L. Treatment of deep wound infection after spinal surgery. Chin J Surg. 043(4): 229–231.
54. Jing L. Treatment of deep infection after thoracolumbar posterior internal fixation. Chin J Surg. 2005;43(20):1325–7.
55. Wang Y. Delayed infection after spinal internal fixation. Chin J Orthop. (08):88–89.
56. Giacomini S. Late-developing infection following posterior fusion for adolescent idiopathic scoliosis. Eur Spine J. 2011;20(1 Supplement):121–7.
57. Qiu G. Abnormalities associated with congenital scoliosis a retrospective study of 226 chinese surgical cases. Spine (Phila Pa 1976). 2012;38(10):814–8.
58. Sheng L. Treatment strategy for early incision deep infection after spinal internal fixation. J Clin Orthop. (5):50–53+59.
59. Haoning Z. Treatment of infection after spinal internal fixation. Chin J Orthop. (015): 1357–1362.
60. Cohen DB. The presentation, incidence, etiology, and treatment of surgical site infections after spinal surgery. Spine (Phila Pa 1976). 2010;35(13):1323–8.
61. Guo X. Debridement with preserving internals combined with vacuum negative pressure sealing drainage to treat early postoperative spinal infection. Chin J Spine and Spinal Cord. 2015;25(12):1123–5.
62. Lee JS. Implant removal for the management of infection after instrumented spinal fusion. J Spinal Disord Tech. 2010;23(4):258–65.
63. Wang X. Treatment of delayed infection after internal fixation of the spine pedicle screw system. Chin J Orthop. 190(20): 1577–1578.
64. Vaccaro A. Is surgical case order associated with increased infection rate after spine surgery. Spine (Phila Pa 1976). 2012;37(13):1170–4.
65. van Middendorp JJ. A methodological systematic review on surgical site infections following spinal surgery: part 1 risk factors. Spine (Phila Pa 1976). 2012;37(24):2034–45.
66. Sosna A. Antibiotic treatment for prevention of infectious complications in joint replacement. Acta Chir Orthop Traumatol Cech. 2006;73(2):108–14.
67. Oliveri G. Prevention of post-operative infections in spine surgery by wound irrigation with a solution of povidone–iodine and hydrogen peroxide. Arch Orthop Trauma Surg. 2011;131(9):1203–6.
68. Zhikui L. Analysis of related factors of incisional infection after single-opening of the posterior cervical spine. Chin J Clin Res. v.31(5): 67–70.
69. Zhisheng L, Feipeng G, Gang C, et al. The causes and treatment of postoperative infection after superior cervical spine surgery. Pract Clin Med, 2013, 014(009): 71–72, 87, cover 3.
70. Dong Y, Zheng X, Honglin G, et al. Treatment of delayed deep infection after spinal internal fixation. Chin J Orthop. 2017;37(18):1150–5.
71. Guo L, Degang T, Wang J, et al. Observation on the therapeutic effects of early debridement and closed negative pressure drainage in the treatment of incisional infection after cervical posterior approach. Zhejiang J Traumatic Surg. 2014;000(004):528–529,530.
72. Nan Z, Faming T, Zihong L, et al. Analysis of effects of wound hedging and drainage for incision infection after cervical posterior approach single-opening surgery. Chin J Medical Guide. 2017;16(4):367–9.
73. Kuibo Z, Tao C, Guo Y, et al. Analysis of risk factors for early surgical site infection after thoracolumbar posterior internal fixation. J Sun Yat-sen Univ. 2013;34(6):986–90.
74. Kim JI, Suh KT, Kim SJ, et al. Implant removal for the management of infection after instrumented spinal fusion. J Spi-nal Disord Tech. 2010;23(4):258–65.
75. Chen SH, Lee CH, Huang KC. et al.Postoperative wound infection after posterior spinal instrumentation: analysis of long-term treatment outcomes. Eur Spine J. 2015;24(3):561–70.
76. Fei C, Lu G, Yijun K, et al. Treatment of deep infection after thoracolumbar posterior internal fixation. Chin J Surg. 2005;43(20):1325–7.
77. Zheng Y, Yu B, Lu S, Xiaoqiang Z. Application of vacuum sealing drainage in the treatment of early wound deep infection after thoracolumbar posterior internal fixation. Orthop Biomech Mater Clin Study. 2013;10(1):35–6.
78. Nenggao F. Zhang Yingbo, Zhang Zhiming, Jiang Cheng, VSD combined with lavage and drainage in the treatment of thoracolumbar incision infection. J Pract Orthop. 2014;20(1):145–8.
79. Xu Y. Analysis of related factors of postoperative wound infection in patients with spinal surgery. Diet Sci 2018 (16).
80. Ke J. Analysis of therapeutic effects of erected "voilet braided sutures" on .postoperative fat liquefaction for obese patients. Chin J Misdiagnostics. 2011;19:4639.
81. Allegranzi B, et al. New WHO recommendations on intraoperative and postoperative measures for surgical site infection prevention: an evidence-based global perspective. Lancet Infect Dis. 2016 Dec;16(12).e288–303.
82. ACS and surgical infection society: surgical site infection guidelines, 2016 Update.

83. Centers for disease control and prevention guideline for the prevention of surgical site infection, 2017. JAMA Surg. Published online May 3, 2017.
84. Guidelines for the prevention of surgical site infections in China. Chin J Gastrointest Surg. 2019;22(4):301–14.
85. Ueno M, Saito W, et al. Triclosan-coated sutures reduce wound infections after spinal surgery: a retrospective, nonrandomized, clinical study. Spine J. 2015 May 1;15(5):933–8.
86. Shani A, Poliansky V, et al. Nylon skin sutures carry a lower risk of post-operative infection than metal staples in open posterior spine surgery: a retrospective case-control study of 270 patients. Srugical Infections. Published online December 31, 2019.
87. Yonggang T, Yi J, Lianping X, et al. Treatment strategies for postoperative spinal infection. Chin J Spine Spinal Cord. 2009;19(9):717–71.

14 Orthopedic Knotting Techniques

Zhongguo Fu and Xiaomin Wu

Abstract

A surgical instrument is a part of a surgeon's hands. Learning how to use surgical instruments is an essential precondition for mastering surgical techniques. In suturing techniques, to meet the approximation requirement of different tissue and organs, the selection of corresponding sutures, suture needles, and needle holders is crucial to suturing quality. Suturing-related instruments are grouped into different categories according to characteristics including specifications, materials, technologies, and special functions, and have their respective application scenarios. We should gain some understanding of such information before suturing. This section will give an overview of the features and application of sutures, suture needles, and needle holders used in orthopedic surgery.

Keywords

Suture · Suture needle · Needle holder

Knotting techniques for surgical suturing can be dated back to fishing and navigation practices ancestors thousands of years ago. Grasping knotting techniques is an essential skill to be possessed by surgeons. If it is failed to effectively sew up and repair the damaged tissue by suture, the whole operation is bound to fail, and all work done concerning the operation is a waste of time and energy and increases the suffering of the patient. Improving knotting techniques is a vital part of continuing education for surgeons.

The ideal suture knotting method shall be meeting the demand of resisting peripheral tissue pulling to the maximum in an easy-to-learn manner with the smallest suture knot. Despite numerous knotting methods of surgical suture documented in literature, so far there is no "universal" suture knot that can cover all suture methods. In clinical practices, surgeons usually select the suture knotting scheme they are most familiar with based upon personal experience and preference.

Though surgeons need not grasp operation techniques of all suture knots, it is necessary to master the operation for some basic suture knots and be familiar with the advantages and disadvantages of them to better meet the demands of clinical work. Learning and training concerning suturing techniques play a vital role during the growth of young surgeons and medical students. Only through consistent practices will surgeons tie surgical suture knots masterly, precisely, and normatively without hesitation during operations.

Orthopedic suturing techniques are commonly applied to reduction and fixation of tendon-to-tendon, tendon-to-bone, ligament-to-bone, and even fracture. Though suture materials and surgical suturing techniques are improving and changing constantly, the main principles of surgical suturing are similar to principles of wound suturing: no tension approximation among sutured tissues, close the dead space; keep tissue in repaired position by virtue of methods including suture, and resist tension acting on sutured tissue until the tissue is healed; take account of postoperative esthetic appearance of sutured skin; and mitigate risks of bleeding and infection.

14.1 Surgical Instruments Concerning Suture Technology

F. U. Zhongguo and W. U. Xiaoming

"A craftsman who wishes to do his work well must first sharpen his tools." In addition to mastering fundamental suturing techniques (such as holding a needle, manipulating

Z. Fu (✉)
Peking University People's Hospital, Beijing, China

X. Wu
Shanghai General Hospital, Shanghai, China

P. Tang et al. (eds.), *Tutorials in Suturing Techniques for Orthopedics*, https://doi.org/10.1007/978-981-33-6330-4_14

a needle, and tying a knot), a superb suture knot closely relies on its matching surgical instruments. The instruments must be thoroughly disinfected before use and carefully maintained after use. In operations, proper suture, needle, and needle holder matching suture needle are selected according to the site of sutured tissue, skin thickness in the site, wound tension, etc.

14.1.1 Surgical suture

Surgical techniques always come first in the course of surgical suturing. Selecting proper sutures according to different features of various sutures will help surgeons achieve the best effect of tissue repair. Unlike implantable medical devices, surgical suture is grouped into Class III sterile medical devices.

1. **Suture specifications** (Table 14.1)

The specifications of suture are represented by numbers and indicate the diameters of suture: starting from above "0", larger number indicates thicker suture (for example: No. 4 suture is thicker than No. 1 suture) and higher tensile strength. In general, there are No. 1–10 sutures. Starting from below "0," more "0" indicates smaller diameter and lower tensile strength. The tensile strength of a suture knot is the strength (in pounds) that it can withstand before breaking.

2. **Materials of suture**

Now domestic surgical sutures are mainly made from materials as follows (Table 14.2):

(a) Silk: widely applied, low-cost, strong, easy to use, occupying the majority of surgical suture market share, with its absorption cycle exceeding 1 year and thus classified into nonabsorbable suture.
(b) Catgut: traditional biological absorbable surgical suture, which has been gradually replaced.
(c) PGA and PGLA synthetic absorbable sutures: more and more widely applied in clinical practices due to favorable biocompatibility and reliable fixation effect.
Absorbable sutures are produced from the collagen of healthy mammals or synthetic polymers. Natural absorbable sutures are degraded by the digestion of enzymes in the human body. Synthetic absorbable sutures are degraded by hydrolysis, in which the water gradually permeates into the suture filaments to cause decomposition of the polymer chain. Compared with the natural absorbable sutures, degradation products of synthetic absorbable sutures after implantation cause lighter tissue reactions.
Absorbable sutures are used for suture embedding without being removed since most of their tensile strength is lost in 60 days. Nonabsorbable suture: normally its tensile strength can be retained for over 60 days, hence it is usually used for tendon suture and sometimes needs to be removed after operation.
(d) Monofilament and multifilament sutures: the monofilament suture is made of a single bunch of filament which encounters less resistance as it passes through the tissue, and can also prevent bacteria from adhering to it. Thus, it is suitable for vascular surgery or contaminated wound suturing. Monofilament sutures are easy to knot, but of less strength, and may break in case of suture folding or curling during ligation.
Refer to Table 14.2 for materials and characteristics of surgical sutures, and Tables 14.3 and 14.4 for suture name, hand feeling in surgery, etc. of absorbable and nonabsorbable sutures accordingly.

3. **Principles and strategies of suture selection**

(a) Principles of suture selection

Table 14.2 Material types and characteristics of surgical sutures

Types of suture	Characteristics	Example
Natural	Digested by enzymes in the human body, greater tissue reaction	Catgut, chromic catgut
Synthetic	Greater tension, smaller tissue reaction	Absorbable suture
Monofilament	Bacteria are not easy to adhere, little tissue pulling	PDS II suture, fishing suture
Multifilament sutures	Easy to knot; good tensile strength; if coated, it has the same characteristics of monofilament	Silk, absorbent braided wire
Absorbable	Nothing remained in body	Predictive absorbent suture
Nonabsorbable	Suitable for wound requiring permanent support	Achilles tendon retention suture

Table 14.1 Conversion of suture diameter specified in United States Pharmacopeia (USP)

USP specifications	10 ~ 0	9 ~ 0	8 ~ 0	7 ~ 0	6 ~ 0	5 ~ 0	4 ~ 0	3 ~ 0	2 ~ 0	1 ~ 0	1	2
EP	0.2	0.3	0.4	0.5	0.7	1.0	1.5	2.0	3.0	3.5	4.0	5.0
Traditional Chinese specifications	–	–	–	–	5 ~ 0	3 ~ 0	1 ~ 0	1	4	7	–	–

Table 14.3 Synthetic absorbable suture

Suture name	Hand feeling in surgery	Tension left	Firmness of knot	Tissue reaction	Absorption time	Clinical application
Vicryl Plus® sutures (Polyglactin 910), multifilament sutures	Good	Tension disappears at fourth week	Good	Slight	56–70 days	Fascia, muscle, and subcutaneous tissue
PDS plus antibacterial sutures (Polydioxanone) monofilament	Fair	Tension retains 50–70% at fourth week	Good	Slight	180–210 days	Fascia, muscle, subcutaneous tissue, or contaminated subcutaneous tissue that requires high strength support
MONOCRYL® plus antibacterial unidirectional suture (Polycaprolactam) monofilament	Good	Tension disappears at third week	Good	Slight	91–119 days	Intradermal continuous suture

Table 14.4 Nonabsorbable suture

Suture name	Type	Hand feeling in surgery	Tension left	Firmness of knot	Tissue reaction	Clinical application
Natural						
Silk	Braided/twisted	Very good	No tension after 1 year	Good	Moderate	Vascular ligation
Synthetic nonabsorbable suture						
Nylon/ETHILON®	Monofilament	Fair	Tension retains 20% after 1 year	Fair	Slight	Skin suturing
PROLENE® (polypropylene)	Monofilament	Fair	Permanent support	Poor	Slight	Skin suture
ETHIBOND® (polyester)	Multifilament	Very good	Permanent support	Good	Slight	Skin suture
Stainless steel suture	Monofilament	Poor	Permanent support	Good	Slight	Bone retention

A desired suture shall be the finest one compatible with the strength of the tissue to be sutured and can provide sufficient tension during healing; it shall have high wear resistance or cutting force and favorable histocompatibility, and will not easily lead to adverse effect (like irritability or carcinogenesis); anti-infectious materials can prevent bacteria from adhering, reproducing, and spreading, and finally be absorbed by the body without leaving any trace. Up to now, no suture can have all these characteristics. In surgery, suture materials with different characteristics need to be selected for tissue suturing in line with the occasion based upon features of the sutured tissue.

Following factors shall be considered first for operation safety concern: ① Tensile strength of the suture shall match up with the tension of sutured tissue to ensure that the wound is healed in a tension-free environment; tensile strength of the suture needs not to exceed the intrinsic tension of the tissue, but shall at least be comparable to that of the sutured tissue. ② Deformability: certain ductility to cope with postoperative tissue edema, and certain flexibility to adapt to postoperative tissue contraction. ③ The suture shall be as fine as possible to minimize rejection reaction in the body, but a fine suture may easily cut the tissue if the wound tension is very high. ④ Comparable to tissue healing speed: decline speed of the suture's tensile strength shall be no faster than the recovery speed of tissue tension. ⑤ Suture quality: suture shall be soft and smooth and feel nice; it shall not drag the tissue during suturing, and be easy to knot and slide; be stored in an aseptic package, and easy to use.

(b) Strategies of suture selection

I. Features of sutured tissue: for slow-to-heal tissues (such as tendons), nonabsorbable sutures shall be selected. For quick-to-heal tissue (skin wounds), absorbable sutures can be taken into consideration. Absorbable sutures are especially good choices for subcutaneous soft tissue since it is easily subject to infection, foreign body reaction, and "thread end extrusion" as a result of poor blood supply.

II. Sutured site: finer absorbable suture with little irritation to tissue, or sutures made from the finest non-reaction monofilament suture materials (such as nylon, polypropylene) can be selected for sutured sites including head and face (eyelid, nose, auricle, lip, etc.) which have lower demands for suture's tensile strength but higher esthetic requirements for the suture and for which foreign body reaction of the suture must be prevented during tissue healing.

Any foreign body in high-concentration crystalloid solution may impel the formation of sediment and stone. Absorbable sutures shall be applied to urinary tract and biliary tract surgery.

Tendon or flap is usually closed under high tension, and hence nonabsorbable sutures are needed in order to retain tensile strength for a long time after the operation.

III. Considerations of clinical treatment (Table 14.5): a suture is a foreign body embedded in the body; hence, it may induce an organism to have a rejection reaction. A suture itself will not cause infection, but it may become a carrier to which bacteria attach. Bacteria will reproduce as soon as they have found a carrier, which may result in infection as a certain amount of bacteria have been reproduced. Besides, a foreign body in the tissue will turn a contaminated wound into an infected one. For an open wound or a contaminated wound having potential risk of infection, some other factors in addition to suture strength shall be considered in selecting a suture, for example, a multifilament suture is easier to become a carrier of bacteria compared with a monofilament. Therefore, monofilaments or absorbable sutures shall be used to suture a contaminated wound that has the potential risk of infection.

14.1.2 Surgical Suture Needle

Materials from which a surgical suture needle is made shall have: sufficient strength and sharpness, and can pass through the tissue with minimal resistance; certain ductility to make sure it will not break under pressure. Since the 1960s, high-nickel stainless steel alloy has been applied to the manufacturing of surgical suture needles in order to meet the requirements of surgical suture needles for high strength and ductility. Stainless steel alloy contains 12% of chromium. A thin protective layer of chromic oxide with good corrosion resistance will take shape on the surface of a suture needle

Table 14.5 Selection of orthopedic sutures

Tissue name	Suture name	Specification	Model	Multifilament absorbable suture	Knotless barbed suture	Characteristics
Achilles tendon	Nonabsorbable polyester suture	2#	W4843			Greater tension, permanent support, less damage
Patellar fracture suture	Nonabsorbable polyester suture	5#	MB66G			Greater tension, sharper orthopedic suture needle, bone-penetrable
Attachment point for tendon and bone	Nonabsorbable polyester suture	2#	X519H			Greater tension, sharper orthopedic suture needle, bone-penetrable
Securing of tendon attachment points around prosthesis	Nonabsorbable polyester suture	5#	MB66G			Greater tension, sharper orthopedic suture needle
Peripheral soft tissue of Achilles tendon	Multifilament absorbable suture	3/0		VCP311H	SXPD2B408	Antibacterial, less foreign body being left in body
Muscle/fascia (thigh)	Multifilament absorbable suture	0#		VCP358H VCP752D	SXPP1A405	Antibacterial, greater tension, absorbable, sharper needle
Muscle/fascia (upper extremity, shank)	Multifilament absorbable suture	2/0		VCP345H VCP751D	SXPP1A404	Antibacterial, greater tension, absorbable, sharper needle
Subcutaneous tissue (upper extremity)	Multifilament absorbable suture	3/0		VCP311H VCP738D VCPB839D	SXPD2B419 SXPP2B419	Absorbable, prevent irritation by foreign body, no thread end extrudes, antibacterial
Subcutaneous tissue (lower extremity)	Multifilament absorbable suture	2/0		VCP345H VCP751D VCPBB839	SXPD2B408 SXPP2B408	Absorbable, prevent irritation by foreign body, no thread end extrudes, antibacterial
Skin	Monofilament absorbable suture	3/0		VCP442H	SXMD2B407	Antibacterial, greater tension, noninvasive, easy to knot
Skin	Polypropylene monofilament nonabsorbable suture	3/0	W8625			Continuously suturing, nonabsorbable, sophisticated reverse cutting needle, esthetic suturing

being exposed to air. Nowadays surgical suture needles are mainly made from stainless steel alloys of high strength and ductility as well as good corrosion resistance.

Surgical suture needles are in different shapes and sizes. The diameter of the needle body matches the dimension of the suture. Up to now, there is no clinical guideline for surgical suture needles. The basic consensus is that the diameter of the needle body shall be as small as possible. Suture needles are selected according to suturing manner, sutured site, and personal experience provided that "suture material is pulled through sutured tissue with minimal trauma."

1. **Structure of suture needle**

   A surgical suture needle is composed of the point, the body, and the swage (Fig. 14.1).

(a) The point: the sharpest section from the sharpest end to the section with the maximum cross-section in the body, which is used to go through the tissue.
(b) The body: the middle section of a suture needle.
(c) The swage: the thickest section of a suture needle where the thread is attached.

2. **Characteristic terms of surgical suture needle**

   Acting force on the point of the suture needle is associated with factors including curvature (diameter) of a needle, geometry of the point, and stainless-steel alloy material. The characteristics are represented by parameters including bending moment, ultimate moment, surgical-yield moment, and needle ductility.

(a) Strength: suture needle's resistance to deformation during passing through tissue; increased needle strength results in decreased tissue trauma; ultimate moment refers to the force required to bend the needle to 90°; surgical-yield moment refers to the maximum external force a needle can withstand in operation before permanent deformation.
(b) Ductility: resistance (of a needle) to breakage under a given amount of deformation or bending.
(c) Sharpness: the ability of the suture needle to penetrate tissue; factors affecting sharpness include the angle (20°–35°) of the point and the body and the taper ratio [i.e., ratio of needle diameter to needle length, usually (1–5): 1]. The needle is sharper if it has a higher taper ratio and a lower angle between the point and the body. The stronger tissue penetrability is, the less collateral damage a needle will cause to the tissue.
(d) Clamping moment: used to evaluate the stability of a suture needle in a needle holder: the interaction of the jaw between the needle and the needle holder.
(e) Chord length: linear distance from needlepoint to swage (Fig. 14.2).
(f) Needle length: curved length of suture needle from needlepoint to swage measured along needle body. The length indicated on the package of a suture is the needle length, not chord length.
(g) Radius: distance from suture needle body to its center of curvature.

3. **Types of suture needle**

(a) According to the shape of cross-section at the needlepoint, suture needles can be classified into: round needle; cutting needle (sharp, usually for skin suturing); taper cutting needle; shovel needle (mainly for ophthalmic surgery); blunt needle.

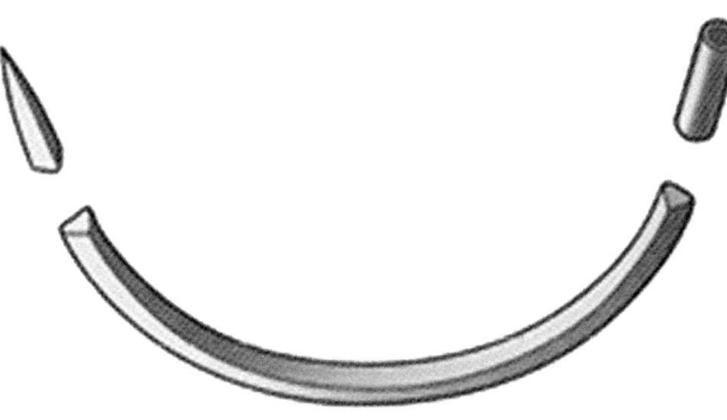

Fig. 14.1 Structure of suture needle

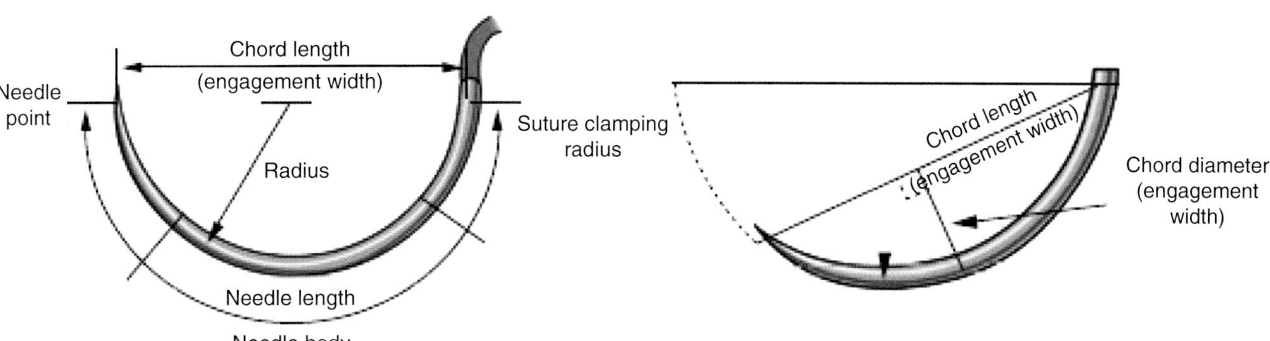

Fig. 14.2 Description of needle characteristics

Table 14.6 Types of needle arc and scope of application

6 types of needle	Applicable site
Straight needle	Gastrointestinal tract/tendon/skin
1/4 arc	Ophthalmic surgery and microsurgery
3/8 arc	Cardiovascular system/pulmonary vascular/skin/ophthalmology
1/2 arc	Gastrointestinal tract/tendon/muscle/cardiovascular system/pulmonary vascular
5/8 arc	Genitourinary tract/cardiovascular system/pelvic cavity/laparoscopic puncture suturing

(b) According to circle arc: 1/2 arc; 3/8 arc (usually for skin suturing); 5/8 arc; straight needle; 1/4 arc (usually for ophthalmic surgery) (Table 14.6).

(c) According to diameter of suture body: the curvature of the body is commonly 2/8 circle, 3/8 circle, 4/8 circle, 5/8 circle, or corresponding needle diameter: 0.25, 0.375, 0.5, 0.625 inch.[1] 3/8 circle (0.375 inch) suture needles are often used for skin suturing, while 4/8 circle (0.5 inch) needles are designed for suturing in confined spaces to adapt to a surgeon's bigger wrist movement.

14.1.3 Needle Holder

1. **Selection of appropriate needle holders**
   (a) The maximum bending moment a suture needle can sustain shall exceed the resultant force of clamping force applied by a needle holder to a suture needle and the force acting on sutured tissue, or otherwise, the needle will be subject to bending and deflection easily during suturing. Suturing tissue with a suture needle being bent out of shape will not only cause extra damage to sutured tissue but also make the needle break easily. Breakage of a suture needle during suturing of deep tissue often means extra time and energy to be spent, and even intraoperative radioscopy needs to be utilized to find the broken needle.
   (b) Compared with a suture needle: if a needle holder is too big, the suture may deform easily during operation and straighten the curved arc of a needle. If a needle is too small, the suture needle will spin along the long shaft of the needle holder.

2. **Mastering the correct method of holding needle**
   (a) Usage of needle holder

Surgeons use needle holders to control suture needles. Jaws of the needle holder shall match up with dimensions of a needle, and the contact point between the needle holder and needle shall be at the thick oval position on the needle body, i.e., 1/3 ~ 1/2 of the needle length, so that the contact area between the needle holder and suture is the biggest, which is favorable for the needle holder to control suture needle stably, and prevent the needle from moving and turning in the course of tissue suturing. The suture needle shall be perpendicular to the needle holder, and the needle holder needs to hold the suture needle until initial engagement and fixation are realized instead of clenching the needle tightly during suturing. Holding the needle holder improperly will easily lead to deformation or breakage of the suture needle during operations.

(b) Mastering the correct method of holding needle holder

Put thumb and ring finger into rings of the needle holder, and index finger on the needle holder to hold it steadily, or grip the whole needle holder in the palm to improve operation flexibility (Fig. 14.3).

3. **Standard operation procedures**
   (a) Keep operational view clear: pull skin by virtue of toothed or toothless skin retractors to reveal operational view steadily and clearly. The suture shall be free from too high tension during suturing to prevent tissue strangulation and necrosis.
   (b) Operational details: angle of needle insertion shall be perpendicular to the skin to reduce the size of needle insertion hole and prevent the skin margin from inverting. Position and depth of needle insertion hole depend on thickness of skin to be sutured. The hole is commonly 1–3 mm away from the wound edge and bilaterally symmetric, and the angle of needle insertion shall be perpendicular to the skin surface.

The needle holder shall keep clamping the needle until the needle is away from the wound. This detail in operation is crucial since earlier unclamping of needle holder may result in small needles dropping in deep wounds.

14.1.4 Selection of Surgical Gloves

Surgeons shall wear cornstarch-free sterile gloves during suturing. Cornstarch commonly used for gloves has been proven to be able to induce wound infection, or result in severe peritoneal adhesion and granulomatous peritonitis, and irritate surgeons' skin to cause latex allergic dermatitis. In 2008, 13 health experts submitted an expert recommendation to the U.S. Food and Drug Administration (FDA) to require cornstarch to be banned on medical gloves.

[1] 1 inch = 2.54 cm

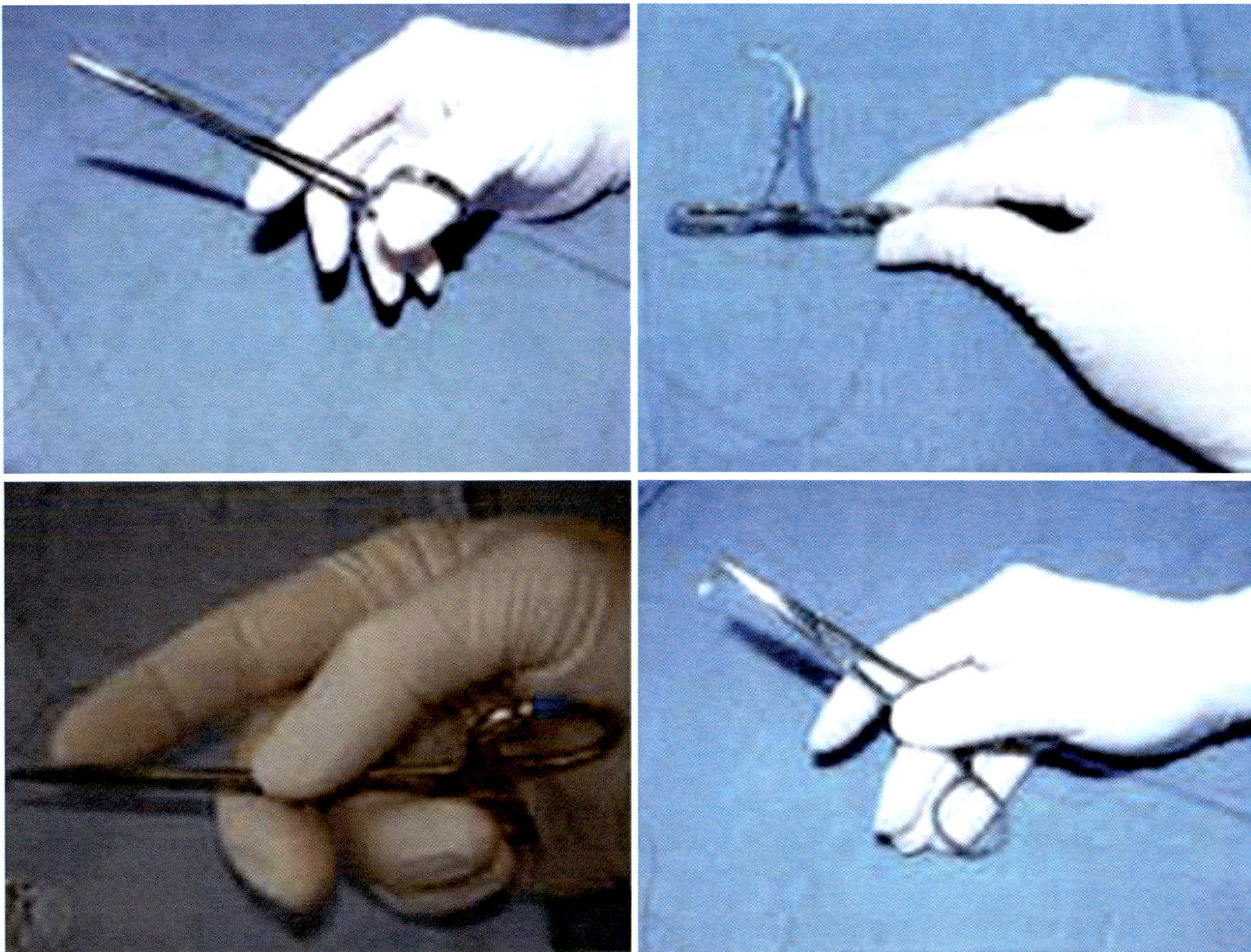

Fig. 14.3 Correct way to hold needle holder

FDA allows holes on 1.5% of surgical gloves in quality control standards of glove manufacturing. As a result, the use of surgical gloves cannot prevent surgeons from directly contacting patients' body fluids, which has increased surgeons' occupational exposure risk of being infected by blood-borne virus. Hospitals can use biogel puncture indicator system to check if there is any hole on gloves or use two pairs of gloves during operations if possible. In surgery, gloves must be replaced timely after being pierced by a suture needle or fracture fragment.

14.2 Common Orthopedic Suture Knots

14.2.1 Structure of a Suture Knot

1. Bight refers to the loose section being bent into a U shape between both ends of a suture. The procedural term "in the bight" implies that a suture has been bent into U shape and is ready for knotting.
2. Both ends of a suture are called limbs or threads, which are working ends of suture knotting.
3. Loop refers to a complete circular ring formed as the working ends of a suture go across the suture.
4. Elbow refers to two intersections taking shape as a complete loop twists for another time. The diameter of a loop depends on the degree of separation among tissue to be sutured.
5. Turn implies that a suture goes across the sutured tissue once, or passes through the sutured tissue from the middle. Round arc forms as a suture goes cross or passes through the sutured tissue twice, and can fully enfold the sutured tissue. Similarly, biarc needs to go across or pass through the sutured tissue three times.
6. Standing end or post limb refers to suture ends in resting state during knotting. A knot-tying line maintains stability since it has been pulled and under tension all the time. The other strand is wrapped with the knot-tying line to form a suture loop for knotting. The standing section lies between a suture knot and post limb.

7. The working end is a post limb to be wrapped with a suture, a suture end involved in the formation of a suture knot, also called "sliding end." "Working section of a suture" lies between a suture knot and working end.
8. A half hitch is a half-complete knot that forms a suture circle by wrapping the sliding end of a suture to the standing end, then the sliding end will pass through the suture circle. A single half hitch is insecure and can be untied easily.
9. Wrap or throw: first wrap one strand of a double-stranded suture with the other to tie an overhand knot, and then continuously tie the same kind or different kinds of overhand knots at the working end. Multiple overhand knots constitute a compact wrap or throw.
10. Neck refers to the transitional section between the suture knot and suture circle.
11. Ears refer to the remaining section at the ends of a suture upon completion of knotting. Too short ears will reduce the stability of the knot, and too long ones may irritate peripheral tissue (Fig. 14.4).

14.2.2 Types of Suture Knot

Knotting techniques can be classified into two kinds: hand knotting and instrument (needle holder) knotting. Operational points for instrument knotting technique: clamp a suture needle with pliers of the needle holder, and form a suture loop around the needle holder, and note to keep tension on both sides of the suture the same all the time.

Common knots used for orthopedic surgery can be roughly classified into: sliding knot (dynamic knot) and non-sliding knot (static knot).

Static knot/non-sliding knot—If a suture cannot slide freely without friction or the tissue to be sutured is relatively loose, pulling the suture heavily to achieve approximation of sutured tissue may result in tissue cutting or suture breakage. In order to avoid such cases, first, make sutured tissue approach and join with each other, maintain stability of the suture by virtue of a static knot to facilitate tissue healing in a tension-free environment.

1. **Square knot**

Also referred to as reef knot, one of the base knots commonly used during operations. Square knots are tied following wrapping both ends of a suture with each other. This knot is easy to tie and will not slip easily (Figs. 14.5, 14.6 and 14.7).

Square knots are often used for ligating smaller blood vessels and direct knotting when suturing tissue of lower tension. For tissue having higher tension, a square knot will be transformed into a half hitch sliding knot to realize tissue approximation in high-tension sites; or a knot loop can be clamped with a needle holder upon completion of the first suture loop to prevent the knot loop from slipping until the second suture loop in the reverse direction is done and tightened. The direction in which the needle holder holds a suture knot loop shall be parallel to the suture knot, and holding the knot in a perpendicular direction will cut the suture.

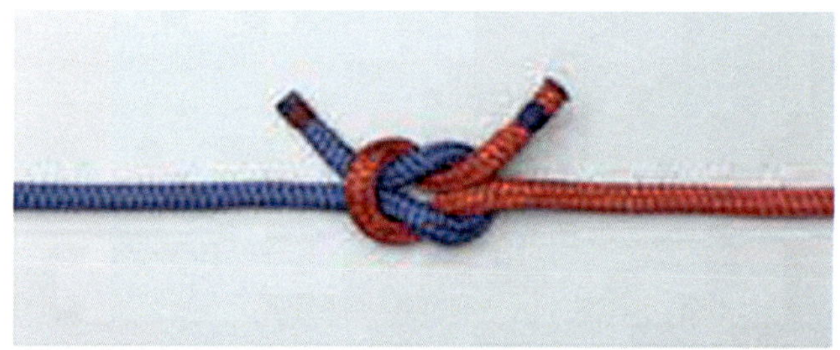

Fig. 14.5 Structure of a square knot

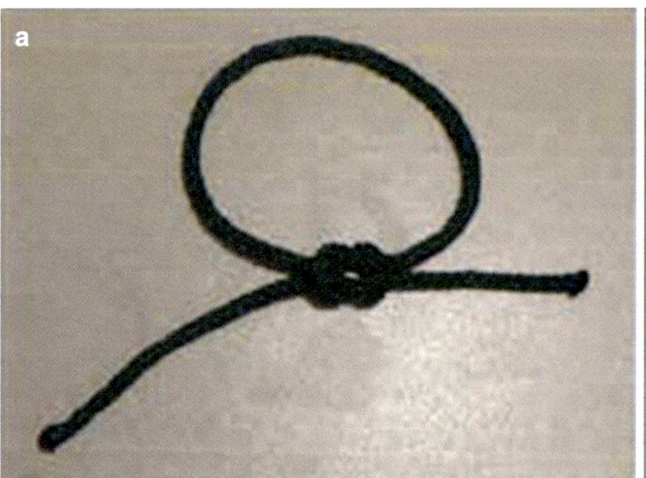

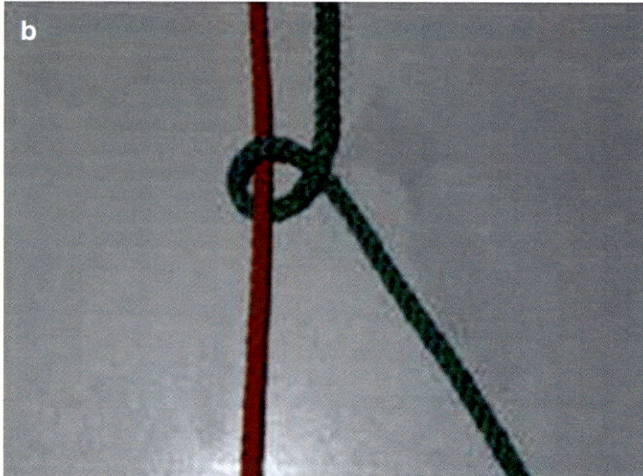

Fig. 14.4 (**a**, **b**) Structure of a suture knot

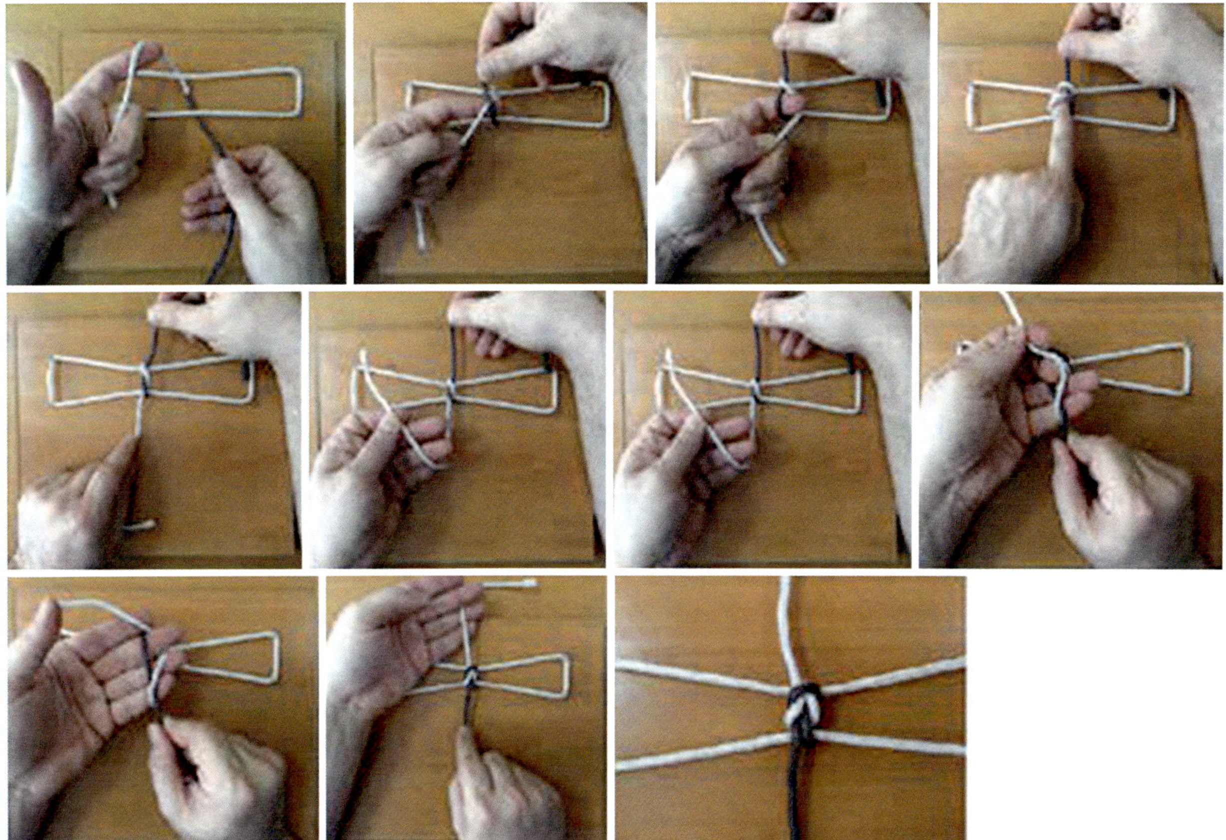

Fig. 14.6 Hand knotting technique for square knot

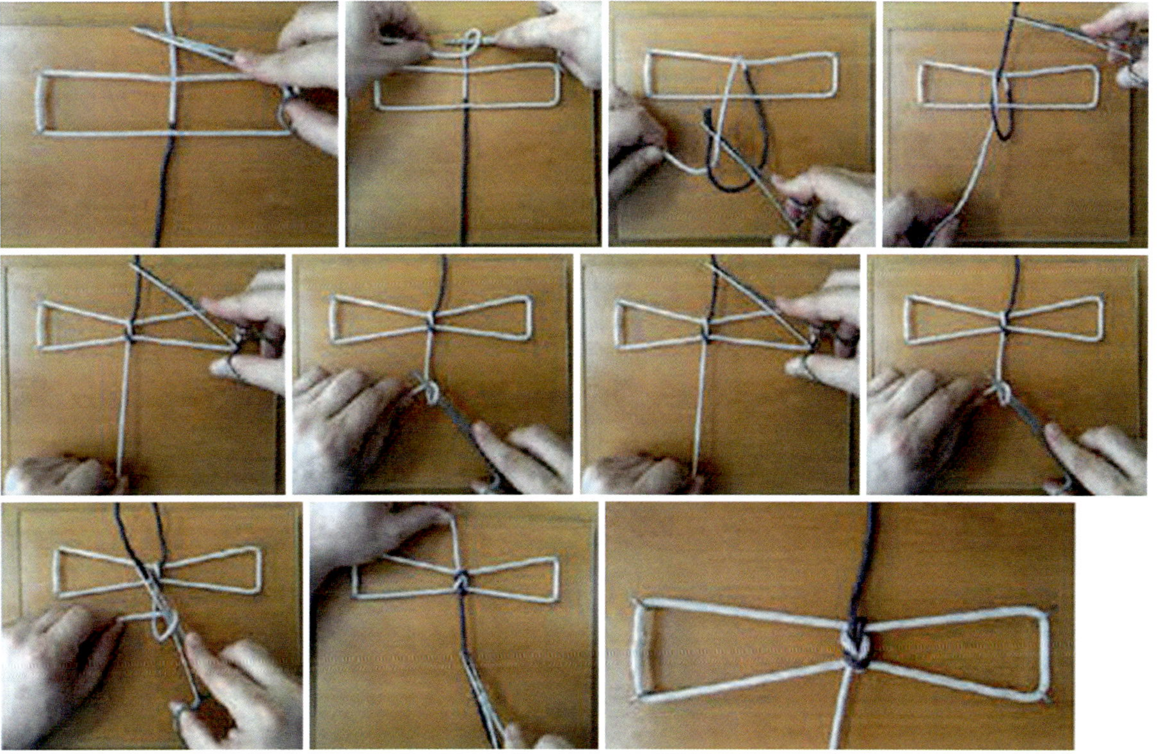

Fig. 14.7 Instrument tie technique for square knot

2. **Surgeon's knot**

As its name implies, a surgeon's knot is the most common knot used by surgeons in suturing wounds. Surgeon's knots have been widely applied in various surgical fields including the department of ENT, gynecology, and obstetrics as well as general surgery. How to improve fixation effectiveness and security during tissue suturing has been a heavily watched topic.

A surgeon's knot is a simplified and improved mode of a square knot, characterized by the sutures being wrapped for another more time when knotting the first basic knot (square knot). Note to wrap strand in correct direction to form a dual overhand knot. Additional suture arc can increase contact area and friction between sutures and the suture knot will not slip or come loose easily when the knot has been tightened. As soon as the first suture loop has been completed and tightened, the wound edges shall be approximated well and tension shall be low among wounds. For local tissue of high tension, another circle can be made. The third suture loop can mitigate the possibility of knot slipping. Surgeon's knots can be used for any kind of suturing of fascia and subcutaneous tissue as well as closing of any skin wound. If a wound raptures, conventional wound closure methods may cause much higher skin tension. Upon completion of the first knot, pull the suture by hands slowly and carefully by turns so that wounds on both sides can approach gradually; or transform a surgeon's knot into a sliding one (Figs. 14.8, 14.9, 14.10 and 14.11).

Keeping sutures parallel and tension on both ends of a suture even during suturing is the basis of fixing a surgeon's knot or square knot successfully.

The suture knot shall be secured after completing a suture loop by wrapping the sutures with each other, and then the suture knot shall be tied in the opposite direction of the former suture knot; otherwise, the suture and suture loop may cross and twist during knotting. It is of great importance to tie each square knot consecutively in a standard manner. Each new knot must be parallel to the last one. After handling the first suture loop, the thread above shall still be above the other when handling the second suture loop, or parallel structure of the suture loop will not be possible, and the knot will become a loose granny knot (Fig. 14.12).

A static knot (square knot or surgeon's knot) can be transformed into a sliding knot by a few simple steps allowing for specific changes in suturing during operations. Tighten the sliding end of a square knot before knot locking, operate two half hitches continuously and the square knot will transform into a sliding slot consisting of two half hitches (Fig. 14.13). Then tie three half hitches by turns on the two strands to lock and secure the knots. Wrap one strand of the suture around the other strand to form two suture loops, which will increase friction between two strands. Some knotting techniques can facilitate security of a square knot as a sliding knot: throughout the knotting process, traction suture shall stay in a tensioned state of being pulled; push the half hitch with the tip of the index finger to the site to be secured, pull the hitch to remove loose section in the suture loop and secure the sliding knot. Then tie several reverse half hitches with the other suture as a sliding line by turns to lock the whole suture knot.

Similarly, a surgeon's knot can be transformed into a sliding knot as well. The surgeon's knot can be advanced to the desired position by index finger or knot pusher once a strand has been secured by pulling. Tension on the pulling line shall be retained all the time in this process. As soon as fracture reduction has satisfactory results, the sliding knot will be locked by the three subsequent alternating half hitches.

3. **Sliding knot**

Sliding knots are usually selected for suturing relatively compact tissue of deep layer or repairing rotator cuff under arthroscope. Sliding knot is a group of different half hitches, forehand/overhand half hitches are fundamental hitches for completing a sliding knot. The knot is characterized by being capable of adjusting tension while knotting, and hence it is also referred to as "dynamic knot." The tissue shall be approximated by pulling suture and then the knot secured by knotting if the tissue to be sutured is dense and the suturing ends are separated from each other. The suture may cut the tissue to be sutured during knotting and fixation firmness of a suture knot will decrease if the suture pulling force is too high or the tissue to be sutured is relatively loose.

Another common mistake occurs in the suturing process of deep tissue. For example, the Revo knot commonly used for arthroscopic surgery is one kind of sliding knot consisting of five half hitches, the knot may retract and the stability of suture knot structure will reduce accordingly if the sliding line is not tightened after the half hitch knots have been advanced to suture knotting position with a knot pusher. In

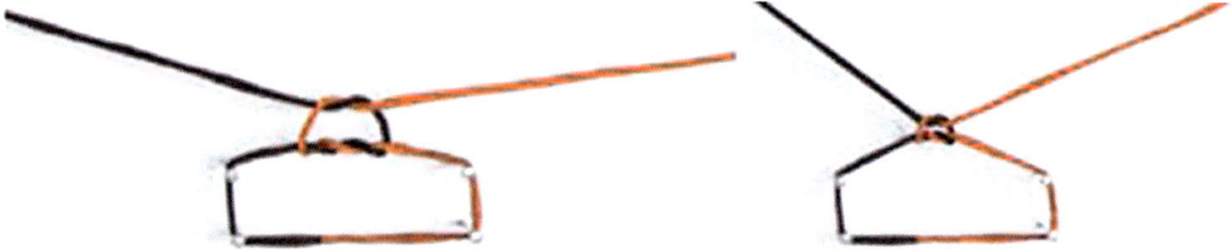

Fig. 14.8 Structure of a surgeon's knot

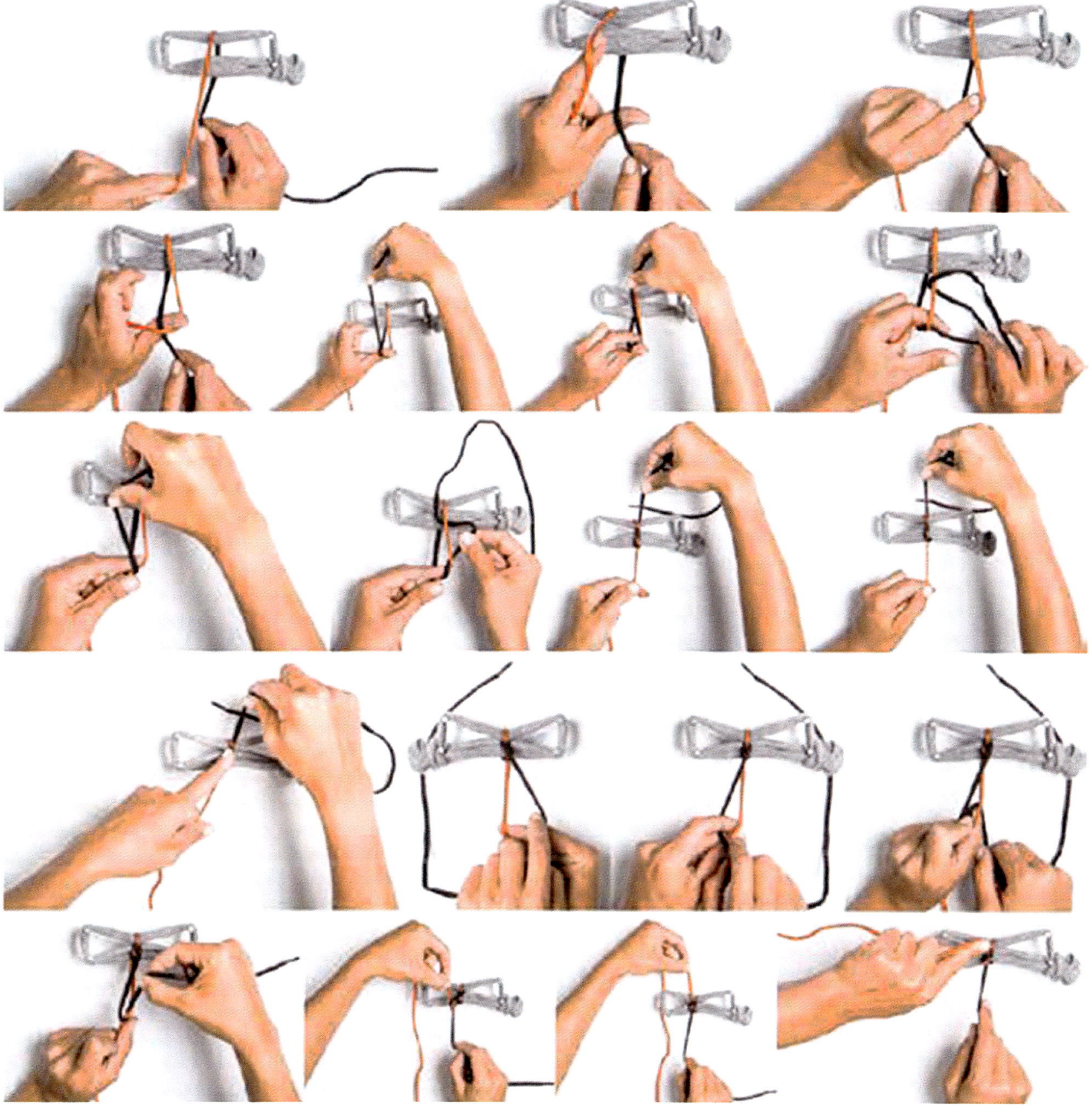

Fig. 14.9 Hand knotting technique for surgeon's knot (I)

order to prevent knot loosening and sliding, it is crucial to ensure that the sliding knot is in the position to be locked. Loosening can be avoided in two ways as follows: tie another non-locking suture loop above the sliding knot which has been completed; lock the sliding knot directly to transform into a non-sliding knot as soon as the sliding knot has been completed.

Sliding knots are usually used for tenodesis or ligaments repair. Besides, to treat an orthopedic trauma, the suture loop technique assisted with sliding knot is vital for assisting reduction and fixation of thrypsis (Fig. 14.14).

Several common sliding knots will be introduced as follows:

(a) Nice knot: invented by Dr. Pascal Boileau, in Nice (France); it was initially used for reducing and fixing greater tubercle for proximal humeral fractures or repairing rotator cuff under arthroscope. The Nice knot is a

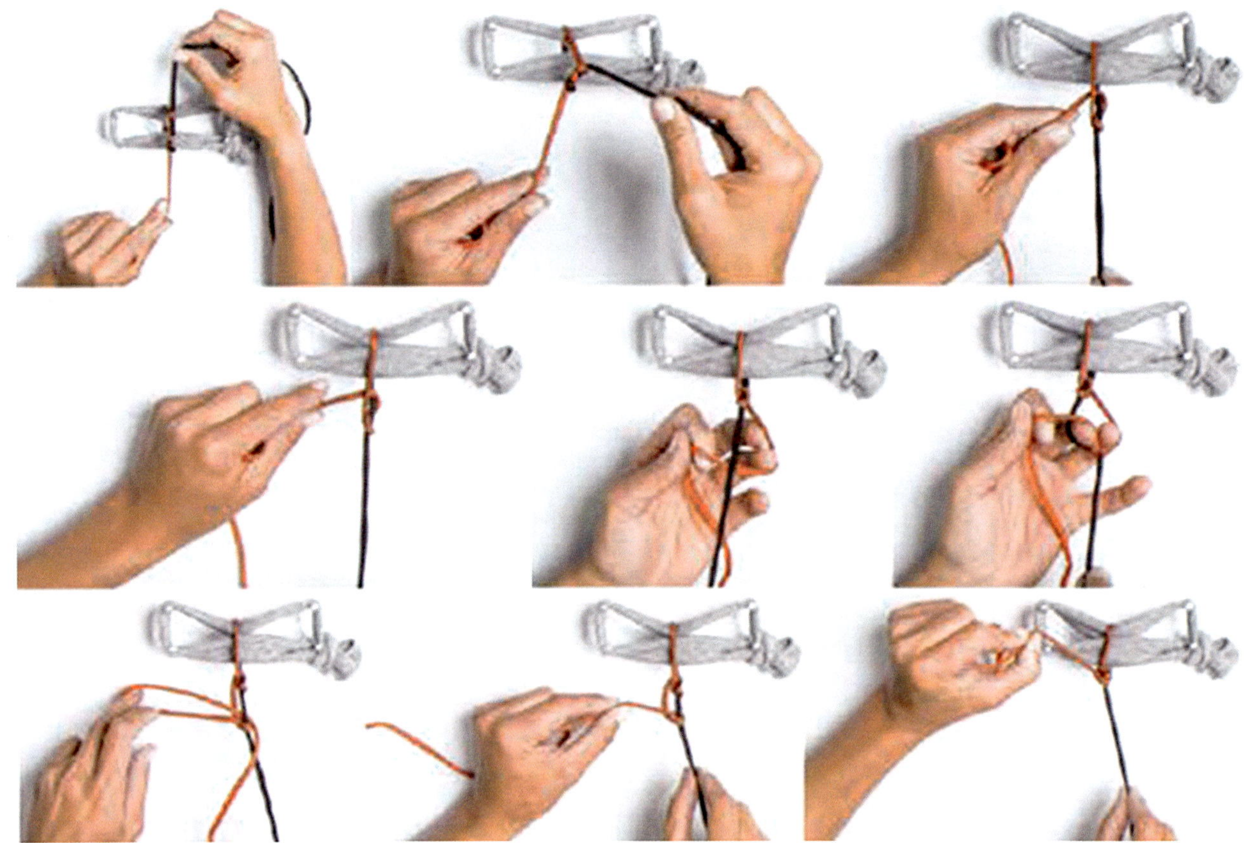

Fig. 14.10 Hand tie technique for surgeon's knot (II)

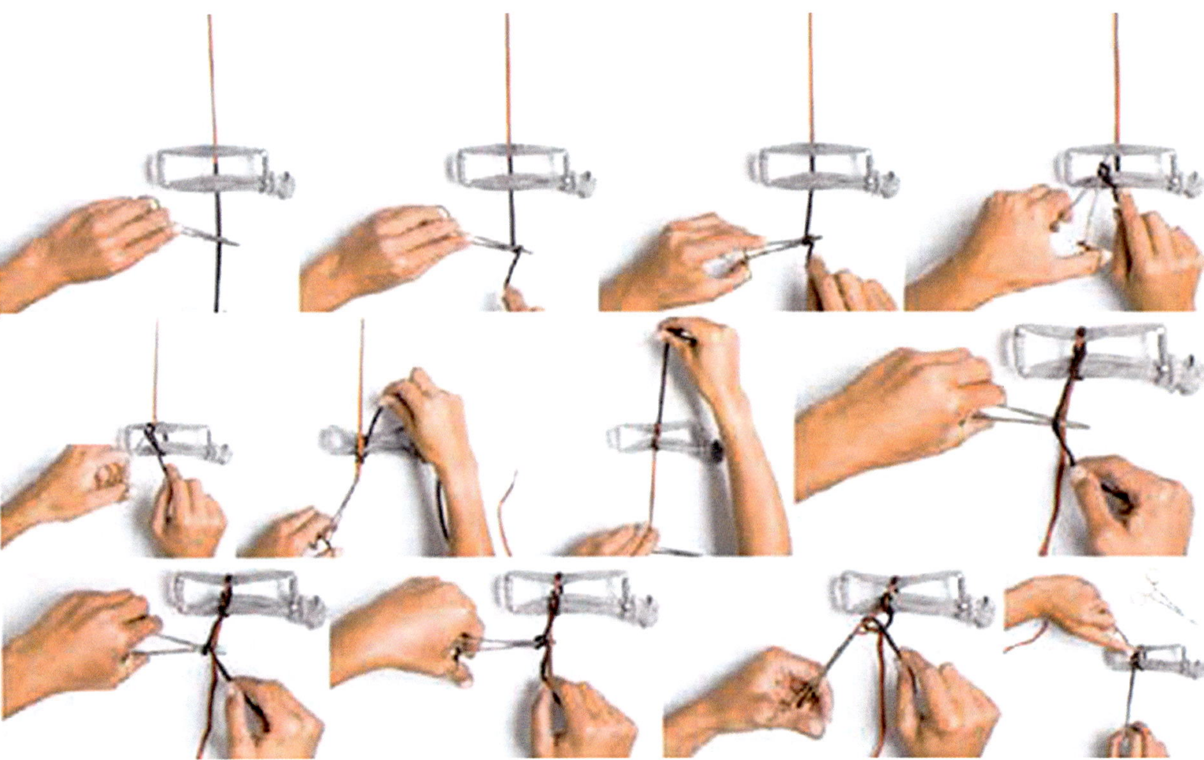

Fig. 14.11 Instrument tie technique for surgeon's knot

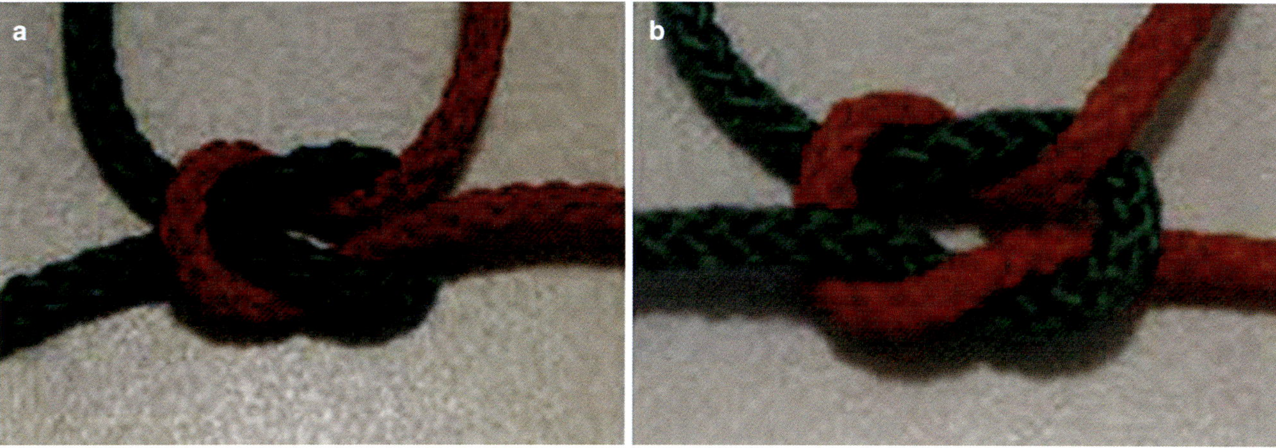

Fig. 14.12 Surgeon's knot. (**a**) Square knot; (**b**) Granny knot

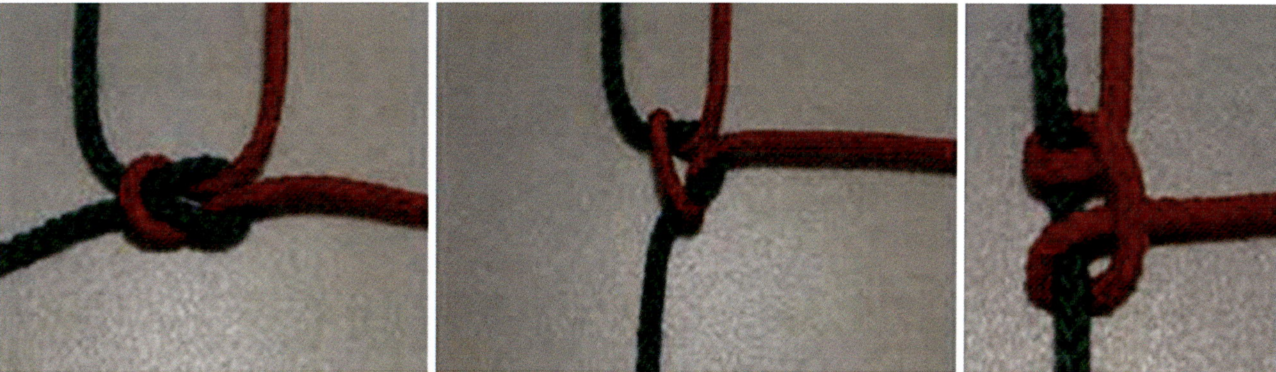

Fig. 14.13 Transformation between square knot and sliding knot

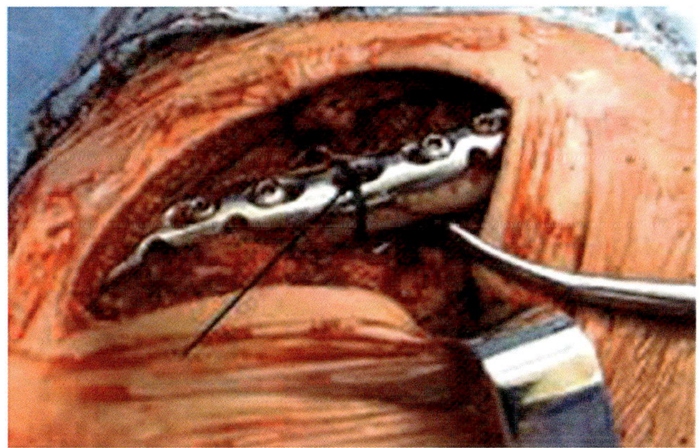

Fig. 14.14 Suture-assisted fixation of clavicle fracture

double-stranded and self-locking high-tension knot. Recent biomechanical studies show that the Nice knot is superior to the surgical knot biomechanically. In practices, the method of "three pairs of alternating half hitches" is often adopted, or the knot can be reduced to two half hitches to ensure that the suture knot will not loosen after being locked.

The knot is of double-stranded structure, with suture end side on the left and bight side on the right. First, wrap the loop side around the suture end side to form an upward overhand knot; then pass the two tail ends of the strand out from the loop; tighten both strands gradually to complete a base knot, and add 3–4 overhand knots if necessary to lock the knot (Figs. 14.15, 14.16, 14.17, 14.18 and 14.19) [6].

(b) Weston knot: described by Dr. Peter Weston, a gynecologist working in San Antonio in Texas, USA in 1991; it can be used as a base knot for continuous suturing. The knot was not initially designed for laparoscopic operation, but now has been used by endoscopists as an elegant sliding knot as it is secure and reliable, small in size, and easy to operate [7].

Knotting method: hold the sliding line with the left thumb and index finger, and knot tying line in the right hand, first adjust the length of a double-stranded suture, a knot-tying line shall twice as long as the sliding line; pass the knot-tying line to the front beneath the straight line, then pass it under the line held in the right hand to complete an upward over-

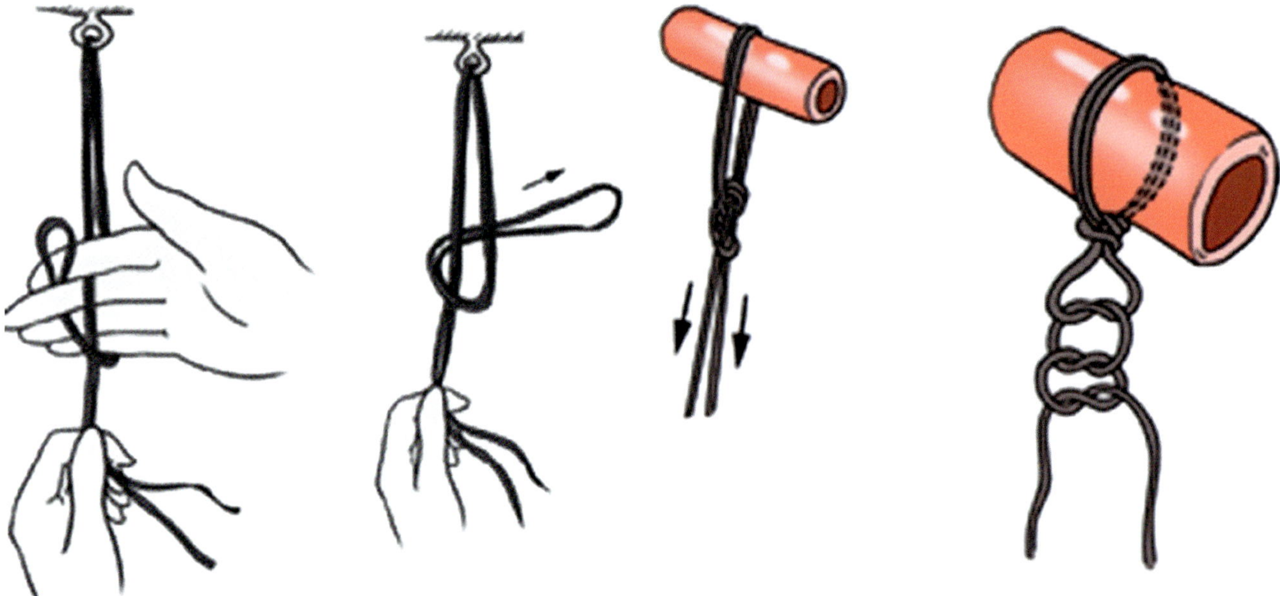

Fig. 14.15 Double-stranded knot, select a long strand for doubling to create the structure characteristic with loop on one side and tie an overhand knot with the two strands

Fig. 14.17 Strain the two tails of the strand gradually so that the knot can slide to tied tissue, then separate the two tail ends, hold one end in each hand and pull hard until the knot is at satisfactory tension, and end the operation by virtue of 3–4 overhand knots

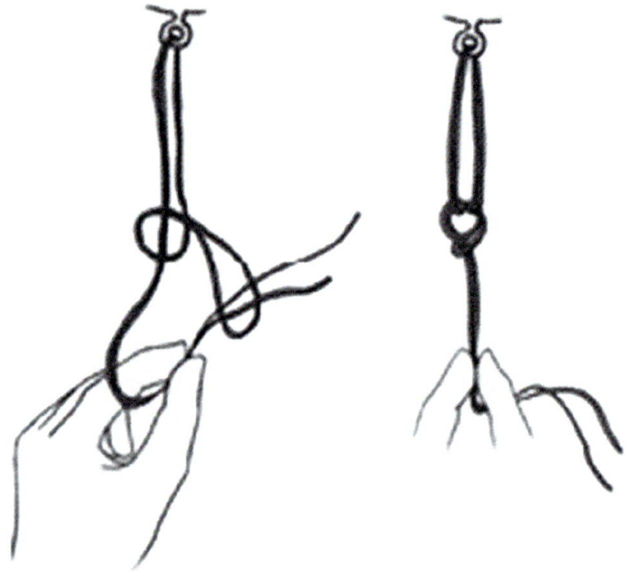

Fig. 14.16 Thread the two tail ends of the strand into the loop to complete the main structure of the knot

hand knot; first wrap the tail end on standing side around the knot-tying line for a half circle anticlockwise, pass it between both lines from front to back, then wrap it around double strands for half a circle clockwise, and pass the tail end through the loop closest to the hand holding the strand from back to front; tighten the suture knot by gradually pulling the straight line in the left hand, with the help of auxiliary knotter, lock the knot by tightening the suture in right hand after pulling the knot to satisfactory tension. Then tie another 3–4 overhand knots to complete final locking (Figs. 14.20, 14.21, 14.22 and 14.23).

During double-row fixation for rotator cuff, first, reduce and fix the lateral structure and then repair medial structure. Weston knot is a low-resistance sliding knot, which is firmer than the Roeder knot if the suture is a braided strand or monofilament (Fig. 14.24).

(c) Hangman's knot: proposed by Seidman et al. in 1999; it is simple yet effective, especially convenient and effective in repairing tissues in small cavities represented by rotator cuff repair [9].

Knotting method: hold the sliding line in the left hand and knot-tying line in the right hand. First, hold a double-stranded line in the left hand and long line in the right hand to make a loop (Fig. 14.25); wrap knot-tying line end along double strands for four circles anticlockwise, and introduce the line end from knot-tying line side (Fig. 14.26); pull the knot-tying line from the line loop close to the side on which the line is held from back to front (Fig. 14.27); gradually tighten the line ends on both sides to lock the loop, and further secure by tying 2–3 overhand knots (Figs. 14.28 and 14.29).

(d) Static surgeon's knot: applicable to repair of tissue structures deep in joints in the lacuna, simple yet effective, and can easily have satisfactory effects [10].

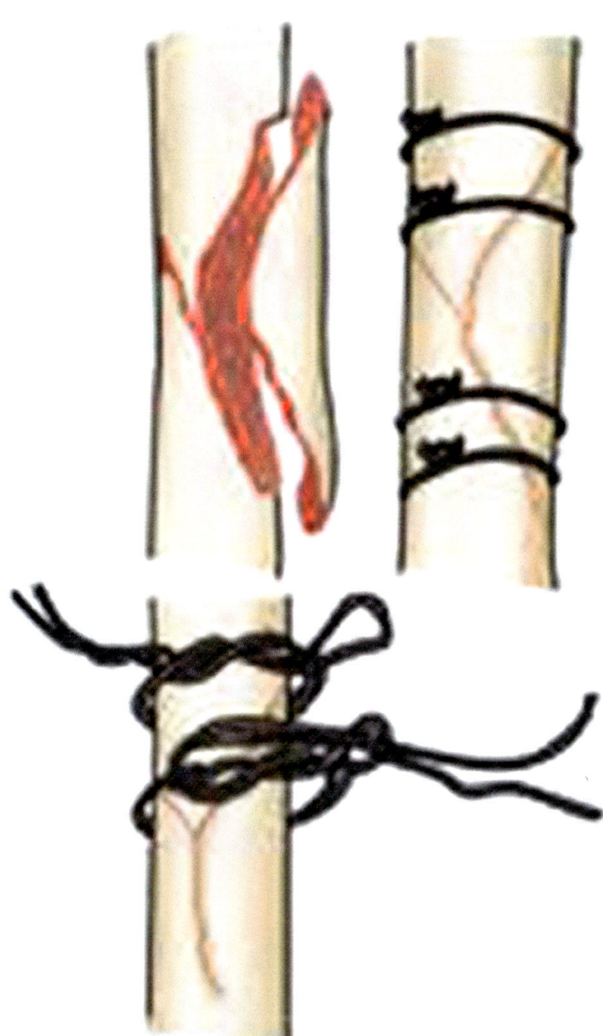

Fig. 14.18 Nice knot-assisted binding of butterfly fracture fragments

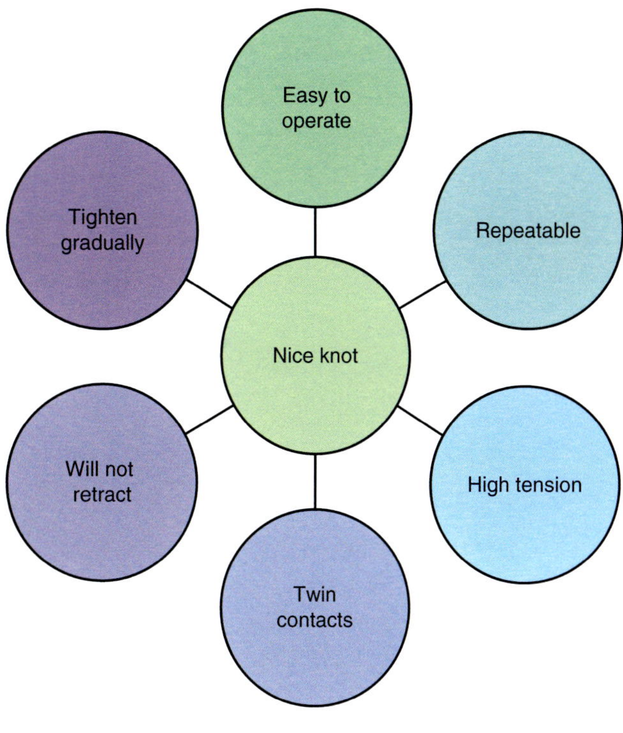

Fig. 14.19 Six features of Nice knot

Knotting method: hold the sliding line in the left hand and knot-tying line in the right hand, wrap the knot-tying line around the sliding line to form three consecutive downward overhand knots (Figs. 14.30, 14.31 and 14.32); then wrap the sliding line around the knot-tying line to make a downward overhand knot and then wrap the knot-tying line around sliding line to make an overhand knot for loop making (Figs. 14.33 and 14.34); and finally wrap sliding line around the knot-tying line to make a downward overhand knot to complete a base knot (Fig. 14.35).

(e) Tennessee Knot: The knot is easy to operate and small in size, suitable for minimally invasive tissue repair in the lacuna [11].

Knotting method: hold the sliding line in the left hand and knot-tying line in the right hand. First, hold the two strands in the left hand, wrap the knot-tying line end along the two

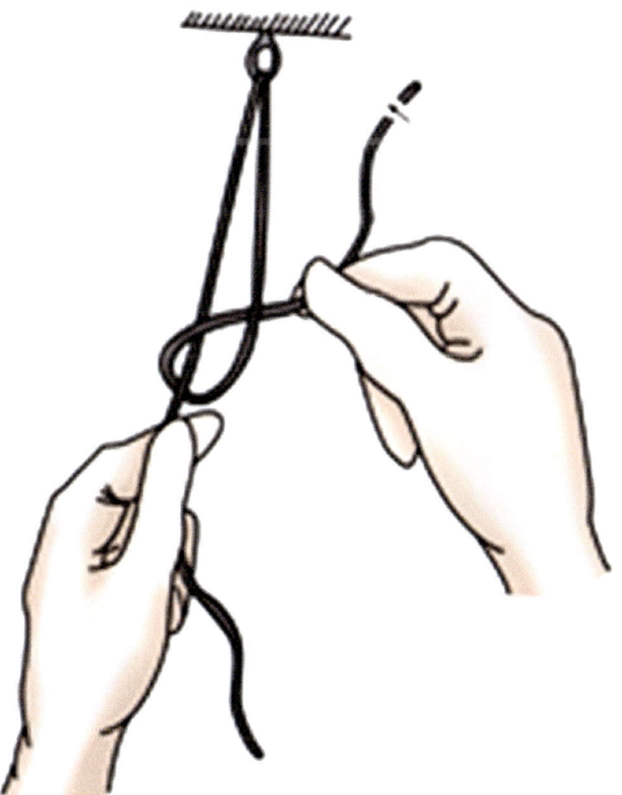

Fig. 14.20 Tie an upward overhand knot with sliding line in left hand and loop line in right hand during knotting

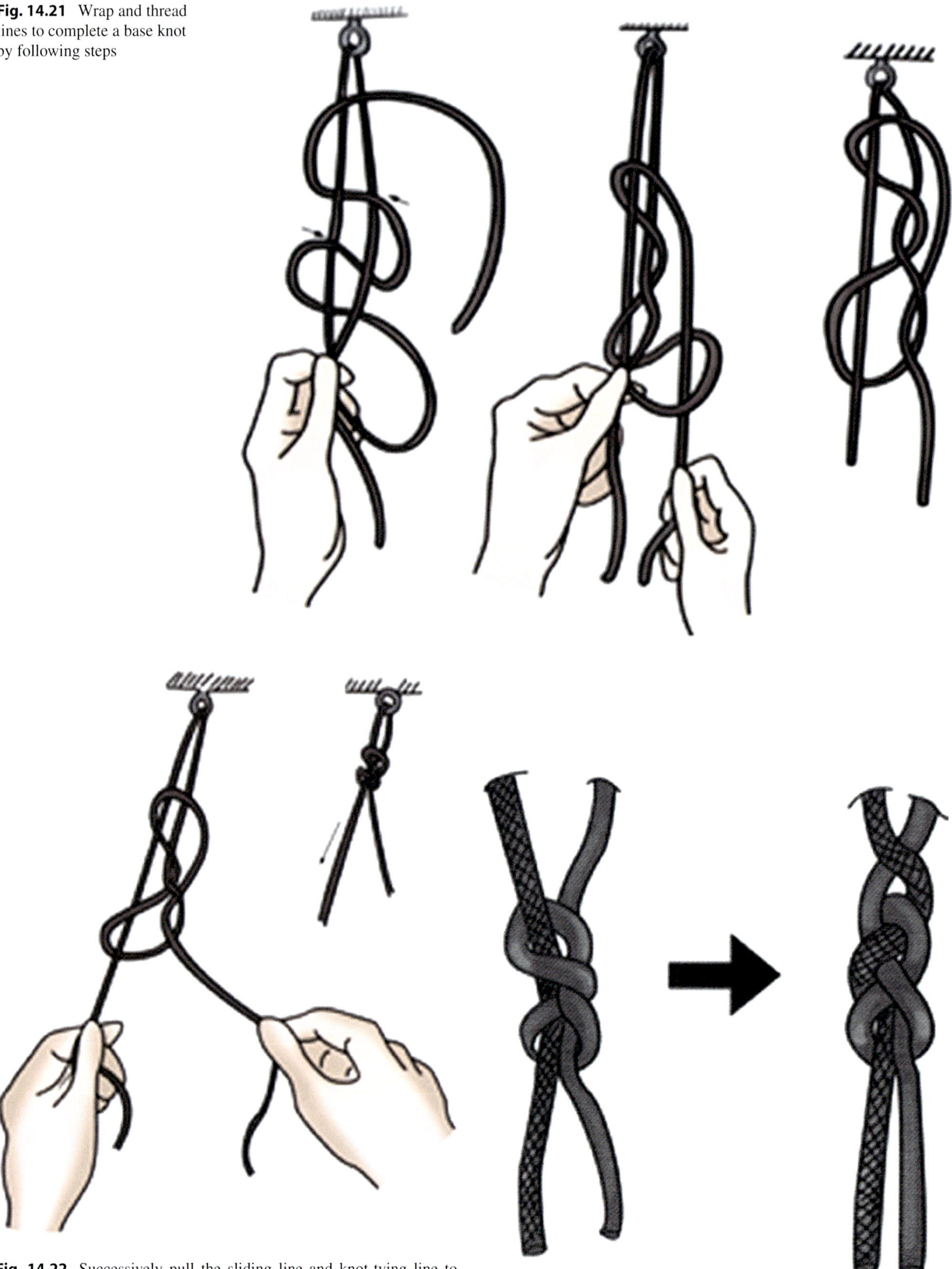

Fig. 14.21 Wrap and thread lines to complete a base knot by following steps

Fig. 14.22 Successively pull the sliding line and knot-tying line to lock the base knot, then tie another 3–4 overhand knots for firm securing

Fig. 14.23 Structure principle of Weston knot

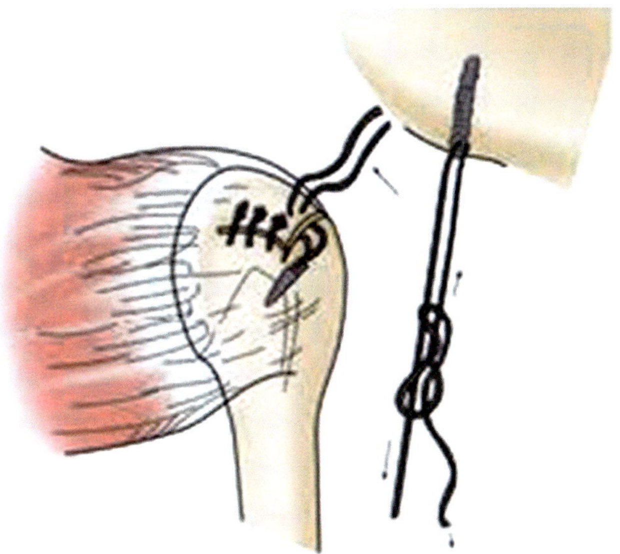

Fig. 14.24 Weston knot is commonly used for repairing rotator cuff injury

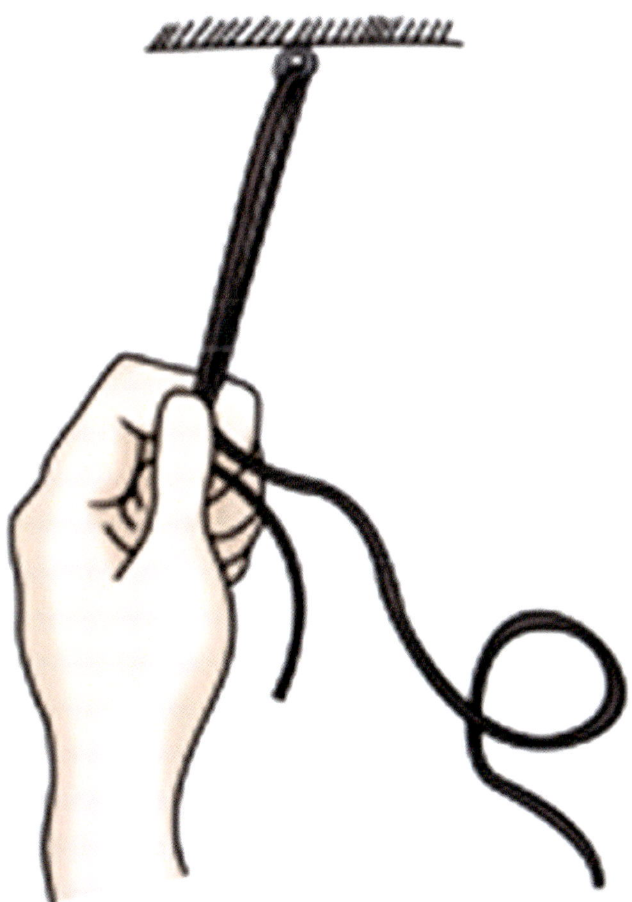

Fig. 14.25 Hold the line by left hand, intend to use knot-tying line for loop

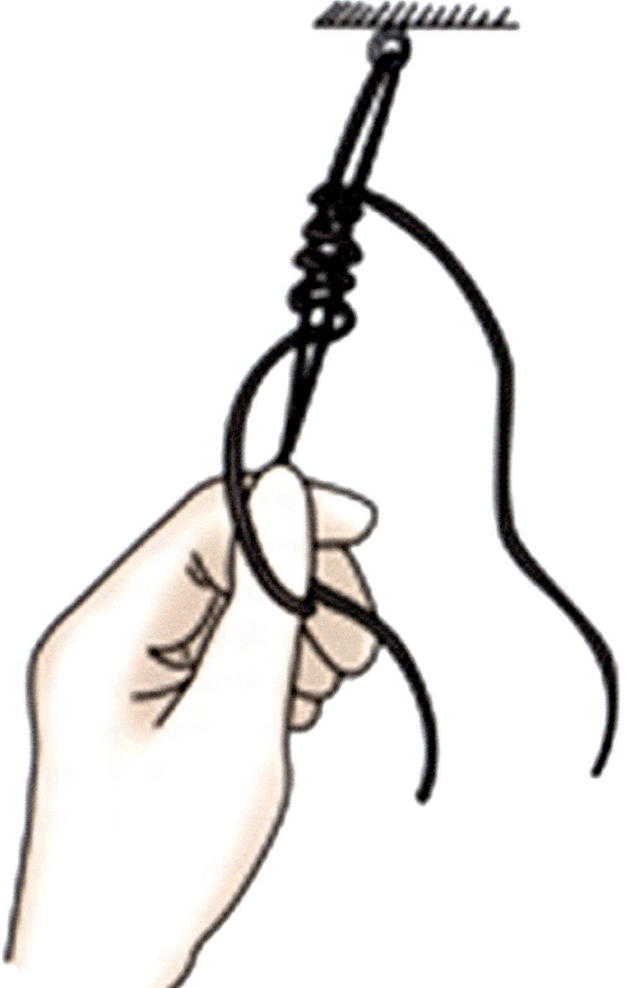

Fig. 14.26 Wrap the knot-tying line around double strands by four circles anticlockwise

strands for one circle clockwise; pass the knot-tying line end from back to front through the two strands. Then pass the knot-tying line end through the first loop on the near-hand side from front to back. Tighten the two strands gradually to complete the base knot. Three to four overhand knots can be performed upon the base knot to achieve securing (Fig. 14.36) [12].

(f) Roeder knot: the earliest slip knot used in arthroscopy surgery; it is simple, effective and practical and there are many improved knotting methods. It is one of the most commonly used knotting methods in surgical operations, more applied in sports medicine.

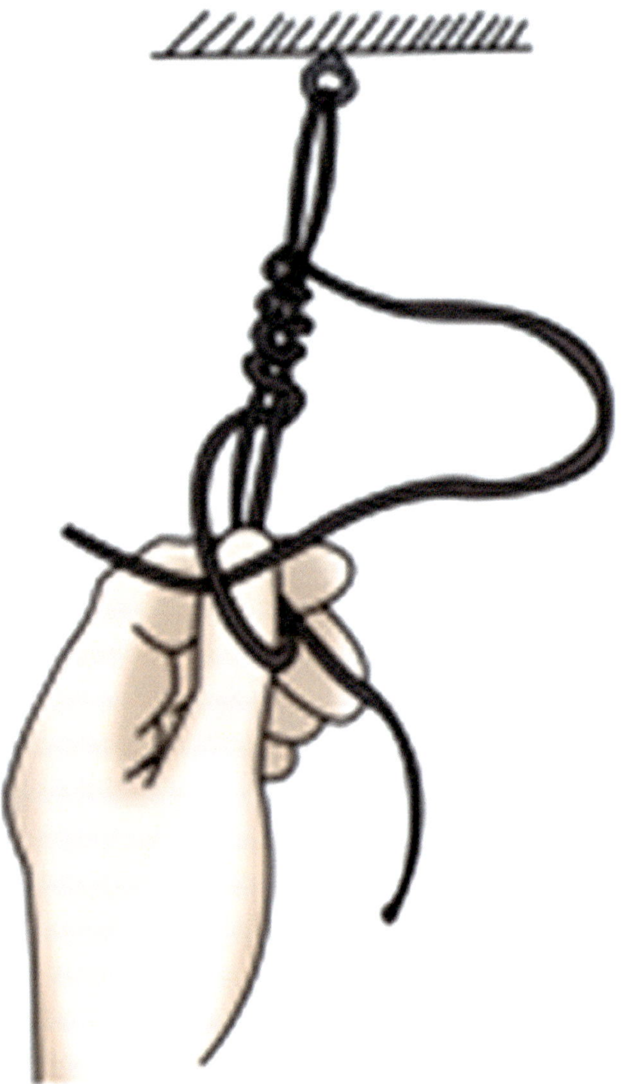

Fig. 14.27 Pass line ends through the loop from top to bottom after wrapping for four circles

Knotting method: hold the sliding line in the left hand and knot-tying line in the right hand. First hold the two strands in the left hand, wrap the tail of the knot-tying line along the two strands for one circle clockwise; pass the tail of the knot-tying line from back to front through the two strands. Then pass the tail of the knot-tying line, further from the other end, through the two strands from front to back. Tighten the two strands gradually to complete the base knot; 3–4 overhand knots can be added upon the base knot to achieve fixation (Fig. 14.37) [13].

(g) SMC knot: first described by Kim SH et al. in a book in 2000; the SMC knot is simple, practical, and is a classic knot in sports medicine. It is also a knot technique used by many well-known domestic experts.

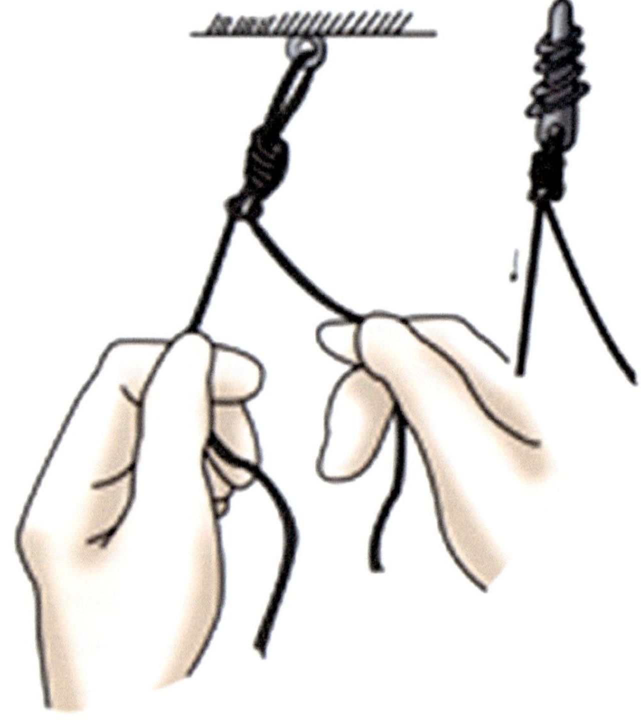

Fig. 14.28 Gradually tighten the straight line to tighten the knot until satisfactory tension is obtained, then pull line end on the other side to lock the knot

Knotting method: hold the sliding line in the left hand and knot-tying line in the right hand. First, wrap the knot-tying line clockwise along the two strands for half a circle, and then pass the knot-tying line end through the gap formed between the sliding line and knot-tying line from back to front. Tighten the two strands gradually to complete the base knot; 3–4 overhand knots can be added upon the base knot to achieve fixation (Figs. 14.38 and 14.39).

(h) Mid-Ship knot: first reported in literature by Frederic Balg et al. in 2005; we believe the stability of this knot is at least equivalent to that of Fisherman's knot. Easy to make and operate, small in size, easy to repeat and teach are its main advantages, and it is a knot technique that is often used in arthroscopic repair surgery [14].

Knotting method: hold the sliding line in the left hand and knot-tying line in the right hand. First, make an upward overhand knot by wrapping the knot-tying line around the sliding line. Wrap the knot-tying line end from the backside of the two strands for half a circle; then pass the knot-tying line end down through the loop surrounding the two strands, tighten the two strands gradually to complete the base knot. Then wrap the knot-tying line around the sliding line to form an upward overhand knot (Figs. 14.40 and 14.41).

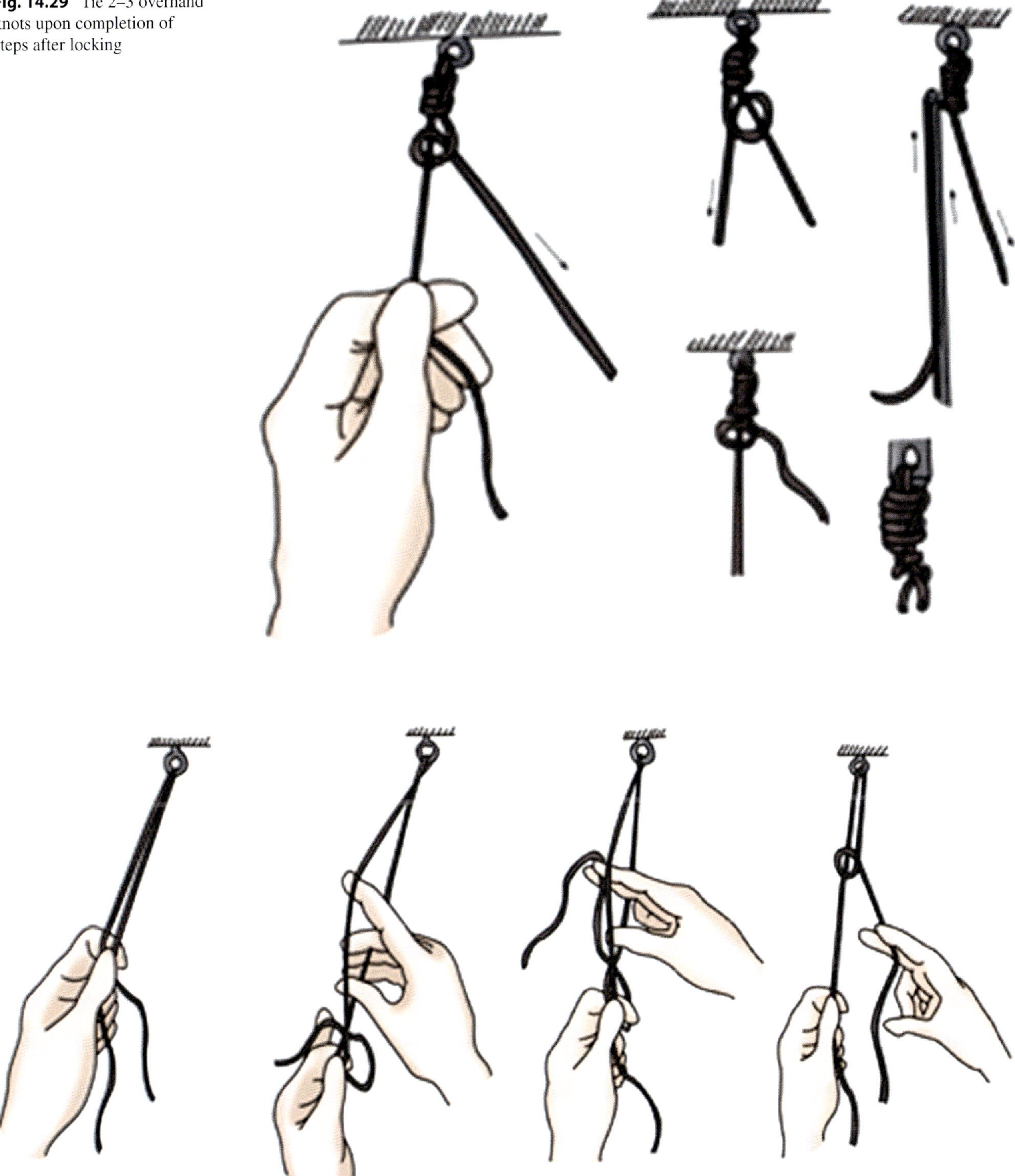

Fig. 14.29 Tie 2–3 overhand knots upon completion of steps after locking

Fig. 14.30 Take sliding line as the base

Fig. 14.31 Guide the knot-tying line downwards by right hand (below the sliding line) to tie an overhand knot

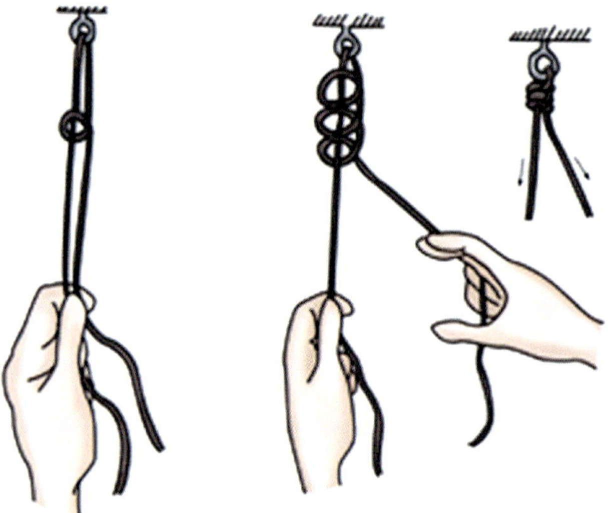

Fig. 14.32 Tie three consecutive downward overhand knots; you can first hold the line in the left hand and gradually pulling knot until ideal tension is obtained, then complete locking by pulling the line in the right hand

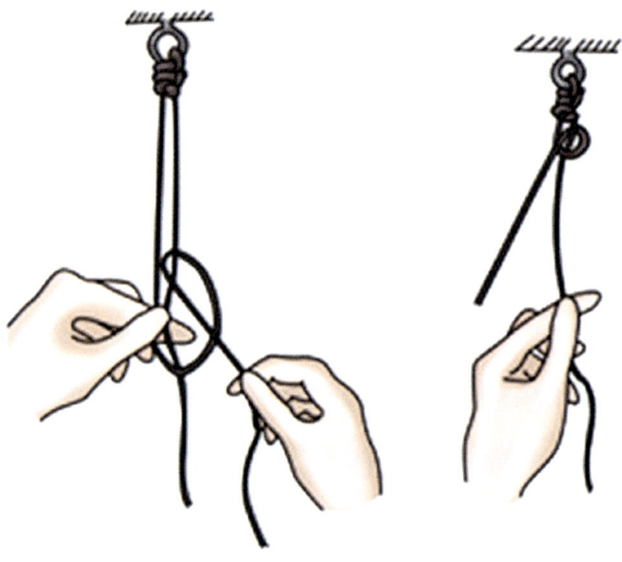

Fig. 14.33 Upon completion of the knot's self-locking, form a downward overhand knot by wrapping sliding line along knot-tying line

(i) MRH knot: first described by Bigon M et al. in 1982; this knot is even simpler in structure, easy to operate, small in size. It is a knot technique frequently used in arthroscopic repair surgery.

Knotting method: The knot is a double-strand structure, the loop side is on the left and the strand end side on the right. First, loop around itself from the loop side, and pass one of the strand ends through the double-stranded loop (Fig. 14.42); then pass the other strand end through the inner loop (Fig. 14.43); tighten the two strands gradually to complete the base knot (Fig. 14.44).

(j) PC knot: The article published by Chris S. Pallia in 2003 described the clinical application of PC knot. The knot structure is simple. It is easy to operate, small in size. It reduces tissue irritation, has a high friction coefficient, strong sliding resistance, and better safety.

Knotting method: hold the knot-tying line in the left hand and sliding line in the right hand. Wrap the knot-tying line around the sliding line clockwise for three circles. Then pass the knot-tying line end from top to bottom through the three loops (Fig. 14.45); tighten the two strands gradually to complete the base knot (Fig. 14.46) [15].

14.3 Application of Suture Technique in Fracture Reduction and Fixation

Fracture reduction and fixation are the main steps of traumatic orthopedic surgery. Similar to the commonly used internal fixation materials such as steel wires (cables), screws, and steel plates, high-strength sutures can also assist fracture reduction and fixation. The suture internal fixation technique is suitable for tendon or ligament avulsion fractures, comminuted fractures, and osteoporotic fractures.

14.3.1 Proximal Humeral Fracture

The reduction and fixation of proximal humeral fractures assisted by the sutures for displacement is a very practical method. Suture fixation can be used for almost all types of proximal humeral fractures.

Take a four-part valgus compression fracture as an example: with the help of sutures, suturing together the compressed humeral head, the greater tubercle, the lesser tubercle, and the upper part of the humeral metaphysis in a way that is similar to "cross" pattern. At the medial and lateral edges of the articular surface, first, use two thick non-absorbable sutures to pass through the rotator cuff tendon–bone junction area, and then pass the sutures through the location where the greater and lesser tubercle fragments are in proximity to the rotator cuff tendon insertion, and reduce the greater and lesser tubercle fractures with the pull of

Fig. 14.34 Form a downward overhand knot by wrapping knot-tying line along sliding line

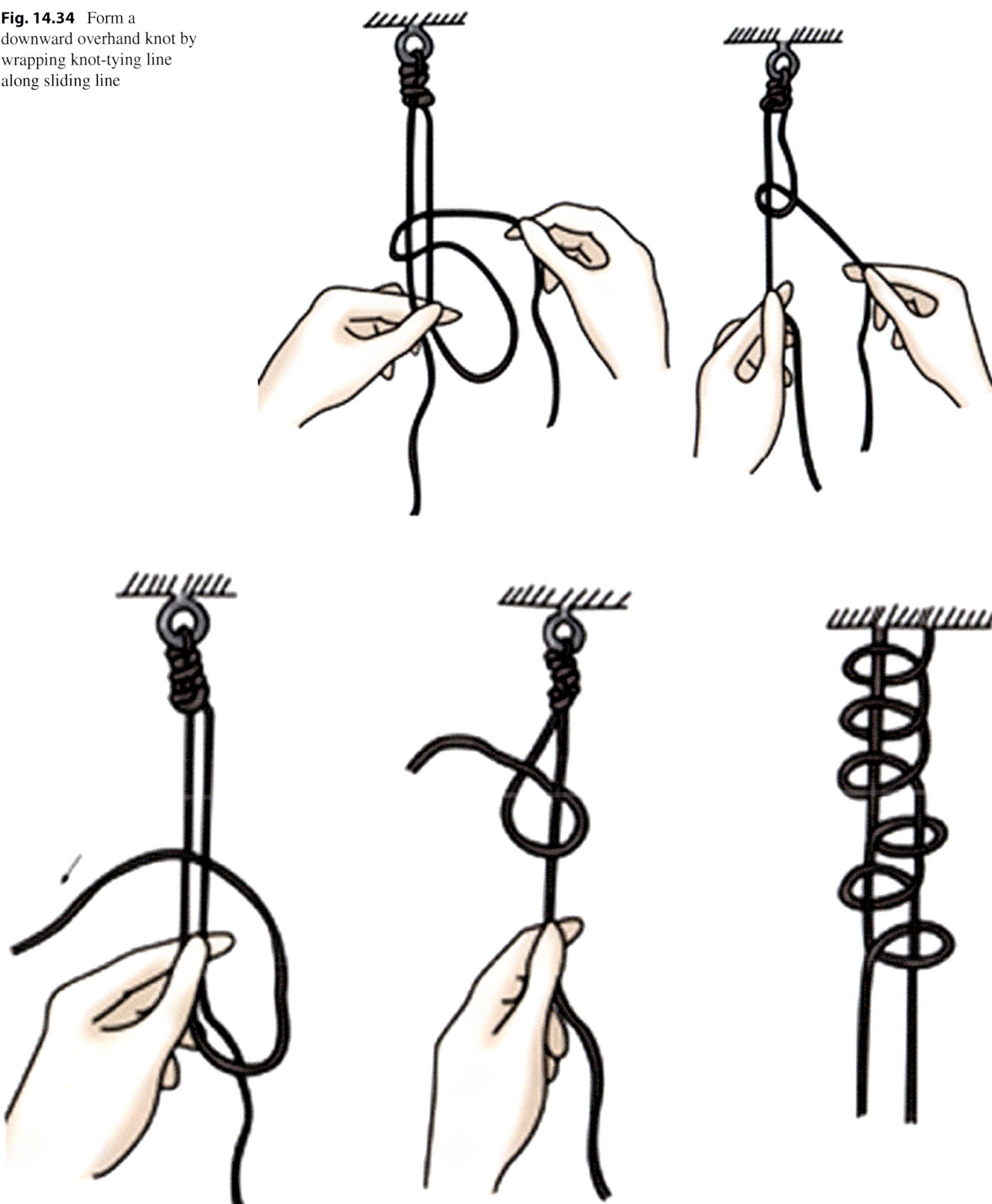

Fig. 14.35 Form a downward overhand knot by wrapping sliding line along knot-tying line

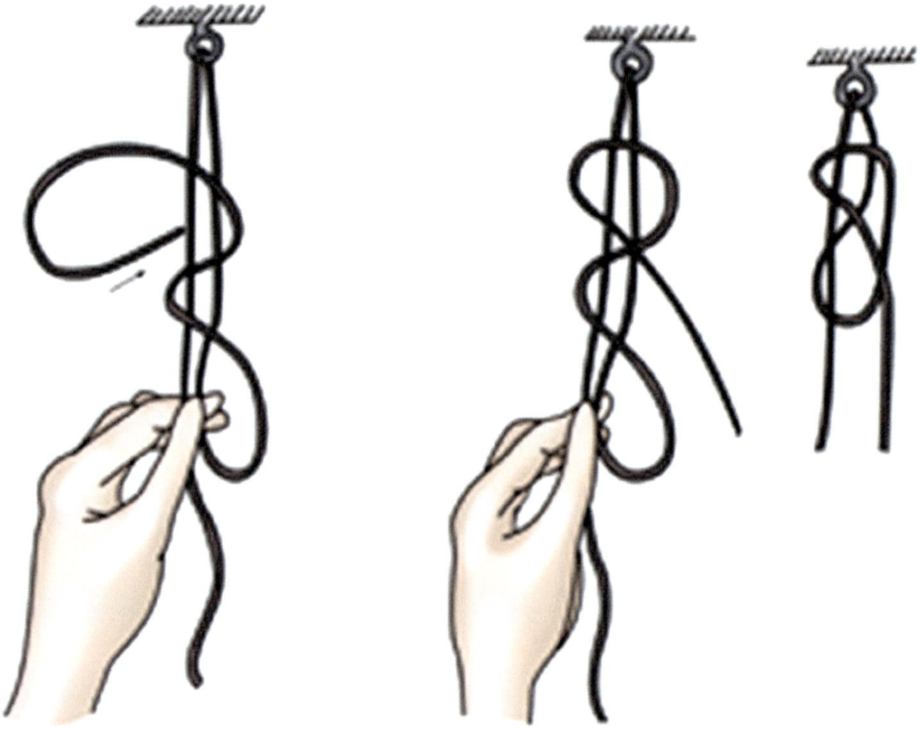

Fig. 14.36 Hold the two strands in the left hand and wrap the knot-tying line counterclockwise for one circle before passing it through the two strands. Finally, thread the end in and out of the loop made initially from front to back, tighten the sliding side of the knot until a satisfactory tension is reached, and then secure it with 3–4 overhand knots

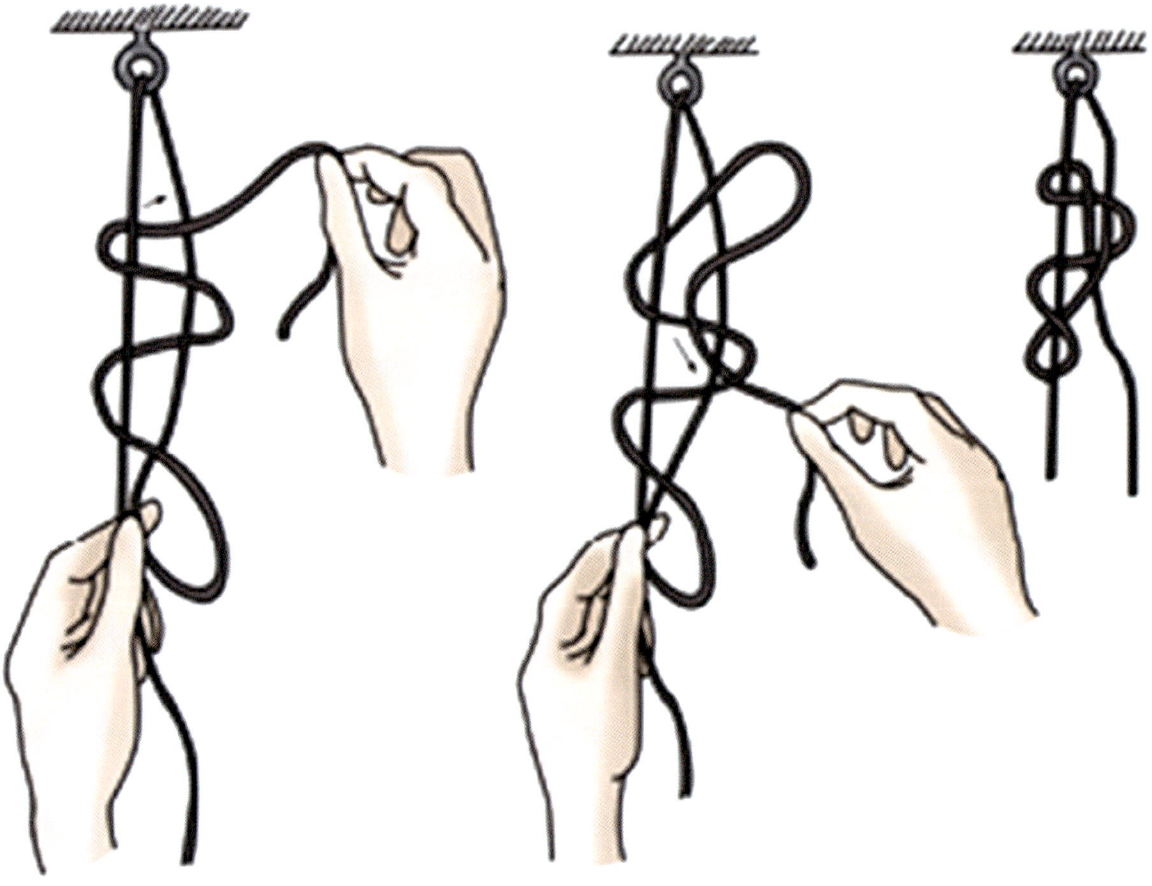

Fig. 14.37 Hold the line in the left hand and wrap the knot-tying line along the two strands counterclockwise. Pass the strand end through the two strands from back to front, and then wrap the end, further from the other end, through the middle structure area from front to back, tighten the sliding side of the knot until satisfactory tension is reached, and then tighten the locking side, and secure it with 3–4 overhand knots

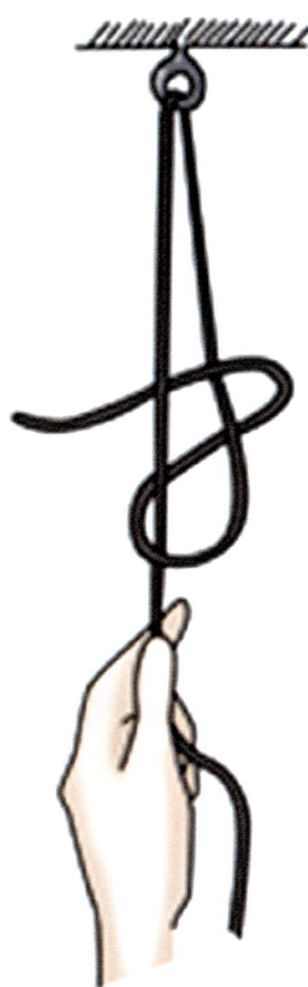

Fig. 14.38 Hold the line in left hand, wrap the thread on the standing side counterclockwise for half a circle along the two strands first, and then wind the knot-tying line end counterclockwise for a circle along the sliding line

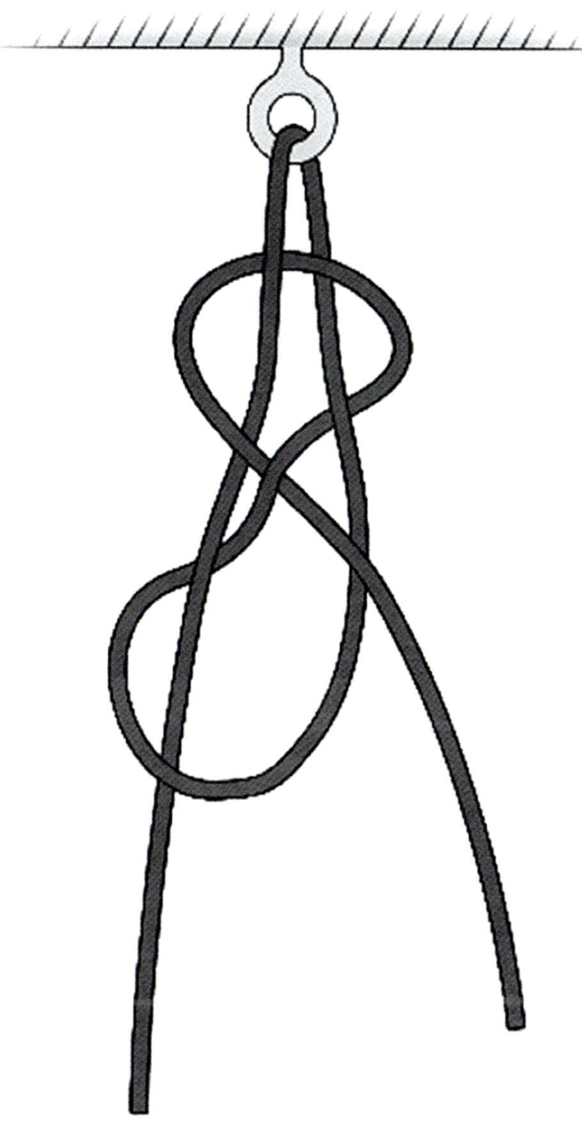

Fig. 14.39 Pass the knot-tying line end from back to front through the gap formed between the sliding line and the knot-tying line to complete the main structure. Tighten the knot gradually from the sliding line side until reaching a satisfactory tension, then tighten it from the locking thread side and fix it with 3–4 overhand knots

suture. After drilling a hole in the lateral cortex of the humeral metaphysis with a 3.5-mm drill bit, pass through two sutures, one from the anterior side of the metaphysis to the greater tubercle fracture tendon–bone junction, the other from the posterior side of the metaphysis to the tendon–bone junction of the lesser tubercle (Fig. 14.47) [16].

When all the sutures are in place, pull the sutures to draw the greater and lesser tubercle fractures closer to the diaphysis, reset the greater and lesser tubercle fractures, and secure them under the humeral head. Knot each pair of sutures first individually, and then cross-knot with each to achieve the purpose of reduction and fixation of the comminuted fracture mass. If found during the operation, that the original knots become loose after the fracture is fixed and compressed with the aid of suture, knot again with the unknotted sutures to achieve fixation.

Both the greater and lesser tubercle fractures contain four sutures to secure them: two sutures fix the tubercle fracture and the humeral metaphysis; two sutures fix the adjacent tubercle fracture. The humeral head is fixated with the proximal humeral shaft by two additional sutures.

In the case of two or three parts of the proximal humerus fracture of the greater tubercle, the displaced greater tubercle is sutured and fixated with the intact lesser tubercle and humeral metaphysis [17].

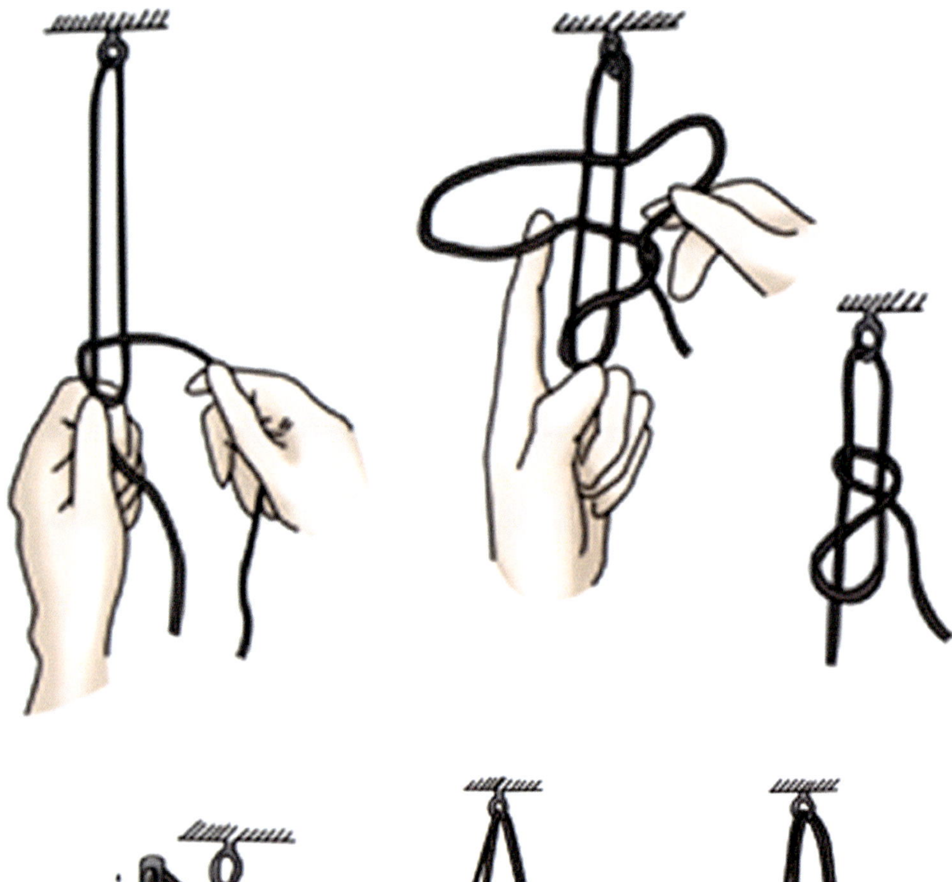

Fig. 14.40 Wrap the knot-tying line around the sliding line to form an upward overhand knot, then wrap the passing out knot-tying line clockwise for a circle around the two strands, and pass the suture end down through the loop surrounding the two strands, and tighten the surrounding strand end gradually to complete the main structure of the knot

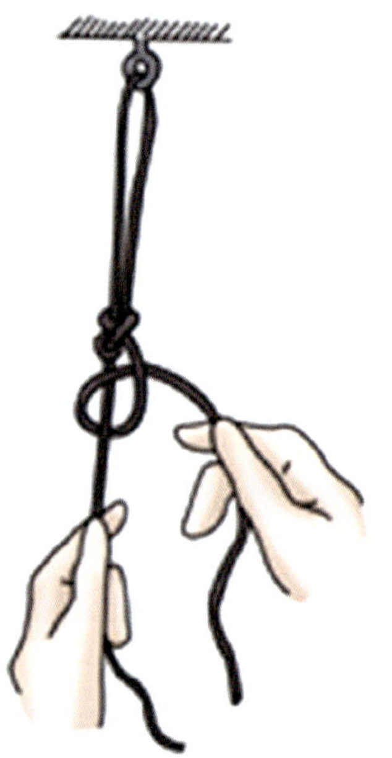

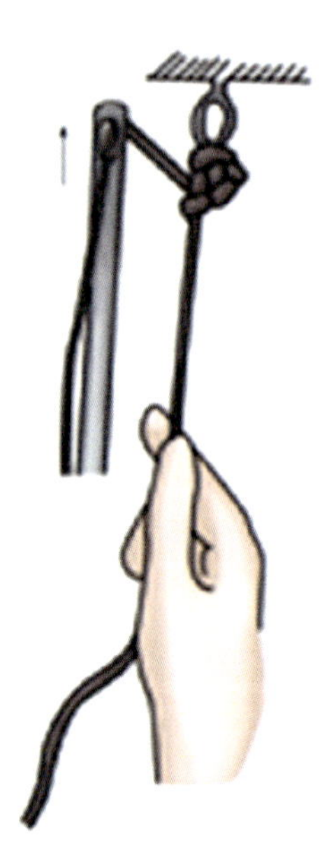

Fig. 14.41 Use the knot-tying line round the sliding line to form an upward overhand knot, tighten the sliding line to complete the final knot structure

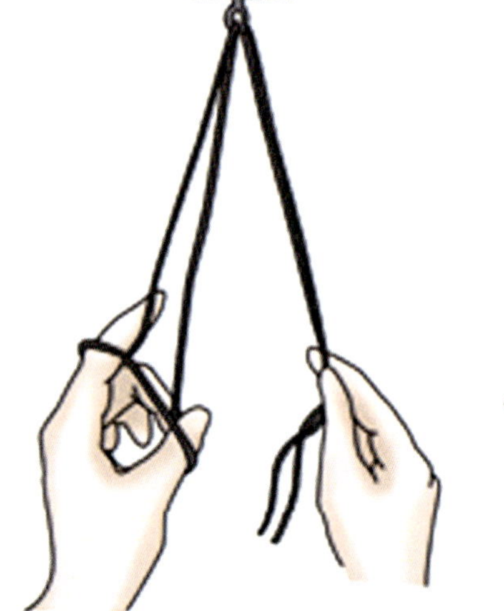

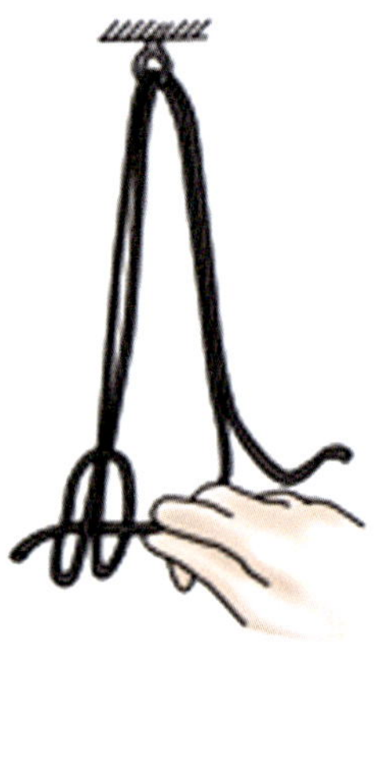

Fig. 14.42 Fold the thread in two, use the left index finger and thumb to form a double loop suture structure, and then pass one of the strand ends through the double loop

When the displaced proximal humerus fracture is small or there is severe osteoporosis, and the risk of failure of using the common methods such as steel plate for internal fixation is high, use the sutures to carry out the reduction and fixation of the displaced greater and lesser tubercle fractures. Among the many suturing methods, the Nice knot is a suture knot method commonly used in the treatment of proximal humeral fractures in recent years. A closed-loop suture with needles that is made of nonabsorb-

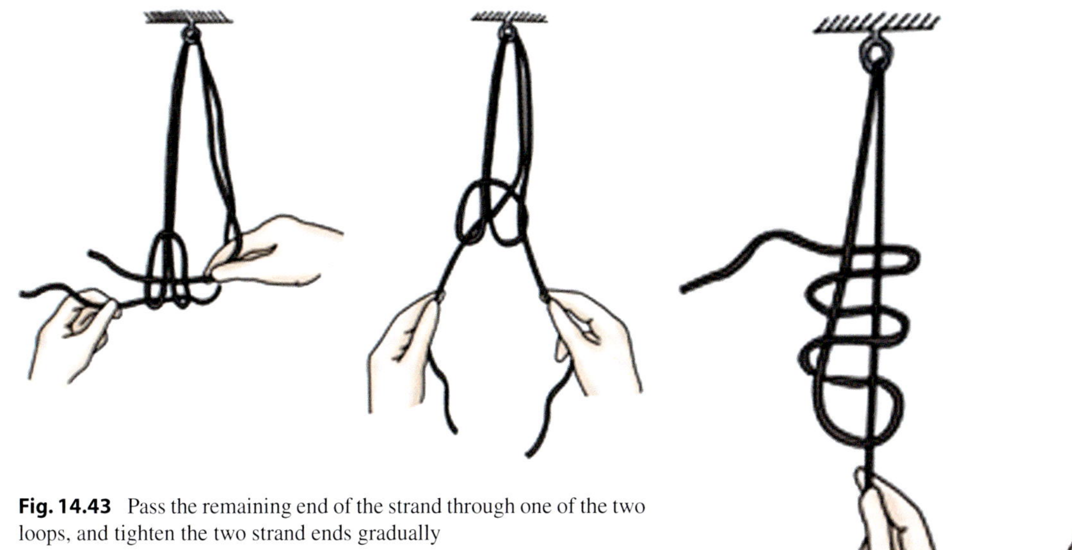

Fig. 14.43 Pass the remaining end of the strand through one of the two loops, and tighten the two strand ends gradually

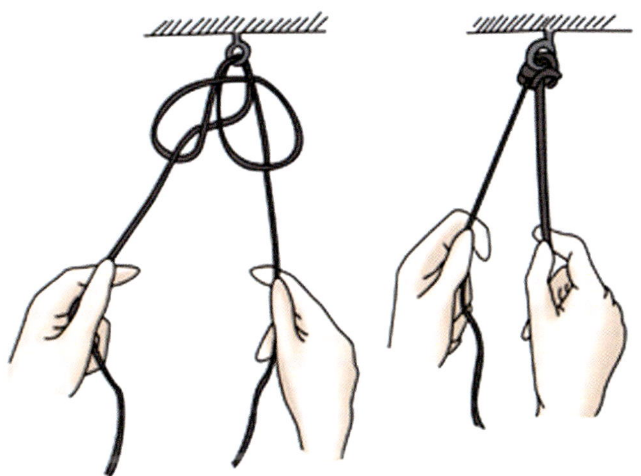

Fig. 14.44 Once the knot is formed with the continuous tightening of the two strands, tighten the end of the thread (sliding line end) that passes through the overhand knot with the help of the suturing device; the knotter helps to apply force to the strand end that passes through the double loop and eventually complete the knot structure

able polyester multi-strand woven material shall be used. During the fixation process, first pass the loop suture through the tissue which is to be fixed with the aid of the suture needle, tie a square knot between the end of the loop suture and the suture end with the needle, then cut off the needle, and pass the two free suture ends through the loop suture. Tighten the loop suture, pull the suture end to complete the fracture reduction, and tie three surgeon's knots between the free ends of the two sutures to complete the lock of the knot, thus preventing the loop from loosening and causing the suture to slip out.

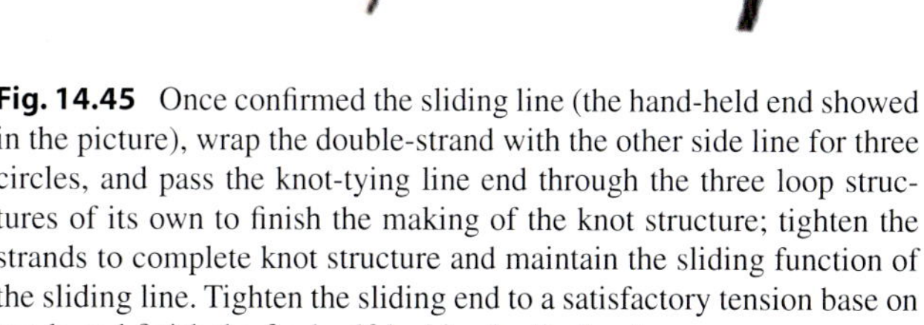

Fig. 14.45 Once confirmed the sliding line (the hand-held end showed in the picture), wrap the double-strand with the other side line for three circles, and pass the knot-tying line end through the three loop structures of its own to finish the making of the knot structure; tighten the strands to complete knot structure and maintain the sliding function of the sliding line. Tighten the sliding end to a satisfactory tension base on needs and finish the final self-locking by the knotter

14.3.2 Avulsion Fracture of ACL (Anterior Cruciate Ligament)

The main advantage of this technique is that the risk of epiphyseal injury is reduced by suture fixation: there is no metal internal fixation penetrates into the metaphysis, therefore avoiding the risk of removing the fixation by reoperation (Fig. 14.48).

14.3.3 Treatment of Butterfly Fragments

As for open reduction and internal fixation of comminuted fractures with plate, the screws may not be able to securely stabilize the smaller butterfly fragments. Although wire or cable cerclage can be used as a supplemental internal fixation for the butterfly fragments, at the regions where soft tissue coverage is not enough (such as clavicle, tibia), there is a risk of irritating thin skin and even secondary skin ulceration or infection if the internal fixation such as wire is applied. A

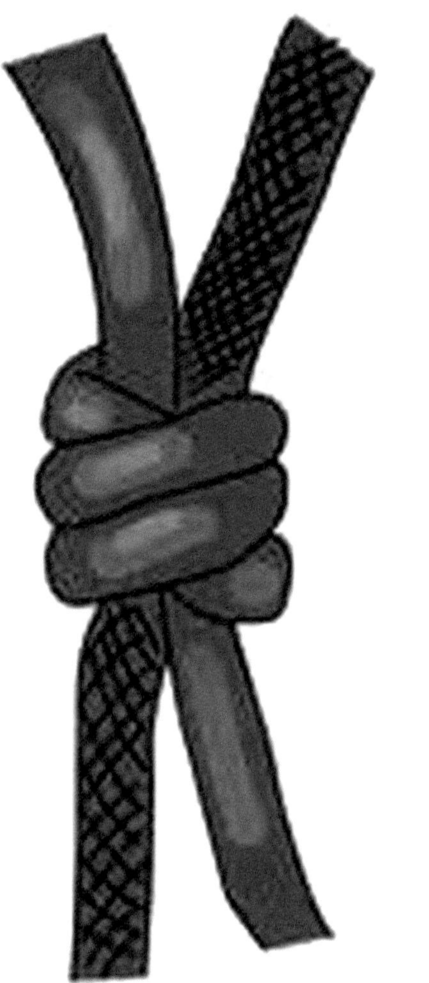

Fig. 14.46 PC knot has a simple structure, stable function, and strong practicability

closed-loop high-strength suture with the needle-like Nice loop can provide an alternative option for the fixation of these bones: it can effectively fix the comminuted fractures and at the same time, reduce the irritation to the soft tissue.

14.3.4 Olecranon Fracture

First, use a 2-mm drill bit to drill two parallel holes on the distal fracture fragment of the olecranon and on both sides of the midline of the ulna. Then drill two more holes on the proximal fracture fragment above the attachment point of the triceps brachii (avoid any damage to the triceps tendon). Pass two nonabsorbable Ethibond sutures through the predrilled bone hole at the distal end to the medullary cavity, and through the fractured part, and then pass through the proximal ulnar bone hole above the triceps tendon insertion. Tie the sutures in a sliding knot, conduct anatomical reduction of the distal and proximal fractures by pulling the sutures, and lock the suture knot under direct sight. Then drill two more holes on the distal fracture fragment, pass the other suture through these bone holes, make a similar of "8" shaped tension band suture, knot outside of the triceps attachment point, and perform pressurization on the fracture end; the working mechanism is similar to that of the traditional cerclage. The first suture is similar to the Kirschner wire, and the second is similar to the tension band suture wound on the Kirschner wire. Its function is to convert the contraction force of the triceps muscle into the compressive stress on the fractured end.

14.3.5 Calcaneus Fracture

Miyamoto et al. introduced a method that combines hollow screws and suture reduction to fix calcaneal tuberosity avulsion fractures. First, pass the suture through the distal part of the Achilles tendon, and achieve fracture reduction by pulling the suture. Use a 4.0-mm hollow screw to fix the calcaneal fracture. Pass the two inner side suture ends to the outer side and the two outer suture ends to the inner side with the aid of wire passer. These sutures are all threaded to the subcutaneous tissue around the calcaneus. Finally, knot and lock the suture with a non-slip knot on the ventral side of the Achilles tendon.

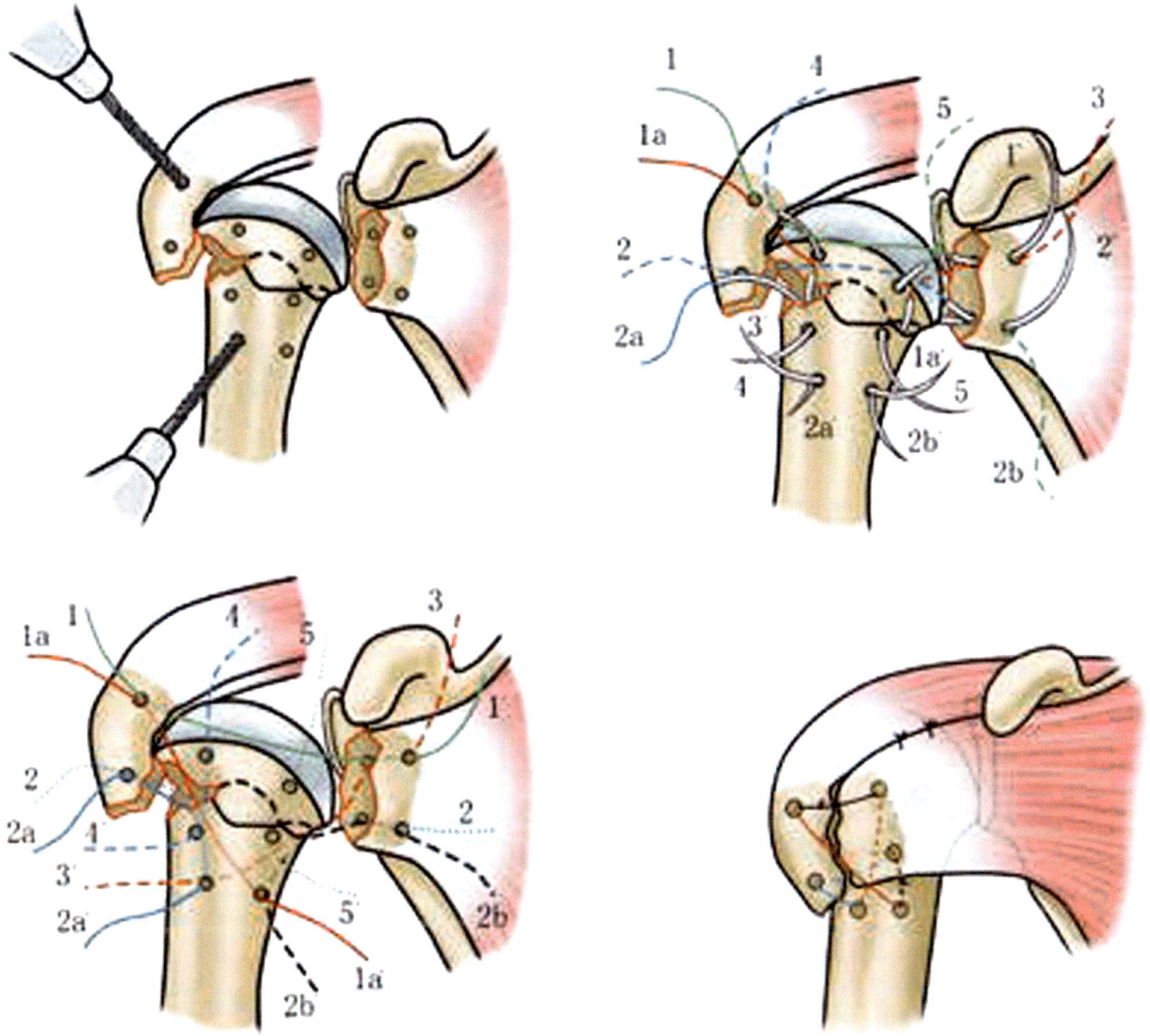

Fig. 14.47 Way to bind and secure sutures for greater and lesser tubercles for proximal humeral fractures

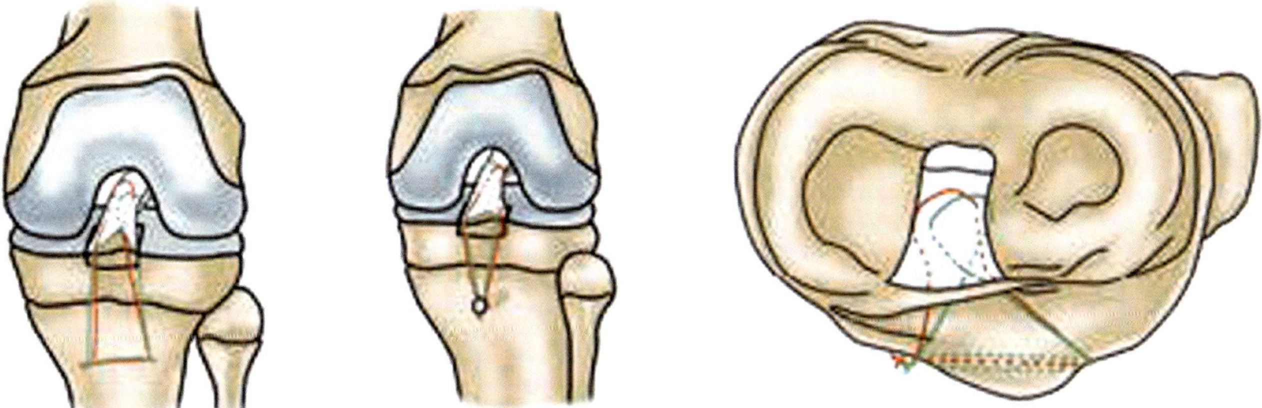

Fig. 14.48 Suture fixation for avulsion fracture of ACL

References

1. Hurt J, Unger JB, Ivy JJ, et al. Tying a loop-to-strand suture: is it safe? Am J Obstet Gynecol. 2005;192(4):1094–7.
2. Galatz LM, Ball CM, Teefey SA, et al. The outcome and repair integrity of completely arthroscopically repaired large and massive rotator cuff tears. J Bone Joint Surg Am. 2004;86-A(2):219–24.
3. Yamaguchi K, Levine WN, Marra G, et al. Transitioning to arthroscopic rotator cuff repair: the pros and cons. Instr Course Lect. 2003;52:81–92.
4. Lieurance RK, Pflaster DS, Abbott D, et al. Failure characteristics of various arthroscopically tied knots. Clin Orthop Relat Res. 2003;408:311–8.
5. Lee TQ, Matsuura PA, Fogolin RP, et al. Arthroscopic suture tying: a comparison of knot types and suture materials. Arthroscopy. 2001;17(4):348–52.
6. Provencher MT, Verma N, Obopilwe E, et al. A biomechanical analysis of capsular plication versus anchor repair of the shoulder: can the labrum be used as a suture anchor? Arthroscopy. 2008;24(2):210–6.
7. Baumgarten KM, Brodt MD, Silva MJ, et al. An in vitro analysis of the mechanical properties of 16 arthroscopic knots. Knee Surg Sports Traumatol Arthrosc. 2008;16(10):957–66.
8. Boileau P, Old J, Gastaud O, et al. All-arthroscopic weaver-Dunn-Chuinard procedure with double-button fixation for chronic acromioclavicular joint dislocation. Arthroscopy. 2010;26(2):149–60.
9. Waitayawinyu T, Martineau PA, Luria S, et al. Comparative biomechanic study of flexor tendon repair using FiberWire. J Hand Surg Am. 2008;33(5):701–8.
10. Behm T, Unger JB, Ivy JJ, et al. Flat square knots: are 3 throws enough? Am J Obstet Gynecol. 2007;197(2):171–2.
11. Nho SJ, Cole BJ, Mazzocca AD, et al. Comparison of ultrasonic suture welding and traditional knot tying in a rabbit rotator cuff repair model. J Shoulder Elb Surg. 2006;15(5):630–8.
12. Boileau P, Brassart N, Watkinson DJ, et al. Arthroscopic repair of full-thickness tears of the supraspinatus: does the tendon really heal? J Bone Joint Surg Am. 2005;87(6):1229–40.
13. Murray TJ, Lajtai G, Mileski RM, et al. Arthroscopic repair of medium to large full-thickness rotator cuff tears: outcome at 2- to 6-year follow-up. J Shoulder Elb Surg. 2002;11(1):19–24.
14. Boileau P, Krishnan SG, Coste JS, et al. Arthroscopic biceps tenodesis: a new technique using bioabsorbable interference screw fixation. Arthroscopy. 2002;18(9):1002–12.
15. Barber FA, Herbert MA, Richards DP. Sutures and suture anchors: update 2003. Arthroscopy. 2003;19(9):985–90.
16. Burkhart SS, Wirth MA, Simonich M, et al. Knot security in simple sliding knots and its relationship to rotator cuff repair: how secure must the knot be? Arthroscopy. 2000;16(2):202–7.
17. Chan KC, Burkhart SS, Thiagarajan P, et al. Optimization of stacked half-hitch knots for arthroscopic surgery. Arthroscopy. 2001;17(7):752–9.

Orthopedic Drainage

15

Wei Su, Xu Gong, Jian Qi, Zekun Zhou, and Shaoyan Li

Abstract

Orthopedic drainage is a surgical means that a certain part of the body and the outside to divert the necrotic tissue, pus, blood, or exudate accumulated in the space between tissues or in the articular cavity to the outside of the body. Among which, drainage is the general term for materials used to create the pathway between the body and the outside for the purpose of drainage, such as cigarette drain and rubber hose; efflux refers to the purulent effusion, hematoma, necrotic tissue, etc.; drainage area refers to the part of the human body to be drained. At present, drainage for therapeutic purpose is widely accepted; however, there exists a major controversy on drainage for preventive purposes.

Keywords

Drainage · Prevention · Treatment · Vacuum sealing

15.1 Overview

Gu Liqiang, Gongxu Suwei, Zhou Zekun and Li Shaoyan

15.1.1 Historical Review

In ancient Rome, human beings had learned to "suck with the mouth" to remove the poisons in the wound; but the real drainage technology began with the catheter drainage described by Hippocrates in ancient Greece [1]. In 1859, Chassagnac began to use the rubber hose as the drainage; in 1882, Kehrer made the first cigarette drain in human beings; in 1895, Kellogg described the prototype of double cannula drainage; in 1898, Heaton developed continuous vacuum aspiration; in 1992, Fleischmann et al. initiated the vacuum sealing drainage technology; at the end of the twentieth century, the basic principles of most drainage technologies had been established and till now, they have been recognized by clinical scholars. There are also records on drainage materials in "Wei Ji Bao Shu," a Chinese medical book: *"If the wound has already festered, it is necessary to make a wick with thick paper and apply it on the wound;"* the "wick" used as the drainage material is a medicated thread made by cutting the mulberry paper, silk wadding paper or copy paper to the appropriate size and rubbing it into a thread [2, 3].

15.1.2 Purpose of Drainage

1. To discharge the pus, necrotic tissue, foreign body, and other efflux from the tissue or articular cavity, reduce pressure, eliminate inflammatory stimulation, reduce the inflammatory reaction, inhibit local bacterial reproduction, prevent spread of infection, and promote regression of inflammation.
2. To ensure the good healing of the wound and reduce the occurrence of complications.
3. To observe the color, quantity, and appearance of the efflux, so as to judge the conditions in the drainage area, such as bleeding and infection.
4. To treat, for example, drainage of superficial and deep abscesses.
5. Drainage by flushing can drain the pus and necrotic tissue in the lesion to the outside of the body. Drainage by flushing applied to the articular cavity can keep the articular cavity lubricated and prevent joint adhesion. Appropriate

W. Su (✉)
Department of Orthopedics, The First Affiliated Hospital of Guangxi Medical University, Nanning, Guangxi, China

X. Gong · Z. Zhou · S. Li
The First Bethune Hospital of Jilin University, Jilin, China

J. Qi
The First Affiliated Hospital, Sun Yat-sen University, Guangzhou, China

P. Tang et al. (eds.), *Tutorials in Suturing Techniques for Orthopedics*, https://doi.org/10.1007/978-981-33-6330-4_15

antibiotics can be added to the flushing fluid to control infection.

6. The drainage can stimulate tissue fluid exudation, and neutralize and dilute toxins. At the same time, stimulation with the drainage can cause fibrinogen to exude, which leads to local adhesion and thus localizes the lesion and eliminates dead space.

15.1.3 Classification of Drainage

According to the Purposes of Drainage: (1) Therapeutic drainage is the drainage of infected lesions, such as drainage after abscess incision, or drainage of body cavity effusion after operation and trauma. (2) Preventive drainage is the drainage intended to prevent hematocele, effusion, and infection.

According to the Drainage Power: (1) Passive drainage utilizes body position, natural pressure difference, such as the pressure difference between the body liquid and the atmosphere, the siphon effect of the drainage, or the gravity of the efflux itself, to achieve the purpose of drainage. (2) Active drainage is the drainage that uses a vacuum aspiration device to drain the efflux.

15.1.4 Common Drainage Materials and Time Limit for Application

1. Drainage strip: Doctors use sterile gauze strips, rubber tubes, or rubber gloves as materials, and cut such materials into the strip or sheet drainage, which is indicated for minor bleeding and exudation in the wound after operation; drainage strip is generally removed in 1–2 days after operation, so as to avoid retrograde infection.
2. Drainage tube connecting vacuum drainage bottle: The indwelling time of the drainage tube should be controlled within 24–48 h as far as possible. For patients with the long indwelling time of drainage tube, attention should be paid when cleaning the drainage tube and the surrounding skin; and broad-spectrum antibiotics can be given at the same time for preventive purposes.
3. Vacuum-assisted wound closure: It is mainly composed of medical foam dressing, semipermeable adhesive film, sucking disc, and pipeline; medical foam dressing is the part of direct contact with the wound surface, and the adhesive film can isolate the wound surface from the outside, and prevent bacterial invasion [4]. Its orthopedic indications include the wounds that cannot be directly closed after debridement, the infected wounds, and the wounds after osteofascial compartment fasciotomy [5]. In addition, vacuum-assisted wound closure can be used as a dressing for fixing free skin graft and treating incision exudation after joint replacement [6]. The US Food and Drug Administration recommends the change of dressing every 2–3 days for vacuum-assisted wound closure; in China, the dressing should be removed in 5–7 days after the operation, up to a maximum of 10 days. If the case of massive exudation, the replacement time should be shortened.

15.1.5 Indications and Common Methods of Orthopedic Drainage

1. After arthroscopy, joint replacement, and fracture repair

The purpose of drainage is to drain the blood, pus, and inflammatory exudation in the intermuscular space and articular cavity to the outside of the body to prevent pooling, secondary infection, swelling, or organization of hematoma, and other adverse complications; at the same time, it can effectively prevent compression as well as irritation to the surrounding skin and is conducive to the healing of the incision.

The placement of drainage tubes during surgery is crucial. If the drainage tube is not placed properly, or the drainage operation is not performed properly, such as inadequate drainage caused by the compression, twist, or angulation of the drainage tube, it will negatively affect the surgical effect and postoperative rehabilitation, and may even lead to infection of the drainage pathway. If the infection is not managed properly, it may prolong the healing of the wound in mild cases, and it may cause operation failure, or it may even induce osteomyelitis in severe cases. The drainage tube should be adjusted timely at dressing change.

However, in recent years, meta-analysis showed that for spinal surgery, especially for spinal fusion, grade 1 and 2 cervical spinal fusion, lumbar discectomy, lumbar decompression or discectomy, and adolescent posterior scoliosis fusion, there was no sufficient evidence to prove that drainage could effectively reduce the incidence of postoperative complications; on the contrary, it might cause some relevant complications due to the drainage.

2. Soft tissue infection and open fracture with concurrent infection

The method of draining infected soft tissue wound is open dressing, fill the incision or wound surface with various gauzes, to achieve the purpose of drainage by the capillary effect of gauzes. Open dressing has drawbacks of contamination and re-infection. Therefore, in recent years, it has been replaced by negative pressure wound therapy (NPWT).

3. Preventive drainage

When it is expected that there will be blood or exudate on the wound surface after surgery, especially when residual cavity may form, it is necessary to place the drainage to avoid hematoma, effusion, and secondary infection; for example, resection of a huge bone or soft tissue tumor, surgical incision with a thick layer of subcutaneous fat, wound with severe soft tissue injury, and contaminated incision. This type of drainage mostly uses open or semi-open tube for drainage; the former is a semi rubber tube for drainage from the incision, and the latter is a drainage tube connected with a disinfection container to collect the efflux. For patients with high risk of postoperative infection, preventive application of NPWT can effectively reduce the incidence of postoperative wound infection compared with traditional dressings.

15.1.6 Precautions for Orthopedic Drainage

1. Deliberate decision must be made on whether to place drainage device or not; unnecessary drainage can increase the incidence of infection.
2. The contraindications of drainage include bone tuberculosis, active bleeding, malignant tumor in the drainage area or long-term use of anticoagulants, and malnutrition.
3. The drainage tube should not be too thin, so as to avoid breaking the drainage tube when removing it.
4. Strict septic operation should be performed when placing the drainage device.
5. Important structures such as tendons, ligaments, blood vessels, and nerves should be bypassed during drainage; if not, natural tissues or non-adhesive dressings can be used to cover the above structures before drainage.
6. The drainage should be placed with the shortest pathway as far as possible; when placing it, make sure it is unobstructed, and avoid distortion and compression.
7. After placing the drainage, its external end should be fixed to prevent it from slipping out or entering the body.
8. The type, number, location, and date of placement of the drainage should be recorded in the operation record.
9. After the operation, the patient should keep an appropriate position to prevent drainage failure due to compression, folding, or pulling of the drainage tube.
10. If the appearance of the efflux is abnormal, corresponding actions should be taken as appropriate; if the efflux is a large amount of blood, surgical exploration should be made again in the drainage area.
11. The drainage material should be removed as early as possible.
12. The outlet of the drainage and the surrounding area should be disinfected and bandaged to prevent retrograde infection.
13. When vacuum sealing drainage is performed, the medical foam dressing should not be cut too small in order to prevent leakage in the wound cavity; forced filling or over-filling in the wound cavity which may injury the tissues should be avoided; regulate the negative pressure for drainage properly to avoid pain in the patient.
14. Perform debridement thoroughly, and drainage cannot replace debridement.
15. Perform hemostasis, especially for patients using NPWT.
16. When using NPWT for drainage, check for the common air leakage sites, and anaerobic bacteria infection should be excluded; meanwhile, determine the timing for dressing replacement based on the amount of exudate and the dressing used.

15.1.7 Time for Removal of Various Drainage Methods

1. Rubber sheet drainage is generally removed in 1–2 days after the operation. The indications of rubber sheet drainage are minor bleeding and exudation in the wound; the duration of drainage should be short because a too long indwelling time may lead to retrograde infection.
2. Cigarette drainage should be removed within 2 days after the operation. Cigarette drainage is generally used for prevention, which uses capillary effect for open drainage and mostly will fail after 48 h.
3. The indwelling time of the rubber tube for drainage should be controlled within 24–48 h as far as possible. Research has shown that the indwelling time of the rubber tube for drainage is positively correlated with the infection rate, and the infection rate increases significantly when the indwelling time is more than 72 h. Once inflammatory reaction occurs around the drainage tube, the drainage tube should be removed immediately. For patients with longer indwelling time of drainage tube, the drainage tube and the surrounding skin should be disinfected, and broad-spectrum antibiotics should be given to prevent infection.
4. For vacuum sealing drainage, US FDA suggests that dressing should be changed every 2–3 days; in China, generally dressing will be removed 5–7 days after operation, and the longest indwelling time should not be more than 10 days. In case of severe exudation, the dressing replacement interval should be shortened, and dressing should be replaced every 2 days.

15.2 Vacuum Sealing Drainage Technology

15.2.1 Vacuum Sealing Drainage

Vacuum sealing drainage (VSD) technology was firstly proposed by Dr. Fleischman of ULM University in Germany in 1993. At first, it was used in orthopedics to treat soft tissue defects and infections [7, 8]. In 1994, Professor Qiu Huade introduced this technology to China [9, 10]. VSD technology is the therapeutic method that uses medical foam material (commonly polyvinyl alcohol or polyurethane) to fill and cover the wound, then uses biological semipermeable film to seal the entire wound surface and lacuna, and provides continuous vacuum aspiration through the vacuum source, so that the wound can be drained thoroughly, thus promoting healing of the wound. VSD technology can facilitate the timely drainage of exudate and liquefied necrotic tissue in the wound and lacuna out of the body, reduce the accumulation of exudate, and promote adequate drainage; VSD technology can effectively isolate the wound from the external environment to reduce the opportunity of infection; VSD technology increases local blood circulation, promotes cell proliferation and growth of granulation tissue, so as to accelerate wound healing. VSD technology has been widely used in the treatment of various wounds at home and abroad [11–14].

15.2.1.1 Technical Principle of VSD

1. *Vacuum:* Continuous and controllable vacuum provides power for active drainage, promotes timely removal of exudates on the wound surface, and eliminates potential lacuna in the wound. The vacuum can form a mechanical traction force. During continuous vacuum aspiration, on the macro level, it can get the two wound edges closer and create conditions for wound closure; on the micro level, the slight change of tissue tension can accelerate the production and renewal of intracellular messenger regulatory proteins to promote cell proliferation and stimulate the growth of granulation tissue. The vacuum can also accelerate local blood circulation, improve local ischemia in muscle and tissue, and is conducive to wound healing [15–17].
2. *Sealing:* Sealing is the prerequisite for maintaining negative pressure on the wound. Sealing can isolate the wound from the outside, restore the integrity of the skin barrier as much as possible, so as to prevent contamination and infection. The closed space creates a relatively low-oxygen or hypoxia and slightly acid environment, which is conducive to cell growth and tissue repair and promotes wound healing [18].
3. *Drainage:* Because of the high plasticity of the VSD material, the negative pressure can reach everywhere of the drainage area, thus achieving thorough drainage. Under the high negative pressure, the drainage tube will not be easily blocked after the segmentation and shaping of VSD material. The local necrotic tissue, bacteria, harmful metabolites, and exudates in the wound can be fully drained, so as to reduce the probability of infection, prevent massive inflammatory mediators from entering the blood circulation, and avoid the "second strike" on the wound and damage to organ functions [19].

15.2.1.2 Application of VSD Technology

With the rapid development of society and economy, open fractures caused by high-energy trauma are more and more common. After debridement and fracture fixation, severe soft tissue avulsion defect often brings great challenges to clinicians during treatment. However, the dressing can easily be infiltrated by exudate and requires frequent replacement, and during the operation, the wound is open or semi-open to the outside. Infection with multidrug-resistant bacteria increases treatment difficulty and healing time, sometimes even results in serious complications, leading to permanent loss of limb function. Wound management with VSD can not only close the wound early and avoid infection, but also enable effective and thorough drainage, improve local blood circulation, promote tissue repair and prevent "second strike." [20] For patients, VSD technology can shorten the duration of treatment, reduce the treatment cost and relieve the pain in patients due to frequent dressing change [21, 22].

1. **Indications**
   (a) Skin defects caused by various reasons, including skin avulsion, degloving injury, local skin necrosis caused by crush injury, exposure of issues such as tendon, nerve, and bone, open fracture combined with the wound that cannot be closed directly, or with soft tissue defect, and decompression with fasciotomy for osteofascial compartment syndrome;
   (b) Various acute and chronic infection wound caused by crush injury, for example, infection after internal fracture fixation, prolonged non-healing of the wound caused by chronic osteomyelitis, and incision wound for drainage caused by articular cavity infection;
   (c) Refractory wound caused by crush injury, for example, diabetic ulcer, pressure sores, etc.
2. **Contraindications**
   (a) Various active bleeding wounds.
   (b) Severe abnormal coagulation function.
   (c) Wound with malignant tumor not excised.
3. **Materials and methods**

The materials required for VSD technology include medical foam material, drainage tube, semipermeable adhesive film, and vacuum source. Among them, medical foam material has direct contact with the wound and other tissues, and the pores between materials are interconnected. There are two commonly used medical foam materials:

(a) *Polyvinyl alcohol (PVA):* White, with relatively small pores, diameter of 0.06–0.27 mm, high tensile strength (522.4 kPa), not easy to break [23].
(b) *Polyurethane (PU):* Black, with relatively large pores, diameter of 0.4–0.6 mm, into which granulation tissue is easy to grow, low tensile strength (111.1 kPa), easy to break. It was once observed that a polyurethane foam fragment remained in the wound and affected healing.

The drainage tube is located in the VSD material and directed to the outside of the body. The semipermeable film covers the surface of the foam material to seal off the drainage area and isolate it from the outside. The vacuum source provides drainage power, so as to ensure the drainage of efflux in the drainage area. After the vacuum is formed, the foam material is fixed with the surrounding tissues to form a closed whole. The negative pressure is generally controlled within −175 ~ −50 mmHg (−23.3 ~ −6.7 kPa) [24], and − 300 ~ −125 mmHg (−40 ~ −17 kPa) [25] for application on the skin outside the incision on limbs or abdominal wall, extraperitoneal wound or body cavity.

4. **Operation of vacuum sealing drainage**

It can be divided into four steps: placement of the drainage; sealing to isolate the drainage area from the outside; connecting vacuum to start drainage; postoperative management and observation.

(a) Placement of the drainage.
   I. *Debridement:* Drainage cannot replace debridement.
   II. *Preparation of the Drainage:* Trim the VSD material according to the length, depth, and shape of the drainage area.
   III. *Filling:* Place the VSD material in the drainage area, ensure full contact of the VSD material with the entire wound surface requiring drainage, and leave no gap.
(b) Sealing: Good sealing is the key to ensuring the drainage effect.
(c) Open negative pressure.

5. **Precautions**
   (a) If wound sealing is not tight, it will lead to air leakage, reduced negative pressure and drainage effects, and obstruction of the tube due to coagulation of blood drainage, which will require flushing with normal saline or frequent replacement of the drainage tube.
   (b) Avoid inappropriate or ineffective negative pressure. Generally, the negative pressure should be kept between −200 and − 125 mmHg. Too high or too low negative pressure will hinder wound healing. Inspect the vacuum conditions regularly. The sign of effective negative pressure is obvious collapse of the wound dressing. If the wound dressing bulges, indicating that the tube is falling off or the semipermeable membrane is loose, it should be treated immediately.
   (c) Avoid inadequate care during the application. It is necessary to observe and record the quantity, nature, and denaturation of drainage fluid during the application of VSD technology. If necessary, the drainage fluid may be sampled for bacterial culture, and appropriate antibiotic treatment may be used. The tube should be replaced once after continuous vacuum sealing for 5–7 days, and should not be distorted or folded. Redness, swelling, and blisters occurring on the skin around the wound indicate that the patient is allergic to the biological semipermeable film, and the use of the film should be stopped in time.
   (d) Avoid too long course of the disease because of unduly insisting on the use of VSD technology blindly. VSD technology has the risk of causing or increasing bleeding. Once a large amount of blood is drained, the use of VSD technology should be discontinued. After 3 weeks of the use of VSD technology, if there is no improvement in wound repair, find out the causes, and use another method for treatment; if the wound worsens, stop the use of VSD technology immediately, and find out the causes and treatment methods.
   (e) Systemic treatment should be considered as well. VSD technology is only local treatment, which cannot replace the holistic treatment. During the clinical application of VSD technology, the overall conditions of the patient should be evaluated. The use of comprehensive treatment can achieve better result with less effort. Improve the general condition, control infection, encourage the patient to have diet with high protein, high vitamin, and high calorie. Deficiency of protein can cause wound edema; deficiency of vitamin C is associated with slow capillary neovascularization and affects the synthesis of collagen fiber; deficiency of vitamin A may affect epithelial regeneration; deficiency of vitamin B complex may affect the function of cell enzymes.

15.2.1.3 Advantages of VSD Technology

1. Polymer foam material is used as an intermediary between the drainage tube and the wound, which is free from the

restriction of body position and enables full wound drainage; the efflux is separated from the drainage tube by the foam material, and will not easily block the drainage tube lumen, making the drainage unobstructed.
2. The biological semipermeable film can isolate the wound from the outside, and constitute a barrier that prevents bacteria from invading the wound, which effectively prevents the contamination and nosocomial cross-infection resulting from routine dressing change and drainage, and maintains a continuous state of high negative pressure.
3. The exudate and necrotic tissue in the drainage area are removed in time, so that the drainage area has "zero accumulation." The wound surface quickly obtains a clean environment and the number of bacteria on the wound surface is reduced, which prevents spread of inspection and absorption of toxins, thus effectively preventing the "second strike" on the body by the reabsorption of toxins.
4. One time sealing drainage can keep effective drainage for 5–10 days without requiring dressing change every day, which alleviates the suffering of patients and the labor of medical staff, and reduces the material consumption caused by multiple dressing changes.
5. Compared with the traditional method, it can shorten the course of treatment by 1/3 ~ 1/2, reduce the bedtime of patients, improve the quality of life of patients, and reduce the use of antibiotics and the medical costs of patients.
6. The operation is simple and easy and can be carried out at the bedside.

15.2.2 Closure of Drainage Port

It is suggested that the drainage port as the contaminated wound should be sutured with Coated VICRYL® Plus Antibacterial Suture (coated polyglactin 910 with triclosan) for closure, which can effectively reduce the risk of surgical site infection.

15.2.3 Precautions for Orthopedic Drainage

1. Deliberate decision must be made on whether to place drainage device or not; unnecessary drainage is harmful and may increase the risk of infection.
2. Would with serious infection should be drained.
3. The drainage should be placed with the shortest pathway as far as possible; when placing it, make sure it is unobstructed.
4. Important structures (blood vessels, nerves, and organs) should be bypassed when placing the drainage device.
5. The drainage should be fixed properly to prevent it from falling off or sliding into the body.
6. The outlet of drainage with passive gravity should be placed as low as possible.
7. If the appearance of the efflux is abnormal, corresponding actions should be taken as appropriate, for example, perform surgical exploration on the drainage area again, withdraw or replace the drainage material.
8. The patency of drainage should be inspected and treated as appropriate in time.
9. The drainage material should be removed as early as possible.

15.2.4 Time for Removal of Various Drainage Methods

The indications of rubber sheet drainage are mild bleeding and exudation on the wound surface. The drainage time should be short, and drainage should be placed on the superficial part. If the indwelling time is too long, there is a possibility of retrograde infection along the drainage sheet. Therefore, it is necessary to remove the drainage early, and removal is generally performed in 1–2 days after operation. Cigarette drainage is an open drainage that utilizes the capillary effect. Generally, it is only intended for the preventive purpose, and mostly it will fail 48 h after placement. Therefore, it should be removed within 2 days after operation. A too long indwelling time of rubber drainage tube is also an important cause of infection. Studies showed that the longer indwelling time of the drainage tube, the greater probability of infection, and the higher chance of local infection. In case that the indwelling time of the drainage tube is longer than 72 h, the infection rate has an obvious trend of increasing. Therefore, it is necessary to clean the skin around the incision and the drainage tube after placing the tube, so as to effectively prevent bacterial contamination. The indwelling time of the drainage tube should be controlled within 24–48 h as far as possible. Once inflammatory reaction occurs around the drainage pathway, the drainage tube should be removed immediately. For patients with long indwelling time of the drainage tube, attention should be paid when cleaning the drainage tube and the surrounding skin, and broad-spectrum antibiotics can be given at the same time for preventive purposes.

References

1. Yongkun Z, Yunjie Z, Yi Z. Clinical puncture and drainage. Jinan: Shandong Science and Technology Press; 2003. p. 5–15.
2. Yu J, He Z. Study on the invention and creation value of external treatment methods in surgery of ancient Chinese medicine. Chengdu: Chengdu University of TCM; 2011. p. 1–120.
3. Riqing L. Surgery of traditional Chinese medicine. Beijing: China Press of Traditional Chinese Medicine; 2007. p. 45–6.

4. Huade Q. Vacuum sealing drainage technology. Beijing: People's Medical Publishing House; 2003. p. 1–40.
5. Webb LX. New techniques in wound management: vacuum-assisted wound closure. J Am Acad Orthop Surg. 2002;10(5):303–11.
6. Scuderi GR. Avoiding postoperative wound complications in Total joint Arthroplasty. J Arthroplast. 2018;33(10):3109–12.
7. Fleischmann W, Strecker W, Bombelli M, et al. Vacuum sealing as treatment of soft tissue damage in open fractures. Unfallchirurg. 1993;96(9):488–92.
8. Fleischmann W, Lang E, Russ M. Treatment of infection by vacuum sealing. Unfallchirurg. 1997;100(4):301–4. German
9. Huade Q. Vacuum sealing drainage technology. Beijing: People's Medical Publishing House; 2003. p. 1–3.
10. Zhiqiang Z, Huade Q, Shiming T, et al. Application of medical foam vacuum sealing drainage in treatment of 29 cases with skin abscess. Mod Gen Surg. 1998;3(1):20–1.
11. Moues CM, Vos MC, van den Bemd GJ, Stijnen T, Hovius SE. Bacterial load in relation to vacuum-assisted closure wound therapy: a prospective randomized trial. Wound Repair Regen. 2004;12:11–7.
12. Yao M, Fabbi M, Hayashi H, Park N, Attala K, Gu G, French MA, Driver VR. A retrospective cohort study evaluating efficacy in high-risk patients with chronic lower extremity ulcers treated with negative pressure wound therapy. Int Wound J. 2014;11:483–8.
13. Huang C, Leavitt T, Bayer LR, Orgill DP. Effect of negative pressure wound therapy on wound healing. Curr Probl Surg. 2014;51:301–31.
14. Schwien T, Gilbert J, Lang C. Pressure ulcer prevalence and the role of negative pressure wound therapy in home health quality outcomes. Ostomy Wound Manage. 2005;51:47–60.
15. Siqueira MB, Ramanathan D, Klika AK, Higuera CA, Barsoum WK. Role of negative pressure wound therapy in total hip and knee arthroplasty. World J Orthop. 2016;7(1):30–7.
16. Glass GE, Murphy GF, Esmaeili A, Lai LM, Nanchahal J. Systematic review of molecular mechanism of action of negative-pressure wound therapy. Br J Surg. 2014;101(13):1627–36.
17. Webb LX, Pape HC. Current thought regarding the mechanism of action of negative pressure wound therapy with reticulated open cell foam. J Orthop Trauma. 2008;22(10 Suppl):S135–7.
18. Borgquist O, Gustafsson L, Ingemansson R, Malmsj M. Micro- and micromechanical effects on the wound bed of negative pressure wound therapy using gauze and foam. Ann Plast Surg. 2010;64(6):789–93.
19. Huang C, Leavitt T, Bayer LR, Orgill DP. Effect of negative pressure wound therapy on wound healing. Curr Probl Surg. 2014;51(7):301–31.
20. Dedmond BT, Kortesis B, Punger K, et al. The use of negative-pressure wound therapy (NPWT) in the temporary treatment of soft-tissue injuries associated with high-energy open tibial shaft fractures. J Orthop Trauma. 2007;21(1):11–7.
21. Yaobin Y, Jiuzheng D, Wei M, et al. A meta-analysis of negative pressure wound therapy versus traditional wound care for open wounds. Chin J Bone Joint Surg. 2014;3:197–201.
22. Kruga E, Bergb L, Leec C. Evidence-based recommendations for the use of negative pressure wound therapy in traumatic wounds and reconstructive surgery: steps towards an international consensus, injury. Int J Care Injured. 2011;42:S1–S12.
23. Bai Lianyang, Bai Xiangjun, Zhang Mao et al. China trauma care training V1. Beijing: People's Medical Publishing House,2019:235–244.
24. Birke-Sorensen H, Malmsjo M, Rome P, et al. Evidence-based recommendations for negative pressure wound therapy: treatment variables (pressure levels, wound filler and contact layer)--steps towards an international consensus. J Plast Reconstr Aesthet Surg. 2011;64 Suppl:S1–S16.
25. Heller L, Levin SL, Butler CE. Management of abdominal wound dehiscence using vacuum assisted closure in patients with compromised healing. Am J Surg. 2006;191(2):165–72.

16 Debridement and Closure of Soft Tissue Injuries

Jie Sun, Xinlong Ma, Fangguo Li, Haotian Qi, Xi Zhang, Yang Yang, Xuelei Wei, and Xin Zhao

Abstract

This chapter introduces the characteristics and mechanism of different soft tissue injuries and briefly demonstrates that for open soft tissue injuries, thorough debridement, and removal and closure of the wound are effective to ensure first-stage wound healing. The appropriate suturing technique can not only prevent infection and promote wound healing, but also reduce systemic trauma reaction and accelerate limb function recovery.

Keywords

Closed wound · Open wound · Crush syndrome
Explosive wound · Suture · Wound · Skin graft and flap

16.1 Soft Tissue Injury Classification and Injury Mechanism

Sun Jie and Jia Jian

16.1.1 Classification

Trauma—refers to mechanical injuries to the human body, generally caused by external mechanical objects contact. Some are caused by the tension imbalance to the tissue structures (such as the injury results from violent muscle contract). The main factor causing trauma is usually called "violent force." Different injuries to different body parts have different characteristics.

Trauma can be classified by objects or violent forces, injury sites, injured tissues and organs, or the pathological changes, etc. According to skin integrity after injury, those with intact skin and no open wounds are called closed injuries, such as contusion, crush injury, sprain, and concussion. Those with damaged skin are called open injuries, such as abrasion, laceration, incised wound, cut wound, and stab wound. In open injuries, it can be further divided into penetrating wound (with both entrance and exit), blind tract wound (with only entrance but no exit), tangential wound (groove-like injuries caused by injury implements rubbing along the tangential direction of the body surface), and rebound wound (with entrance and exit at the same point).

16.1.1.1 Closed Trauma

1. **Contusion** is the most common soft tissue trauma, which is caused by blunt objects or other blunt forces. It does not break the skin but causes injury to subcutaneous fat, small vessels, and muscle tissues with low anti-cracking strength.
2. **Sprain** is a common trauma that occurs when limb dynamics are out of balance. The main reason is that one side of the joint is under excessive tension, and the joint may be temporarily subluxated, and the related ligament, tendon, or muscle may be torn. After the limbs regain their balance, the joints will be reset immediately, but it will take some time for soft tissue injuries to heal. Some sprains can leave the weakness of ligaments or joint capsules, resulting in repeated sprains. Severe sprain can also be accompanied by articular cartilage injury, bone flap avulsion, etc.
3. **Crush injury** refers to the mechanical or ischemic injury to the muscles caused by prolonged crushing of heavy objects on limbs, trunk, and other muscle-rich parts. Severe cases can lead to life-threatening complications characterized by myoglobinuria, hyperkalemia, acidosis, and acute renal failure, which is called crush syndrome [1]. It can be seen that the former is simple and direct injuries to muscles caused by crushing, while the latter is a series of systemic reactions caused by muscle cell injury after pressure is released.

J. Sun (✉) · X. Ma · F. Li · H. Qi · X. Zhang · Y. Yang · X. Wei
X. Zhao
Tianjin Hospital, Tianjin, China

P. Tang et al. (eds.), *Tutorials in Suturing Techniques for Orthopedics*, https://doi.org/10.1007/978-981-33-6330-4_16

The main pathophysiological changes of crush syndrome include direct injury of muscle tissue and ischemia-reperfusion injury [2–4]. Continuous mechanical extrusion force causes injuries to muscle cells and microvessels, while low perfusion causes hypoxia and edema of muscle cells. If this situation continues longer than 2.5 h, irreversible necrosis of skeletal muscle fibers will occur. Hypoxia can also cause abnormal cell metabolism, destruction of cell membrane integrity, and release of potassium ions, lactic acid, creatine kinase, and various inflammatory mediators and toxins. When the crushing force is removed, the blood supply is restored to the ischemic limb, and excessive liquid is accumulated in the osteofascial compartment, which on the one hand causes the decrease of effective circulating blood volume, leading to hypovolemic shock; on the other hand, the recovery of blood supply will start the mechanism of ischemia-reperfusion injury, resulting in intracellular calcium overload and massive release of free radicals and myoglobin, etc. When myoglobin enters the blood circulation, it is filtered by the glomerulus, and forms cast in the renal tubules, blocking the renal tubules, causing injury to the proximal renal tubular epithelial cells, and in severe cases, causing renal ischemic infarction. The above pathophysiological changes will eventually lead to acute consequences such as hypovolemic shock, electrolyte disturbance represented by hyperkalemia, metabolic acidosis, and malignant arrhythmia, and long-term complications such as acute renal failure, coagulation dysfunction, adult respiratory distress syndrome, and sepsis.

16.1.1.2 Open Trauma

1. **Bruise** It is the most superficial open trauma, caused by tangential motion friction between injury implements and the skin surface. Bruise leads to the exfoliation of skin cells, with a small amount of blood constituent effusion, which may cause a mild inflammatory reaction. At present, "moist healing theory" is widely used in clinical practice to treat skin bruises. Moist healing means covering the wound with moist dressing or ointment, which makes the surface of the wound form a wet environment. A relatively stable environment can protect the nerve endings at the wound surface, so as to avoid effusion and adhesion when changing dressings, and reduce the sensation of pain [5–7]. A moist environment can finally speed up the healing, reduce the scar formation of the wound, and relieve the pain of patients in the process of diagnosis and treatment.
2. **Tension blister** Refers to the superficial injury caused by internal tangential movement acting on the skin, which is common in local skin excessive swelling and prolonged pressure. Due to blood circulation disorder of local skin, the obstruction of venous reflux, local venous blood stasis, and increased permeability of blood vessels result in small blisters on the epidermis. If tension blisters are not treated in time, blisters may break and easy to cause infection. Simply withdrawing the blister fluids is accompanied with a high recurrence rate. A study showed that [8] the incidence of tension blisters in all lower limb fractures was 7.2%; among them, 47% were bloody, 43% were clear, and 10% of them appeared simultaneously. Another study found that [9] the incidence of postoperative complications in bloody tension blisters was higher than that in clear blisters.
3. **Stab wound** It is caused by sharp objects penetrating into tissues. The diameter of the stab wound is small, and it is easy to be blocked by clots; the depth of the wound is much greater than its diameter, which is directly proportional to the force, so it may injury multiple layers of tissues. This wound condition is prone to be complicated with infection, especially anaerobic infection.
4. **Incised and cut wounds**. Incised wound is caused by cutters or other sharp objects. The linear movement of the object on the tissue can cut open the tissue without using great force. The length and depth of the wound depend on the contact surface between the injury implement and the tissue, and its edges are neat. Incised wound generally has no injury and stimulation to noncontact tissues. Therefore, the severed blood vessels often lack a contraction response and bleed more. Cut wound is also the trauma caused by cutters. The difference between the cut wound and the incised wound is that the cutters causing the cut wound are heavier or/and the acting force is larger, with almost vertical movement applying to the body, so the wound is deeper and may hurt the bones. If the cutting edge of the cutters is blunt, the wound edge will be rough, the noncontact tissue may be damaged, and the inflammatory reaction after injury is obvious.
5. **Laceration** It is caused by the traction of some parts of the human body by running vehicles and machines, etc. The forces are more violent so the injury can be more serious. Most of the lacerated wounds caused by oblique tension are petaloid, and in severe cases, the skin is torn off in pieces; those caused by parallel tension are linear fracture; most of those caused by multidirectional tension are stellate. One of the characteristics of wounds is the appearance of filaments, which are collagen-rich fibrous tissues with strong anti-cracking strength. In addition, wound contamination is often serious. Those who are injured by high energy impact often have deep tissue injuries, including fracture, muscle fracture, nerve and blood vessel fracture, and avulsion. Because of the serious injury, it is easy to make a diagnosis.
6. **Explosive injury** When an explosive takes place, it releases energy instantaneously, causing mechanical or chemical injuries to the body, which is called explosive injury, and is characterized by high disability and mortal-

ity [10]. Explosives can be divided into low-order and high-order explosives. The energy released by low-order explosives (gunpowder) occurs at subsonic speed, and its essence is the "combustion" of certain materials. The explosion of high-order explosives (C4 and TNT explosives) can quickly transform explosives into high-pressure gas and release energy at supersonic speed [11]. Epidemiological investigation shows that the current explosive injury includes four grades, and the typical characteristic of the first-grade explosive injury is caused by the shock wave acting on the surface tissue and hollow viscus of the body, resulting in anatomical and physiological changes; the second-grade explosive injury is the penetrating injury and the rare blunt instrument injury caused by explosive fragments hitting the body; the third-grade explosive injury refers to fracture, limb disconnection, craniocerebral injury, and other penetrating injuries caused by a large number of high-heat airflow, that is, explosive wind, impacting the body; the fourth-grade explosive injury is independent of the first-, second-, and third-grade injury mechanisms, and its injuries, discomfort, and pathological changes include complications and the complexity of existing conditions, involving thermal or chemical burns, radiation exposure, inhalation injury caused by dust or toxic gas exposure, etc. [12] Considering that explosive injuries are mostly those in different grades of combination, the diagnosis and treatment measures also have their particularity and complexity. It is of great scientific value to fully understand the possible injuries caused by various injury mechanisms and realize accurate assessment and individualized diagnosis and treatment.

7. **Gunshot injury** It is caused when the human body tissues are shot by bullets or shrapnel from rifles, pistols, and shotguns. Firearms produce high-velocity tremendous kinetic energy, which is transformed into pressure, heat, etc. after entering the tissue, causing special trajectory, and serious injury to noncontact tissue. Medical staff should adopt multidisciplinary comprehensive disease assessment in the early stage of treatment, especially pay attention to the prevention and treatment of acute complications such as respiratory arrest, cardiac arrest, acute renal failure, and acute respiratory syndrome, which is of great significance to reduce the death risk of patients with multiple injuries and firearms injuries.

16.1.2 Morel-Lavallée Injury

Morel-Lavallée injury is a closed degloving injury of skin subcutaneous tissue and fascia layer, which was first proposed by French doctor Morel-Lavallée in 1863. Morel-Lavallée injury in the traditional sense refers to the closed subcutaneous hematoma in the posterolateral side of the greater trochanter of femur and fat necrosis secondary to soft tissue degloving injury [13]. Such serious soft tissue injury is often secondary to pelvic or acetabular fractures. Literature reports that the incidence is 2.5–8.3%, and the ratio of male to female is 2-1 [14]. Clinically, due to the lack of sufficient understanding of such injury, the rates of missed diagnosis and misdiagnosis often increase relatively. Inappropriate early treatment, in addition to affecting the definitive treatment of fractures, may also cause local skin and soft tissue necrosis, infection, or posttraumatic pseudo-cysts, and other complications.

16.1.2.1 Injury Mechanism and Pathological Process

Shear force causes the subcutaneous tissue to separate from the fascia layer, forming a closed space, and the subcutaneous tissue moves and separates from the deep fascia layer. The perforating artery and lymphatic vessel in the fascia layer break, which leads to the accumulation of hematoma, lymph, soft tissue fragments, and fat particles, followed by fat necrosis, and finally produces pseudo-cysts [15]. The pseudo-cysts are filled with low coagulation, high molecular weight, and thin lymph, which is the main factor hindering posttraumatic self-absorption [16].

The pathological process is mainly divided into four stages: the first stage: the formation of potential space due to the separation of subcutaneous tissue and fascia layer; the second stage: the rupture of the perforator vessel and the lymphatic vessel, and accumulation of the blood lymph and necrotic fat tissue, etc.; the third stage: the reabsorption of blood cells in the cavity, residues of plasma fluid, lymph, and other tissue fluids; the fourth stage: the formation of fibrous pseudo-cysts caused by local aseptic inflammation [17].

Prognosis: (1) Organization of hematoma, adhesion of cyst wall dissection, and self-healing of injury; (2) Difficulty in self-absorption of the large amount of effusion, hindering healing of subcutaneous tissue and fascia, resulting in formation of pseudo-cysts; (3) Hematoma and liquefied fat are good media, and even if there is no open wound, it is easy to cause hematogenous infection. In severe cases, it may be complicated with septic shock. Hak, et al. reported that 46% of bacteria culture before debridement showed positive [18]; (4) Primary and secondary effusions destroy local skin blood supply, which is easy to cause skin necrosis.

16.1.2.2 Clinical Symptoms

Early local skin swelling, cyanosis or pale, ecchymosis, abrasion, and hypoesthesia, among which local hypoesthesia or sensory loss can be distinguished from common contusion; some early symptoms are not noticeable, with only local skin mobility increases, and the early fluctuation after injury may also be not shown until several days after the injury as the gradual increase of hematoma; local puncture may suck out bloody liquid mixed with fat particles; it may be accompanied by pain, contraction, or local contour change. As the disease progresses, there may be redness and necrosis on the skin surface, mainly manifested by local pain and progressive swelling, which evolves into inflammatory reaction and fibrous pseudo-cysts around the cavity [19].

Morel-Lavallée injuries are mostly located at bony processes. It usually occurs in the greater trochanter of femur, lumbosacral part, and proximal thigh, among which it is reported that greater trochanter of femur and buttocks account for 30.4%, thigh 20.1%, pelvis 18.6%, lumbosacral part 3.4%, near buttock end 6.4%, around joints 15.7%, calf 1.5%, abdomen 1.5%, head 0.5%, and others 2% [20].

16.1.2.3 Imaging Examination

X-ray examination often shows no special findings, and the density of soft tissue can present irregular images. CT shows the dark liquid area between subcutaneous tissue and muscular layer, which is helpful to evaluate the local injury of the deep fascia plane, but sometimes lacks characteristic imaging findings. Ultrasound often shows flat or fusiform anechoic areas or hypoechoic areas in the subcutaneous fascia layer, with irregular boundary in acute phase and smooth boundary in chronic phase, which is helpful for rapid diagnosis, and soft tissue contusion of patients may limit examination. Multiple sequences are sensitive to soft tissues, which can be used for diagnosis and classification. Acute, subacute, and chronic diseases show different imaging findings. Mellado et al. divided the injuries into the following six types according to the shape of the injuries, the presence or absence of fibrous pseudo-capsule, the signal characters, and enhancement characteristics on T1WI and T2WI (Fig. 16.2, Table 16.1) [21].

Table 16.1 MRI classification of Morel-Lavallée injuries

Type	Content	T1W1	T2W1	MRI finding
I	Serum-like fluid	Low	High	Occasional capsule, no enhancement, layered and streaked
II	Subacute hematoma	High	High	Thin capsule, various forms of enhancement, oval and fusiform
III	Chronic hematoma	Mix	Mix	Thick capsule, internal or marginal enhancement, oval and fusiform
IV	Closed laceration	Low	High	No capsule, no enhancement, liner
V	Quasi-circular pseudonodule	Multiple signals	Multiple signals	Thick or thin capsule, internal or marginal enhancement, round
VI	Coinfection	Multiple signals	Multiple signals	Thick capsule, which may be accompanied by sinus tract formation, and internal or marginal enhancement

16.1.2.4 Treatment Methods

Once a diagnosis is determined, it is advisable to perform thorough debridement of the hematoma and all necrotic tissues as soon as possible, and the operation timing should be at least no later than the definitive treatment of the fracture.

So far, there are no unified guidelines for the early treatment of Morel-Lavallée, and the treatment sequence of Morel-Lavallée injury and fracture is still controversial. First, the treatment of Morel-Lavallée injury may delay the time of internal fixation of the fracture, and it is more difficult to treat fracture. If the internal fixation is performed first, the risk of infection may increase. Individualized treatment should be proposed based on comprehensive consideration of injury and clinical manifestations.

1. Simple local pressure dressing, which is only suitable for acute injury involving the periphery of knee joint with a small scope.
2. Local pressure dressing combined with percutaneous aspiration, which is suitable for patients with early detection and limited lesion scope. The therapeutic effect should be closely assessed. If poor effectiveness or ineffectiveness is observed, surgery should be performed as early as possible. The recurrence is as high as 83% when the volume of effusion is more than 50 ml. Nickerson et al. recommends percutaneous aspiration for cases with volume of effusion less than 50 ml [22].
3. Injection of drugs to promote adhesion of the cavity gaps: The drugs that can be administered include tetracyclines and talcum powder, etc. The pathological process of this method is that adhesion-promoting substances promote the aggregation of neutrophils, macrophages, and mesothelial cells, and producing inflammatory and cellulosic reactions, thus promoting scar formation. However, for large-scale injuries, the residual cavity is inevitable, which results in incomplete healing of injuries. Some researchers have reported that infection occurs after surgery with this method. Nickerson et al. recommended using it when the volume of effusion is less than 400 ml [22]. When there are fibrous pseudo-cysts, the effectiveness is poor. For large-scale injury, the residual cavity is inevitable, which makes the injury unable to heal completely.
4. Tseng, Tornetta et al. recommended early percutaneous limited incision, debridement and irrigation, vacuum aspiration, and catheter drainage. Closure of the cavity

gaps is essential during surgery, and the drainage tube should be withdrawn when the drainage volume is less than 30 ml/24 h [23].

5. Arthroscopic debridement and percutaneous suturing, which features with small surgical trauma, and is helpful to protect the blood supply of soft tissues and promote wound healing. It is suitable for patients with early diagnosis. It is very important to close the cavity during surgery.
6. Incision, thorough debridement and internal suture, thorough removal of necrotic substances, elimination of dead space, and primary or secondary closure of wounds. Carlson reported 22 patients who underwent thorough debridement and internal suture, with primary closure of wounds, and no infection or recurrence. For those who have clear evidence of infection, incision, debridement, drainage and secondary relaxation suture are performed [24].

To sum up, Morel-Lavallée injuries should be treated as a potential or hidden open fracture. Early diagnosis and timely treatment can basically prevent the ischemia and necrosis of skin and soft tissue, secondary infection of hematoma, or formation of pseudo-cysts. Choosing appropriate treatment timing and surgical methods according to injury pathology is the key to obtain satisfactory efficacy. While dealing with soft tissue injury, necessary surgery should be performed on fracture within a time limit. Percutaneous closed drainage is suitable for subjects with early diagnosis; the surgery ≤3 days after injury has less trauma, which is helpful to protect the blood supply of soft tissues and promote wound healing; incision and drainage is suitable for patients with huge lesion range, severe systemic symptoms, or delayed diagnosis. Hematoma and necrotic tissue are completely removed during surgery, and the use of the VSD technique for continuous vacuum sealing drainage after surgery is helpful to eliminate dead space and promote wound healing; pseudo-cysts incision, cyst wall clearance, and interlaminar suture are suitable for patients with chronic diseases, mature cyst wall and ineffective treatment by the above methods.

16.2 Treatment of Open Fracture with Soft Tissue Injury

Sun Jie and Jia Jian

16.2.1 General Treatment of Traumatic Patients

Appropriate treatment is based on a good understanding of the injury mechanism. High-energy forces often lead to more serious soft tissue injuries. Although some patients do not have open injuries, they should still be treated according to the principle of open injuries, such as acute arterial injuries or osteofascial compartment syndrome in calves and forearms [25, 26].

1. **Treatment of single limb injuries**

For the first physical examination, the wound size, and the conditions of skin, muscle, bone, nerve, and blood vessel must be recorded in detail, and then use sterilized dressing to cover the wound. After transferred to the operating room, the dressing should be removed. If the open wound is large or there is active bleeding, it is advisable not to carry out examination until the arrival of the senior doctor or the consultant of relevant departments, so as to reduce the exposure of the open wound and secondary injuries. Wounds less than 1 cm are mostly caused by the broken end of fracture piercing the skin from inside to outside, and then the broken end of fracture retracts into the skin. Such wounds need thorough debridement under anesthesia and is even more necessary for patients who are injured in swamps, wetlands, bathrooms, and other similar places. When the broken end of the fracture is exposed, avoid putting it back into the skin until debridement is performed. During physical examination, the skin temperature, color, and capillary filling degree of limbs should be compared with those of healthy limbs. In the initial evaluation, X-rays should be performed on the injured part, and besides bone tissue injury, attention should also be paid to whether there are imaging findings of foreign bodies in soft tissues.

For patients with a single closed limb injury, special attention should be paid to the degree of limb swelling and blood supply. Prolonged compression of limbs, such as crushing injury without fracture and lithotomy postural operation, can lead to severe swelling of limbs, soft tissue ischemia, and then osteofascial compartment syndrome, which is often overlooked in clinical practice. Misdiagnosis of osteofascial compartment syndrome is one of the most common medical dispute lawsuits in North America [27]. The most credible signs of osteofascial compartment syndrome are pains inconsistent with the degree of injury and passive traction pain of involved muscle groups. The greatest challenge of treating osteofascial compartment syndrome is making the decision regarding the timing to perform surgical decompression [28]. Once the diagnosis is made, fascial compartment incision and decompression should be performed.

Arterial injury is a serious complication, which can cause limb necrosis and amputation. Single limb injury accompanied by arterial injury is easy to be overlooked, especially for closed dislocation. Supracondylar fracture of humerus in children can cause brachial artery injury, and knee dislocation can cause popliteal artery injury [29]. When the arterial injury is suspected, the vascular ultrasound is feasible. The advantage of ultrasonography is that it can quickly and accurately locate the plane of vascular injury and buy time for saving limbs. The disadvantage is poor visualization for the surgeons. CT angiography is an important method to judge vascular injury, which can directly display the course and injury plane of the artery, but its operation is time-consuming. Because the contrast agent is injected into blood vessels under pressure, there is the possibility of false-negative, and a few patients are allergic to contrast agents. Once limb artery injury is found, the emergency surgery should be performed immediately.

2. **Handling of Multiple Injuries**

Multiple injuries are mostly caused by high-energy forces, which often cause open fractures of limbs accompanied by injuries to the abdominal/pelvic organs and brain. The omission diagnosis rate of patients with multiple injuries admitted to hospital within 24 h can be as high as 12% [30, 31].

For patients with multiple injuries, the treatment strategy in ATLS (Advanced Trauma Life Support) standard [32] should be followed. Key monitoring indexes include vital signs, pulse oxygen content, intake and output volume, arterial blood gas, hematocrit, and central venous pressure. Traumatic patients are divided into three categories, Grade I trauma, Grade II trauma, and nontraumatic service admission (Table 16.2), and high-grade patients should be treated preferentially. The evaluation should be rapid and accurate, without delaying effective treatment due to unclear diagnosis. The principle of resuscitation is to put saving lives first, preserve or repair injured tissues and organs as much as possible, recover functions, and actively prevent and treat systemic and local complications.

Table 16.2 Grading of traumatic patients

Grade I trauma	Grade II trauma
SPB ≤ 90 and/or receiving blood transfusion in transfer	11 < GCS ≤ 14
GCS ≤ 12 or further deterioration of GCS	Age ≤ 5 or ≥ 65
RR > 30 or < 8	Fall height > 20 feet
RTS (trauma correction score) ≤ 11	Trauma of automobile to pedestrians, trauma in cab
Gunshot wound to head	Incised wound near wrist/ankle joint
Open pelvic fracture	Trauma accompanied by burn
Penetrating injury near knee/elbow joint	Multiple fractures/open fractures
No pulse at the extremities	Pelvic fracture/crush injury
Traumatic paralysis	Projectile/tilting vomiting occurs
Patients with abnormal airway or tracheal intubation	Inter hospital referral, trauma occurring ≤24 h
Flail chest	Patients with warfarin/pregnancy trauma

The ABCDE-based evaluation and treatment process

A: Airway with cervical protection. The treatment measures include lifting the jaw, removing foreign bodies in the respiratory tract, establishing an established artificial airway (orotracheal/nasopharynx endotracheal intubation, cricothyroidotomy).

B: Breathing and ventilation. Common causes of acute ventilation dysfunction include tension pneumothorax, flail chest with lung contusion, massive hemothorax, and open pneumothorax. During the physical examination, the respiratory rhythm and depth are observed carefully, observing whether there are cyanosis and subcutaneous emphysema and whether respiratory sounds decrease at auscultation, etc. Treatment should be performed by giving high-concentration oxygen (oxygen therapy should be given to all traumatic patients), relieving tension pneumothorax (acupuncture decompression/placement of chest catheter), and closing open pneumothorax.

C: Circulation and bleeding control. External/internal bleeding with hypovolemic shock, massive hemothorax, and pericardial tamponade are the common causes of acute circulatory disorder. It is necessary to identify the source of external bleeding and the potential source of internal bleeding in time. It is very important to establish a good venous access. In the emergency clinic, local pressure dressing should be used firstly for the injured limb to control bleeding, and external fixation braces should be used to temporarily stabilize the fracture.

D: Neurological state. Whether pupils are equal in size and sensitive to light should be evaluated, and arrange brain CT examination in time.

E: Exposure/Environment control. Hypothermia is a fatal complication of traumatic patients, so active measures should be taken to keep constant body temperature, and the liquid used during resuscitation should be used after heated by a liquid heating device to avoid iatrogenic hypothermia.

Placement of urinary catheter can not only preliminarily eliminate the possibility of urethral injury, but also roughly evaluate the degree of fluid supplement according to urine volume. After resuscitation, patients should be evaluated again. Special attention should be paid to electrolyte balance and the acid–base balance disorder should be actively corrected. Lactic acid is often used as a marker of hypoperfusion, which can be used as one of the indicators of injury severity and prognosis, and liver and kidney function should also be monitored at the same time. Blood routine, blood coagulation routine, blood type, cross-matching, and other hematological examinations are very important. Blood transfusion treatment can maintain hemodynamic stability. If necessary, an emergency infusion of platelets or fresh frozen plasma can be given. Bedside X-rays are performed to confirm the fractures in all parts of the body, and bedside B-ultrasound to confirm the injuries of abdominal parenchymal organs such as liver, spleen, and kidney. When there is a pelvic ring injury, a rectovaginal examination should be performed to rule out open wounds. After receiving the corresponding resuscitation measures, traumatic patients reestablish the stability of the internal environment. When the general condition permits, early fracture treatment can bring benefits to patients and avoid complications caused by long-term immobilization

16.2.2 Debridement and Routine Treatments in Trauma Rooms

For seriously contaminated open wounds, during the preliminary examination, preliminarily wash and disinfect the wound, and carefully remove foreign matters and obviously necrotizing soft tissues. Normal saline is preferable as the flushing fluid to avoid inducing excessive pain and unnecessary bleeding and aggravating inflammatory reactions for patients. Arterioles with noticeable active bleeding can be ligated using sutures; in case of active bleeding of large arteries, hemostasis can be achieved using gauze packing or small vascular clamp; during the patient's transfer from the emergency department to the operating room, the number of gauzes and vascular clamps in the body should be informed to relevant persons, so as not to leave them inside the patient.

16.2.3 Bacterial Culture, Anti-Infection, and Tetanus

1. **Bacterial culture**

During the initial wound assessment, the swab bacterial culture of tissue in the wound is carried out in a strictly sterile environment. However, most surgeons prefer to perform wound swab examination in the operating room and cut off several pieces of representative wound tissues at the same time, so as to create a suitable microbial environment. Before and after the debridement of wounds, the swab operation is performed to determine whether the debridement is complete or not. The wound secretion culture and drug sensitivity test at different times are also effective references for the adjustment of antibacterials.

2. **Anti-infection**

Although there are controversies about the types and duration of antibiotics, the systematic use of antibiotics for open fractures is still considered a standard treatment. The most effective way to prevent open fracture infection is to use antibiotics according to experience as early as possible (0.5–1 h before the operation) for a short term (24–48 h). Early use of antibiotics can reduce risk factors of open fracture infection by 59% [33]. Bacterial test results are an important basis for guiding the application of antibiotics, but we cannot get the test results at the first time, so we can only use them by experience. Therapeutic antibiotics should be used according to the results of bacterial culture. The wound contamination of open fractures is dominated by Staphylococcus, and cephalosporins against *Staphylococcus aureus* are selected. Staphylococcus is the main pathogen of orthopedic infection, and the first-generation cephalosporins are generally preferred [34].

The guidelines of prophylactic antibiotics for open fractures in China are divided into two levels, Level 1 recommendations: (1) Antibiotics against Gram-positive bacteria should be used as early as possible after injury; (2) Aminoglycoside antibiotics are used in combination for Gustilo III open fracture contaminated by Gram-negative bacteria; (3) For patient wounds with fecal and potentially Clostridium contamination (such as agricultural-related injuries), high-dose penicillin should be used in combination; (4) Antibiotics have no advantages over aminoglycosides and cephalosporins, which have adverse effects on fracture healing and increase the infection risk of Gustilo III open fracture. Level 2 recommendations: (1) The use of antibiotics should last for 72 h for open fractures, and should not exceed 24 h for patients with wounds covered by soft tissue; (2) The use of aminoglycosides antibiotics once a day is safe and effective for Gustilo II and III open fractures [35].

3. **Tetanus**

Tetanus is a specific infection causing muscle spasm by Clostridium tetani invading the human body through the skin or mucous membrane wounds. The diagnosis of tetanus mainly depends on the history of trauma and clinical manifestations, with limited mouth opening, sardonic facies, and increased muscle tension as the characteristic manifestations, and high sensitivity and specificity of the tongue depressor test. When diagnosis based on the above symptoms is difficult, the laboratory diagnosis method can be considered. Positive clostridium tetani culture or PCR assay in wound tissues can confirm tetanus, but negative results cannot rule out the diagnosis. Serum tetanus IgG antibody can protect the body when its concentration is >0.1 U/ml [36, 37].

Laboratory test is not a routine method, for it cannot be implemented in most hospitals in China at present. Human beings have no natural immunity to tetanus and need artificial immunity. Active immunization is very important for tetanus prevention. Tetanus Toxoid vaccine (TT) can be used as a monovalent antigen vaccine alone or combined with diphtheria toxoid or diphtheria toxoid and pertussis vaccine [38]. At present, there are refined tetanus antitoxin (TAT), equine tetanus immunoglobulin, and human tetanus immunoglobulin (HTIG). The dosage of HTIG is 3000–6000 U, and that of TAT is (50,000–200,000) U [39]. The main principles of tetanus treatment: sedation and analgesia and muscle relaxation to control spasm, correction of autonomic nerve dysfunction to avoid exhaustion; thorough debridement and anti-Clostridium tetanus treatment; neutralization of toxins in the circulatory system; and symptomatic support treatment [40, 41]. Early and thorough debridement after injury is one of the key measures. Antibiotics play an auxiliary role in the treatment of tetanus, so it is recommended to give antibiotics to inhibit the proliferation of Clostridium tetani in wounds. The first-line medications recommended are metronidazole and penicillin. Pay attention to nutritional supplements (high calorie and high protein) and maintain the balance of water and electrolyte, for tetanus patients consume more calories and moisture every day because of repeated paroxysmal convulsions and massive sweating, and try to adopt enteral nutrition support for animal injuries.

At present, open fractures caused by animal bites are common [42, 43]. The main pathogens from animal bites are oral flora of the animal and human skin flora. Capnocytophaga (a Gram-negative bacterium requiring complex nutrition) caused by dog bite can lead to bacteremia and fatal sepsis after dog bite, especially in patients without spleen, those with long-term alcohol abuse, and those with basic liver diseases [44, 45]. Rabies is a fatal disease, and there is no prohibition on human rabies vaccination after exposure [46]. It is very important to wash the dog bite wounds thoroughly and effectively. Primary wound closure can be adopted for simple laceration wounds. In the early treatment of susceptible patients, it is necessary to conduct wound cleaning and debridement of inactivated tissues, open and drain bite wounds, change dressing regularly, and delay wound closure according to the wound condition after 72 h of injury [47].

16.2.4 Wound Dressing

Open wounds should be bandaged with sterile dressing after being examined by doctors in the clinic. The thickness of the dressing should not be too thin to avoid blood extravasation and internal and external communication, thus increasing the risk of infection. Elastic compression bandages should be used locally to bandage open wounds. When there is active bleeding, tourniquet should not be used at the proximal end of limbs as much as possible, which may easily cause long ischemia time at the distal end of limbs. Limbs are temporarily fixed by a splint or brace, which is convenient for patient handling and examination.

16.3 Principles of Debridement of Soft Tissue Injury

Sun Jie and Jia Jian

16.3.1 Debridement and Suturing

Debridement is to clean and decontaminate fresh and open stained/contaminated wounds, remove blood clots and foreign bodies, cut off dead tissues, and then close wounds, so as to minimize contamination, even turn them into clean wounds, thus achieving healing by first intention and facilitating the recovery of the function and morphology of injured parts.

The complete concept of debridement of contaminated wounds should be attributed to Pierre Joseph Desault (1744–1795), Director of Surgery, French Charity Hospital. He advocated trimming the wound edge and removing all inactivated tissues and foreign bodies. In 1878, Carl Reyher published the treatise *Initial Debridement of Gunshot Wounds*, stating that debridement and antimicrobial agents could significantly reduce the mortality and amputation rate of the wounded. He advocated that after debridement, the wound should only be filled with dressing, and the granulation tissue should be allowed to grow gradually to close the wound without delayed suturing. His correct ideas about early debridement were not recognized until the First World War. In 1898, Friederic in Leipzig, Germany, confirmed through animal experiments that the most effective time limit for debridement of contaminated wounds was 6 h after injury. He also proved the importance of removing necrotic muscle tissue and found that the presence of necrotic tissue in the wound would aggravate the infection. His articles attracted wide attention and supported the importance of early debridement with scientific experiments.

In 1916, Tuffier published a paper on delayed suturing at an international academic conference, which was agreed by the most. In 1917, at the meeting of the allied countries on the principles of war injury treatment, it was determined that the principles of war injury treatment were: cutting off necrotic tissue, removing foreign bodies, opening wounds without suturing. Initial suturing is only suitable for wounds within 8 h. Later, scholars all advocated that open fracture and amputation wounds should not be sutured at the initial stage, thus determining the principles of treatment of war wounds.

16.3.2 Debridement Procedures

16.3.2.1 Washing

Choose sterile dressing to cover the wound, wash the skin around the wound, shave off the hair, remove the grease stains with gasoline, then wash with soapy water, and finally wash with distilled water. Wash the wound after washing the surrounding skin. First rinse with isotonic saline simply, then rinse with hydrogen peroxide solution, and then rinse with isotonic saline repeatedly. Rinsing can be carried out under pressure, commercial wound flushers can cause pulse or pressure rinsing, and unconditional grass-roots units can use sterile plastic bottles as simple flushers. It is recommended to use enough normal saline for low-pressure rinsing. According to Gustilo typing, it is recommended to use 3, 6, and 9 L of normal saline for wound rinsing for type I, II, and III, respectively [48–51]. The skin is disinfected after the wound is rinsed. At present, iodophor disinfectant is commonly used, which has little irritation to the skin and can be used in the wound. After disinfection, sterile drapes are laid as usual.

16.3.2.2 Cleaning

Skin debridement: Cut off the inactivated skin, and trim the irregular skin with blood supply by cutting off the contaminated area of 1–2 mm along the edge of the wound.

Subcutaneous tissues: thoroughly remove contaminated, inactivated, and non-bleeding subcutaneous tissues.

Subcutaneous fat: it has a poor blood supply and is easy to cause infection; therefore, some more fat tissues can be removed.

Muscle debridement: Inactivated muscles should be removed completely; severely contaminated and completely broken tendon ends should also be removed; in treating muscles, it is necessary to observe the "4C signs", namely, Color, Contractibility, Consistency, and Capacity of blood.

Blood vessel debridement: The adventitia is removed after contamination without fracture; important blood vessels with complete rupture, contusion, and thromboembolism need to be anastomosed or transplanted after resection to ensure blood supply of limbs; small vessels with severe contusion should be excised, and the broken ends can be ligated.

Nerve debridement: For those that are lightly contaminated, lightly swab with normal saline cotton balls, and those who are seriously contaminated, carefully peel off and remove the contaminated epineurium and keep its branches as much as possible.

Tendon debridement: Tendons that are severely cracked, contaminated, and lose vitality should be removed, and uninjured tendons should be carefully protected.

Debridement of fracture end: The depth of treatment for periosteal cortex contamination usually does not exceed 0.5–1.0 mm, and the penetration of cancellous and marrow cavity can reach 1 cm; contaminants entering the marrow cavity can be scraped off with a curette; small free bone flaps that have lost contact with surrounding tissues should be removed as appropriate.

Recleaning: After thorough debridement, the wound is rinsed with sterile normal saline 2–3 times; then soaked or put a wet compress with 0.1% active iodine for 3–5 min, and rinsed off with saltwater; if the wound is heavily contaminated and has a long time after injury, it can be washed with 3% hydrogen peroxide and then rinsed with saltwater; surgical instruments and gloves are replaced, a layer of sterile drape is spread around the wound, and the tissue is to be repaired.

16.3.2.3 Repairing

Treatment of fracture: After debridement, the fracture should be reconstructed under direct vision. If it is stable after reduction, plaster support or continuous bone traction can be used for external fixation. Fixation can be considered in the following cases: (1) Those with anastomosis and repair of vascular and nerve injuries; (2) After fracture reduction, the broken end is extremely unstable; and (3) Multiple fractures and segmental fractures.

Fixation by external fixator: (1) External fixator technique is simple, safe, and convenient, with little blood loss. (2) It has advantages when injury control is needed, such as type IIIC open fracture and unstable patients with multiple injuries [52]. (3) External fixator can protect the blood supply of the fracture site, avoid local soft tissue injury or increased pressure in the compartment caused by implants, and can be used for fractures with severe soft tissue injury and severe wound contamination [53, 54]. (4) It is used for temporary external fixation, which is convenient for the second stage of internal fixation treatment. For patients with serious injury contamination and potential infection risk, it can be used as a terminal fixation method [55].

Internal fixation: (1) Intramedullary nail fixation: Patients have good tolerance, with early weight-bearing time, low reoperation rate, and low malalignment incidence [56]. Gustilo types I and II, including a small number of type III of open fractures for the long shaft of lower limbs, can be fixed with intramedullary nails in case of thorough debridement and good soft tissue coverage. Reaming is not recommended for patients with open long bone fractures. Reaming is not recommended for patients with multiple injuries [57]. (2) Plate fixation [58–60]: The following situations can be considered to be treated by plate fixation: Intra-articular and metaphyseal fractures; Thorough debridement and good coverage of the wound at the same time.

Factors to be considered in fracture fixation: Anatomical location and characteristics of fracture; surrounding skin and soft tissue conditions, including the location and extent of open wounds; degree of contamination; general condition of other patients with combined injuries.

The principles of fracture fixation are as follows: intra-articular fractures should be anatomized and reduced; for fracture of diaphysis and metaphysis, only need to restore limb length and alignment; the surgical approach and the placement of internal fixation or external fixation should be designed reasonably so as not to affect the follow-up operation.

Vascular repair: After debridement, the important vascular injuries should undergo primary anastomosis without tension. If there are many defects, autologous vascular graft repair is feasible.

Nerve repair: After nerve fracture, strive for primary suture repair. If there is a defect, the distal and proximal ends of the nerve can be dissociated or the adjacent joints can be flexed, so that the two broken ends can be sutured together. If the defect is larger than 2 cm, an autologous nerve graft can be performed. If conditions do not permit, it can be left to the second stage.

Tendon repair: The tendon with sharp tool cut, flat end, and no tissue contusion can be sutured after debridement.

16.4 Wound Closure

Sun Jie and Jia Jian

Complete debridement is the basis for treating open soft tissue injuries. On the basis of complete debridement, reliable measures must be taken to close and cover the wound.

16.4.1 Wound Treatment Concept

The treatment goal of open fracture decades ago was to fix the fracture quickly, firmly and conduct primary closure of wounds, but the current treatment principle is repeated debridement and staged operation of delayed wound closure, which can reduce the complications of wound healing and promote limb salvage of complex limb trauma.

16.4.2 Patient Assessment and Wound Assessment

The assessment of patients and wounds must be comprehensive, systematic, and evidence-based. Primary closure can be achieved in most trauma wounds. However, a considerable number of wounds involve the reconstruction of tissue defects, from simple debridement and suture, skin grafting to complex tissue flap transplantation. Therefore, the assessment of patients and wounds is very important for the formulation of treatment protocols.

Patients with wounds should receive comprehensive medical history collection and physical examination, including systematic review. Medical history collection includes current and previous trauma history, and also includes the patient's occupation, interests, and treatment expectations; at the same time, patients' treatment compliance should also be evaluated. The systemic factors related to patients with poor outcomes include diabetes, obesity, peripheral arterial occlusive disease, malnutrition (lack of protein and vitamin C, etc.), chronic renal failure, taking steroids or other immunosuppressant drugs, scar diathesis, connective tissue diseases (such as Ehlers–Danlos syndrome, Marfan syndrome, osteogenesis imperfecta).

Medical history collection and physical examination include:

1. **Injury time** For assessment of primary or secondary closure, the traditional view is that wounds within 6 h of injury are considered to have low contamination level of pathogenic microorganisms, which is the "golden time" for wound suture; pathogenic microorganisms have begun to reproduce and spread in wounds within 6–12 h of injury, but they have not reached a significant level, so primary suture can also be performed after debridement; a large number of pathogenic microorganisms have reproduced within wounds that have been injured for more than 12 h, which greatly increases the probability of infection. Therefore, sutures are generally not recommended for wounds that have been injured for more than 12 h [61]. However, some studies in recent years have shown that for wounds less than 19 h, as long as there are no visible signs of infection and severe skin and soft tissue crush and inactivation, they can also be sutured [62, 63]. Therefore, at present, for wounds within 19 h, it is necessary to comprehensively consider whether to conduct primary suture according to the wound position, blood supply, soft tissue condition, contamination degree, and the patient's own situation [64].
2. **Injury mechanism and energy** Identify whether there are foreign bodies in the wound, and predict the occurrence of infection or scar formation. Wounds caused by sharps have little injury to surrounding tissues, and the risk of infection and significant scar formation is relatively low. Skin laceration can produce wounds with irregular edges and damage surrounding tissues, and the risk of infection and scar formation is moderate [63]. Direct stress injury (such as beating and explosive injury) can lancinate the skin and damage the adjacent soft tissue, usually forming radial laceration; these wounds have the highest risk of infection [65]. It is necessary to pay attention to whether there is a closed degloving injury of tissue, that is, Morel-Lavallée injury, if there is shear force injury.

3. **Location and size of wound** It is important to identify the conditions at the bottom of the wound for the formulation of the treatment protocol, such as the fracture under laceration or the deep structure injury that penetrates the joint space when the finger is lacerated. When examining the wound, it should be evaluated whether there are tissue exposure and defects, tissue ischemia or necrosis, and whether there are signs of inflammation and infection.
4. **Foreign bodies** Not all foreign bodies can be found by direct visual examination of the wound, especially if the bottom of the wound cannot be seen. If the foreign body is radiopaque, radiological evaluation is helpful, which is an appropriate auxiliary means for visual observation [66, 67]. When properly trained ultrasound doctors perform bedside ultrasound, it is also helpful to detect foreign bodies, including radiation-permeable substances.
5. **Neurovascular or tendon injuries** Careful evaluation of peripheral circulation and extremity sensory can determine whether there is neurovascular injury. Examination of the nervous system for conscious and cooperative patients can easily identify the related motion or sensory loss. For unconscious or uncooperative patients, attention should be paid to gross functional loss. For any wound on the tendon, tendon function should be evaluated and the bottom of the wound should be carefully explored to determine the condition of the tendon injury. The position of the body part at the time of injury must be considered during assessment. The end of the tendon that has been completely severed may retract, and thus cannot be detected.

After summarizing all kinds of examination results needed for clinical decisions, the complex interrelationships among all these factors should be analyzed to formulate the optimal treatment protocol. The treatment protocol may be a conservative, nonsurgical protocol, or a complex protocol that requires staged reconstructive surgery.

16.4.3 Preoperative Plan and Selection of Operation Timing

16.4.3.1 Preoperative Plan

The formulation of a preoperative plan is an important treatment specification. When making a detailed preoperative plan, surgeons will carefully evaluate various feasible plans, so as to better evaluate the advantages and disadvantages of surgical treatment and benefit the whole surgical team. Traditional preoperative plan tools include drawing, photo, X-ray, CT, and MRI, etc. At present, the application of many modern tools, such as surface scanners, micro-scanners, and computer simulation technologies, can accurately simulate each surgical step. We should first consider the method with the highest success rate and better postoperative effect, rather than the simplest one. A perfect preoperative plan should take into account the function, good-looking, and appropriate surgical difficulty. The following several basic principles should be followed when formulating an operation plan before any reconstructive surgery of soft tissues [68].

Principle 1: Similar Tissues are Selected as Substitutes
When repairing tissue defects, the same tissue should be preferred to replace the defect part, that is, skin replaced by skin, fat replaced by fat, muscle replaced by muscle, and bone tissue replaced by bone tissue, so as to restore the normal function and appearance of the tissue to the greatest extent.

Principle 2: Selection of Donor Site
The human body itself is a precious "tissue bank," but the available tissue resources are limited. In the preoperative planning of soft tissue repair, while considering the recovery of the function of the recipient site, the tissue injury of the donor site should also be fully considered. The principle of operation is to ensure that the injury to the donor site caused is not more serious than the original defect. In patients requiring amputation, amputated limbs can provide valuable tissue for reconstructive surgery.

Principle 3: Function and Good-Looking
Esthetic factors are not as important as facial repair when repairing limb trauma. In preoperative planning, the recovery of the function of the weight-bearing area must be considered first, and the incision position should be carefully designed to avoid scar in the pressure area.

Principle 4: Alternate Plan
There is a certain risk of failure in any reconstructive surgery of tissues, so there must be an alternate operation plan. If unexpected surgical results before surgery are encountered during and after surgery, it is necessary to adjust the original plan and re-implement the new surgical protocol.

16.4.3.2 Selection of Operation Timing

After the surgical protocol is determined, the next step is to determine the operation timing. In the past, due to the different nature and time of debridement of soft tissues, there were some controversies about the operation timing of closing the wound in different medical centers. Active debridement and early closure of lower limb wounds with myocutaneous flaps can reduce the incidence of osteomyelitis, nonunion, and amputation. Most reconstructive surgeries of tissues are allowed to be delayed for 1–2 days, which should be used to improve the operation plan and treat various comorbidities, such as low protein and hyperglycemia, as much as possible. If the tissue reconstruction involves different professional disciplines, it is necessary for the teams of different disciplines to fully communicate with each other about the surgical protocol, and determine the treatment sequence and the optimal operation timing.

16.4.4 Primary and Secondary Closure of Wounds

Wound closure is quite challenging in trauma treatment. The objectives of wound treatment include: (1) control bleeding; (2) reduce the risk of infection; (3) obtain the optimal healing; (4) minimize the discomfort and loss of function caused by treatment; and (5) get the optimal cosmetic result.

The ideal way of wound closure is primary or early wound closure. The decision to perform primary suturing on the wound, make the wound heal through secondary suturing, or delay primary suturing depends on the time of injury, the mechanism, and the degree of contamination. Inflammatory signs (redness, fever, swelling, and pain) are the absolute contraindications for wound suturing. If there are no such signs, it is necessary to decide whether to suture the wound according to clinical judgment. There is no exact treatment method to ensure success. When the first treatment fails, other treatments should be considered.

Traditionally, the wound healing process after tissue injury is divided into three main phases: inflammation and exudation phase, granulation tissue hyperplasia phase, and scar formation and remodeling phase. However, with the rapid development of molecular biology, people have gradually deepened their understanding of wound repair. Now, the healing process after tissue injury is regarded as a process of proliferation, differentiation, migration, apoptosis, and disappearance of various repair cells, and it is also the result of network interaction formed by a series of different types of cells, structural proteins, growth factors, and protein kinases. The inflammatory phase and proliferative phase will be shortened if primary or early closure of the wound can be achieved, so as to obtain ideal wound healing and functional recovery.

16.4.4.1 Primary Wound Closure

After debridement, the surgeon should decide whether to close the wound immediately according to clinical experience. Failure of primary wound closure will bring more injuries and worse clinical results than delayed or secondary wound closure.

1. **Indications**

In general, the primary closure can usually be achieved for wounds that can be closed by drawing the wound edge close or skin transplantation or flap transfer. For open wounds with internal fixation of fractures, it is still controversial whether to keep them open and delay primary closure or perform primary closure at the first debridement. The absolute contraindications of primary closure wounds include severe contaminated wound (wastewater, farm, etc.), a large area of soft tissue defect (high energy weapon wound, gunshot wound, and explosive wound), excessive wound tension, and stab wound. Relative contraindications include wound opening time longer than 12 h, bite by humans and animals, foreign body residue, deep fracture, and acute fasciotomy decompression wound.

When deciding whether to carry out primary wound closure, the influence of various systems of the whole body and related conditions should also be considered, including the followings: current medical history and injury mechanism, accompanying injury to the body, patient age, blood vessel status, blood glucose status, immune function, and coagulation function.

The primary wound closure should not be adopted if adjacent tissues may lead to delays and a large amount of inactivation, and multiple debridement must be performed before wound closure, especially in the following situations: blast injury, explosive wound, thermal burn, and electric shock wound.

The biggest obstacle of primary wound closure is the excessive tension of the skin margin of the wound. When it is difficult to judge the tension of the wound, the judgment that tends to have high tension should be chosen. It is best to open the wound and wait for the second stage operation to close the wound. An accurate approximation of subcutaneous fascia helps to reduce the skin tension during the primary wound closure. When the wound is sutured, it is found that the skin margin between sutures turns white, indicating that the tension is too high.

2. **Timing**

The length of time from injury to operation is another important factor that affects the decision of primary wound closure. Generally speaking, after thorough debridement, most of the wounds 6–8 h after injury can achieve primary wound closure. For those over 8 h, the possibility of infection increases. For those over 24 h, infection is usually difficult to avoid, the debridement and primary wound closure is not suitable. At this time, there has been mass propagation of bacteria and the wound has been infected, so debridement can destroy the formed granulation tissue barrier and cause the infection to spread. Contamination degree is a very important factor that affects the time limit of debridement and determines the primary wound closure. If the contamination is serious, the wound can be infected within 3–4 h. On the contrary, the wound with light contamination can also be completely debrided even after more than 24 h. Wounds that exceed 24 h in winter can sometimes be debrided for primary closure.

3. **Suture materials**

Absorbable sutures are generally used to suture fascia, subcutaneous layer, and joint capsule, while nonabsorbable sutures are used to suture skin and tendon. In 2003, a new generation of absorbable sutures containing antimicrobial agents (triclosan) was launched. Retrospective analysis showed that the use of absorbable sutures containing antimicrobial agents (triclosan) significantly reduced the incidence of surgical site infection (SSI) in orthopedic surgery compared with ordinary sutures.

4. **Basic principles of suturing**
   (a) Ensuring good approximation of sutured wounds. Suturing should be performed in layers according to the anatomical level of the tissue. Fascia closure is usually performed, and the subcutaneous tissue is sutured to close the dead space, and other tissues are not involved or sutured to prevent effusion, hematocele, and infection. Dermal suturing can achieve good surface approximation and relieve tension, so that the epidermis can be closed on the premise of obtaining a good appearance. The stitch edge and length of the wound must be uniform, so as to keep the wound good-looking, tightly sutured as well as in consistent stress and shared tension.
   (b) Maintain proper tension inside the stitching. Tension of suture should be based on the close contact of incision edges. Excessive tension can easily cause tissue curling and overlapping, damage local blood supply, and even tissue cutting and ischemic necrosis. When the tension is too loose, it will leave dead space, which will easily lead to hematoma and infection. Relaxation suturing should be performed when the wound tension is high. The operator needs to consider that tissue edema will be accompanied after trauma or operation, so the skin tension will increase in the first few days after wound closure, which needs to be considered in advance when the wound is sutured. This should be considered in advance when suturing the wound. If the defect is too large, flap transposition coverage or skin graft may be considered.
   (c) Interrupted suture is used instead of continuous suture when closing open wounds. The main reasons include two aspects: possible soft tissue edema and wound contamination. In case of hematoma formation, local wound inflammation, and infection, some knots can be removed at intervals to reduce tension.
   (d) Select appropriate sutures and suture needles

Skin staples close wounds quickly. For severe traumatic patients with heavy bleeding, long operation period, large dosage of anesthetics, and poor systemic status, in order to end the operation as soon as possible, the wound closing speed becomes extremely important. The speed advantage of staple is obvious. However, the staples need to be removed within the specified time, which will easily cause the wound widening and secondary wound dehiscence, and eventually form bad-looking scars. Meanwhile, the staple is expensive.

With regard to suture removal, it is generally recommended that the suture of limb parts be removed 10–14 days after surgery. In some critical or special parts, such as thighs or calcaneus, the suture may be removed after 3 weeks. When the primary wound closure cannot be achieved, delay closure can be considered.

16.4.4.2 Secondary Wound Closure

Secondary wound closure describes the healing of a wound after being dissected or a defect being formed, including a complex process of tissue regeneration, granulation tissue proliferation, and scar formation, with which the synergistic effect is reflected in multiple healing processes. Secondary closure occurs in wounds with large defect, irregular wound edge, dehiscence, infection, or in which the wound edges cannot be approximated.

For fasciotomy or traumatic wounds under high tension, the primary wound closure cannot be attained. Some alternative methods of closure can be applied, for example, the large surgical wound can be approximated and closed by elastic tension sutures, which can help reduce the swelling. For fasciotomy wounds, the tension suture can be placed without the need of skin graft. Another technique for tension wound closure is the rubber strip which can gradually approximate the wound edges with its elasticity. This method can avoid dragging of the skin. When the swelling subsides, under the natural elasticity of the rubber strip, the wound edges can be tightened and approximated (Fig. 16.1).

The methods conducive to facilitating the secondary wound closure include: negative pressure wound therapy; elevation of the affected limb for elimination of swelling; the application of an A-V impulse system, etc. The disadvantages of the secondary wound closure include: delayed wound closure; high risk of infection; large scar formation, etc.

16.4.5 The Method for Closure of Some Special Wounds

1. **Wounds that cannot bear tension**: the requirements for the suture technique are different for some special wounds. For example, skin avulsion wound, post-tension reduced incision wound, and suture of skin flap, if they are completely closed for good approximation and

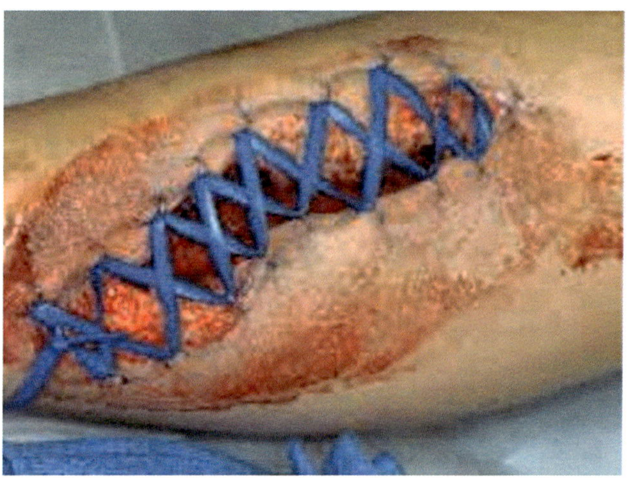

Fig. 16.1 Relaxation treatment of wounds by rubber strips

eversion like common wounds, it is highly likely that the blood supply will be affected by the excessive tension on the wound edge, resulting in local or even large area necrosis. Therefore, for such wounds, considering that the wound cannot bear the tension after being closed, it is usually stitched in the position where the skin naturally relaxes, and the gap of the skin edge is partially reserved for secondary healing, while the larger wound can be covered by skin grafting.

If such wounds are closed by direct suture, the method of knotting and cutting the suture after the needle is removed is also different from the conventional one. In knotting, the "clockwise–counterclockwise" sliding knot should be tied rather than the usual "clockwise–counterclockwise–clockwise" square knot. When cutting the suture, the tail of the suture should be left longer, with the advantage that once the swelling of local skin and soft tissue occurs postoperatively resulting in large tension at the suture and subsequently affecting the blood supply of the skin, forceps or scissors can be used to relax the suture knot to relieve tension without causing the knot becoming unraveled.

2. Wounds with irregular shape: For triangular wounds, diagonally direct suture is not allowed, because it will affect the blood supply of skin at the tip of the triangle and cause skin necrosis here. The correct suture method is to bite from one side of the triangle, through underneath the skin at the tip of the triangle, and then withdraw from the other side of the triangle. Similarly, for a Y-shaped wound, the needle should be bitten from one obtuse angle of the Y-shape, through underneath the skin at an acute angle, and then withdrawn from another obtuse angle.

   For wounds in more irregular shapes, it can be firstly trimmed into a more regular shape by enhanced debridement and then sutured.

   For wounds with unequal skin length on both sides, one end of the wound is aligned firstly for interrupted suture until the end of the wound is reached, which will eventually lead to the phenomenon of "dog ear." Under such circumstances, the "dog ear" cannot be cut off from the bottom of the "dog ears" with scissors, which will in turn create a new "dog ear" for the following suture. The correct way is to cut one side of the "dog ear" along the front sutured wound with a scalpel, then spread the "dog ear" and cut off the other side along the wound [69].
3. Multiple parallel adjacent wounds: Sometimes, clinically, there are multiple parallel wounds in one area, and only narrow skin strips exist between the wounds. Such trauma is common in women who slash their wrists, and they will tentatively make multiple cuts on their wrists. However, due to pain and women's timidity and weakness, the wounds are generally not deep. Under such circumstance, if the interrupted suture is conducted directly in two or more adjacent wounds, respectively, the blood supply of narrow skin strips between the wounds will be affected due to the tension caused by the dense sutures, which is likely to cause necrosis. The correct way is: if the skin strip is very narrow, it can be cut off directly, so that two adjacent wounds can become a large wound, and then sutured. Finally, the phenomenon of "dog ear" may occur at both ends of the wound, and the "dog ear" can be removed according to the above method. Another method can also be taken: Bite from outside the skin on one side of the wound, through underneath the skin under the skin strip between the wounds, and then exit from the skin on the opposite side of the wound on the other side, tie the knot; in such a way the two wounds can be sutured together. This method can also be used for more parallel adjacent wounds.
4. Z-plasty: For the wounds perpendicular to the knuckle print on the palmar side of the finger, direct suture will cause scar contracture in the later stage, affecting the flexion and extension function of the finger. It is required to adopt Z-plasty to close the wounds: An incision is made with the same length as the wound respectively on both sides of the wound at an angle of 60° with both ends of the longitudinal wound, the two incisions are parallel, and subcutaneous tissues are dissected to make them become two equilateral triangular flaps. Cross-suture of the two flaps can change the vertical wound ends by 75%, so that they are no longer perpendicular to the knuckle prints [70].

16.5 Wound Coverage

Sun Jie and Jia Jian

16.5.1 Wound Assessment

The two types of wounds should be carefully identified: Those without exposed bones, tendons, and major nerves and vessels in wounds, and those with exposed bones, tendons, and major nerves and vessels in wounds. The former can be covered by skin grafting, while the latter needs to be covered by skin flap.

16.5.2 Skin Grafting and Skin Substitutes

Skin graft, skin substitute, and tissue flap with or without skin graft have been routinely used in soft tissue repair, which greatly expand the ability of plastic surgeons to perform reconstruction surgery and improve the outcome and quality of life of traumatic patients.

Skin grafts include autologous skin grafts, allogeneic skin grafts, and xenogenic skin grafts. Autologous skin graft refers to the transplantation of the same patient's skin from the donor site to the recipient site. Autologous skin graft is the most commonly used graft in skin reconstruction of various indications. Skin transplantation between two different individuals of the same species is called allogeneic skin grafting. Allogeneic skin graft can be a freshly collected graft or a frozen cadaveric skin graft preserved with glycerol. Application of allogeneic skin graft on superficial split-thickness wounds can relieve pain to the greatest extent and promote re-epithelialization. Allogeneic skin grafts are generally used only in burn centers. Xenogenic skin graft refers to skin transplantation between two different individuals of two different species, which is taken from a species unrelated to human beings and can be used to temporarily cover wounds, especially large-area burns. At present, only porcine skin grafts are used [71, 72]. Xenogenic skin graft is generally readily available, but it may not be as effective as an allogeneic skin graft.

16.5.2.1 Skin Grafting

The biological materials and biosynthetic materials are taken as skin substitutes to temporarily cover the wound. Biological dressing is used to cover and debride the wound, so as to avoid the wound from being dehydrated, and the neoepithelium will separate it from the wound.

In general, any wounds filled with granulation tissue can be covered by a skin graft. However, for wounds in which granulation tissue is not formed or bone and cartilage are obviously exposed, the tissues with autologous blood supply (skin flap) is required to be transplanted for surgical repair.

1. **Autologous skin graft**

Autologous skin grafts can be razor-thin skin graft, split-thickness skin graft (STSG), or full-thickness skin graft (FTSG) (Fig. 16.2). The grafted skin graft has no blood supply and initially survives by absorbing the plasma exuded from the recipient site [73]. In the following 48–72 h, new blood vessels are formed by the capillaries of the skin graft bed to supply the blood. Complete blood circulation is restored within 4–7 days.

(a) Split-thickness skin graft (STSG)

Also known as partial-thickness skin graft, is a portion of the skin of the donor site for transplantation, which contains both the epidermis and the underlying partial dermis. With the remaining skin components, the donor site can heal spontaneously. STSG is most commonly used in tissue coverage. It contains epidermis and dermis with different thickness, ranging from 8/1000 inch (0.196 mm) to 12/1000 inch (0.294 mm).

When large area coverage is needed, the surface area of STSG can be enlarged by using a skin graft mesher (Fig. 16.3). The gap (i.e., mesh) of the mesh skin graft allows the liquid to freely flow out, thus improving the success rate of skin grafting. The proportion of skin graft meshing depends on the amount of skin graft in the donor site.

Skin grafting and fixation

Before skin grafting, the wound bed should be debrided to ensure no hematoma, exudation, and infection. The STSG is transplanted with the dermis face down to the recipient site and fixed. Skin grafts can be fixed with staples, sutures, or tissue glue.

Staple is the fastest way to fix the skin graft to the wound. This technology is simple and straightforward and inexpensive. If the wound surface is irregular in shape, multiple sutures can also be used for tacking suture. After STSG is fixed, appropriate dressing is required to stabilize the skin graft.

(b) Full-thickness skin graft (FTSG)

FTSG refers to the full-thickness skin grafting. Therefore, there is no dermis or epidermis left in the donor site, and the wound must be closed by pushing and advancement of the adjacent skin locally or using another local flap. FTSG is thicker, so it takes longer for revascularization than STSG.

Placement and fixation of skin graft: Tissue wounds should be debrided, and there must be no hematoma, exuda-

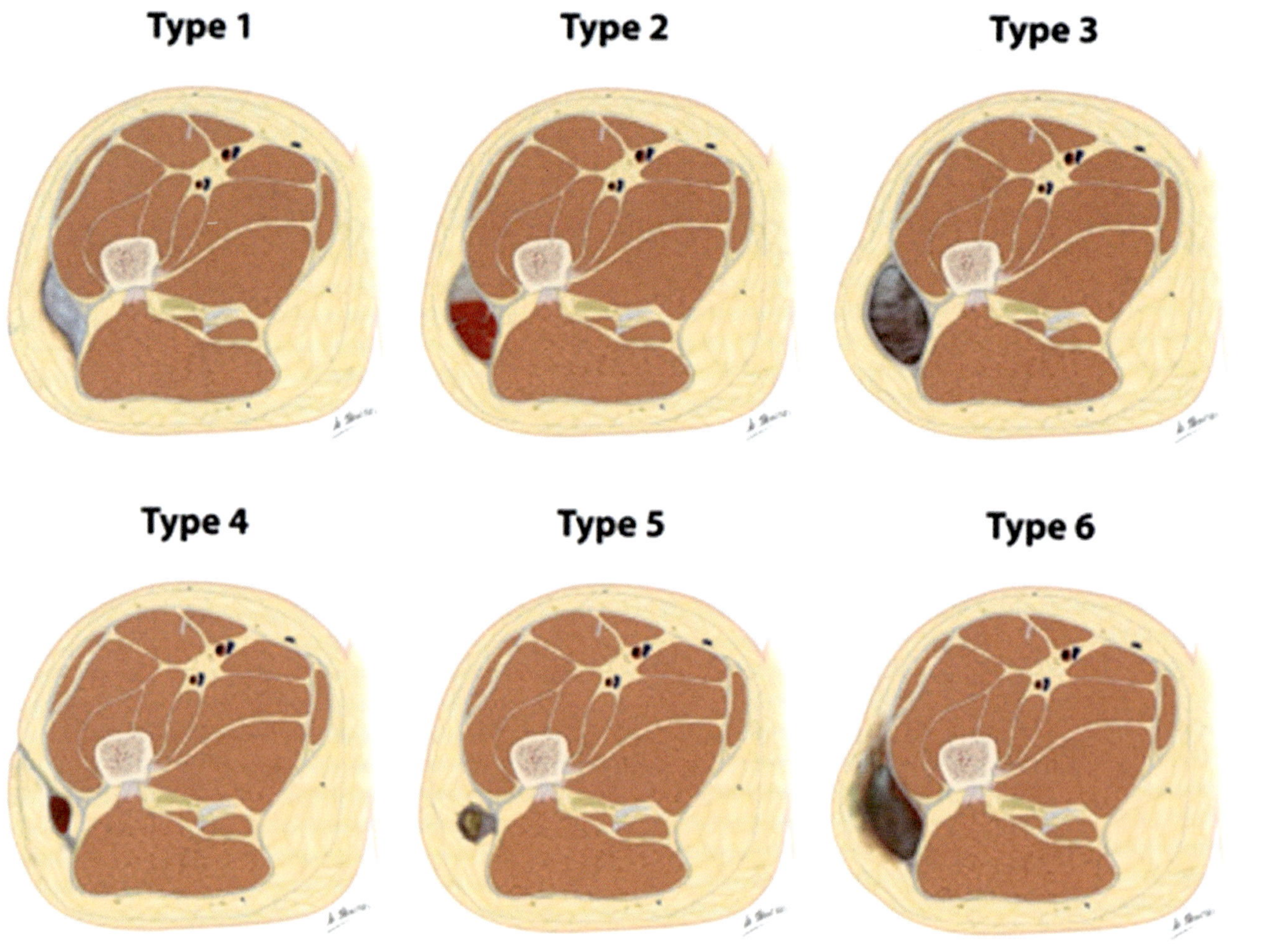

Type 1 Type 2 Type 3

Type 4 Type 5 Type 6

Fig. 16.2 Structural diagram of autologous skin graft

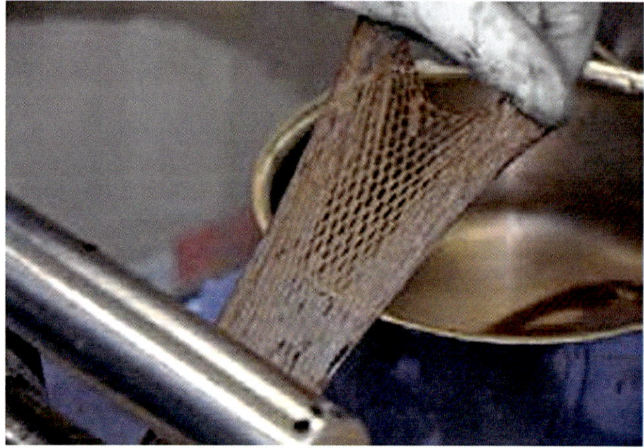

Fig. 16.3 Production of mesh skin graft

tion, and infection. FTSG is implanted into the recipient site and sutured with a fast-absorbing fine suture. The skin graft can be fixed to the recipient site by mattress suture. Some small holes can be punctured on FTSG to promote bloody exudate discharge without destroying skin graft integrity.

(c) Principles for selection of autologous skin graft
   I. For the parts with low requirements for wear resistance on the dorsal side, the split-thickness skin graft can be used, the depth of which does not exceed the dermis, and portion of the dermis is remained in the basal wound, without subcutaneous soft tissue exposed. In such a way, the donor site can naturally heal by vaseline gauze coverage and pressure dressing, and the wound can also be directly sutured for healing by primary intention.
   II. For the parts with high requirements for wear resistance on the palmar side, the full-thickness skin graft, containing full epidermis and dermis, should be used as far as possible. The basal wound of the donor site is subcutaneous soft tissue, and the wound of the donor site needs to be sutured. However, hair follicles will be included in the full-thickness skin

graft, which will cause unnecessary hair on the palmar side.

III. For granulation wounds, the ultrathin skin graft, only containing epidermis, without the dermis, is usually used. The donor site can heal naturally. For donor sites with thinner skin graft, the healing is mainly achieved by epithelialization of hair follicles, with little dermal regeneration. The thicker the skin graft, the better the quality of the skin in the recipient site after survival, and the thicker skin graft can also increase the probability of the re-domination and sensory recovery of the Markel's complex in the recipient site. Of course, the thicker the skin graft, the worse the healing of the donor site is [74].

16.5.2.2 Skin Substitutes

Sometimes the number of skin for transplantation is insufficient during autotransplantation, which affects the completion of skin grafting; however, the life span of allografted and xenografted skin grafts is limited. Besides, allograft also has the potential risk of carrying virus infection. Biosynthetic skin substitutes (dermal regeneration template) give surgeons more choices in reconstruction. These skin substitutes are used to provide dermal components at the reconstruction site to improve skin flexibility and restore the functions of normal skin [75].

16.5.2.3 Skin Flap Grafting

There are many kinds of skin flaps, from simple to complex, which can be divided into the following categories.

1. Local skin flap
   (a) Advancement flap: A small defect can be covered by an advancing skin flap. On fingers, such advancement flap has a special name—Moberg flap. This flap includes bilateral neurovascular bundles, and the cutting range of the flap to the proximal can span one or two joints according to the length of the longitudinal axis of the wound. In the process of dissection, please note that each perforating branch of the digital artery should be cut off and ligated [76].
   (b) VY flap: The defect can also be covered with a VY flap, which can be a single VY of the finger pulp or double VY of both sides of fingers. There are many variations for VY flaps: From the single VY flap of the finger pulp invented by Atasoy in 1935, to the double VY flap with bilateral blood vessels designed by Kutler in 1947, and then to the elongated VY flap with one side digital artery designed by Venkataswamy and Segmüller in 1976, so as to cover a larger area of the wound [77–80].
   (c) Rotation flap: A wide range of skin flaps need to be dissected.
      I. Two special rotation flaps for rhomboid wound: Limberg flap and Dufourmentel flap [81].
      II. Flag flap: A flag flap with a narrow pedicle can be designed with an arterial branch as the pedicle, and the flap can rotate in a wider range with the root of the "flagpole" as the rotation point. This flap is actually an island flap [82].

2. **Cross-finger flap**

For the skin and soft tissue defect on the palmar side of the middle and distal segment of the finger, if the adjacent finger is intact, the "["-shaped flap can be lifted from its dorsal side to cover the wound on the palmar side of the affected finger with split-thickness skin graft in the donor site. The general principle is that the wound of the index finger is covered by the middle finger, that of the middle finger is covered by the ring finger, and that of the ring finger is covered by the little finger, because this is the rest position of the finger, and the position is comfortable after suturing. Of course, the wound of the single finger can also be covered in reverse order according to specific conditions [83].

3. **Distal pedicled flap**

For cases of wounds with more skin and soft tissue defects or multi-finger, dorsal palmar side wounds, the distal pedicled flap is a safe and reliable choice. Including cross-chest flap, cross-arm flap, abdominal flap/tubular flap/buried flap, etc.

(a) Cross-arm flap is suitable for skin and soft tissue defects of fingers. Its appearance and texture are close to those of fingers, but it will limit the movement of healthy limbs.
(b) Cross-chest flap, similar to cross-arm flap, will not affect the movements of the contralateral limb but will leave scars on the exposed parts of the chest, so it is necessary to communicate with patients before surgery.
(c) Abdominal flap, which is suitable for large defect of palm and dorsum of the hand.
(d) Abdominal tubular flap, which is used for the coverage of the wounds of degloving injury and avulsion amputation injury of thumb.
(e) Abdominal buried flap, which is used for a large area of skin and soft tissue coverage of hand degloving injury, and the operation should be conducted several times [84].

4. **Island flap**
   (a) Neurovascular bundle island flap
      I. Anterograde neurovascular bundle island flap: It is usually taken from the ulnar side of the middle finger and the radial side of the ring finger, the neurological bundle of one side of the finger is taken as the pedicle, the rotation point

is the common digital artery from the superficial palmar arch, and the donor site needs to be covered with skin grafts. This flap is often used to cover the wound on the palm side of the thumb, which can resolve its feeling, appearance, and wear resistance, but the disadvantage is that the feeling of donor fingers would be sacrificed [85].

II. Retrograde digital artery island flap: It is taken from the proximal of the same finger side, with the digital artery of this side as the pedicle, with or without the digital nerve, and the rotation point does not exceed the point where the distal perforating branch of the middle phalanx originates. If the flap area is small, the donor site can be sutured directly. This flap is often used to cover the defect on one side of the finger pulp or distal segment of the index-little finger. The advantages are simple operation, high survival rate, and good recovery of wear resistance. The disadvantages are that sometimes the skin flap is slightly thicker and the digital artery needs to be sacrificed [86].

III. First dorsal metacarpal artery island flap: It takes the first dorsal metacarpal artery and branches of the superficial branch of the radial nerve as the pedicle, and is often used to cover the dorsal thumb wound to the lunar side [87].

(b) Perforator flap: Perforator flap does not include well-known arteries, which relies on artery perforating branch for blood supply.

I. Finger dorsal island fascia flap: It does not contain well-known arteries and is usually taken from the dorsal side of fingers. The radial dorsal side or ulnar axis is taken as the pedicle, and the dorsal and rotational points do not exceed the point where the distal perforating branch of the middle phalanx originates. The donor site should be covered with skin grafts. This flap is often used to cover the dorsal or lateral dorsal wounds of the middle and distal thumb-little finger. The advantage is that there is no need to sacrifice the digital artery, and the skin flap is thinner, while the disadvantages are scar left on the bare backside and adhesion between skin graft and extensor tendon [88].

II. Radial/ulnar retrograde island flap of the first metacarpal bone: The nutrient vessel of radial nerve superficial branch is taken as the pedicle. If the flap area is not large, the donor site can be sutured directly. This flap is often used to cover the wound on the dorsal thumb or toward one side [89].

III. Retrograde dorsal metacarpal artery island flap: The dorsal metacarpal artery is taken as the pedicle, and the perforating branch at the finger web is taken as the rotation point to cover the wound near the middle part of the middle index-little finger. The donor site does not need skin grafting [90].

IV. Forearm island fascia flap: The donor site is located on the dorsal forearm, and the superficial branch of radial nerve or cutaneous nerve superficial branch of lateral forearm and its nutrient vessels are taken as the pedicle. Skin grafting is needed in the donor site. It can cover a large area of defects on the dorsal or radial side of the hand. The disadvantage is that an obvious skin grafting scar is left in the bare forearm, and some feelings need to be sacrificed [91].

V. Flap of suprawrist cutaneous branch of ulnar artery: The donor site is located on the ulnar forearm, and the suprawrist cutaneous branch of the ulnar artery is taken as the rotation point, which can cover a large area defect of palm and dorsal ulnar side [92].

(c) Perforator propeller flap: It is an improvement of the perforator flap. After crossing the rotation point, the pedicle of the perforator flap can be extended and dissected a little to form a bilobed flap with the perforator as the axis, the donor end, and near the recipient end as the rotation point. After rotating 180°, it covers the wounds of the recipient site and the donor site near the pedicle, respectively [93].

5. **Free flap**

Free flap is a flexible and diverse choice for cases with proximal flap or pedicled flap unavailable for coverage due to objective conditions. There are many donor sites in the whole body where the flap can be collected, and commonly used clinically are as follows:

(a) Anterolateral thigh (ALT) free flap: The perforating branch of the lateral circumflex femoral artery is taken as the blood supply pedicle, which can be used to cover a large area of wounds in extremities [94].

(b) Forearm vein free flap: It is located on the medial side of the proximal forearm or the palmar side of the distal forearm. The flap contains two veins without arteries, which are respectively anastomosed with the arteries and veins in the wound to provide blood supply and venous reflux of the flap. The key point of this operation is to destroy and ligate the small communicating branch between the two veins in the flap, and only keep the larger communicating branch at the distal end of the flap, so as to avoid the arteriovenous shunt just after the arterial blood enters the flap, which will affect the blood perfusion of most flaps. This flap can cover small- and medium-sized wounds in the hands [95].

(c) Free latissimus dorsi flap: It is located in the chest and back, with the thoracodorsal artery as the pedicle, the flap can cover a large area of wounds in extremities. The key point of this operation is to avoid the injury of the thoracodorsal nerve, so as to avoid the occurrence of intercostal muscle paralysis. This flap can be made into a myocutaneous flap containing latissimus dorsi when necessary [96].

(d) Toe pulp-free flap: It is taken from the first and second toe pulp, including arteria digitalis, vena digitalis, and digital nerve. Because of the similarity of skin texture and appearance, this flap is specially used to cover the wounds of the finger pulp, which can obtain satisfactory appearance, feeling, and texture effect [97].

(e) Free hallux nail flap: It is taken from the skin and soft tissue of the dorsal (including nail bed), lateral and partial plantar sides of the hallux, while the skin and soft tissue of the medial hallux need to be preserved. The flap contains the first dorsal metatarsal artery—dorsal digital artery on the fibular side of the hallux, superficial dorsal vein, and digital nerve. The donor site can be covered by shortened suture or other flaps. This flap is used to cover the degloving injury of the thumb, which can recover the appearance, feeling, and texture of the thumb well [98].

(f) Dorsalis pedis free flap: The flap is taken from the dorsum of the foot, with the dorsalis pedis artery as the blood supply pedicle, and is often used to cover the wound on the back of the hand. This flap can contain the extensor digitorum pedis longus muscle tendon, which can cover the wound and meanwhile be transplanted to repair the defect of the extensor tendon of the hand [99].

Flap summary: It mainly includes five categories: local transfer flap, cross-finger flap, distal pedicled flap, island flap, and free flap. Further subdivided, local transfer flaps include advancement flaps, VY flaps, rotation flaps, etc. Distal pedicled flaps include cross-arm flaps, cross-chest flaps, abdominal flaps (buried, tubular), island flaps include island flaps with major neurovascular bundles, and fascia flaps without major neurovascular bundles.

16.5.2.4 Decision on Wound Coverage

When the operator faces a wound, he/she firstly debrides and enlarges the wound into a neat wound, and then judges whether there are deep tissues (bones and tendons, major nerves and vessels) exposed, if not, skin grafting can be used for coverage. If there is deep tissue exposed in the wound, it is necessary to further judge the size of the area: if the area is small, it can be covered with a local transfer flap; if the area is larger, it should be covered with a cross-finger flap and island flap. If the local conditions close to the skin and soft tissue or close to fingers do not permit, it should be covered with a distal pedicled flap; if the defect area is larger or other objective conditions are not suitable for the distal pedicled flap, the free flap should be considered for coverage [100].

At present, there are two ideas about flap selection: one is the straight ladder theory: it advocates that the flaps should be selected in the order from simple to complex, and simple and low-risk flaps should be used as far as possible, and if conditions do not allow, the flaps should be selected step by step according to the complexity. Secondly, elevator theory: it advocates "what is lacking should be supplemented," and the skin flap donor site should be selected according to the appearance and texture required by the recipient site [101, 102].

References

1. The INSARAG Medical Working Group. The medical management of the entrapped patient with crush syndrome. Geneva: United Nations; 2011.
2. Gonzalez D. Crush syndrome. Crit Care Med. 2005;33(1s):S34–41.
3. Reis ND, Better OS. Mechanical muscle-crush injury and acute muscle-crush compartment syndrome: with special reference to earthquake casualties. J Bone Joint Surg Br. 2005;87(4):450–3.
4. Gillani S, Cao J, Suzuki T, et al. The effect of ischemia reperfusion injury on skeletal muscle. Injury. 2012;43(6):670–5.
5. Junker JPE, Kamel RA, Caterson EJ, et al. Clinical impact upon wound healing and inflammation in moist, wet, and dry environments. Adv Wound Care. 2013;2(7):348–56.
6. Svensjö T, et al. Accelerated healing of full-thickness skin wounds in a wet environment. Plast Reconstr Surg. 2000;106(3):602–12.
7. Shim Y, Hong G, Choi S. Autogenous healing of early-age cementitious materials incorporating superabsorbent polymers exposed to wet/dry cycles. Materials. 2018;11:2476.
8. Strauss EJ, Petrucelli G, Bong M, et al. Blisters associated with lower-extremity fracture: results of a prospective treatment protocol. J Orthop Trauma. 2006;20(9):618–22.
9. Glordano CP, Koval KJ. Treatment of fracture blisters: a prospective study of 53 cases. J Orthop Trauma. 1995;9(2):171–6.
10. Hamele M, Poss WB, Sweney J. Disaster preparedness, pediatric considerations in primary blast injury, chemical, and biological terrorism. World J Crit Care Med. 2014;3(1):15–23.
11. Elsayed NM, Atkins JL. Explosion and blast-related injuries. 1st ed. Singapore: Elsevier; 2010. p. 1–26.
12. Wang DW, Liu Y, Jiang MM. Review on emergency medical response against terrorist attack. Mil Med Res. 2014;1:9–12.
13. Morel-Lavallée M. Decollementstraumatiques de la peau et des couches sousjacentes. Arch GenMed. 1863;1:20–38.
14. Shen C, Peng J, Chen X. Efficacy of treatment in peri-pelvic Morel-Lavallee lesion: a systematic review of the literature. Arch Orthop Trauma Surg. 2013;133(5):635–40.
15. De Coninck T, et al. Imaging features of Morel-Lavallée lesions. J Belg Soc Radiol. 2017;101(S2):15.
16. Liang Y, Li WZ, Jia J. Surgical treatment of unstable pelvic fractures associated with Morel-Lavallee injuries. Orthopedic J China. 2012;22(22):2098–101.
17. John A, Scolaro MD, et al. The morel-Lavallée lesion: diagnosis and management. J Am Acad Orthop Surg. 2016;24(10):667–72.

18. Hak DJ, Olson SA, Matta JM. Diagnosis and management of closed internal degloving injuries associated with pelvic and acetabular fractures: the Morel-Lavallee lesion. Trauma. 1997;42(6):1046–51.
19. Kohler D, Pohlemann T. Operative treatment of the peripelvic MorelLavallée lesion. Oper Orthop Traumatol. 2011;1:15–20.
20. Vanhegan IS, Dala-Ali B, Verhelst L, et al. The Morel-Lavallee lesion as a rare differential diagnosis for recalcitrant bursitis of the knee: case report and literature review. Case Rep Orthop. 2012;593193:2012.
21. MelladoJ M, Bencardino JT. Morel-Lavalléelesion: review with emphasison MR imaging. Magn Reson Imaging ClinN Am. 2005;13(4):775–82.
22. Nickerson TP, et al. The Mayo clinic experience with morel-lavallee lesions: establishment of a practice management guideline. J Trauma Acute Care Surg. 2014;76(2):493–7.
23. Tseng S, Tornetta P. Percutaneous management of Morel-Lavallée lesions. J Bone Joint Surg Am. 2006;1:92–6.
24. Carlson DA, Simmons J, Sando W, et al. Morel-lavalee lesions treated with debridement and meticulous dead space closure: surgical technique. J Orthop Trauma. 2007;21(2):140–4.
25. Regel G, Bayeff-Filloff M. Diagonosis and immediate therapeutic management of limb injuries. A systematic review of literature. Unfallchirurg. 2004;107(10):919–26.
26. Hayden JW. Compartment syndromes: early recognition and treatment. Postgrad Med. 1983;74:191–202.
27. Templemen D, Varecka T, Schmidt R. Economic costs of missed compartment syndromes, paper 212, 60th annual meeting, AAOS, San Francisco, CA, Feb, 1993.
28. Field CK, Se Kowsky J, Holler LH, et al. Fasciotomy in vascular trauma: it is too much, too offen? Am Surg. 1994;60:409–11.
29. Darabos N, Gusic N, Vlahovic T, et al. Staged management of knee dislocation in polytrauma injured patients. Injury, Int J Care Injured. 2013;44(S3):S40–5.
30. Chan RN, Ainscow D, Sikorski JM. Diagnostic failure in the multiple injury. J Trauma. 1980;20:684–7.
31. Buduhan G, McRitchie DI. Missed injuries in patients with multiple trauma. J Trauma. 2000;49:600–5.
32. Vasconez HC, Nicholls PJ. Management of extremity injuries with external fixator or Ilizarov devices cooperative effort between orthopedic and plastic surgeons. Clin Plast Surg. 1991;18(3):505–13.
33. Okike K, Bhattacharyya T. Trends in the managerment of open fractures. A critical analysis. J Bone Joint Surg(Am). 2006;88:2739–48.
34. Sf M. Perioperative rational use of antibiotics in orthopaedic inpatients: analysis of 994 cases. Sichuan Med J. 2011;32(7):1138–40.
35. Lu J, Zhang M. Guidelines of prophylactic antibiotics for open fractures. Chin J Emerg Med. 2012;21(2):174.
36. Tetanus:information for health professionals. Effective date 30 June 2015.
37. Thwaites CL, Beeching NJ, Newton CR. Maternal and neonatal tetanus. Lancet. 2015;385(9965):362–70.
38. Liang JL, Tiwari T, Moro PJ, et al. Prevention of pertussis, tetanus, and diphtheria with vaccines in the United States: Recommendations of the Advisory Committee on Immunization Practices (ACIP). MMWR Recomm Rep, 2018, 67(No. ILg-2): 1–44.
39. Tetanus vaccines: WHO position paper-February 2017. Wldy Epidemiol Rec. 2017;92(6):53–76.
40. Rodrigo CJ, Fernando D, Rajapakse S. Pharmacological management oftetanus: an evidence-based review. Crit Care. 2014;18(2):217.
41. Thwaites CL, Yen LM. Tetanus. In: Longo DL, ASJ F, Kasper DL, et al., editors. Harrison's principles of internal medicine. 18th ed. McGraw Hill: NewYork; 2011. p. 1197–200.
42. Ellis R, Ellis C. Dog and cat bites. Anl Fanl Phvsician. 2014;90(4):239–43.
43. Ambro BT, Wright RJ, Heffefinger RN. Management of bite wounds in the head and neck. Facial Plast Surg. 2010;26(6):456–63.
44. Munnynck K, Voorde W. Forensic approach offatal dog attacks: a case report and literature review. Int J Legal Med. 2002;116(5):295–300.
45. Rogan TV, Bratton SL, Dowd MD, et al. Severe dog bites in children. Pediatrics. 1995;96(5):947–50.
46. WHO Expert consultation on Rabies, third report: Oh yeah, oh WOW WHO technical series report no.1012, Geneva, 2018.
47. Xiaowei Z, Wei L, Xiaowei H, et al. Comparison of primary and delayed wound closure of dog-bite wounds. Vet Comp 0rthop Traumatol. 2013;26(3):204–7.
48. Gustilo RB, Mendoza RM, Williams DN. Problems in the management of type III (severe) open fractures: a new classification of type III open fractures. J Trauma. 1984;24(8):742–6.
49. FLOW Investigators, Bhandari M, Jeray KJ, et al. A trial of wound irrigation in the initial management of open fracture wounds. N Engl J Med. 2015;373(27):2629–41.
50. Anglen JO. Comparison of soap and antibiotic solutions for irrigation of lower-limb open fracture wounds. A prospective, randomized study. J Bone Joint Surg Am. 2005;87(7):1415–22.
51. Sprague S, Petrisor B, Jeray K, et al. Wound irrigation does not affect health-related quality of life after open fractures: results of a randomized controlled trial. Bone Joint J. 2018;100-B(1):88–94.
52. Pape HC, Tornetta P 3rd, Tarkin I, et al. Timing of fracture fixation in multitrauma patients: the role of early total care and damage control surgery. J Am Acad Orthop Surg. 2009;17(9):541–9.
53. Marsh JL, Nepola JV, Wuest TK, et al. Unilateral external fixation until healing with the dynamic axial fixator for severe open tibial fractures. J Orthop Trauma. 1991;5(3):341–8.
54. Edwards CC, Simmons SC, Browner BD, et al. Severe open tibial fractures. Results treating 202 injuries with external fixation. Clin Orthop Relat Res. 1988;230:98–115.
55. Sirkin M, Sanders R, DiPasquale T, et al. A staged protocol for soft tissue management in the treatment of complex pilon fractures. J Orthop Trauma. 1999;13(2):78–84.
56. Henley MB, Chapman JR, Agel J, et al. Treatment of type II, IIIA, and IIIB open fractures of the tibial shaft: a prospective comparison of unreamed interlocking intramedullary nails and half-pin external fixators. J Orthop Trauma. 1998;12(1):1–7.
57. Roberts CS, Pape HC, Jones AL, et al. Damage control orthopaedics: evolving concepts in the treatment of patients who have sustained orthopaedic trauma. Instr Course Lect. 2005;54:447–62.
58. Benirschke SK, Agnew SG, Mayo KA, et al. Immediate internal fixation of open, complex tibial plateau fractures: treatment by a standard protocol. J Orthop Trauma. 1992;6(1):78–86.
59. Kregor PJ, Stannard JA, Zlowodzki M, et al. Treatment of distal femur fractures using the less invasive stabilization system: surgical experience and early clinical results in 103 fractures. J Orthop Trauma. 2004;18(8):509–20.
60. Moed BR, Kellam JF, Foster RJ, et al. Immediate internal fixation of open fractures of the diaphysis of the forearm. J Bone Joint Surg Am. 1986;68(7):1008–17.
61. Hamer ML, Robson MC, Krizek TJ, et al. Quantatative bacterial analysis of comparative wound irrigations. Ann Surg. 1975;181:819–22.
62. Burke WA, Osbourne DD, Taylor DD, et al. Evaluation of the "Golden period" for wound repair: 204 cases from a third world emergency department. Ann Emerg Med. 1988;17(5):496–00.
63. Javaid M, Feldberg L, Gipson M, et al. Primary repair of dog bites to the face: 40 cases. J R Soc Med. 1998;91:414–6.
64. Alan S, Peterson MD. The "Golden period" for wound repair. J Lanc Gen Hosp. 2010;5(4):134–5.

65. Stamou SC, Maltezou HC, Psaltopoulou T, et al. Wound infections after minor limb lacerations: risk factors and the role of antimicrobial agents. J Trauma. 1999;46:1078.
66. Russell RC, Williamson DA, Sullivan JW, et al. Detection of foreign bodies in the hand. J Hand Surg Am. 1991;16:2.
67. Donaldson JS. Radiographic imaging of foreign bodies in the hand. Hand Clin. 1991;7:125.
68. Principlization of plastic surgery. by D. Ralph Millard. 1986.
69. Yd G, et al. Hand surgery. Shanghai Scientific & Technical Publishers. 2002;12:238–41.
70. Ian AM. The Z-Plasty in hand surgery. J Bone Joint Surg Br. 1967;49-B(3):448–57.
71. Song IC, Bromberg BE, Mohn MP, et al. Heterografts as biological dressings for large skin wounds. Surgery. 1966;59:576.
72. Elliott RA, Hoehn JG. Use of commercial porcine skin for wound dressings. Plast Reconstr Surg. 1973;52:401.
73. Ratner D. Skin grafting. Semin Cutan Med Surg. 2003;22:295.
74. SW W, et al. Green's operative hand surgery, vol. 1. 6th ed. Philadelphia: Elsevier Churchill Livingstone; 2010. p. 1645–6.
75. van der Veen VC, van der Wal MB, van Leeuwen MC, et al. Biological background of dermal substitutes. Burns. 2010;36:305.
76. Macht SD, Watson HK. The Moberg volar advancement flap for digital reconstruction. J Hand Surg Am. 1980;5(4):372–6.
77. Atasoy E, Loakimidis E, Kasdan ML, et al. Reconstruction of the amputated finger tip with a triangular volar flap. A new surgical procedure. J Bone Joint Surg Am. 1970;52:921–6.
78. Weston PA, Wallace WA. The use of locally based triangular skin flaps for the repair of finger tip injuries. Hand. 1976;8(1):54–8.
79. McGregor IA, McGregor AD. Fundamental techniques of plastic surgery: and their surgical applications. 9th ed. Edinburgh: Churchill Livingstone; 1995. p. 206–11.
80. Kutler W. Clinical notes, suggestions and new instruments: a new method for finger tip amputations. JAMA. 1947;133:29–30.
81. Chasmar LR. The versatile rhomboid (Limberg) flap. Can J Plast Surg. 2007 Summer;15(2):67–71.
82. Iselin F. The flag flap. Plast Reconstr Surg. 1973;52(4):374–7.
83. Megerle K, Palm-Bröking K, Germann G. The cross-finger flap. Oper Orthop Traumatol. 2008;20(2):97–102.
84. Yd G, et al. Hand surgery, vol. 12. Shanghai: Shanghai Scientific & Technical Publishers; 2002. p. 238–41.
85. Littler JW. In: Wallace AB, editor. Neurovascular skin island transfer in reconstructive hand surgery. London: Transactions of the International Society of Plastic Surgeons, Second Congress; 1959. p. 175–8.
86. Lai CS, Lin SD, Yang CC. The reverse digital artery flap for fingertip reconstruction. Ann Plast Surg. 1989;22(6):495–00.
87. Tränkle M, Sauerbier M, Heitmann C, et al. Restoration of thumb sensibility with the innervated first dorsal metacarpal artery island flap. J Hand Surg Am. 2003;28(05):758–66.
88. Keramidas E, Rodopoulou S, Metaxotos N, et al. Reverse dorsal digital and inter-commissural flaps used for digital reconstruction. Br J Plast Surg. 2004;57(1):61–5.
89. Koray CO, Hifzi V, Ahmet K. Reversed neurofas-ciocutaneous flaps based on the superficial branches of the radial nerve. Ann Plast Surg. 1999;43(4):367–73.
90. Earley MJ, Milner RH. Dorsal metacarpal flaps. Br J Plast Surg. 1987;40(4):333–41.
91. Soutar DS, Tanner NSB. The radial forearm flap in the management of soft tissue injuries of the hand. Br J Plast Surg. 1984;37(1):18–26.
92. Oppikofer C, Büchler U, Schmid E. The surgical anatomy of the dorsal carpal branch of the ulnar artery: basis for a neurovascular dorso-ulnar pedicled flap. Surg Radiol Anat. 1992;14:97–101.
93. Shimpei O, Kevin CC, Sandeep JS, et al. Clinical applications of perforator-based propeller flaps in upper limb soft tissue reconstruction. J Hand Surg Am. 2011;36(5):853–86.
94. Agostini T, Russo GL, Zhang YX, et al. Adipofascial anterolateral thigh flap safety: applications and complications. Arch Plast Surg. 2013;40:91–6.
95. Malrey L, Young-Keun L, Dong-Hee K. The clinical result of arterialized venous free flaps for the treatment of soft tissue defect of the fingers. Medicine. 2019;98(23):e16017.
96. Quillen CG, Shearin JC, Georgiade NG. Use of the latissimus dorsi myocutaneous island flap for reconstruction in the head and neck area: case report. Plast Reconstr Surg. 1978;62(1):113–7.
97. Jyoshid RB. Free toe pulp flap for finger pulp and volar defect reconstruction. Indian J Plast Surg. 2016;49(02):178–84.
98. Morrison WA, O'Brien BM, MacLeod AM. Thumb reconstruction with a free neurovascular wrap-around flap from the big toe. J Hand Surg Am. 1980;5(6):575–83.
99. Kwang SL, Sang WP, Hak YK. Tendocutaneous free flap transfer from the dorsum of the foot. Microsurgery. 1994;15(12):882–5.
100. Jeffrey BF, Leonid IK, Nicholas BV. Soft tissue reconstruction of the hand. J Hand Surg Am. 2009;34(6):1148–55.
101. Gottlieb LJ, Krieger LM. From the reconstructive ladder to the reconstructive elevator. Plast Reconstr Surg. 1994;93:1503–4.
102. Erin AM, Jeffrey F. Soft tissue coverage of the hand and upper extremity: the reconstructive elevator. J Hand Surg Am. 2016;41(7):782–92.